Development of Self-Awareness and Wellbeing:

Global Learning Challenges in a Shifting Society

Margaret Hiro Kimishima
International Center of Transdisciplinary Research, Japan

Frederic Andres
National Insitute of Informatics, Japan

IGI Global
Scientific Publishing
Publishing Tomorrow's Research Today

Vice President of Editorial	Melissa Wagner
Director of Acquisitions	Mikaela Felty
Director of Book Development	Jocelynn Hessler
Production Manager	Mike Brehm
Cover Design	Jose Rosado

Published in the United States of America by
IGI Global Scientific Publishing
701 East Chocolate Avenue
Hershey, PA, 17033, USA
Tel: 717-533-8845
Fax: 717-533-7115
Website: https://www.igi-global.com E-mail: cust@igi-global.com

Library of Congress Cataloging-in-Publication Data

Names: Kimishima, Margaret Hiro, editor. | Andres, Frederic, 1962- editor.
Title: Development of self-awareness and wellbeing : global learning challenges in a shifting society / Edited by Margaret Kimishima, Frederic Andres.
Description: Hershey, PA : IGI Global Scientific Publishing, [2025] | Includes bibliographical references and index. | Summary: "The book delves into the complex interplay between personal development, self-awareness, and overall well-being in an ever-evolving world. As educational systems and learning environments face unprecedented challenges, this book highlights the necessity of fostering these critical aspects of human growth amidst dynamic societal, technological, and cultural changes"-- Provided by publisher.
Identifiers: LCCN 2024060566 (print) | LCCN 2024060567 (ebook) | ISBN 9798337303604 (hardcover) | ISBN 9798337303611 (paperback) | ISBN 9798337303628 (ebook)
Subjects: LCSH: Education--Social aspects--Cross-cultural studies. | Self-consciousness (Awareness)--Cross-cultural studies. | Well-being--Cross-cultural studies. | Education and globalization--Cross-cultural studies.
Classification: LCC LC191 .D52 2025 (print) | LCC LC191 (ebook) | DDC 306.43--dc23/eng/20250213
LC record available at https://lccn.loc.gov/2024060566
LC ebook record available at https://lccn.loc.gov/2024060567

British Cataloguing in Publication Data
A Cataloguing in Publication record for this book is available from the British Library.

Table of Contents

Detailed Table of Contents

This chapter explores how sustainable well-being and a renewal of modern life can be achieved through an integrative understanding of ikigai, inochi, and Zen mindfulness. In today's society, rapid technological advancement, information overload, and a fading sense of purpose have heightened the need for self-awareness and well-being. Amidst this, the Japanese concept of ikigai has gained global attention. Commonly described as the intersection of what one loves, is good at, what the world needs, and what one can be paid for, in Japan ikigai often emphasizes purpose and service to others over monetary reward. At its core lies inochi—the Japanese view of life as interconnected with nature and society, rooted in the gratitude of living in the present moment. Zen and mindfulness practices help cultivate this awareness and promote mind-body harmony. Together, ikigai, inochi, and Zen mindfulness form a holistic framework that nurtures both personal fulfillment and social balance.

The concept of "Mutual Nurturing" derived from the indigenous Law of Origin, emphasizing its significance in reshaping global education systems and fostering sustainable communities. Drawing on the ancient wisdom of American indigenous cultures, the study integrates perspectives on complex, transdisciplinary thinking advocated by modern initiatives like UNESCO's "Seven Necessary Knowledges for the Education of the Future." The Eagle's Vision metaphor is central to this discussion, illustrating the balance of context-awareness and precise action. The article examines the interplay of three "mind-souls"—body, reason, and emotion—and their role in achieving alignment and coherence in human experience. By revisiting ancestral philosophies and practices, the paper proposes a paradigm shift in education, public policy, and human behavior to restore harmony between humanity and the planet. The authors call for a transcultural dialogue and the reorientation of societal values towards mutual upbringing, enabling sustainable and equitable futures.

The study explores the intersection of neuroscience, neurophilosophy, and indigenous knowledge systems to address systematic and empirical evidence about the interface between visible and invisible - unseen world - phenomena by examining the Pakasqa Nuna (subconscious) at the ancestral medical practices, providing highlights in the integration of indigenous knowledge into contemporary biomedical and neurocognitive paradigms. Drawing on ethnomedicine practices, the paper proposes a consilient and trandisciplinary approach that bridges cultural and scientific perspectives. It emphasizes the health and wellness as rooted in the interrelation of human, natural, and sacred communities. The study also critiques the limitations of reductionist views in neuroscience and psychiatry, advocating for the reconceptualization of mental health disorders. By exploring altered states of consciousness and their neurophenomenological impacts, the research offers new pathways for integrating spiritual dimensions into global health paradigms and science development.

This document is a profound and a systematization of indigenous knowledge and ceremonial practices centered on the teachings of the Gunadule people and their relationship with Mother Earth that turns into Bachelor's Program in Pedagogy of Mother Earth at the University of Antioquia which delves deeply into the spiritual and symbolic dimensions of human life, presenting the womb as a sacred space of origin and a living memory that informs the wisdom of all beings, offering a pedagogy that celebrates community, relationality, and the cyclical nature of existence. The document also emphasize its role in fostering ecological consciousness and spiritual resilience. This work contributes to broader discourses on education from first source of ancestral wisdom as vital pathways for addressing ecological and spiritual crises in the modern world. It invites readers to reconnect with their origins, embrace the principles of Mother Earth, and participate in collective healing through silence, sweet words, and good hearts

Section 2
Practices and Pedagogies for Personal and Collective Growth

The chapter explores the integration of mindfulness into parenting and education as a transformative approach to addressing child anxiety and fostering emotional resilience. The analysis highlights the role of mindfulness in mitigating the challenges faced by children and adolescents, particularly in the post-COVID-19 era, where stressors have amplified mental health concerns. Grounded in cultural sensitivity, the chapter examines the interplay of parenting styles, educational practices, and sociocultural influences, advocating for mindful parenting and classroom strategies that enhance self-awareness, emotional balance, and adaptive coping mechanisms. Through a synthesis of theoretical insights and practical applications, it emphasizes mindfulness as a culturally adaptable tool for nurturing children's well-being and resilience in a rapidly evolving global society. This holistic approach not only addresses the immediate symptoms of anxiety but also promotes long-term psychological stability, making a case for integrating mindfulness into broader child development frameworks.

This study analyzed the author's own recovery process from a decade of social withdrawal from the perspective of mindfulness, wellbeing, and a holistic approach. In particular, it focused on the internal transformation and gradual process of social participation that occurred as a result of a change in outlook on life and death at the age of 39, and explored the recovery mechanism. The analysis revealed that mindfulness practice enabled the individual to distance himself from anxiety about the past and future, that the five elements of the PERMA theory developed while influencing each other, and that the integration of physical, mental, and social approaches promoted comprehensive recovery. These results indicate that a combination of internal awareness and gradual social participation is effective for recovery from long-term withdrawal, and present the possibility of a new support approach.

traditional Japanese introspective practices, drawing inspiration from the aesthetic and philosophical elements of Zen Buddhism, Shugendō, calligraphy, the tea ceremony, and karesansui (dry landscape) gardens. Rooted in profound spiritual experiences—particularly through practices such as waterfall meditation (*takigyō*) and conch shell blowing in Shugendō—Arai's work offers a compelling counterpoint to the existential and psychological challenges of the digital age. It highlights the enduring importance of introspection and well-being in contemporary life. This study critically examines the philosophical foundations of Arai's artistic practice, assessing its potential to cultivate a deeper sense of interconnectedness and to promote a more integrative and reflective mode of engagement in an increasingly AI-driven world. The analysis situates Arai's approach within broader discourses on the interrelations among truth, human flourishing, nature, and technology.

Our research study has many targets and research goals that aim to achieve, but the main one is to unveil the psychological consequences that the pandemic brought with it due to the restrictions made to minimize the chances of getting infected and spreading the virus on and on. The main goal of this research is set to evaluate the presence of anxiety and depression symptoms as mental health issues, as consequences due to the pandemic COVID-19 lifestyle and social relation changes, in adult population. In this study, 900 people responded willingly to the three questionnaires that evaluated the social & lifestyle changes during the outbreak, and the presence of anxiety (CPAS-15) and depressive symptoms (PHQ-9). Throughout this research, we were able to prove that people are highly anxious (63.62%), and also (36.38%) out of them show the presence of depression. These two variables have been proven to correlate with one another positively, including the lifestyle changes and social relationship changes during the pandemic.

In a world overwhelmed by negative narratives and relentless information, human sensitivity is diminishing, turning individuals into indifferent beings. Despite this decline, hope remains in fostering genuine human values through discussions and

Foreword

In a world that is mutating more rapidly than ever—technologically, ecologically, and socially—there is a growing recognition that our external and collective challenges are deeply tied to our internal states. Our inner conflicts have a deep impact in the outer world, and especially those due to a reduction of the human being to a binary and conditioned machine whose behavior must adapt to materialistic and competitive world. Going beyond duality, human being is here described in all his complexity: body and soul connected to his environment, able to modify and protect nature, towards a collective evolution.Amidst this shift, the pursuit of self-awareness and well-being is not a luxury, but a necessity. This book arrives at a critical moment, offering a diverse and powerful collection of voices that illuminate how human flourishing can be cultivated even in the most complex global conditions.

Development of Self-Awareness and Well-Being: Global Learning Challenges in a Shifting Society is more than a book. It is a collective meditation on how we, as individuals and as communities, can adapt and thrive in the face of adversity. The chapters span cultures, continents, and disciplines—bringing together thought leaders and practitioners who understand that self-awareness is the foundation of both personal transformation and societal evolution. However, self-awareness is not only a solitary and comfortable path.

While crossing what we may call, the dark night of the soul, companions may mirror the issue towards light and meaning, in certain cases we may even speak of a rebirth process from inside out, towards a journey of interdependency and integration of a collective intelligence, a collective intelligence that may be more careful and loving for our future.

From the exploration of prenatal memory and mindfulness in education to the wisdom of indigenous philosophies and the challenges of modern workplaces, this book invites the reader to consider well-being as a multidimensional, lifelong practice. Each chapter stands as a testament to the idea that learning—when rooted in empathy, reflection, and cultural sensitivity—can be a healing transformative force.

What sets this work apart is its integrative nature. Science meets spirituality. Art meets activism. Tradition meets innovation. The result is a volume that not only bridges disciplines but also connects the mind, body, and spirit in the search for meaningful and creative living.

This book will resonate with educators, leaders, students, and seekers alike. It challenges institutions to become more human, caring, cooperative and it empowers individuals to go deeper in their journey and become more authentic. In a time when many feel disoriented or disconnected, it reminds us that returning to ourselves—with compassion, clarity, and courage—is the most radical act of all. That can only be done through dialogue and together.

We mirror one another, as we mirror the universe. We shall become what is being mirrored to us.

We encourage you to read this book slowly, reflectively, and with an open heart. Let it be a companion on your journey toward self-understanding and collective well-being.

Mariana Thieriot Loisel
Université Laval, Canada

Preface

In an era defined by rapid technological transformation, social disruption, and psychological uncertainty, the need to reconnect with ourselves—and one another—has never been more urgent. This book, *Development of Self-Awareness and Well-Being: Global Learning Challenges in a Shifting Society*, emerges from a collective effort to explore the inner landscapes of human experience, emotional resilience, and the evolving nature of well-being in diverse global contexts.

The chapters compiled here are authored by educators, philosophers, psychologists, healers, and practitioners who span continents and cultures. Each contributor brings a unique lens to the shared pursuit of self-awareness and collective flourishing. The book begins with foundational insights into emotional intelligence and prenatal memory, which serve as gateways to understanding the roots of consciousness and human connection. These early explorations establish a bridge between ancient wisdom and emerging psychological science.

As the narrative progresses, the book turns to real-world applications, from mindfulness in parenting and recovery to storytelling and pedagogical strategies that promote empathy, empowerment, and engagement. Whether through spiritual traditions, artistic inquiry, or integrative education, each chapter addresses the complex question of how we learn to live fully in ourselves while relating meaningfully to others.

This journey would not be complete without confronting the challenges we face in society today—from the silent crises of mental health and social withdrawal to the institutional pressures placed on educators and professionals. Here, our contributors do not shy away from the darkness, but rather seek light through dialogue, reflection, and healing practices rooted in culture, nature, and inner truth.

In the final part of the book, we examine well-being through the lens of the workplace, where burnout, alienation, and disconnection are increasingly common. Yet, as our contributors reveal, organizations that foster happiness, emotional intelligence, and a sense of purpose can become powerful incubators of growth, inclusion, and innovation.

This book is not a prescription, but an invitation: to reflect, to feel, to remember, and to act with awareness. It is for anyone seeking to navigate the shifting terrain of our times with greater clarity, compassion, and courage. We hope the insights offered here serve not only as guidance but also as inspiration to embrace the full potential of human life—rooted in self-awareness and guided by the pursuit of well-being for all.

Margaret Hiro Kimishima
International Center of Transdisciplinary Research, Japan

Frederic Andres
National Insitute of Informatics, Japan

Acknowledgment

We thank all the contributors and reviewers who made this book possible. In addition, we thank Allie Jeanne Wilson, Mei Saegusa, Tomohiro Matsumoto for their great contributions to this book.

Introduction

You're about to read our anthology, *Development of Self-Awareness and Well-Being: Global Learning Challenges in a Shifting Society*. It is a book about a new era: An era of exploring new values and educational systems. When a baby is born into this world, they certainly expect to enter a world that can offer them a variety of experiences. They surely expect to have exciting dreams and hopes to accomplish for their future. As these babies grow up, they face various challenges (gender, race, economic disparity, educational disparity, spirituality, religion, economic disparity, regional disparity) that stand in their way and leave them at a loss. However, with the guidance of the adults who came before them, they have built a sense of well-being appropriate to their time. We are about to face coexistence with a creature like AI, something humanity has never encountered before.

This book consists of 19 chapters written by top experts in a variety of disciplines including AI, coronavirus, education, religion, spirituality, traditional medicine, western medicine, data science, indigenous studies, and writing. Throughout the anthology, you will encounter experiences that have never guided you before.

TIMELESS INSIGHTS FOR TRANSFORMATIVE TIMES

Bridging Ancient Wisdom and Modern Realities

This anthology brings to light timeless insights—threads of wisdom that have endured quietly beneath the surface of mainstream culture, often suppressed or overlooked due to their misalignment with dominant values and societal norms. For centuries, voices and perspectives from diverse traditions and communities were marginalized, not because they lacked value, but because they challenged the prevailing narratives of power, conformity, and identity.

As we step into the complexities of the 21st century, a global shift in consciousness is unfolding. We are beginning to embrace the full spectrum of human diversity—across age, ethnicity, gender, ability, race, religion, socio-economic background, and more. This new era calls for the reintegration of the very knowledge we once ignored: the deep, intuitive, holistic understanding of life and nature that our ancestors cultivated across civilizations.

Yet, as history often moves not in straight lines but in spirals, humanity finds itself revisiting old patterns with new intensity. The current social and ecological upheavals are not isolated incidents but reflections of a greater systemic imbalance. What we witness today is not merely political or environmental disruption—it is the echo of a deeper polarity, a call for equilibrium.

The wisdom traditions collected in this book speak to that need for balance. They remind us that within the dualities of life—light and dark, stillness and movement, reason and intuition—lies a trustworthy center. This center is not fixed; it evolves as we grow in self-awareness. It is our compass in a world of constant flux, and it helps us navigate uncertainty with courage, compassion, and curiosity.

Ancient knowledge is not a relic of the past—it is a key to unlocking the present and reimagining the future. It offers fresh perspectives, creative solutions, and alternative paths to healing, sustainability, and meaningful coexistence. From indigenous approaches to nature and resource management to timeless philosophies of inner peace and social harmony, these teachings offer vital contributions to solving contemporary challenges—especially those concerning environmental sustainability, mental health, and cultural fragmentation.

The Intersection of Tradition and Innovation in Human Well-Being

To cultivate well-being in a rapidly evolving world, we must expand our understanding of human nature beyond conventional frameworks. Today's society is increasingly defined by dualities: material and spiritual, human and machine, tradition and innovation. As we explore new paradigms of learning, healing, and coexistence, it becomes essential to embrace non-binary, holistic views of identity, growth, and wisdom.

This book offers a space where such exploration can begin—especially as we face the unprecedented challenge of raising and educating future generations in an age of artificial intelligence. In a world where machines may soon match or surpass human capabilities in many domains, we must protect and nurture the uniquely human: our stories, values, beliefs, lived experiences, and emotional intelligence.

The COVID-19 pandemic served as a collective wake-up call. An invisible force reshaped our values and social structures in profound ways. In its aftermath, many of us began to focus more on well-being, relationships, purpose, and the non-material dimensions of life. The pandemic also exposed a deeper, more insidious "invisible enemy"—a loss of connection, community, and meaning.

As AI systems grow increasingly complex and autonomous, the line between the human and the artificial becomes harder to draw. It is now more urgent than ever to ask oneself: What makes us human? What values do we want our technologies to reflect? Whose ethics will shape the algorithms that influence our lives?

Cultural differences are not obstacles—they are the diverse expressions of a shared human spirit. This anthology seeks to find the common ground where cultures, disciplines, and generations converge. It brings together thinkers, educators, healers, and visionaries from around the world to identify and articulate the universal values that unite us. In doing so, we offer a blueprint for aligning emerging technologies with deeply human principles—especially the one thing machines cannot replicate: love and empathy.

Through these pages, may you rediscover what it means to be human. May you be inspired to reflect, question, connect, and contribute to a world where both ancient wisdom and modern innovation serve the greater good.

Section 1
Foundations of Self-Awareness and Well-Being

Chapter 1
The Role of Emotional Intelligence in Self-Awareness and Well-Being

Frederic Andres
https://orcid.org/0000-0002-5003-7579
National Institute of Informatics, Japan

ABSTRACT

Emotional intelligence (EI) is crucial for fostering self-awareness and promoting well-being in today's complex world. This chapter examines the relationship between EI, self-awareness, and well-being, highlighting their role in personal growth, emotional resilience, and life satisfaction. By analyzing EI components—self-awareness, self-regulation, motivation, empathy, and social skills—the study emphasizes self-awareness as the foundation for managing emotions, recognizing triggers, and improving decision-making. It explores EI's positive impact on mental and physical well-being, including stress reduction, emotional regulation, and purpose. Case studies and research offer practical strategies to develop EI and self-awareness, advocating for their integration into education, workplaces, and community programs to empower individuals in navigating challenges with confidence and emotional balance.

DOI: 10.4018/979-8-3373-0360-4.ch001

1. INTRODUCTION

Emotional intelligence (EI in the following of the chapter) is increasingly recognized as a fundamental skill for navigating the complexities of modern life. In a world characterized by rapid technological advancements, shifting societal dynamics, and heightened emotional stress, the ability to understand and manage one's emotions is more critical than ever (Ishi, 2017). EI enables individuals to cultivate self-awareness, regulate their emotions, and build meaningful relationships—skills that are essential not only for personal well-being but also for professional success and social harmony (Gunderman et al., 2011). Research suggests that individuals with high EI tend to exhibit greater resilience, improved mental health, and stronger interpersonal connections, making EI a key factor in both individual fulfillment and collective well-being (O'Connor et al., 2019).

To fully grasp the significance of EI, it is essential to define its core components and their interrelated roles. Emotional intelligence encompasses five key elements: self-awareness, self-regulation, motivation, empathy, and social skills (Antonopoulou, 2024). Among these, self-awareness serves as the foundation, allowing individuals to recognize their emotions, understand their triggers, and reflect on their behaviors. This self-knowledge enables better decision-making, emotional control, and the capacity to respond to challenges with clarity and confidence. Furthermore, well-being including mental and physical level is deeply influenced by EI, as emotional regulation and resilience play a crucial role in stress management, life satisfaction, and overall health.

This chapter explores the intricate relationship between EI, self-awareness, and well-being, emphasizing their collective impact on personal growth and emotional resilience. It delves into how EI enhances life satisfaction by fostering mindfulness, emotional balance, and a sense of purpose. Through a detailed analysis of the five EI components, the discussion highlights the essential role of self-awareness in managing emotions effectively. The chapter also presents case studies and research-based strategies that illustrate practical approaches to developing EI, advocating for its integration into education, workplaces, and community programs. By equipping individuals with the tools to enhance their emotional intelligence, society can cultivate a culture of emotional well-being, empowering people to navigate life's challenges with confidence and composure.

2. UNDERSTANDING EMOTIONAL INTELLIGENCE (EI)

"Emotional intelligence is the ability to make our emotions work for us, instead of against us." — Peter Salovey

2.1 Historical Background and Theoretical Foundations

The concept of Emotional Intelligence (EI) (Filice et al., 2024) has evolved over the past century, rooted in psychological theories of intelligence, emotion, and social behavior. Early research on intelligence primarily focused on cognitive abilities, such as logical reasoning and problem-solving. However, psychologists began recognizing that emotional and social competencies play a crucial role in human success and well-being (Occhipinti et al., 2023). One of the earliest contributions to EI can be traced back to Edward Thorndike who introduced the concept of "social intelligence" (Thorndike et al., 1937), emphasizing the ability to understand and manage people. Later, Howard Gardner introduced the theory of multiple intelligences, focusing on the idea of interpersonal and intrapersonal intelligence (Gardner, 1983), acknowledging the importance of emotional and social understanding.

The modern framework of Emotional Intelligence was formally introduced by Peter Salovey and John Mayer, who defined EI as the ability to perceive, understand, manage, and regulate emotions in oneself and others (Salovey et al., 1990). This concept gained widespread recognition after the publication of the book *Emotional Intelligence* (Goleman, 1995), which highlighted its significance in personal and professional success. Goleman expanded on Salovey and Mayer's work by categorizing EI into five key components: self-awareness, self-regulation, motivation, empathy, and social skills, which remain central to EI research and application today.

Building on these foundations, *Emotional intelligence: Implications for personal, social, academic, and workplace success* (Brackett et al., 2011) provides a compelling and integrative overview of how emotional intelligence shapes critical life outcomes. With clarity and depth, the authors have bridged theoretical foundations with practical applications, demonstrating that emotional intelligence is a dynamic and influential factor across diverse contexts. Their work underscores the relevance of EI not only as a psychological construct but also as a key contributor to human flourishing. Emotional intelligence is influenced by both innate cognitive-emotional abilities and environmental factors such as parenting, education, social interactions, and workplace culture. Brackett et al. (2011) emphasize that EI can be enhanced through targeted interventions—especially in educational and organizational settings—that foster emotional skills like empathy, regulation, and interpersonal communication. These efforts can strengthen individuals' capacities to navigate complex emotional situations, thereby supporting personal development and social effectiveness.

Looking at later research, the article *The Ability Model of Emotional Intelligence: Principles and Updates* (Mayer et al., 2016) provides a comprehensive and thoughtful update to one of the most foundational models of emotional intelligence. By refining the conceptual clarity and reinforcing the cognitive underpinnings of EI as an ability, the authors make a valuable contribution to both research and practice. The discussion effectively bridges theory with application, offering nuanced insights into how EI skills—such as perceiving, using, understanding, and managing emotions—can be assessed and developed. Emotional intelligence is influenced by both individual factors (e.g., cognitive development, personality traits) and external influences (e.g., environment, education, life experiences). According to the ability model, EI can be enhanced through cognitive training, emotional awareness exercises, and feedback mechanisms that improve a person's ability to process and use emotional information effectively. This Mayer et al. model emphasizes that EI is not static but can evolve over time through intentional learning and reflective experiences.

2.2 Components of Emotional Intelligence

EI is composed of five core elements (Cooper et al., 2023), each contributing to a person's ability to navigate emotions effectively:

Self-awareness is the ability to recognize and understand one's emotions, thoughts, and behavioral patterns. It serves as the foundation of EI, as it allows individuals to identify emotional triggers and assess their impact on decision-making and interactions. Self-aware individuals are more likely to engage in self-reflection, leading to greater emotional control and personal growth.

Self-regulation refers to the ability to manage and control emotional responses in different situations. It involves skills such as impulse control, adaptability, and maintaining emotional balance under stress. Individuals with strong self-regulation can respond to challenges rationally rather than react impulsively, fostering resilience and effective problem-solving.

Motivation within EI goes beyond external rewards and refers to an intrinsic drive to achieve goals, overcome obstacles, and maintain a positive outlook. Emotionally intelligent individuals are often self-motivated, proactive, and persistent in their pursuits, displaying optimism and resilience even in the face of difficulties.

Empathy is the ability to understand and share the feelings of others, enabling deeper interpersonal connections. It plays a crucial role in effective communication, conflict resolution, and compassionate leadership. People with high empathy can recognize nonverbal cues and perspectives, leading to stronger relationships and improved social harmony.

Social skills encompass the ability to build and maintain relationships, communicate effectively, and navigate social interactions with confidence. Strong social skills contribute to teamwork, leadership, and emotional connection, making them essential for both personal and professional success. EI-driven social skills enhance collaboration, negotiation, and the ability to influence others positively.

2.3 The Interplay Between EI and Personal Development

Emotional intelligence is deeply intertwined with personal development, influencing various aspects of an individual's life, from decision-making and stress management to relationship-building and career growth. High EI enables individuals to:

- Develop a deeper understanding of themselves and their emotions.
- Cultivate resilience and adapt to life's challenges with emotional balance.
- Enhance communication skills and build stronger, more meaningful relationships.
- Improve leadership abilities (White et al., 2023), teamwork, and professional success.
- Foster mental and physical well-being by reducing stress and promoting positive emotions.

By strengthening EI, individuals can unlock greater self-awareness, emotional control, and interpersonal effectiveness, ultimately leading to a more fulfilled and balanced life. This chapter further explores how EI can be cultivated and applied in various contexts, empowering individuals to navigate challenges with emotional resilience and confidence.

3. SELF-AWARENESS: THE CORE OF EMOTIONAL INTELLIGENCE

"He who knows others is wise; he who knows himself is enlightened." —Lao Tzu

This timeless insight from Taoist philosophy highlights self-awareness as not just a psychological skill but a spiritual path toward inner clarity and enlightenment—echoing the central role it plays in emotional intelligence.

Self-awareness is the foundation of Emotional Intelligence (EI) and plays a crucial role in personal development, emotional regulation, and well-being. It is the ability to recognize and understand one's emotions, thoughts, and behaviors, enabling individuals to make conscious decisions, manage stress, and build healthier relationships. Without self-awareness, it is challenging to regulate emotions, empathize with others, or develop meaningful social connections. Advances in neuroscientific research have provided deeper insights into how the brain supports self-awareness and emotional intelligence, reinforcing its significance in cognitive and emotional processes.

3.1 Definition and Significance of Self-Awareness

Self-awareness is the ability to recognize and understand our own emotions, thoughts, and behaviors, and to appreciate how they influence both ourselves and those around us. This process encompasses two dimensions: internal and external self-awareness.

Internal self-awareness involves a deep understanding of our personal values, strengths, and emotions. It enables us to be attuned to our inner experiences, which shapes our choices and actions. On the other hand, external self-awareness focuses on how we are perceived by others. This awareness helps us navigate social interactions and respond in ways that align with our social context, facilitating more meaningful and effective connections.

From a neuroscientific perspective, self-awareness is closely tied to certain regions of the brain, particularly the prefrontal cortex, with a special emphasis on the medial prefrontal cortex (mPFC). The mPFC plays a pivotal role in processes like introspection, emotional regulation, and self-referential thinking. Alongside the mPFC, other brain areas contribute to self-awareness. For example, the anterior cingulate cortex (ACC) is involved in monitoring conflicts and regulating emotions, while the insular cortex is essential for interoception – the ability to sense internal body states, which significantly influences emotional awareness. Additionally, the default mode network (DMN), a network of brain regions activated during self-reflection, plays a crucial role in the ability to think about ourselves and our experiences in a more introspective and holistic manner.

In essence, self-awareness is not just a mental concept, but a complex neurological process that shapes how we understand ourselves, interact with others, and manage our emotional and social lives.

Neuroscientific studies, particularly those using fMRI and EEG, have provided valuable insights into the biological underpinnings of self-awareness. These studies reveal that increased activity in brain regions like the prefrontal cortex, anterior cingulate cortex, and insular cortex is linked to higher emotional intelligence (EI), improved decision-making, and enhanced stress management. By understanding these neurological connections, we gain a deeper appreciation for the importance of self-awareness in personal growth and development.

The significance of self-awareness within the framework of emotional intelligence is profound. First, it enables **improved emotional regulation**, as individuals with heightened self-awareness are better able to recognize and manage their emotions, leading to more controlled emotional responses. This awareness also enhances **decision-making**; when we are attuned to the emotional influences shaping our thoughts, we can make more rational and deliberate choices. Furthermore, self-awareness strengthens **relationships** by fostering better communication skills and the ability to resolve conflicts in a constructive manner. Finally, it cultivates **greater resilience**, as being aware of one's emotional state allows for greater adaptability and emotional balance, particularly in challenging situations. In all these ways, self-awareness plays a crucial role in fostering emotional intelligence and promoting overall personal development.

Developing self-awareness is a **lifelong process** that enhances both personal and professional growth. It serves as the **first step toward mastering emotional intelligence**, as individuals who understand their own emotions are better equipped to regulate them and respond effectively to others.

3.2 Recognizing Emotions and Identifying Triggers

To develop self-awareness, individuals must first recognize their emotions and understand the factors that trigger them. Emotions often arise in response to external events, internal thoughts, or subconscious associations. Recognizing these emotions is a vital first step in emotional regulation and personal growth.

From a neuroscientific perspective, emotional recognition involves key brain regions, particularly the amygdala, which is responsible for processing emotions such as fear and anger. However, effective emotional regulation requires higher-order brain regions, such as the prefrontal cortex, to mediate the amygdala's responses and prevent impulsive reactions. Studies in affective neuroscience have shown that emotionally intelligent individuals tend to exhibit stronger connectivity between the prefrontal cortex and the limbic system, which allows them to quickly recognize emotions, assess their significance, and choose appropriate responses.

Recognizing emotions and understanding what triggers them is a vital part of building emotional intelligence and self-awareness. The process begins with the ability to accurately label one's feelings. Rather than using vague expressions like "I feel bad," it's more constructive to name emotions clearly—identifying whether one feels angry, sad, excited, anxious, or something else. This clarity helps to make sense of what's going on internally.

Over time, tracking how emotions change throughout the day can reveal patterns and connections between experiences and emotional responses. By becoming more observant, individuals can begin to notice the specific situations, interactions, or even times of day that tend to provoke certain feelings. This kind of emotional journaling or reflection offers valuable insights into one's emotional dynamics.

It is also helpful to distinguish between primary and secondary emotions. Often, what we initially feel is not the root emotion but a reaction to it. For instance, anger might be the surface-level response, while the underlying feeling could be hurt, fear, or a sense of being misunderstood. Understanding these deeper emotions allows for more thoughtful responses and better emotional regulation.

In addition to recognizing emotions, identifying emotional triggers is essential for managing them effectively. These triggers generally fall into three main categories. **Situational triggers** arise from external circumstances—such as particular environments, events, or social interactions—that prompt an emotional reaction. **Cognitive triggers** stem from within, including thoughts, beliefs, or memories that influence how one feels. Lastly, **physical triggers** relate to the body's condition: fatigue, hunger, illness, or discomfort can all significantly impact emotional states.

Together, these practices not only deepen one's understanding of emotional patterns but also pave the way for more intentional, compassionate, and constructive reactions to life's challenges.

Individuals can better anticipate their reactions, prevent impulsive behavior, and cultivate healthier emotional responses by having a self awareness of their emotions and identifying the triggers that provoke them. It allows for a more thoughtful and controlled approach to emotions, contributing to overall emotional intelligence and well-being.

3.3 The Role of Self-Reflection in Emotional Regulation

Self-reflection is a powerful tool for enhancing self-awareness and improving emotional regulation. It involves examining one's thoughts, emotions, and behaviors in order to gain deeper insight into personal experiences. By reflecting on our actions and reactions, we can better understand the underlying emotions that drive our behavior and make more conscious choices in the future.

From a neuroscientific standpoint, self-reflection is facilitated by the default mode network (DMN), which becomes active during introspection and mind-wandering. Key brain regions, including the prefrontal cortex, anterior cingulate cortex (ACC), and insula, are involved in processing self-referential information, evaluating past experiences, and making adjustments for future actions. Research using functional MRI has shown that practices such as mindfulness meditation (Ariño et al., 2023) and journaling can increase the activity and connectivity of these brain regions, leading to enhanced emotional regulation and self-awareness.

Engaging in self-reflection offers numerous benefits that significantly contribute to mental health and emotional resilience. Regular self-reflection enhances mindfulness and presence, allowing individuals to become more attuned to their thoughts and emotions, thereby reducing distractions and improving focus. It also aids in identifying personal strengths and areas for improvement, facilitating targeted personal development. By processing emotions through self-reflection, individuals can manage stress more effectively, leading to reduced emotional strain. Additionally, analyzing past experiences through self-reflection enhances problem-solving skills, providing valuable insights for navigating future challenges and making informed decisions.

To practice self-reflection effectively, several techniques can be employed. Journaling allows individuals to articulate their emotions and experiences, helping to identify recurring patterns and gain clarity on emotional responses. Mindfulness meditation (Hölzel et al., 2011) involves observing thoughts and feelings without judgment, fostering greater awareness of emotional states and cultivating a sense of calm. Seeking feedback from trusted individuals offers valuable perspectives on personal strengths and areas for growth. Lastly, conducting daily self-check-ins by assessing one's emotions and mental state throughout the day helps individuals stay attuned to their feelings and respond thoughtfully. By cultivating self-awareness through emotional recognition and self-reflection, individuals can gain greater control over their emotional responses, build emotional resilience, and approach challenges with confidence and clarity. This practice ultimately fosters a deeper understanding of oneself, promoting emotional growth and healthier interactions with others.

Developing self-awareness—the ability to recognize and understand one's own emotions—is a foundational element of emotional intelligence and plays a pivotal role in shaping an individual's overall well-being. As highlighted by (Sánchez-Álvarez et al, 2016) in their meta-analytic investigation, higher emotional intelligence, particularly in the domain of emotional awareness, is consistently associated with greater levels of subjective well-being. Self-awareness enables individuals to accurately identify their emotional states, which in turn supports more effective emotional regulation, better interpersonal relationships, and a clearer sense of personal meaning. These capacities contribute directly to enhanced life satisfaction and emotional balance, suggesting that cultivating self-awareness is not only a pathway to emotional growth but also a critical determinant of psychological well-being.

4. EMOTIONAL INTELLIGENCE AND WELL-BEING

"When we are no longer able to change a situation, we are challenged to change ourselves." — **Viktor E. Frankl**

This quote emphasizes the power of internal emotional regulation—a core part of emotional intelligence—as essential to maintaining well-being in the face of life's challenges.

Emotional Intelligence (EI) plays a vital role in promoting **mental health, emotional resilience, and overall well-being**. Individuals with high EI can effectively manage their emotions, cope with stress, and maintain **healthy social relationships**, all of which contribute to greater life satisfaction. Scientific research has demonstrated strong links between EI and **mental, emotional, and physical health**, highlighting its role in fostering purpose and fulfillment.

This section explores **how EI enhances mental resilience, reduces stress, supports physical health, and contributes to a meaningful life**.

4.1 How EI Contributes to Mental Health and Emotional Resilience

Emotional resilience refers to an individual's ability to adapt and recover from stress, adversity, and emotional challenges. Emotional intelligence (EI) provides the essential skills needed to navigate life's difficulties with greater stability and confidence. By cultivating EI, individuals are better equipped to face emotional challenges and emerge stronger from them.

Engaging in self-reflection offers numerous benefits that significantly contribute to mental health and emotional resilience. Regular self-reflection enhances mindfulness and presence, allowing individuals to become more attuned to their thoughts and emotions, thereby reducing distractions and improving focus. It also aids in identifying personal strengths and areas for improvement, facilitating targeted personal development. By processing emotions through self-reflection, individuals can manage stress more effectively, leading to reduced emotional strain. Additionally, analyzing past experiences through self-reflection enhances problem-solving skills, providing valuable insights for navigating future challenges and making informed decisions.

Following (Self-reflection, 2012) effectively, several techniques can be employed. Journaling (Sawhney et al., 2018) allows individuals to articulate their emotions and experiences, helping to identify recurring patterns and gain clarity on emotional responses. Mindfulness meditation involves observing thoughts and feelings without judgment, fostering greater awareness of emotional states and cultivating a sense of calm. Seeking feedback from trusted individuals offers valuable perspectives on personal strengths and areas for growth. Lastly, conducting daily self-check-ins by assessing one's emotions and mental state throughout the day helps individuals stay attuned to their feelings and respond thoughtfully.

Neuroscientific studies support these findings, showing that higher activity in the prefrontal cortex (which is associated with decision-making and emotional control) and lower reactivity in the amygdala (responsible for fear and stress responses) are linked to both higher emotional intelligence and greater resilience. These brain activity patterns help individuals manage emotional challenges effectively, contributing to enhanced mental health and emotional stability.

4.2 The Impact of EI on Stress Reduction and Emotional Balance

Chronic stress can have detrimental effects on both mental and physical health (e.g. nurse domain (Huang et al., 2019)), but emotional intelligence (EI) provides valuable tools for managing stress and maintaining emotional stability. By developing EI, individuals are better equipped to cope with life's pressures and reduce the harmful impact of stress on their well-being. Emotional intelligence (EI) plays a pivotal role in mitigating stress and promoting emotional balance. Individuals with high EI possess self-awareness, enabling them to identify and understand the sources of their stress. This awareness (Malekar, 2007) allows them to proactively address or mitigate these stressors, fostering a sense of control over their environment. Moreover, their adeptness at emotional regulation helps them manage their reactions in challenging situations, maintaining composure and preventing overreactions. This ability to stay calm under pressure enhances their capacity to think clearly and handle stress effectively. Furthermore, emotionally intelligent individuals are skilled in the healthy expression of emotions. Rather than suppressing their feelings, they process and express them constructively, preventing emotional buildup and reducing stress. Their adaptive problem-solving skills also contribute to stress reduction; by analyzing situations thoughtfully, they can navigate challenges more effectively and make informed decisions. These competencies collectively enable individuals with high EI to manage stress more efficiently, leading to improved emotional well-being and resilience.

4.3 The Science Behind EI and Stress Management

Research suggests that the physiological response to stress is less intense in individuals with higher EI. The hypothalamic-pituitary-adrenal (HPA) axis, which governs the body's stress response, is less reactive in these individuals, resulting in lower levels of cortisol, the stress hormone. This means that emotionally intelligent people are better able to manage stress, both mentally and physically.

Additionally, mindfulness-based EI training (Sousa et al., 2021) has been shown to increase gray matter density in brain regions responsible for self-regulation and emotional control. These brain changes contribute to greater stress resilience, allowing individuals to remain calm and composed during stressful situations.

"Can emotional intelligence be trained? A meta-analytical investigation" (Mattingly et al, 2019) provides a rigorous and insightful synthesis of empirical studies, convincingly demonstrating that emotional intelligence is not only a measurable construct but also a trainable skill. By integrating findings across multiple interventions, Mattingly et al highlight the effectiveness of structured training programs in enhancing key EI components, such as emotional awareness, regulation, and empathy. Emotional intelligence is typically trained through experiential learning techniques such as role-playing, feedback sessions, mindfulness practices, coaching, and cognitive-behavioral strategies. These programs often target self-awareness, self-regulation, motivation, empathy, and social skills. Effective EI training also includes reflection exercises, group discussions, and real-life scenario analysis to help individuals better recognize, understand, and manage emotions in themselves and others.

By cultivating emotional intelligence, individuals can maintain emotional balance, preventing stress from overwhelming their mental and physical health. With the ability to regulate emotions, express them healthily, and approach stress with adaptability, emotionally intelligent people (Robinson, 2024) are better able to navigate life's challenges without compromising their well-being.

4.4 Connections Between EI, Physical Health, and Life Satisfaction

Emotional Intelligence (EI) plays a vital role not only in shaping our mental well-being but also in influencing our physical health and overall life satisfaction. Research increasingly shows that individuals with high EI experience a range of health benefits that extend far beyond emotional balance.

For instance, emotionally intelligent people often enjoy better cardiovascular health. This connection is attributed to their ability to manage stress more effectively and make healthier lifestyle choices, which in turn can lead to lower blood pressure and a reduced risk of heart disease. Similarly, strong emotional regulation helps reduce chronic stress—one of the key factors known to weaken the immune system—thus supporting stronger immune function.

In addition, individuals with high EI are more likely to adopt and maintain healthier lifestyle habits. They tend to exercise regularly, follow balanced diets, sleep better, and avoid harmful coping mechanisms such as smoking or excessive alcohol use. These habits collectively contribute to improved physical well-being over time.

Beyond physical health, EI is closely linked to life satisfaction. People with high emotional intelligence typically experience more positive emotions in their daily lives and build stronger, more meaningful relationships that enhance their overall happiness. They also tend to feel a greater sense of control and purpose, allowing them to face life's challenges with a growth-oriented mindset rather than feeling overwhelmed or defeated.

Longitudinal studies support these observations, revealing that individuals with higher levels of EI consistently report greater happiness, fulfillment, and satisfaction with life. These findings highlight the powerful role of emotional intelligence as a key factor in achieving both physical health and holistic well-being.

4.5 Purpose and Fulfillment Through Emotional Intelligence

Emotional intelligence (EI) plays a pivotal role in helping individuals discover a deeper sense of purpose and fulfillment in life. By fostering alignment between emotions, values, and actions, EI empowers people to pursue goals that are both personally meaningful and professionally rewarding.

One of the key ways EI contributes to a sense of purpose is by enabling individuals to understand and align their emotions with their core values. This emotional awareness helps clarify what truly matters, guiding life choices and goal-setting in a more authentic and intentional direction. Rather than relying on external validation, emotionally intelligent individuals are often driven by intrinsic motivation—they find satisfaction and meaning from within.

Furthermore, EI strengthens interpersonal relationships through empathy, active listening, and effective communication. These meaningful connections foster a sense of belonging and social purpose, reinforcing the idea that fulfillment often stems from how we relate to others and contribute to our communities.

Emotional intelligence also supports continuous personal growth. By promoting self-reflection and resilience, EI helps individuals adapt to challenges, learn from experiences, and strive for improvement—key elements in the pursuit of long-term satisfaction and purpose.

Scientific evidence reinforces the link between EI and life purpose. Neurological studies indicate that emotionally intelligent individuals tend to have higher levels of dopamine and serotonin, neurotransmitters associated with motivation and well-being. Moreover, research shows that practices like mindfulness, self-reflection, and nurturing positive social interactions—core aspects of EI—are consistently associated with a stronger sense of life purpose.

In essence, emotional intelligence is not only a guide for emotional balance but also a catalyst for living a meaningful, purpose-driven life.

5. DEVELOPING EMOTIONAL INTELLIGENCE AND SELF-AWARENESS

Knowing yourself is the beginning of all wisdom." — **Aristotle**

This quote reflects the core of self-awareness, which is foundational to emotional intelligence. It speaks to the timeless spiritual and philosophical understanding that self-knowledge is key to growth, clarity, and wise living.

Developing emotional intelligence (EI) and self-awareness is a **lifelong process** that enhances personal growth, resilience, and overall well-being (Rasri et al., 2024). By actively cultivating self-awareness, individuals can better understand their emotions, behaviors, and thought patterns, leading to improved emotional regulation and decision-making. This section explores **effective strategies for developing self-awareness, practical techniques to enhance EI, and the role of emotional regulation in personal and professional growth**.

5.1 Strategies for Cultivating Self-Awareness

Self-awareness—the ability to recognize and understand one's own emotions, thoughts, and behaviors—is the cornerstone of emotional intelligence. It enables individuals to become more attuned to their internal states, helping them identify emotional triggers, unconscious biases, and habitual reactions. With greater self-awareness comes increased self-control, allowing people to respond to life's challenges with intention rather than impulse.

Developing self-awareness begins with introspection and self-reflection. By consciously examining how they think and feel in different situations, individuals can begin to recognize patterns in their emotional responses. Asking reflective questions such as "What triggered my reaction?" or "How could I have responded more constructively?" helps deepen this awareness and paves the way for growth.

Another powerful strategy involves seeking feedback from others. Trusted friends, mentors, or colleagues can offer honest perspectives on how one's emotions and behaviors affect those around them. In professional settings, structured feedback tools like 360-degree evaluations can help uncover blind spots, offering insights into interpersonal dynamics that might otherwise go unnoticed.

Emotional check-ins throughout the day are also valuable. Taking brief pauses to assess current emotional states—and examining whether these emotions stem from the present moment or are shaped by past experiences or distorted thinking—can help individuals stay grounded and better manage their responses.

Mindfulness practices offer yet another path to cultivating self-awareness. By fostering present-moment awareness and observing emotions without judgment, mindfulness allows individuals to better understand their internal experiences and reduce emotional reactivity. Instead of getting lost in regrets about the past or anxieties about the future, mindfulness brings clarity and calm to the now.

Neuroscientific research supports the importance of these practices. Studies show that areas of the brain such as the anterior cingulate cortex and prefrontal cortex—key regions involved in emotional regulation and self-awareness—are activated and even strengthened through regular meditation and reflective practices. These changes in brain structure enhance emotional insight and increase one's capacity for self-regulation.

In cultivating self-awareness, individuals lay the groundwork for all other aspects of emotional intelligence, leading to more intentional, resilient, and fulfilling lives.

5.2 Practical Techniques for Enhancing Emotional Intelligence

Developing emotional intelligence (EI) is a lifelong journey that can be significantly enriched through intentional, structured practices. One of the most effective approaches is mindfulness and meditation. These practices train individuals to observe their emotions as they arise, without reacting impulsively. Over time, mindfulness enhances the function of the prefrontal cortex, the brain region responsible for self-control and resilience.

Techniques like Mindfulness-Based Stress Reduction (MBSR) (Grossman et al., 2010) have been shown to reduce stress, anxiety, and emotional reactivity, helping people respond more calmly and effectively in everyday situations.

Journaling and expressive writing also offer a powerful path to emotional growth. By articulating thoughts and emotions on paper, individuals can gain clarity, identify recurring emotional patterns, and process difficult experiences. Simple journaling prompts such as "What emotion dominated my day?" or "How did I handle a difficult conversation?" encourage reflection and support emotional regulation and problem-solving skills.

Cognitive reframing (Pipas, 2021), a cornerstone of Cognitive Behavioral Therapy (CBT), helps individuals shift their perspective on challenging situations. This technique teaches people to reinterpret negative thoughts in more constructive ways. For example, instead of thinking, "I failed at this task, so I must not be good enough," one might reframe the thought as, "This was a learning opportunity, and I can improve next time." Such shifts in perspective reduce self-criticism and build emotional resilience.

Active listening and empathy-building exercises are also central to EI development. These practices encourage individuals to truly hear others without rushing to judgment or formulating a response. By mirroring the speaker's emotions or paraphrasing their message, listeners can foster deeper understanding and connection—key ingredients of empathy and emotional attunement.

Finally, role-playing and social simulations provide hands-on opportunities to practice emotional responses in realistic scenarios. Whether navigating workplace conflict or responding to constructive criticism, simulated environments—sometimes supported by virtual reality (VR) or AI tools—allow individuals to refine their emotional and social skills in a safe, controlled setting.

Together, these techniques offer practical and accessible ways to strengthen emotional intelligence. With consistent practice, individuals can build greater emotional insight, foster healthier relationships, and navigate life's complexities with confidence and compassion.

These techniques are widely applied in personal development, therapeutic settings, and leaderships (Durham et al., 2023). Citizens from all types of life can cultivate their emotional skills by engaging in proven techniques that enhance emotional regulation, empathy, and self-awareness.

5.3 The Role of Emotional Regulation in Personal Growth

Emotional regulation—the ability to effectively manage and respond to emotional experiences—is a cornerstone of emotional intelligence and a vital driver of personal growth. It empowers individuals to remain calm under pressure, make thoughtful decisions, and handle social situations with poise and clarity.

At the heart of emotional regulation lies the capacity to understand emotional triggers. This involves identifying specific situations, environments, or individuals that consistently provoke strong emotional reactions. By keeping an emotion journal, individuals can recognize recurring patterns, uncover underlying causes, and begin to anticipate and better manage their emotional responses.

Developing healthy coping mechanisms is another essential component. Rather than resorting to emotional suppression, social withdrawal, or harmful habits like substance use, emotionally intelligent individuals adopt positive strategies. These might include deep breathing exercises, physical activity, journaling, or engaging in creative or relaxing hobbies—all of which help process emotions in a healthy and constructive way.

Striking a balance between emotional expression and self-control is also key. Emotional regulation does not mean bottling up feelings; rather, it involves expressing emotions constructively without becoming reactive or overwhelmed. Assertive communication plays an important role here, allowing individuals to articulate their needs and boundaries clearly, without aggression or passivity.

Cultivating a growth mindset further supports emotional regulation by encouraging individuals to view challenges not as threats, but as opportunities for learning and development. This mindset shift fosters resilience and allows for self-compassion in the face of setbacks, reducing harsh self-criticism and enhancing long-term emotional well-being.

From a neuroscientific perspective, emotional regulation involves specific brain regions. Training in emotional intelligence has been shown to decrease activity in the amygdala—the brain's alarm system—leading to reduced stress responses. At the same time, the prefrontal cortex, responsible for rational thinking and impulse control, becomes more active, enhancing our ability to respond to stress thoughtfully rather than reactively.

Together, these insights reveal that emotional regulation is not just about controlling emotions but using them wisely. It enables individuals to move through life with greater confidence, resilience, and purpose, making it a fundamental skill for anyone seeking personal growth and emotional mastery.

6. EMOTIONAL INTELLIGENCE IN DIFFERENT LIFE DOMAINS

"The greatest ability in business is to get along with others and influence their actions." — **John C. Maxwell**

This quote emphasizes the role of emotional intelligence in professional and social domains, highlighting its importance in fostering positive relationships and effective interactions across different areas of life.

Emotional Intelligence (EI) is a versatile skill that influences various aspects of life, from education and work to broader societal well-being. Integrating EI in different domains fosters personal development, social harmony, and professional success. This section explores how EI enhances learning environments, strengthens workplace dynamics, and contributes to healthier communities.

6.1 Education: Integrating EI in Learning Environments

The role of emotional intelligence (EI) in education extends far beyond test scores and academic achievement. By nurturing emotional and social competencies, educational systems can empower students to manage their emotions, build meaningful relationships, and develop resilience—essential skills for thriving both inside and outside the classroom.

Research has consistently shown that students with higher levels of EI not only perform better academically but also exhibit greater empathy, improved mental health, and enhanced social behavior. When emotional intelligence is integrated into the learning environment, it creates a foundation for more compassionate, focused, and emotionally resilient learners.

One of the most immediate benefits of EI in education is improved academic performance. Emotionally intelligent students are better equipped to handle stress, maintain focus, and stay engaged in their studies. Skills such as emotional regulation and self-awareness enhance critical thinking and problem-solving—core competencies that translate directly to better learning outcomes.

Beyond academics, EI contributes significantly to positive classroom behavior and stronger social interactions. Students who develop emotional intelligence tend to collaborate more effectively, resolve conflicts peacefully, and demonstrate respect for diversity. Schools that embed EI into their curricula often report lower rates of bullying, fewer disciplinary issues, and stronger peer relationships.

Emotional intelligence also plays a vital role in supporting students' mental health. EI-based programs reduce anxiety and depression, increase self-esteem, and build coping skills that help students navigate both academic and personal challenges. Initiatives such as (Social and Emotional Learning, 2014) have proven especially impactful, showing long-term reductions in emotional distress and aggressive behavior while fostering a greater sense of well-being.

To successfully integrate emotional intelligence in education, several practical strategies can be adopted. Teaching emotional literacy—helping students to recognize, name, and express their emotions in healthy ways—is a foundational step. Mindfulness and reflection practices, such as journaling and deep breathing exercises, can promote self-awareness and emotional regulation. Empathy-based learning methods, including storytelling, role-playing, and group discussions, help students develop compassion and perspective-taking.

Equally important is equipping educators with emotional intelligence skills themselves. When teachers model emotional awareness, empathy, and effective communication, they create a positive emotional climate in the classroom and become role models for emotionally intelligent behavior.

One inspiring example comes from Finland, where emotional intelligence is deeply embedded in the education system. Through the integration of Social Emotional Learning-based programs, Finnish schools have seen notable improvements in both academic success and students' emotional well-being—highlighting how powerful EI can be in shaping a more holistic and human-centered educational experience.

In essence, emotional intelligence is not a peripheral addition to education—it's a transformative force that fosters academic success, emotional health, and lifelong interpersonal skills. By integrating EI into learning environments, we prepare students not just to pass exams, but to thrive as thoughtful, resilient, and emotionally capable individuals.

6.2 Workplaces: Enhancing Leadership, Teamwork, and Professional Growth

In modern professional settings, emotional intelligence (EI) has emerged as a crucial skill set that complements—and often amplifies—the value of technical expertise. In an era defined by rapid change, global collaboration, and complex interpersonal dynamics, EI enables professionals to lead with empathy, communicate with clarity, and thrive in diverse teams.

Emotionally intelligent leadership has a profound impact on organizational culture and performance (Bashir, 2016). Leaders who possess high EI inspire and motivate their teams, foster trust, and guide decision-making with both empathy and strategic thinking. Such leaders are not only skilled communicators but also adept at navigating conflict, managing team morale, and creating inclusive environments where every voice is valued.

Teamwork also flourishes in emotionally intelligent workplaces. When team members are attuned to their own emotions and sensitive to the emotional cues of others, collaboration becomes smoother and more effective. High-EI teams are better equipped to handle disagreements constructively, communicate across cultural and personality differences, and build relationships rooted in mutual respect. This emotional awareness contributes significantly to cohesive, innovative, and high-performing teams.

Another key benefit of emotional intelligence in the workplace is its role in boosting employee engagement and reducing burnout. By equipping individuals with the tools to manage stress, stay resilient, and adapt to change, EI fosters a more positive work experience. Organizations that prioritize EI see higher levels of job satisfaction, improved well-being, and lower turnover rates—outcomes that directly contribute to long-term success (Côté, 2014).

To cultivate EI within professional environments, several strategies have proven effective. Offering targeted EI training for both leaders and employees is a foundational step. These coaching programs help individuals develop core competencies such as self-awareness, empathy, and emotional regulation. Communication and feedback workshops are also valuable, encouraging practices like active listening, assertiveness, and constructive dialogue.

Mentorship and peer support systems can create emotionally supportive workplace cultures where individuals feel seen, heard, and valued. Additionally, introducing mindfulness and work-life balance programs helps employees manage emotional fatigue and sustain their performance over time.

One notable example of integrating EI into professional development is Google's "Search Inside Yourself" program. This initiative combines mindfulness practices with emotional intelligence training, empowering employees to enhance self-awareness, manage stress, and cultivate meaningful workplace relationships. The program has been praised for improving productivity and employee satisfaction, illustrating how EI can transform not only individuals but entire organizational ecosystems.

Key Takeaways

Emotional intelligence is not a soft skill—it is a strategic advantage. By embedding EI into leadership models, team practices, and organizational culture, workplaces can nurture more resilient, collaborative, and effective professionals equipped for the challenges of a dynamic world.

6.3 Communities: Promoting Emotional Intelligence for Societal Well-Being

Emotional intelligence (EI) plays a foundational role in shaping the health, harmony, and resilience of society. When individuals are emotionally aware, empathetic, and socially responsible, communities become more cohesive, compassionate, and equipped to face both everyday challenges and large-scale crises.

At the heart of emotionally intelligent communities are stronger social bonds. EI fosters open, respectful communication and constructive approaches to resolving conflict, enabling individuals to navigate differences without hostility. Communities rich in emotional intelligence tend to be more inclusive, peaceful, and responsive to the needs of their diverse members.

Empathy and social responsibility are also deeply embedded in emotionally intelligent cultures. Individuals with high EI are more likely to volunteer, participate in civic initiatives, and champion social justice causes. Their actions contribute to a shared sense of purpose and responsibility, strengthening the moral and ethical fabric of society. When emotional awareness becomes a community norm, prosocial behaviors flourish and collective well-being rises.

In times of crisis—whether personal, local, or global—EI becomes a critical factor in resilience. Community programs centered on emotional intelligence provide essential support networks, reduce stigma around mental health, and help individuals process trauma. Societies that cultivate EI are better prepared to respond to disasters, economic instability, and collective grief with compassion and strength.

To promote emotional intelligence on a societal level, a range of strategies can be implemented. Community-based EI education—delivered through schools, public forums, and local organizations—equips people of all ages with essential emotional skills. Empathy and diversity programs, including cultural exchanges and social awareness workshops, foster understanding across differences and nurture inclusive mindsets.

Integrating EI training into social services can further amplify its impact. When caregivers, counselors, and community workers are emotionally attuned, they provide more effective, compassionate support to those in need. Meanwhile, public initiatives focused on emotional well-being—such as mental health campaigns and resilience-building activities—create environments where emotional literacy and support are widely accessible.

A striking example of these principles in action is found in Denmark's national initiative to teach empathy in schools. This long-term investment in emotional education has contributed to greater happiness, stronger social cohesion, and even a reduction in crime rates—highlighting how emotional intelligence, when cultivated early and consistently, can transform the very fabric of society.

Ultimately, emotionally intelligent communities are not merely desirable—they are essential. As we navigate increasingly complex social and global challenges, EI offers a path toward more harmonious, just, and resilient societies grounded in empathy and mutual respect.

7. CASE STUDIES AND RESEARCH-BASED INSIGHTS

"In the middle of difficulty lies opportunity." — Albert Einstein

This quote speaks to the value of research and case studies, suggesting that even in complex or challenging situations, there are valuable insights to be found—mirroring the purpose of examining real-world examples to understand emotional intelligence in action.

Understanding Emotional Intelligence (EI) through **real-world applications and scientific research** provides valuable insights into its **practical benefits and transformative impact**. This section explores **case studies and empirical research** highlighting how EI fosters **self-awareness, resilience, and well-being** across different settings.

7.1 Real-World Examples of EI Fostering Self-Awareness and Resilience

Case Study 1: EI Training for Healthcare Professionals

In high-stress environments such as hospitals and clinics, emotional intelligence (EI) is not just an asset—it's a necessity. Healthcare professionals constantly navigate emotionally charged situations, from managing patient suffering to communicating with distressed families, all while maintaining clinical precision. In this demanding context, EI becomes a vital skill that enables practitioners to deliver compassionate care without compromising their own mental health (Jiménez-Picón et al, 2021).

A compelling example of EI's impact in healthcare comes from a study conducted at a major hospital, where doctors and nurses participated in a structured emotional intelligence training program. The results were significant: participants reported stronger emotional regulation, improved communication with patients and colleagues, and notably lower levels of burnout. This transformation underscores a powerful insight—when healthcare workers are equipped with emotional intelligence skills, they become more resilient to compassion fatigue and better able to maintain their emotional balance.

Beyond individual well-being, EI training contributes directly to patient care. Emotionally intelligent healthcare professionals listen more attentively, express empathy more genuinely, and respond to complex emotional dynamics with greater sensitivity. These qualities not only improve patient satisfaction but also foster trust, which is fundamental to effective healing and treatment adherence.

Ultimately, integrating EI training into medical education and professional development helps build a healthcare workforce that is both emotionally resilient and deeply attuned to the human side of healing (Sahney et al, 2024). In a field where emotional exhaustion is a constant risk, emotional intelligence offers a sustainable path forward—enhancing both care quality and caregiver well-being.

Case Study 2: Emotional Intelligence in Leadership – Initiate by Google's "Search Inside Yourself" Program

Google's innovative approach "Search Inside Yourself" to enhance leadership and workplace well-being through emotional intelligence (EI) initiated a powerful corporate cultural edge around the world. This program created in 2007 is a mindfulness-based EI training initiative designed to help employees develop self-awareness, empathy, and emotional regulation. The program was not just about personal development but aimed at improving leadership effectiveness and fostering a positive work environment.

Through this program, participants learned to recognize and manage their emotions, enhancing their capacity to lead with empathy and communicate more effectively. As a result, employees reported increased job satisfaction, decreased levels of workplace stress, and improved collaboration within teams. The program's emphasis on mindfulness also allowed individuals to become more attuned to their own emotional states and the needs of those around them.

The success of the "Search Inside Yourself" program highlighted a key takeaway: EI-driven leadership cultivates a work culture grounded in trust, respect, and mutual understanding. In turn, this leads to higher productivity, stronger interpersonal connections, and a more engaged workforce. By integrating emotional intelligence into leadership practices, Google demonstrated how cultivating these skills not only benefits individual leaders (Caporale-Berkowitz et al., 2021), but also creates a healthier, more harmonious workplace environment for all.

Case Study 3: EI and Student Success – The RULER Approach in Schools

The RULER program[1], developed by Yale University from 2005, is a groundbreaking initiative that integrates emotional intelligence (EI) into school curricula to foster improved student outcomes. By teaching students how to Recognize, Understand, Label, Express, and Regulate their emotions, RULER empowers them to navigate both their academic and social lives more effectively.

Schools that have implemented the RULER program have witnessed a significant transformation in students' emotional regulation, academic performance, and peer relationships. Students became more adept at managing their emotions, which helped reduce instances of bullying, anxiety, and disciplinary actions. As a result, there was an overall improvement in the school environment, making it more supportive and conducive to learning.

The success of the RULER program (South et als., 2022) underscores a key takeaway: incorporating emotional intelligence into education not only enhances self-awareness and emotional resilience but also promotes long-term personal growth. By equipping students with the tools to manage their emotions effectively, RULER fosters a foundation for academic success, stronger relationships, and overall well-being.

7.2 Research Findings on the Impact of EI in Various Settings

EI and Mental Health: A Neuroscientific Perspective

Recent studies in neuroscience provide compelling evidence that Emotional Intelligence (EI) plays a critical role in mental health by promoting emotional regulation, reducing stress, and fostering resilience. Research has consistently shown that individuals with higher EI tend to experience lower levels of stress, anxiety, and depression, highlighting the significant impact of EI on overall psychological well-being.

One of the key mechanisms behind these benefits lies in the brain's prefrontal cortex. Neuroscientific studies have demonstrated that EI is closely linked to enhanced functioning of this region, which is responsible for complex cognitive processes such as emotional regulation, decision-making, and self-control. The prefrontal cortex helps individuals manage their emotions, assess situations rationally, and avoid impulsive reactions. Enhanced prefrontal cortex activity is associated with a greater ability to regulate negative emotions and engage in proactive coping strategies during stressful events, which is crucial for maintaining mental health.

Furthermore, individuals with high EI exhibit improved cognitive flexibility, meaning they are better equipped to adapt their thinking and behaviors in response to changing circumstances. This flexibility is a cornerstone of emotional resilience—the ability to bounce back from setbacks and navigate through challenging emotional experiences. Research has shown that when faced with stressful situations, emotionally intelligent individuals can reframe negative thoughts, manage emotional reactions, and maintain positive coping mechanisms. This ability to regulate emotions and thoughts not only reduces vulnerability to mental health disorders like anxiety and depression but also enhances emotional resilience, allowing individuals to thrive in the face of adversity.

Key Takeaways

Neuroscientific research underscores the significant impact of Emotional Intelligence on mental health. By strengthening the prefrontal cortex and improving cognitive flexibility, Emotional intelligence enables individuals to regulate emotions more effectively, reduce the impact of stress, and enhance their overall emotional resilience. These findings offer valuable insights into how cultivating EI can act as a protective factor against mental health challenges and promote long-term psychological well-being.

EI in the Workplace: Research on Leadership and Job Performance

Emotional Intelligence (EI) has become a vital skill in the workplace, influencing leadership effectiveness, employee satisfaction, and organizational success. Research consistently underscores the significant role EI plays in shaping workplace dynamics and improving overall job performance (Alferaih, 2017). A meta-analysis of over 100 studies conducted by leading researchers (Hongjiang, 2018) in the field found that leaders with high EI consistently outperform their peers in key areas such as team management and decision-making. Ikart in hisresearch (Ikart, 2023) pointed out that leaders with strong EI are better equipped to navigate complex interpersonal dynamics, foster positive work environments, and make informed decisions that benefit both individuals and teams. Their ability to recognize and manage their own emotions, as well as empathize with others, enables them to respond more effectively to challenges, resolve conflicts more efficiently, and maintain strong team morale, even in high-pressure situations. As a result, these leaders are viewed as more approachable, trustworthy, and motivating, leading to higher levels of employee satisfaction and team performance.

Beyond leadership, employees with high EI also experience a range of benefits that positively impact their work experience. Studies show that these employees exhibit greater job satisfaction, lower levels of stress, and a stronger sense of engagement with their work. One of the primary reasons for these outcomes is that emotionally intelligent employees are better at managing workplace stressors, navigating social dynamics, and building positive relationships with colleagues. Their ability to regulate their own emotions helps them stay calm and focused during difficult situations, leading to higher productivity and a more collaborative work environment. Furthermore, emotionally intelligent employees are less likely to experience burnout, which leads to lower turnover rates and greater organizational loyalty. High EI also improves an employee's ability to offer constructive feedback and receive criticism, making them more adaptable and open to professional development opportunities.

Organizations that prioritize the development of EI among their employees also see significant improvements in their overall performance. Companies investing in EI training programs report increased employee engagement, better teamwork, and higher levels of productivity. These programs help employees develop key EI skills such as emotional regulation, empathy, and conflict resolution, which enhance their interpersonal effectiveness and ability to collaborate. When employees are trained to be more emotionally intelligent, they are better equipped to handle the challenges of the modern workplace, leading to improved organizational communication and employee retention. Additionally, emotionally intelligent employees are more likely to take initiative, work autonomously, and contribute positively to a company's innovation and growth. As a result, companies that integrate EI into their culture not only see improvements in internal dynamics but also experience a more resilient and productive workforce.

Key Takeaways

EI plays a critical role in workplace success, influencing everything from leadership effectiveness to employee satisfaction and organizational productivity. The research shows that emotionally intelligent leaders are better equipped to manage teams, make decisions, and foster a healthy work environment, while employees with high EI enjoy greater job satisfaction, workplace harmony, and long-term career success. Furthermore, organizations that invest in EI development see tangible benefits, including increased productivity, lower turnover, and a more engaged workforce. As the workplace continues to evolve, EI will remain a key factor in shaping organizational culture and driving long-term success.

EI in Education: Enhancing Learning and Emotional Well-Being

Emotional Intelligence (EI) has a profound impact on the educational experience (Bar-On, 2007, influencing both academic achievement and emotional well-being. Research consistently supports the importance of EI in promoting positive student outcomes. Studies show that students with high EI tend to score higher on standardized tests and exhibit stronger interpersonal skills compared to their peers. These students are better equipped to handle the pressures of academic life, including time management, goal-setting, and overcoming challenges, thanks to their enhanced ability to regulate emotions and focus on tasks. Moreover, emotionally intelligent students can manage stress more effectively, leading to better academic performance and improved cognitive functioning during exams and assignments. The emotional awareness and self-regulation that EI fosters allow students to stay calm under pressure, make thoughtful decisions, and engage more deeply in complex academic tasks.

In schools where EI-focused curricula have been implemented, behavioral problems such as bullying, aggression, and disengagement tend to decrease significantly. These schools report a more positive school climate, with students demonstrating better social skills, empathy, and conflict resolution abilities. Students with higher EI are less likely to act impulsively, are better at managing their emotions, and more likely to engage in proactive problem-solving. As a result, there is a noticeable reduction in disciplinary issues, which creates a more conducive learning environment. Furthermore, these students tend to have more positive relationships with their peers and teachers, fostering a sense of belonging and emotional security within the school community. By incorporating EI into the curriculum, schools can create an environment that nurtures both academic and emotional growth, encouraging students to develop as well-rounded individuals.

The integration of EI into education has long-lasting benefits that go beyond academic success. When schools focus on developing emotional intelligence, they not only enhance students' academic outcomes, but also contribute to their social-emotional development. EI promotes self-awareness, self-regulation, empathy, and social skills, which are essential for students' success both in and outside the classroom. Research shows that these skills help students build stronger peer relationships, better handle conflicts, and make responsible decisions. Moreover, students who develop EI are more likely to experience higher levels of well-being, greater emotional resilience, and a stronger sense of purpose in life. They are also better prepared to face the challenges of adulthood, from managing career pressures to maintaining healthy relationships and emotional balance. By incorporating EI into educational practices, schools can help students grow into emotionally intelligent, responsible, and well-adjusted individuals who can succeed academically while also thriving emotionally.

Key Takeaways

EI in education plays a critical role in fostering both academic success and emotional well-being. Research supports the fact that emotionally intelligent students outperform their peers in both standardized testing and interpersonal relationships. Schools that integrate EI into their curricula see a reduction in behavioral problems, improved student engagement, and a positive, nurturing school environment. Most importantly, EI integration enhances social-emotional development, preparing students for lifelong success both in their academic careers and in navigating the complexities of adult life.

7.3 Lessons Learned from EI-Focused Programs and Interventions

Key Lessons from Successful EI Programs

Emotional Intelligence (EI) programs have shown to be highly effective in fostering both personal and professional growth across various domains. The key lessons learned from successful EI programs highlight the importance of early development, mindfulness practices, and creating supportive organizational cultures.

Early EI Development is Critical

One of the most important lessons is that developing EI from an early age can have significant long-term benefits. Programs such as Social and Emotional Learning (SEL) in schools have demonstrated positive, lasting impacts on students' academic success, mental health, and interpersonal relationships. Research shows that early exposure to EI-focused curricula equips students with essential emotional regulation and social skills that stay with them throughout their lives. This foundational EI development not only enhances students' ability to navigate challenges during their school years but also prepares them for success in their personal lives and professional careers. By embedding EI into education systems early on, young people gain a head start in developing critical emotional and social competencies, setting them on a path toward greater well-being and resilience in adulthood.

Mindfulness Enhances EI

Mindfulness practices are increasingly recognized as powerful tools for enhancing EI. Programs that incorporate mindfulness—such as meditation, deep breathing, and focused attention exercises—have been shown to significantly improve self-awareness, emotional regulation, and cognitive function. Regular mindfulness practices help individuals develop a greater awareness of their emotions, which is essential for self-regulation. By learning to observe their emotional responses without judgment, individuals can more effectively manage reactions to stressors and difficult situations. This improved emotional control leads to better decision-making, increased cognitive flexibility, and enhanced ability to handle interpersonal conflicts. Mindfulness, as part of an EI development program, can be a transformative tool, offering individuals a way to build emotional resilience and maintain a balanced, focused mindset both at work and in personal life.

Organizational Culture Matters

Successful EI programs also emphasize the role of organizational culture in shaping outcomes. In workplaces where EI is integrated into leadership training and teamwork strategies, the overall professional relationships improve, and employees experience lower stress levels and greater collaboration. Companies that prioritize EI in their leadership development initiatives create environments where leaders are not only emotionally intelligent themselves but also encourage the growth of EI within their teams. This leads to improved communication, more effective conflict resolution, and a greater sense of trust among colleagues. When EI is embedded in an organization's culture, it fosters an atmosphere of mutual respect, emotional support, and psychological safety, allowing employees to feel valued and empowered. This, in turn, translates into enhanced teamwork, increased productivity, and improved employee well-being, contributing to a more positive and cohesive workplace culture.

Key Takeaways

The success of EI programs highlights three key lessons: the importance of early development through programs like SEL in schools, the transformative effects of mindfulness practices on emotional intelligence, and the critical role of organizational culture in fostering strong relationships and reducing stress in the workplace. By investing in EI development at various stages of life and within organizational settings, individuals and organizations alike can experience profound benefits, from improved emotional resilience to enhanced collaboration and productivity.

Challenges and Areas for Improvement

While the benefits of Emotional Intelligence (EI) programs are widely recognized, several challenges remain in ensuring their effectiveness and broad application. These challenges highlight areas where further research, adaptation, and innovation are needed to maximize the potential of EI in improving personal and professional outcomes. Scaling EI Programs Across Diverse Populations: One of the primary challenges in implementing EI programs is scaling them across diverse populations, especially when considering cultural and economic differences. What works in one context or culture may not always be directly transferable to others. For example, cultural norms around emotional expression and social interaction can significantly affect how EI is understood and applied. In some cultures, emotional expression is more open and encouraged, while in others, there may be a greater emphasis on emotional restraint. These differences may influence the way individuals engage with EI training and how effective it is in promoting self-awareness, emotional regulation, and social skills. Additionally, economic disparities can limit access to quality EI programs, especially in underprivileged areas. To address this challenge, it is essential to adapt EI programs to different cultural contexts and make them accessible to all populations, ensuring that people from various backgrounds can benefit from emotional intelligence development.

Long-Term Impact Studies

Another critical area for improvement is the need for long-term impact studies to assess the sustainability of EI interventions across different sectors. While short-term results from EI programs often show positive outcomes, there is still limited research on how these interventions affect participants over time. Understanding the long-term benefits of EI training is crucial to ensuring its lasting impact on personal development, mental health, and workplace productivity. Furthermore, evaluating the effectiveness of these programs over time can provide valuable insights into how to improve and refine EI interventions. Long-term studies will help identify whether the gains in emotional regulation, stress reduction, and social skills endure, and whether these benefits contribute to lasting changes in behavior, performance, and overall well-being. Without this evidence, it can be difficult to justify the investment in EI programs in the long term.

Bridging Neuroscience and EI Applications

Finally, a significant opportunity for improving EI programs lies in bridging neuroscience with practical EI applications. While we know that EI is associated with emotional regulation and cognitive flexibility, a deeper understanding of the neuroscientific basis of these processes can enhance the evidence-based approach to EI training. Neuroscience can provide insights into how brain structures and neural pathways are involved in emotional responses, decision-making, and interpersonal interactions. By integrating this knowledge with EI training techniques, educators and practitioners can design more targeted and effective interventions that align with how the brain processes and regulates emotions. This interdisciplinary approach has the potential to enhance the efficacy of EI programs, making them more personalized and scientifically grounded. Furthermore, understanding the neurological mechanisms behind emotional intelligence could lead to the development of new training methods that optimize brain function, ultimately improving the outcomes of EI development.

8. FUTURE DIRECTIONS AND CONCLUSION

As the world becomes increasingly complex and interconnected, Emotional Intelligence (EI) will continue to play a pivotal role in shaping personal development, professional success, and societal well-being. Let us explore the future of Emotional Intelligence, practical ways to integrate Emotional Intelligence into daily life, and a final reflection on its profound significance for individuals and communities.

8.1 The Evolving Role of EI in a Rapidly Changing World

The Need for EI in the Age of AI and Automation

As we move deeper into the age of AI and automation, the landscape of work is shifting dramatically. While artificial intelligence is automating many routine tasks, it is also creating new demands for uniquely human skills. Emotional intelligence (EI) remains one of the most essential traits that technology cannot replicate, particularly in roles that require adaptability, empathy, and human connection. In an increasingly automated world, those who excel in emotional intelligence will be better equipped to navigate change, respond to new challenges, and maintain a human-centered approach in their interactions with machines and other people.

Jobs that require high levels of emotional intelligence—such as in leadership, healthcare, and education—are expected to be in greater demand. These fields rely on the ability to understand, motivate, and connect with others on an emotional level, something that machines simply cannot do. As AI and automation take over more technical tasks, human workers will increasingly be called upon to add value through their emotional awareness, problem-solving skills, and collaborative abilities. As such, future workplaces may see a greater emphasis on EI training, alongside the development of technical skills, to ensure employees are prepared to thrive in this new environment.

EI in the Digital Era: Managing Virtual Communication and Social Media

With the rise of remote work, virtual interactions, and digital communication, new challenges are emerging for emotional intelligence. The way we communicate and interact has shifted from face-to-face exchanges to predominantly digital mediums, such as emails, video calls, and social media. These platforms, while convenient, often lack the non-verbal cues and emotional context that we rely on in face-to-face interactions. This creates a challenge for recognizing emotions, interpreting tone, and fostering meaningful connections.

EI plays a crucial role in overcoming these barriers. In virtual settings, individuals with high emotional intelligence can use their empathy and social awareness to better understand and respond to the emotional needs of others. They are more attuned to subtle cues in digital communication, such as word choice or timing, and are adept at managing misunderstandings or conflicts that may arise online. As the digital world continues to expand, there may be a growing need for digital well-being initiatives that integrate EI-based strategies to reduce stress, foster positive online interactions, and help prevent conflicts in virtual environments. These strategies can improve mental health and overall well-being in a world that increasingly operates through screens.

EI and Global Challenges: Climate Change, Mental Health, and Social Cohesion

The pressing global challenges of our time—such as climate change, mental health crises, and political polarization—demand new solutions that prioritize emotional resilience and cooperative problem-solving. Emotional intelligence can serve as a foundational tool in addressing these crises, fostering resilience, cooperation, and constructive dialogue in times of uncertainty. As societies grapple with climate disasters, escalating mental health issues, and divisions within communities, the ability to manage emotions, work together, and find common ground becomes more critical than ever.

EI-based interventions can enhance collective well-being and contribute to more effective conflict resolution in response to these global challenges. For instance, in the face of climate change, fostering empathy and understanding across different cultures and perspectives can encourage collaborative efforts in sustainability and environmental protection. Similarly, in addressing mental health issues, promoting emotional awareness and resilience can support individuals in navigating the psychological toll of these crises.

EI can also play a significant role in promoting social cohesion in times of political and social unrest. By integrating emotional intelligence into community programs, policymaking, and crisis response efforts, we can create environments that encourage dialogue, foster inclusivity, and help resolve conflicts in a more ethical and compassionate manner. Schools and workplaces that integrate EI into their curricula and practices can contribute to promoting diversity, inclusivity, and ethical decision-making, ensuring that emotional intelligence becomes a cornerstone of collective problem-solving and social progress (OECD, 2015) in the face of global challenges.

8.2 Integrating EI Development into Daily Life

Practical Approaches for Individuals

Integrating Emotional Intelligence (EI) into daily life requires consistent, practical efforts that can gradually enhance self-awareness, emotional regulation, and interpersonal relationships. For individuals seeking to develop their EI, there are several approaches that can be seamlessly incorporated into their routines. These practices not only help individuals grow emotionally but also contribute to more meaningful interactions, improved decision-making, and better mental well-being.

Mindfulness Practices

One of the most effective ways to integrate EI into daily life is through regular mindfulness exercises. Mindfulness (Ho) helps individuals become more aware of their emotions as they occur in the moment, fostering a deeper connection with their feelings. By practicing mindfulness—whether through meditation, focused breathing, or body scans—individuals can heighten their self-awareness, allowing them to better recognize emotional responses before they escalate. This awareness helps to regulate emotions, reducing impulsivity and promoting more thoughtful decision-making. Mindfulness also improves an individual's ability to be present and attentive, which is essential for practicing empathy and building emotional resilience. Over time, these practices help individuals gain better control over their emotions, leading to more balanced and composed reactions to challenges.

Journaling

Another valuable approach to integrating EI development into daily life is journaling. By regularly reflecting on their emotions and experiences, individuals can gain a better understanding of their emotional triggers and personal growth. Journaling provides an opportunity to process feelings in a non-judgmental way, promoting self-reflection and emotional insight (Liu et al., 2024). Writing down emotions allows individuals to express what they are feeling, track emotional patterns, and gain clarity on how they respond to various situations. This practice is particularly helpful for cultivating self-awareness, as it enables individuals to identify recurring emotional reactions and take proactive steps to manage them. Journaling also supports the development of emotional regulation by giving individuals a structured space to reflect and recalibrate their emotional responses.

Active Listening

Active listening is an essential skill that enhances emotional intelligence and strengthens interpersonal relationships. Practicing active listening in everyday conversations helps individuals develop empathy—a crucial EI component. Active listening involves fully focusing on the speaker, understanding their emotions, and responding thoughtfully. This approach requires an individual to listen without judgment or interruption, allowing the other person to express themselves fully. By practicing this kind of listening, individuals become more attuned to the emotions of others, improving their ability to empathize and respond appropriately. It also deepens social skills, as it fosters open, meaningful communication and promotes a sense of connection and trust. Active listening in both personal and professional settings helps to build stronger, more supportive relationships, reducing misunderstandings and fostering emotional balance.

Emotional Check-Ins

Simple yet effective, emotional check-ins are a powerful practice for cultivating emotional awareness throughout the day. By pausing at regular intervals—whether in the morning, during breaks, or before important decisions—individuals can take a moment to assess their current emotional state. This practice of checking in helps individuals become more mindful of their feelings and identify any emotional shifts that may need attention. Emotional check-ins are particularly useful for improving self-awareness, as they allow individuals to recognize whether they are feeling stressed, anxious, or calm. Understanding their emotional state enables them to respond more appropriately to external events, make better decisions, and adjust their behavior accordingly. Regular emotional check-ins also promote a sense of control and balance, contributing to improved mental health and emotional resilience.

Incorporating these practical approaches into daily life can significantly enhance one's emotional intelligence, fostering deeper self-awareness, better emotional regulation, and more meaningful relationships. By integrating mindfulness practices, journaling, active listening, and emotional check-ins, individuals can strengthen their EI and apply it in a variety of contexts, from personal growth to professional success. These habits not only empower individuals to navigate their emotions more effectively but also foster emotional balance and social harmony in their everyday lives.

Strategies for Families, Schools, and Workplaces

Building Emotional Intelligence (EI) in individuals is not only a personal effort but can be supported by the environments in which people live, learn, and work. Families, schools, and workplaces play key roles in fostering emotional intelligence, each contributing uniquely to the development of self-awareness, emotional regulation, and interpersonal skills. By implementing targeted strategies, these sectors can create environments where EI is cultivated, leading to improved emotional resilience, better communication, and enhanced collaboration.

Families are often the first place where emotional intelligence is nurtured. Parents and caregivers have a unique opportunity to shape their children's emotional development by encouraging open emotional communication. When children feel safe to express their emotions without judgment, they learn to identify and understand their feelings, which is the foundation of self-awareness. Parents can model healthy emotional regulation by demonstrating how to manage frustration, sadness, or anger constructively. Additionally, empathy can be taught by encouraging children to understand others' perspectives and feelings. Simple activities, like discussing emotions at the dinner table or offering comfort when a child is upset, can help children learn how to handle their emotions and understand the emotions of those around them. Family dynamics that promote emotional openness provide the groundwork for developing a high level of EI, fostering children who grow into emotionally intelligent individuals capable of handling life's challenges with balance and empathy.

In the domain of education, schools are crucial environments for shaping and nurturing emotional intelligence from a young age. Implementing Social-Emotional Learning (SEL) programs is one of the most effective ways to cultivate EI in students. SEL programs help students develop essential skills in self-awareness, self-regulation, empathy, and social interactions. By incorporating SEL into the curriculum, students are not only taught academic content but also emotional competencies that will serve them throughout their lives. These programs can take many forms, from classroom discussions on emotions to activities that teach problem-solving and conflict resolution skills. Research has shown that schools that implement SEL programs experience reductions in behavioral problems, improved academic performance, and stronger relationships among students. Moreover, students who develop EI early are more likely to manage stress, collaborate effectively, and engage in healthy social interactions. Teaching EI in schools prepares students to navigate a complex world with resilience, empathy, and self-regulation, equipping them for success in both their academic and personal lives.

In term of workplace, emotional intelligence plays a critical role in fostering collaboration, productivity, and a healthy work environment (Takong et al., 2021). Organizations can support the development of EI by integrating it into leadership programs and training initiatives. Leaders who demonstrate high EI are better equipped to manage teams, resolve conflicts, and motivate employees effectively. By prioritizing EI in leadership development, workplaces can cultivate leaders who are attuned to the emotions of their teams, fostering emotionally intelligent teams that collaborate seamlessly and handle stress with resilience. EI training can also be offered to employees at all levels to help them improve their communication skills, understand emotional triggers, and manage stress. A workplace that values EI creates a culture of empathy and mutual respect, improving job satisfaction, reducing turnover, and increasing productivity. Additionally, organizations that focus on EI can help employees navigate interpersonal conflicts with greater ease, fostering an environment where employees feel understood, valued, and emotionally supported. In the long run, these efforts contribute to a more positive workplace culture, where employees are empowered to work together effectively and bring their best selves to work.

By integrating emotional intelligence development strategies into family settings, schools, and workplaces, we can foster individuals who are better equipped to handle the emotional demands of modern life. These environments provide vital support for building EI, which ultimately contributes to healthier relationships, greater personal fulfillment, and a more cohesive society. Whether through encouraging emotional expression at home, implementing SEL programs in schools, or fostering emotional intelligence in leadership at work, each sector plays an essential role in empowering individuals to navigate their emotions with balance, empathy, and self-awareness.

Leveraging Technology for EI Growth

As technology continues to shape our lives in profound ways, it offers powerful tools for fostering Emotional Intelligence (EI) development. By integrating advanced technologies, individuals can enhance their self-awareness, emotional regulation, and interpersonal skills in innovative and accessible ways. From AI-powered coaching apps to virtual reality simulations and wearable technology, these tools provide dynamic opportunities for individuals to cultivate EI skills in both personal and professional settings. Below are key examples of how technology can support and enhance emotional intelligence growth.

AI-Powered Emotional Coaching or Personality Development Service

This type of service can track mood and emotions over time (Pempho, 2024), offer personalized feedback and exercises to help individuals reflect on their feelings, identify emotional patterns, and build self-awareness. By analyzing emotional data, these services can suggest guided self-reflection exercises, mindfulness practices, and other activities tailored to the user's emotional needs (Nagaraj, 2024). For instance, TherapAI mood-tracking prompts users to reflect on what triggered a particular emotion, enabling them to better understand their emotional responses and develop more effective emotional regulation strategies (Lal, 2024). Over time, users can track their emotional growth, identify patterns, and develop healthier coping mechanisms for managing their emotions. This kind of service makes EI development more accessible, providing users with on-the-go emotional coaching at their fingertips. With the support of AI, individuals can make more informed, conscious decisions about how to manage their emotions and interactions with others.

Virtual Reality Simulations

Virtual reality (VR) has been revolutionizing emotional intelligence development in the field of cyberpsychology (Ancis, 2020) by providing immersive, real-world emotional scenarios for individuals to practice EI skills (Shadiev, 2021). VR simulations can simulate challenging emotional situations such as workplace conflicts (Himanshu, 2023), difficult conversations, or emotionally charged, offering users a safe space to practice conflict resolution, empathy (Weng et al., 2024), and other essential EI skills (Papoutsi, 2021). For example, in a VR-based scenario, a user might step into the shoes of a manager who must navigate a tense conversation with an employee, allowing them to practice empathy, active listening, and emotional regulation in real-time. These simulations provide immediate feedback, enabling individuals to assess their emotional responses and improve their decision-making in real-world situations. VR also allows users to experience different perspectives including as therapy (Garcia-Gutierrez et al., 2025), which enhances empathy—a key component of EI. By offering a fully immersive, interactive experience, VR can accelerate EI development and help individuals apply their emotional intelligence in education (Wang, 2025) or improving their mental health (Gkoumas et al., 2024) in a variety of contexts, both personal and professional.

Wearable Technology

Wearable devices like smartwatches (Halder et al., 2024), fitness trackers, and biofeedback sensors (Bhatt et al. 2024), are increasingly being used to support emotional regulation and stress management. These devices can monitor physiological indicators such as heart rate, body temperature, and skin conductivity, providing users with real-time data on their emotional state. For example, if a wearable detects increased heart rate or elevated stress levels, it can alert the user, offering prompts for deep breathing exercises or mindfulness practices to help them regulate their emotions. This biofeedback allows individuals to develop a greater awareness of their emotional triggers and the physical manifestations of stress, helping them manage their responses more effectively . Over time, users can learn to recognize early signs of emotional distress and take proactive steps to calm themselves before stress escalates. By combining real-time monitoring with actionable insights, wearable technology enables users to be more proactive in managing their emotional well-being, enhancing both emotional regulation and self-awareness (Arabian 2023).

By leveraging the power of technology, individuals can take a more proactive and personalized approach to developing their emotional intelligence. Whether through AI-powered services for emotional tracking and reflection (Rebouillat et al., 2020), virtual reality scenarios for real-world practice, or wearable devices offering biofeedback and stress management, technology provides innovative tools to enhance EI skills. These technological advancements can empower individuals to better understand and regulate their emotions, improve interpersonal relationships, and cultivate greater emotional resilience—ultimately leading to improved mental well-being and overall life satisfaction. The integration of these tools into everyday life ensures that emotional intelligence development is not only accessible but also engaging, making it easier for individuals to continue their EI growth journey in an increasingly complex and digital world.

9. CONCLUSION

EI as a Lifelong Skill (Rasni, 2024) for Personal Growth Emotional intelligence (EI) is not a fixed trait, but rather a dynamic and evolving skill that can be cultivated throughout life. It requires continuous learning, practice, and self-reflection to develop fully. By prioritizing EI, individuals can experience profound personal growth, achieving higher levels of emotional resilience, self-awareness, and a deeper sense of purpose. EI empowers individuals to navigate life's challenges with greater emotional balance and a heightened ability to manage relationships effectively. As citizens face personal and societal shifts in this 21st century, fostering emotional intelligence equips individuals with the tools to adapt and thrive, both personally and professionally. This lifelong investment in EI not only strengthens personal well-being but also enhances overall quality of life.

The influence of Emotional Inteligence extends far beyond the individual—it has the potential to reshape entire societies. Communities that prioritize emotional intelligence in education (Chen 2020), leadership, and community programs tend to experience greater social harmony, ethical decision-making, and an overall sense of emotional well-being for for all generations of citizens (for example, teanager generation (Mavroveli, 2007)). The positive ripple effects of EI reach all corners of society, fostering a culture of empathy, cooperation, and mutual understanding. As the world faces growing challenges—whether they be social, economic, or environmental—EI acts as a powerful tool for navigating uncertainty. In a world that increasingly demands collaboration and adaptability, the integration of EI into everyday life enhances the ability to build stronger relationships (Al-Mualm, 2023), resolve conflicts with understanding (Irawan, 2024), and maintain resilience in the face of adversity. In this way, emotional intelligence contributes not only to personal well-being but to the collective well-being of society (Ibrahim et al., 2022) as a whole.

The importance of emotional intelligence cannot be overstated, and its cultivation must be a priority for individuals, educators, organizations, and policymakers alike. Actively integrating EI development into our personal lives, educational systems, workplaces, and public institutions can lead to a more emotionally aware and resilient society. This involves fostering environments where emotional intelligence is valued and nurtured, from childhood through adulthood. By embracing and promoting emotional intelligence, this strategy enables to tackle the opportunity to build a future where self-awareness, emotional resilience, and human connection are at the forefront of our collective consciousness. This, in turn, will lead to healthier individuals, stronger communities, and a more compassionate, empathetic world (Singh et al. 2024). It is important to commit to making emotional intelligence an integral part of our personal growth and societal development, ensuring that the future is one where emotional well-being thrives for all.

REFERENCES

Al-Mualm, J. A. (2023). Effects of ethical leadership and emotional intelligence on organization commitment. *Journal of Global Social Sciences*, *4*(14), 119–146. DOI: 10.58934/jgss.v4i14.156

Alferaih, A. (2017). Conceptual model for measuring Saudi banking managers' job performance based on their emotional intelligence (EI). *The International Journal of Organizational Analysis*, *25*(1), 123–145. DOI: 10.1108/IJOA-10-2014-0807

Ancis, J. R. (2020). The age of cyberpsychology: An overview. *Technology, Mind, and Behavior*, *1*(1). Advance online publication. DOI: 10.1037/tmb0000009

Antonopoulou, H. (2024). The value of Emotional Intelligence: Self-awareness, self-regulation, motivation, and empathy as key components. *Technium Education and Humanities*, *8*, 78–92. DOI: 10.47577/teh.v8i.9719

Arabian, H., Abdulbaki Alshirbaji, T., Schmid, R., Wagner-Hartl, V., Chase, J. G., & Moeller, K. (2023). Harnessing wearable devices for emotional intelligence: Therapeutic applications in digital health. *Sensors (Basel)*, *23*(19), 8092. Advance online publication. DOI: 10.3390/s23198092 PMID: 37836923

Ariño, P., Yang, C. C., Pérez, Ó., Brown, L. L., Hernández, S. E., Barrós, A., & Picó, M. (2023). Psychological benefits and neural correlates of an 8-week mindfulness training: A resting-state functional connectivity MRI study. *Neuroscience Applied*, *2*(103652), 103652. DOI: 10.1016/j.nsa.2023.103652

Bar-On, R. (2007). The impact of emotional intelligence on giftedness. *Gifted Education International*, *23*(2), 122–137. DOI: 10.1177/026142940702300203

Bashir, N. A. (2016). Leadership connection to emotional intelligenceand stress at workplace. *Journal of Management Research*, *9*(1), 43. DOI: 10.5296/jmr.v9i1.9338

Bhatt, C., Tasleem, A., Rawat, N., Singh, S., Bahuguna, T., & Singh, T. (2024, July 26). SentiSense: Pioneering emotional intelligence through advanced detection technology. *2024 Asia Pacific Conference on Innovation in Technology (APCIT)*, 1–5. Presented at the 2024 Asia Pacific Conference on Innovation in Technology (APCIT), MYSORE, India. DOI: 10.1109/APCIT62007.2024.10673585

Brackett, M. A., Rivers, S. E., & Salovey, P. (2011). Emotional intelligence: Implications for personal, social, academic, and workplace success. *Social and Personality Psychology Compass*, *5*(1), 88–103. DOI: 10.1111/j.1751-9004.2010.00334.x

Caporale-Berkowitz, N. A., Boyer, B. P., Lyddy, C. J., Good, D. J., Rochlen, A. B., & Parent, M. C. (2021). Search inside yourself: Investigating the effects of a widely adopted mindfulness-at-work development program. *International Journal of Workplace Health Management, 14*(6), 593–604. DOI: 10.1108/IJWHM-08-2020-0139 PMID: 38283264

Chen, J., & Guo, W. (2020). Emotional intelligence can make a difference: The impact of principals' emotional intelligence on teaching strategy mediated by instructional leadership. *Educational Management Administration & Leadership, 48*(1), 82–105. DOI: 10.1177/1741143218781066

Cooper, J., Davis, L., & Norton, F. R.Jr. (2023). A literature review of the influence of Emotional Intelligence (EI) and the Big Five personality traits on leadership effectiveness. *Journal of Leadership, Accountability and Ethics, 20*(5). Advance online publication. DOI: 10.33423/jlae.v20i5.6658

Côté, S. (2014). Emotional intelligence in organizations. *Annual Review of Organizational Psychology and Organizational Behavior, 1*(1), 459–488. DOI: 10.1146/annurev-orgpsych-031413-091233

de Sousa, G. M., de Lima-Araújo, G. L., de Araújo, D. B., & de Sousa, M. B. C. (2021). Brief mindfulness-based training and mindfulness trait attenuate psychological stress in university students: A randomized controlled trial. *BMC Psychology, 9*(1), 21. DOI: 10.1186/s40359-021-00520-x PMID: 33526085

Durham, M. R. P., Smith, R., Cloonan, S., Hildebrand, L. L., Woods-Lubert, R., Skalamera, J., & Killgore, W. D. S. (2023). Development and validation of an online emotional intelligence training program. *Frontiers in Psychology, 14*, 1221817. DOI: 10.3389/fpsyg.2023.1221817 PMID: 37663347

Filice, L., & Weese, W. J. (2024). Developing emotional intelligence. *Encyclopedia, 4*(1), 583–599. DOI: 10.3390/encyclopedia4010037

Garcia-Gutierrez, A., Montesano, A., & Feixas, G. (2025). Using virtual reality to promote self-identity reconstruction as the main focus of therapy. *Journal of Clinical Psychology, 81*(5), 345–354. DOI: 10.1002/jclp.23771 PMID: 39826102

Gkoumas, C., Bourikas, L., Mantadelis, T., & Karakasidou, E. (2024, October 21). Advancing mental health with immersive virtual reality: Benefits, challenges, and emerging trends. *2024 IEEE International Symposium on Mixed and Augmented Reality Adjunct (ISMAR-Adjunct)*, 273–280. Presented at the 2024 IEEE International Symposium on Mixed and Augmented Reality Adjunct (ISMAR-Adjunct), Bellevue, WA, USA. DOI: 10.1109/ISMAR-Adjunct64951.2024.00064

Goleman, D. (1995). *Emotional intelligence*. Bantam Books, Inc.

Grossman, P., Niemann, L., Schmidt, S., & Walach, H. (2010). Mindfulness-based stress reduction and health benefits: A meta-analysis. *Focus on Alternative and Complementary Therapies*, *8*(4), 500–500. DOI: 10.1111/j.2042-7166.2003.tb04008.x

Gunderman, R. B., & Brown, T. (2011). Emotional intelligence. *Journal of the American College of Radiology*, *8*(5), 298–299. DOI: 10.1016/j.jacr.2011.02.007 PMID: 21531303

Halder, N., Setu, J. H., Rafid, L., Islam, A., & Amin, M. A. (2024, June 3). Smartwatch-based human stress diagnosis utilizing physiological signals and LSTM-driven machine intelligence. *2024 Advances in Science and Engineering Technology International Conferences (ASET)*, 01–08. Presented at the *2024 Advances in Science and Engineering Technology International Conferences (ASET)*, Abu Dhabi, United Arab Emirates. DOI: 10.1109/ASET60340.2024.10708730

Himanshu, K. (2023). The role of emotional intelligence in building effective workplace: A quantitative study. (2023). *Journal of Cardiovascular Disease Research*. Advance online publication. DOI: 10.48047/jcdr.2021.12.04.347

Hölzel, B. K., Lazar, S. W., Gard, T., Schuman-Olivier, Z., Vago, D. R., & Ott, U. (2011). How does mindfulness meditation work? Proposing mechanisms of action from a conceptual and neural perspective. *Perspectives on Psychological Science: A Journal of the Association for Psychological Science, 6*(6), 537–559. DOI: 10.1177/1745691611419671

Hongjiang, L. V., Chengxuan, H. A. N., & Daojin, W. (2018). The relationship between emotional intelligence and leadership effectiveness: A meta-analysis. *Xinli Kexue Jinzhan*, *26*(2), 204. DOI: 10.3724/SP.J.1042.2018.00204

Huang, H., Liu, L., Yang, S., Cui, X., Zhang, J., & Wu, H. (2019). Effects of job conditions, occupational stress, and emotional intelligence on chronic fatigue among Chinese nurses: A cross-sectional study. *Psychology Research and Behavior Management*, *12*, 351–360. DOI: 10.2147/PRBM.S207283 PMID: 31191056

Ibrahim, N., Mohamed, A., Mahmud, M., & Abdullah, S. R. (2022). Emotional intelligence, spiritual intelligence and psychological well-being: Impact on society. *Malaysian Journal of Society and Space*, *18*(3). Advance online publication. DOI: 10.17576/geo-2022-1803-06

Ikart, E. M. (2023). *Emotional intelligence: Why its matters in change leadership and innovation in the 21st century styles of work*. DOI: 10.34624/IJBI.V2I4.34732

Irawan, M. B. (2024). Exploring emotional intelligence's role in workplace conflict resolution: A mixed-methods study. *Acta Psychologica, 3*(3), 88–99. DOI: 10.35335/psychologia.v3i3.62

Ishii, Y. (2017). Emotional Intelligence: How to Measure and Promote. The Proceedings of the Annual Convention of the Japanese Psychological Association.

Jiménez-Picón, N., Romero-Martín, M., Ponce-Blandón, J. A., Ramirez-Baena, L., Palomo-Lara, J. C., & Gómez-Salgado, J. (2021). The Relationship between Mindfulness and Emotional Intelligence as a Protective Factor for Healthcare Professionals: Systematic Review. *International Journal of Environmental Research and Public Health, 18*(10), 5491. DOI: 10.3390/ijerph18105491 PMID: 34065519

Lal, A., Dhadwal, P., Gade, D., & Joy, J. (2024, December 6). TherapAI: AI-powered therapy chatbot with sentiment analysis, mood tracking, and automated reporting for enhanced mental health support. *2024 International Conference on Communication, Control, and Intelligent Systems (CCIS)*, 1–8. Presented at the 2024 International Conference on Communication, Control, and Intelligent Systems (CCIS), Mathura, India. DOI: 10.1109/CCIS63231.2024.10932101

Liu, Y., Chen, Z., Xie, X., Hu, Y., Zhang, L., Xu, D., & Wang, Y. (2024, September 30). MoodMonster: Integrating AI and Art for Emotional Journaling. *2024 Artificial Intelligence x Humanities, Education, and Art (AIxHEART)*, 92–97. Presented at the 2024 Artificial Intelligence x Humanities, Education, and Art (AIxHEART), Laguna Hills, CA, USA. DOI: 10.1109/AIxHeart62327.2024.00022

Malekar, S. (2007). Emotional Intelligence-Self Awareness. *Review of Professional Management- A Journal of New Delhi Institute of Management, 5*(2), 46. DOI: 10.20968/rpm/2007/v5/i2/100966

Mattingly, V., & Kraiger, K. (2019). Can emotional intelligence be trained? A meta-analytical investigation. *Human Resource Management Review, 29*(2), 140–155. DOI: 10.1016/j.hrmr.2018.03.002

Mavroveli, S., Petrides, K. V., Rieffe, C., & Bakker, F. (2007). Trait emotional intelligence, psychological well-being and peer-rated social competence in adolescence. *British Journal of Developmental Psychology, 25*(2), 263–275. DOI: 10.1348/026151006X118577

Mayer, J. D., Caruso, D. R., & Salovey, P. (2016). The Ability Model of Emotional Intelligence: Principles and Updates. *Emotion Review, 8*(4), 290–300. DOI: 10.1177/1754073916639667

Nagaraj, G. A. M., Khan, A. A., Sathish, Ritika, & Mohiuddin, A. (2024, August 7). EMOWELL: Emotional well-being web application for better understanding using NLP techniques. *2024 5th International Conference on Electronics and Sustainable Communication Systems (ICESC)*, 861–865. Presented at the 2024 5th International Conference on Electronics and Sustainable Communication Systems (ICESC), Coimbatore, India. DOI: 10.1109/ICESC60852.2024.10689904

O'Connor, P. J., Hill, A., Kaya, M., & Martin, B. (2019). The measurement of emotional Intelligence: A critical review of the literature and recommendations for researchers and practitioners. *Frontiers in Psychology*, *10*, 1116. DOI: 10.3389/fpsyg.2019.01116 PMID: 31191383

Occhipinti, J.-A., Hynes, W., Geli, P., Eyre, H. A., Song, Y., Prodan, A., & Hickie, I. B. (2023). Building systemic resilience, productivity and well-being: A Mental Wealth perspective. *BMJ Global Health*, *8*(9), e012942. DOI: 10.1136/bmjgh-2023-012942 PMID: 37748793

OECD. (2015). *Skills for Social Progress: The Power of Social and Emotional Skills, OECD Skills Studies*. OECD Publishing., DOI: 10.1787/9789264226159-

Papoutsi, C., Drigas, A., & Skianis, C. (2021). Virtual and Augmented Reality for Developing Emotional Intelligence Skills. *International Journal of Recent Contributions from Engineering* [iJES]. *Science & IT*, *9*(3), 35–53. DOI: 10.3991/ijes.v9i3.23939

Pempho, J., & Melvin, M. (2024). Mental health support app with mood tracking and resources. *I-Manager s Journal on Mobile Applications and Technologies*, *11*(1), 5. DOI: 10.26634/jmt.11.1.20662

Pipas, C. F., & Pepper, E. L. (2021). Building Community Well-being Through Emotional Intelligence and Cognitive Reframing. *Family Practice Management*, *28*(1), 23–26. PMID: 33433184

Rasri, W., Promduea, S., Bamrungchai, S., & Kanyarat, M. (2024). Holistic learning: Integrating Knowledge for Lifelong Benefit Through Natural Human Learning Processes. *Journal of Education and Learning Reviews*, *1*(3), 33–44. DOI: 10.60027/jelr.2024.767

Rebouillat, S., Steffenino, B., Lapray, M., & Rebouillat, A. (2020). New AI-IP-EI trilogy opens innovation to new dimensions; Another chip in "the innovation wall", what about emotional intelligence (EI)? *Intelligent Information Management*, *12*(04), 131–182. DOI: 10.4236/iim.2020.124010

Robinson, M. D. (2024). Ability-related emotional intelligence: An introduction. *Journal of Intelligence, 12*(5), 51. DOI: 10.3390/jintelligence12050051 PMID: 38786653

Sahney, R., Malhotra, P., & Mohanan, A. (2024). Elevating healthcare with emotional intelligence: Lessons from the COVID-19 pandemic. *Current Medicine Research and Practice, 14*(4), 181–185. DOI: 10.4103/cmrp.cmrp_34_24

Salovey, P., & Mayer, J. D. (1990). Emotional intelligence. *Imagination, Cognition and Personality, 9*(3), 185–211. DOI: 10.2190/DUGG-P24E-52WK-6CDG

Sánchez-Álvarez, N., Extremera, N., & Fernández-Berrocal, P. (2016). The relation between emotional intelligence and subjective well-being: A meta-analytic investigation. *The Journal of Positive Psychology, 11*(3), 276–285. DOI: 10.1080/17439760.2015.1058968

Sawhney, N., Graver, C., & Breitkopf, E. (2018, June 19). Audio journaling for self-reflection and assessment among teens in participatory media programs. *Proceedings of the 17th ACM Conference on Interaction Design and Children.* Presented at the IDC '18: Interaction Design and Children, Trondheim Norway. DOI: 10.1145/3202185.3202752

Self-reflection. (2012). *SpringerReference.*, DOI: 10.1007/SpringerReference_223827

Shadiev, R., Wang, X., & Huang, Y.-M. (2021). Cross-cultural learning in virtual reality environment: Facilitating cross-cultural understanding, trait emotional intelligence, and sense of presence. *Educational Technology Research and Development. Educational Technology Research and Development, 69*(5), 2917–2936. DOI: 10.1007/s11423-021-10044-1

Singh, S., & Srivastava, N. (2024). Self Compassion and Emotional Intelligence among working and non-working women. *International Journal For Multidisciplinary Research, 6*(5), 28696. Advance online publication. DOI: 10.36948/ijfmr.2024.v06i05.28696

Social and Emotional Learning *The SAGE Encyclopedia of Classroom Management.*, DOI: 10.4135/9781483346243.n314

South, C. L., & DeJarnette, N. (2022). RULER: A social emotional learning program's impact on school climate. *Education. Society and Human Studies, 3*(1), 52. DOI: 10.22158/eshs.v3n1p52

Takong, A. J., Abdul Latip, H. B., & Apoi, A. (2021). The impacts of emotional intelligence and individual performance on work-life balance. *International Journal of Academic Research in Economics and Management Sciences*, *10*(3). Advance online publication. DOI: 10.6007/IJAREMS/v10-i3/10578

Thorndike, R. L., & Stein, S. (1937). An evaluation of the attempts to measure social intelligence. *Psychological Bulletin*, *34*(5), 275–285. DOI: 10.1037/h0053850

Wang, Y., & Pan, L. (2025). Immersive virtual reality in education: Impact on the emotional intelligence of university students. *Education and Information Technologies*, *30*(4), 5283–5299. DOI: 10.1007/s10639-024-13013-2

Weng, H.-C., Huang, L.-Y., & Lin, W.-Y. (2024, January 26). Empathetic skills through virtual reality: A new frontier in emotional training. *2024 IEEE 7th Eurasian Conference on Educational Innovation (ECEI)*. Presented at the 2024 IEEE 7th Eurasian Conference on Educational Innovation (ECEI), Bangkok, Thailand. DOI: 10.1109/ECEI60433.2024.10510873

White, B. A. A., & Quinn, J. F. (2023). Personal Growth and Emotional Intelligence: Foundational Skills for the Leader. *Clinics in Sports Medicine*, *42*(2), 261–267. DOI: 10.1016/j.csm.2022.11.008 PMID: 36907624

ENDNOTES

1 https://rulerapproach.org/

Chapter 2
Application of Prenatal Memory to the Development of Self-Awareness and Wellbeing

Akira Ikegawa
https://orcid.org/0000-0002-0447-2799
Ikegawa Clinic, Japan

ABSTRACT

This chapter explores Prenatal Memory Education (PME) as a groundbreaking framework for enhancing self-awareness and well-being from the earliest stages of life. By integrating traditional Japanese Taikyo practices with cutting-edge neuroscience, epigenetics, and psychology, PME redefines the fetus as a sentient being with emotions and awareness. The approach emphasizes empathetic, two-way communication between parents and the fetus, fostering stronger maternal-fetal bonds, reducing maternal stress, and supporting the child's emotional and cognitive development. PME advocates for interdisciplinary research to validate its potential, offering practical insights into transforming pregnancy into a collaborative journey that nurtures lifelong emotional resilience, social adaptability, and happiness. It positions pregnancy not just as a biological process but as a critical period for establishing trust, empathy, and positive family dynamics that shape future generations.

DOI: 10.4018/979-8-3373-0360-4.ch002

INTRODUCTION

"Education cannot improve without improvements in childbirth." This statement by Masatoshi Taguchi highlights the fundamental connection between childbirth and education (Ikegawa, 2020). Despite growing recognition of prenatal development's critical role, interdisciplinary collaboration between medicine and education remains limited (Verny, 1981; Chamberlain, 1998). This paper aims to bridge these gaps by presenting research into prenatal memory and its potential to transform self-awareness and well-being.

Addressing the challenges of prenatal development and its long-term effects requires a robust interdisciplinary approach. Medicine, education, and psychology have traditionally operated in silos, limiting the exchange of insights and practical applications. However, recent advancements in prenatal memory research demonstrate the need for collaborative frameworks that integrate these disciplines.

Medicine: Obstetricians and pediatricians play a crucial role in monitoring and safeguarding maternal and fetal health. Their expertise provides the biological foundation for understanding prenatal development and its implications for health and well-being (WHO, 2016).
Education: Educators and developmental psychologists contribute by designing and implementing early childhood programs that build on the insights from prenatal research. Recognizing the prenatal period as a critical stage in human development, they advocate for practices that promote emotional bonding and cognitive growth from an early age (Shichida & Tsunabuchi, 1998).
Psychology: Prenatal psychology bridges the gap by exploring the emotional and cognitive dimensions of fetal development. Research into prenatal memory and maternal-fetal bonding highlights the importance of addressing emotional well-being alongside physical health (Chamberlain, 1998).
Collaborative Frameworks: Interdisciplinary collaboration facilitates a comprehensive approach to prenatal care and education. Initiatives such as joint research projects, cross-disciplinary training, and shared knowledge platforms enable professionals from diverse fields to work toward common goals. For example, integrating prenatal education into obstetric practices can enhance maternal engagement, while psychological insights can inform educational strategies for parents.

By breaking down disciplinary barriers, interdisciplinary collaboration paves the way for holistic approaches to prenatal care, fostering well-being and self-awareness from the earliest stages of life.

1. WHEN DOES LIFE BEGIN?

Prenatal memories are typically considered non-existent. However, numerous accounts suggest otherwise, with recollections not only of the womb but also of birth, infancy, and even pre-conception—a period when no physical body exists. Many women also report a firm belief in their pregnancy even before taking a pregnancy test (Carman & Carman, 2019).

Despite the difficulties in empirical validation, these phenomena can be explained by assuming the presence of an unseen consciousness inhabiting the womb, capable of nonverbal communication (Verny, 2020). This concept is extensively discussed in *Cosmic Cradle* (Carman & Carman, 2019), where the authors documented prenatal memories from children and adults across 25 countries, introducing the idea of a "Spirit Baby." This term refers to a pre-born soul maintaining a connection with its mother and family during pre-conception, pregnancy, or even postpartum. A similar concept is articulated by Kumiko Ito as "Wonder Baby" (Ito, 2024).

The term " " (Tainaikioku), meaning "prenatal memory," is widely recognized in Japan. Thomas R. Verny explored the scientific basis of such phenomena in *The Embodied Mind* (Verny, 202.0). His work discusses the possibility of memories being retained not only in neural cells but also in somatic cells, and how these memories might influence gene expression, enabling adaptation to environmental changes. This research underscores the significant impact of maternal conditions during pregnancy on the fetus (Verny, 1981).

Carman and Carman's *Cosmic Cradle* also discusses the concept of Spirit Babies, proposing that life begins even before conception (Carman & Carman, 2019). Similarly, Kumiko Ito's notion of "Wonder Baby" aligns with this view, offering a novel perspective on the commencement of life (Ito, 2024).

Traditionally, life has been thought to begin after birth. However, research on prenatal memory and Verny's findings increasingly highlight the substantial impact of the prenatal period—from conception to birth—on an individual's later life (Chamberlain, 1998). This perspective validates the belief that the prenatal environment has profound implications for lifelong development.

The traditional view that fetuses lack awareness and emotions risks neglecting the psychological and relational dynamics of pregnancy, childbirth, and parenting. Conversely, recognizing fetuses as entities with awareness and emotions enables the early establishment of parent-child relationships, fostering love and communication during pregnancy (Shichida & Tsunabuchi, 1998). This approach not only supports the child's healthy development but also enhances the quality of parent-child bonds and promotes socio-emotional growth. As evidenced by numerous studies, addressing well-being from the prenatal stage lays a critical foundation for a fulfilling life (Verny, 1981).

2. PERSPECTIVES ON MATERNAL AND FETAL HEALTH

Educational approaches supporting the health and development of mothers and fetuses include prenatal care, prenatal training, and " " (Taikyo), a Japanese practice that emphasizes creating a positive emotional and physical environment during pregnancy. These approaches share the common goal of reducing maternal stress and promoting maternal and fetal health for optimal development.

Prenatal Care

Prenatal care focuses on the medical management of maternal and fetal health, the early detection of complications, and risk mitigation. It is primarily a medically driven approach, characterized by evidence-based methods that prioritize the lives of both the mother and the fetus (WHO, 2016).

Prenatal Training

Prenatal training aims to maintain physical fitness, prepare for childbirth, and reduce stress during pregnancy. This approach provides practical techniques to support physical and mental preparation for a positive birth experience. Examples include yoga and breathing exercises (Field, 2008).

Taikyo

Taikyo emphasizes the emotional development of the fetus and the formation of parent-child bonds. It uniquely views the fetus as an entity with emotions and intentions, emphasizing communication between the mother and fetus (Shichida & Tsunabuchi, 1998). Through activities like talking to the fetus, playing music, and meditating, Taikyo seeks to foster the fetus's emotional development and strengthen the parent-child bond (Chamberlain, 1998).

Comparative Overview

While all three approaches share the overarching goal of maternal and fetal health, they differ significantly in their conceptualization of the fetus and intervention methods. Prenatal care treats the fetus as a biological entity, prenatal training focuses on stabilizing the mother's physical and mental state, and Taikyo uniquely engages the fetus as a sentient being. These distinctions are summarized in Table 1.

3. THE HISTORY OF TAIKYO

The origins of Taikyo trace back to ancient China during the Western Han Dynasty (206 BCE–8 CE), where *The Greater Dai's Book of Rites* described fetal education as part of moral cultivation (Liu, 200 BCE). This text proposed that a fetus is influenced by the mother's behavior and mental state, highlighting the importance of maternal conduct for fetal development. In ancient China, it was widely believed that maternal attitudes significantly impacted fetal growth. However, in modern times, the lack of scientific evidence led to skepticism and declining acceptance of such views.

In the 1960s, advancements in medical technology, such as ultrasound, revealed that fetuses respond to sound, spurring research into fetal sensory perception (Liley, 1969). The Tibetan medical text *The Four Medical Tantras* (8th century) documented the detailed process of development from conception to birth, suggesting that fetuses could develop conflicting emotions toward the mother by the 37th week. Similarly, *The Mahāratnakū a Sūtra (Volume 55: Chapter on Dwelling in the Womb), as presented in A Treasury of Mahāyāna Sūtras, describes the fetus acquiring sensory perception within seven days, suggesting a deep understanding of fetal experiences that surpasses contemporary insights (Chang, 1983).*

Modern scientific exploration of prenatal memory began with Thomas Verny's *The Secret Life of the Unborn Child* (1981) and David Chamberlain's *Babies Remember Birth* (1988). In Japan, Masaru Ibuka initiated early childhood education efforts in 1969, establishing a foundation for Taikyo (Ibuka, 1969). The 1990s witnessed a surge in interest, with Makoto Shichida publishing books emphasizing the importance of fetal and early childhood education (Shichida, 1990).

However, the 1995 Aum Shinrikyo incident led to widespread criticism of activities associated with spiritual practices, including yoga and meditation, causing Taikyo to fall into disrepute temporarily (Reader, 2000). In recent years, renewed scientific interest in the sensory and emotional capacities of fetuses has revitalized the appreciation of Taikyo, affirming its significance in fostering maternal-fetal bonds and long-term well-being (Ikegawa, 2020).

4. RESEARCH ON THE CONSCIOUSNESS OF FETUSES

Investigating whether fetuses possess consciousness is fundamental to understanding the origins of human awareness and the formation of memory. Rose (1991) conducted a groundbreaking study by interviewing children aged 2.5 to 3.5 about their memories of birth and the prenatal period. This study is considered the first to investigate the existence of prenatal memories in children, marking a groundbreaking step in psychological and neuroscientific research. Rose's work expanded the scope of memory research by venturing into the unexplored domain of mental states during the perinatal and prenatal periods. Similarly, Vlcek (2017) proposed, based on personal experiences, that consciousness exists even before birth, suggesting that human evolution and growth are driven by a creative process rooted in consciousness.

After a period of limited investigation into prenatal memory, interest was reignited by Akira Ikegawa's 2005 study, which suggested the potential existence of fetal memories and significantly influenced subsequent research (Ikegawa, 2005). In Japan, Ohkado and Ikegawa (2014) conducted further research, while internationally, Carman and Carman (2019) contributed independent studies, gradually building a body of evidence supporting prenatal memory.

The practical application of these findings can be seen in prenatal memory education(PME), which integrates research insights into parenting practices. This approach reevaluates traditionally disregarded memories, including those from the fetal period, peri-conception, and early infancy, and incorporates them into childcare strategies. Chamberlain (1998) noted that this method aims to enhance psychological stability and strengthen parent-child bonds, particularly for children who retain prenatal memories. Understanding how these memories influence home environments and parenting practices could significantly advance education and social welfare (Verny, 1981).

Conceptual frameworks such as the "spirit baby" and "wonder baby" further explore the idea of a pre-conception soul-like presence (Clare, 2020; Makichen, 2008). The spirit baby concept suggests that parental bonds begin even before conception, implying that prenatal consciousness and memory may hold critical insights into the mysteries of life itself.

Scientific debates continue regarding the origins of consciousness. While some argue that consciousness begins at birth, shortly thereafter, or around the first year of life (Kagan, 2004), emerging hypotheses suggest that consciousness may exist even earlier—potentially pre-conception. Although modern science has not yet fully validated this idea, an increasing body of evidence from prenatal memory research supports its plausibility.

These developments expand the understanding of memory and prompt a reevaluation of the nature of life and consciousness. They encourage deeper reflection on awareness and its profound meanings, paving the way for transformative explorations into the mysteries of consciousness (Penrose, 1994).

5. PME BASED ON THE PREMISE OF FETAL CONSCIOUSNESS

PME is an innovative educational method based on the premise that fetuses possess consciousness and intention. Unlike traditional Taikyo, which involves unidirectional interaction from parents to the fetus, PME emphasizes bidirectional communication, treating the fetus as an active participant. The term "education" was intentionally added to "prenatal memory" to highlight the application of this concept as a structured approach to deepen the bond between parents and their fetus, enhance parent-child relationships, promote psychological stability, and foster harmony within the family.

While the hypothesis of fetal consciousness and memory is not yet fully proven by science, PME is grounded in the belief that its potential social value outweighs the need to wait for complete scientific validation. Sharing this knowledge in a flexible and open manner, alongside ongoing scientific exploration, is considered the most effective approach.

It is especially important to convey this information to expectant parents even before scientific evidence fully confirms the hypothesis. Many parents-to-be seek more than just a scientific perspective on childbirth; they also desire an experience that enriches their inner emotional and spiritual lives. For these individuals, the concept of PME provides meaningful insights and practices, regardless of the current limitations of scientific validation.

In recognition of this need, the PME Association (PREMEA) was established in 2017 to develop standardized programs and train instructors. Today, over 300 certified instructors are actively working to disseminate PME concepts, primarily to parents navigating pregnancy, childbirth, and early parenting. PREMEA also leverages an e-learning platform to make PME accessible to a broader audience globally.

By addressing the aspirations of expectant parents for a deeper connection with their unborn children, PME bridges the gap between scientific thinking and the emotional and spiritual dimensions of childbirth. This integrated approach not only aligns with the values of families but also holds the potential to contribute significantly to societal well-being.

6. THE FOUNDATIONS OF MODERN SCIENCE AND THE POSITION OF PME

Modern science is rooted in the rise of early modern science in the 17th century, where René Descartes proposed mind-body dualism, asserting the independence of mind and body as separate entities (Descartes, 1641). Descartes' dualism played a foundational role in establishing scientific thought, allowing for the clear distinction between physical and mental phenomena. However, his contemporary, Baruch Spinoza, criticized this view and argued for monism, viewing mind and body as inseparable aspects of a single substance. Spinoza's philosophy profoundly influenced subsequent debates on the relationship between mind and body.

David Hume further critiqued Cartesian dualism with his "bundle theory of perception," positing that the human mind is not an independent entity but merely a collection of sensations and perceptions (Hume, 1739). This perspective lent support to monistic approaches, leading to a gradual philosophical shift from dualism to monism. As science evolved, it increasingly focused on observable and measurable phenomena. Consequently, Descartes' notion of the "mind" became less relevant in scientific inquiry, as it was deemed unobservable and unmeasurable (Daston & Galison, 2010). Over time, non-measurable phenomena were often dismissed as "unscientific," sidelining research on consciousness and subjective experiences.

Despite the success of materialistic science, it has limitations, particularly in explaining consciousness and subjective experiences (Nagel, 1974). Against this backdrop, PME emerges as an approach that integrates new perspectives, blending concepts from quantum mechanics, traditional dualistic thought in Japanese philosophy, and modern scientific ideas. For instance, the PF Theory proposed by Takashi Taneichi draws on quantum mechanics to suggest that human existence comprises both a physical body in three- or four-dimensional spacetime and a conscious entity in extra dimensions (Taneichi, 2018; Ikegawa, 2020).

While monistic frameworks attempt to explain consciousness within the physical realm, PME adopts a dualistic perspective. This approach views the mind as a non-material entity distinct from the body, emphasizing the importance of subjective experiences and free will. This dualistic framework aligns with many traditional religious and spiritual concepts, resonating with intuitive human understandings of existence.

Recent developments in neuroscience, particularly in the study of the Default Mode Network (DMN), provide further insight into these discussions. Research indicates that the DMN, which governs self-referential thought, memory, and imagination, begins to form in the fetal stage and shows significant development in neonates (Gao et al., 2015; Liu et al., 2020). These findings challenge traditional views that considered such networks exclusive to postnatal development. Studies utilizing fMRI(Functional Magnetic Resonance Imaging), MEG (Magnetoencephalography), and 1H-MRS (Proton Magnetic Resonance Spectroscopy) have revealed the presence of early neural activity and connectivity indicative of DMN formation in utero and in newborns, highlighting the profound potential of prenatal life in shaping consciousness (Barta et al., 2022; Thomason et al., 2021).

These breakthroughs underscore the need to reconsider traditional paradigms of pregnancy, childbirth, and parenting. Prenatal experiences and maternal interactions may influence the early formation and activity of the DMN, thus impacting cognitive and emotional development. Building on these insights, the framework of PME which integrates ancient Japanese practices with modern neuroscience, offers promising pathways to foster a holistic approach to pregnancy and early parenting. PME emphasizes maternal mindfulness, communication with the fetus, and the nurturing of a positive intrauterine environment, aiming to support the nascent DMN and overall neural development.

By stepping beyond the limitations of traditional materialistic science, the integration of PME and DMN research provides a compelling vision for future research and practice. This interdisciplinary approach bridges science and spirituality, offering new opportunities to explore the profound connections between consciousness, development, and the human experience.

7. THE NECESSITY OF TAIKYO WITH BIDIRECTIONAL COMMUNICATION

Here, traditional Taikyo is referred to as Taikyo1.1. This practice is characterized by a unidirectional approach where the mother is the primary participant in interacting with the fetus. It involves activities such as playing music, maintaining emotional calmness, and speaking to the fetus. These practices aim to positively influence the fetus's emotional development, perceiving it as a passive entity that responds to external stimuli (Shichida & Tsunabuchi, 1998). The designation "1" in Taikyo1.1 signifies the unidirectional communication from the mother to the fetus, highlighting the focus on the mother as the central figure in this interaction. The ".1" further emphasizes the singular role of the mother in this traditional practice.

In contrast, PME is referred to as Taikyo2.3, reflecting its transformative evolution by incorporating the concept of bidirectional communication. The "2" in Taikyo2.3 signifies this shift towards mutual interaction, where communication flows both ways between the fetus and others, recognizing the fetus as an active participant. This advanced approach redefines the fetus as an active participant with emotions and intentions, emphasizing dynamic interactions among the fetus, the mother, and the father (Ikegawa, 2015). The ".3" in Taikyo2.3 symbolizes the triadic relationship where the fetus, mother, and father are seen as co-creators of meaningful prenatal communication. Fathers, and when possible, other family members, are encouraged to engage actively, thus enriching the prenatal experience and creating a more inclusive framework.

Taikyo2.3 goes beyond the unidirectional nature of Taikyo1.1 by fostering reciprocal interactions. Parents are encouraged not only to communicate with the fetus but also to perceive and respond to its reactions. For instance, fetal movements are interpreted as potential responses, which deepen emotional bonds and build trust between the parents and the fetus (DeCasper & Spence, 1986). Practical methods within Taikyo2.3 include sharing emotions where parents express love and gratitude to the fetus, imagining and acknowledging its emotional responses to foster mutual understanding. Fathers and family members are also invited to engage in tactile interactions, such as speaking to the fetus, touching the mother's abdomen, or playing music to create physical and emotional connections (Ikegawa, 2015). Additionally, families are encouraged to visualize the health and happiness of the fetus while sharing positive energy, further reinforcing their bond. The differences between Taikyo1.1 and Taikyo2.3 are summarized in Table 1, highlighting their key features and distinctions.

Scientific evidence supports the principles of Taikyo 2.3. Studies in neuroscience demonstrate that fetuses can recognize and remember their mother's voice during late pregnancy, an ability that continues after birth. This suggests that prenatal auditory experiences significantly influence later development (DeCasper & Spence, 1986). Moreover, research indicates that maternal stress during pregnancy induces epigenetic changes in the fetus, potentially leading to long-term health impairments and even affecting subsequent generations. For example, prenatal exposure to famine has been linked to persistent epigenetic modifications associated with adverse health outcomes (Heijmans et al., 2008). Additionally, maternal behaviors and stress levels are known to shape fetal gene expression and stress responses, highlighting the critical importance of maternal care and mental well-being during pregnancy (Meaney & Szyf, 2005). Furthermore, studies reveal that prenatal environmental exposures—such as stress, malnutrition, and toxins—affect the placental epigenome, triggering molecular changes that can propagate across generations (Lapehn & Paquette, 2022; Cutfield et al., 2007). These findings underscore the necessity of mitigating maternal stress during pregnancy to protect the health of both current and future generations. While both Taikyo1.1 and Taikyo2.3 share the goal of enhancing prenatal development and establishing strong parent-child bonds, their approaches diverge significantly. Taikyo1.1 focuses on the mother's role and perceives the fetus as a receptive being, while Taikyo2.3 expands this perspective by acknowledging the fetus's active participation and involving the entire family.

The evolution from Taikyo1.1 to Taikyo2.3 represents a broader understanding of prenatal communication and its impact on family dynamics. Taikyo2.3 not only reduces maternal stress and fosters secure parent-child relationships but also creates a cooperative environment where fathers and other family members actively participate. Placing hands on the pregnant mother's belly to engage in bidirectional communication with the fetus is considered a particularly important practice. This is because the warmth, vibrations, and presence of caregivers or close family members, conveyed through touch, are believed to strengthen the fetus's connection with the external world. This enhances bidirectional communication between the fetus and the surrounding environment, further enriching the prenatal experience. This inclusive approach offers a richer prenatal experience and lays the foundation for long-term emotional well-being, underscoring its transformative potential in redefining prenatal care (Ikegawa, 2015; Verny, 1981).

8. COMPARISON BETWEEN TAIKYO AND PME

Taikyo and PME share commonalities in their emphasis on the significance of the prenatal period for human development and personality formation. Both approaches recognize that a mother's behavior and interactions with the fetus during pregnancy can profoundly influence the child's later life (Shichida & Tsunabuchi, 1998). Activities such as maintaining emotional calm, engaging in conversations with the fetus, playing music, and reading are believed to promote emotional development and foster healthy growth (Chamberlain, 1998). Both methods stress the importance of establishing parent-child bonds during pregnancy, actively engaging with the fetus's emotions and consciousness to create deeper connections.

Additionally, both Taikyo and PME treat the fetus not as a mere biological entity but as a being with emotions and consciousness. This perspective encourages families to respect the fetus and provide a calm and nurturing environment (Verny, 1981). For instance, Taikyo emphasizes the positive influence of maintaining maternal positivity and talking to the fetus, while PME advocates for treating the fetus as an entity with memory and intent, underscoring the significance of these early interactions (Ikegawa, 2020).

Despite their similarities, significant distinctions exist between Taikyo and PME. While Taikyo views the fetus as a receptive being influenced by maternal emotions and actions, PME goes further, positing the fetus as an autonomous entity with memory and intent (Chamberlain, 2003). This philosophical divergence shapes their respective approaches to understanding fetal development and the origins of life.

Moreover, Taikyo traditionally operates under the assumption of the fetus as a physical being. In contrast, PME adopts a dualistic view, suggesting that consciousness coexists with the body and may even precede its physical formation (Taneichi, 2018). Taneichi, a quantum physicist, posits that human consciousness could be an undiscovered fermion existing in extra dimensions, potentially interacting with the physical body through quantum phenomena. This aligns with Penrose's theory that consciousness arises from quantum processes occurring within the microtubules of brain cells, suggesting a non-computational mechanism underlying awareness (Penrose, 1994).

Such theories propose that the fundamental nature of consciousness may not be confined to the material world but rather exists in a quantum realm where it interacts with spacetime and matter. This perspective broadens the scope of PME, allowing it to incorporate concepts such as pre-conception awareness and intermission memories, which resonate with the multidimensionality of quantum states. For instance, Penrose's hypothesis that quantum superposition and objective reduction (OR) are key to consciousness provides a framework for understanding how the fetus's consciousness could emerge before the body fully forms.

By integrating these quantum mechanical and metaphysical perspectives, PME offers a holistic approach to understanding fetal development and awareness. It challenges traditional paradigms by suggesting that the fetus's consciousness may operate on a quantum level, influencing and being influenced by the physical world even before birth. Through this lens, PME posits that the resonance of emotions and intentions between parents and their fetus—facilitated by quantum-level interactions—can foster empathy and mutual understanding during pregnancy. This shared emotional connection is hypothesized to lay the groundwork for the fetus to develop a sense of self-acceptance and even experience early forms of happiness by the time of birth. Such a framework envisions pregnancy as a transformative period where the emotional and quantum interactions between parents and their unborn child contribute to lifelong psychological resilience and well-being.

9. BENEFITS OF TRANSITIONING TO PME

Understanding memories from the prenatal stage helps children gain a profound understanding of their origins and purpose (Chamberlain, 1998). This awareness supports their psychological stability and lays a foundation for motivation, self-fulfillment, and the development of self-esteem. It is hypothesized that by recognizing their early connections and sense of belonging, children may cultivate a strong sense of self-worth and positive identity, contributing to their overall emotional well-being.

Furthermore, prenatal memory-based methods may help mitigate unconscious trauma, promoting harmony within families and strengthening familial bonds (Verny, 1981). By involving fathers and siblings, PME cultivates a family-wide culture of acceptance and support for the fetus, enhancing connections within the family (Klaus & Kennell, 1993).

The implementation of PME also profoundly impacts parents' behaviors and attitudes during pregnancy. This approach encourages parents to engage in meaningful interactions with their fetus, enriching the pregnancy and childbirth experience. For parents, these practices have the potential to lead to personal growth and increased happiness. For instance, engaging in a dialogue with the fetus provides parents with unique insights and allows them to approach pregnancy and childbirth as transformative life events. This process is valuable not only for mothers but also for fathers and other family members, making it a shared experience.

PME also has the potential to advance obstetrics and midwifery by integrating new perspectives into the existing framework of Taikyo. Incorporating bidirectional communication fosters a more active and holistic approach to fetal interaction, inspiring innovative strategies in childbirth and parenting. This enhanced framework is believed to strengthen the parent-child relationship during pregnancy, potentially yielding better outcomes for both.

In education and healthcare, PME has the potential to serve as a new practice. It may provide a foundation for developing tailored educational programs that enhance self-awareness and social skills among children. In healthcare, it offers a foundation for patient-centered care, addressing individual physical and psychological challenges. For example, by treating the fetus as a conscious being and conveying positive emotions and messages, a foundation can be established for children to understand themselves positively after birth, fostering a sense of self-worth and confidence (Chamberlain, 2013).

In addressing modern societal challenges such as weakened parent-child relationships and children's mental health issues, similar to fetal psychology, this approach treats the fetus as a being with prenatal memory, capable of forming connections and experiencing awareness even before birth. PME offers a vital perspective by promoting the reevaluation of the value of life and human connections, ultimately strengthening familial bonds and contributing positively to the broader society.

10. PROPOSING CHILDBIRTH WITH HAPPINESS AS THE GOAL

Japan's obstetrics is among the most advanced in the world. As of 2020, the perinatal mortality rate was 3.2 per 1,000 births, and maternal mortality was 4 per 100,000 births (WHO, 2020; Ministry of Health, Labour and Welfare, 2020). These figures position Japan as one of the safest countries globally. These achievements reflect the high standards of medical care and technology, ensuring the safety of mothers and infants. However, these successes prompt a critical question: Is being healthy the same as being happy?

While medical advancements have safeguarded lives, the often-overlooked aspect of "happiness" warrants attention. Modern obstetrics primarily focuses on ensuring the physical health of mothers and babies, leaving the pursuit of their happiness unaddressed. This gap calls for reflection from all involved in childbirth.

Happiness extends beyond the absence of illness or injury. It encompasses emotional stability, fulfillment, harmonious relationships, and a sense of purpose (Ryff & Singer, 1998). In the context of childbirth—a pivotal life event—happiness for both mother and child involves not only physical health but also emotional security and deeper family bonds. Recognizing this dimension has the potential to transform childbirth into a more enriching experience.

Although modern obstetrics prioritizes minimizing risks through advanced techniques, this focus on efficiency sometimes overshadows the intrinsic value of childbirth. For example, the emphasis on specialization and streamlined medical processes can neglect the emotional needs of mothers and families (Gaskin, 2013). In such environments, the opportunity to pursue happiness through childbirth may diminish.

"Childbirth with happiness as the goal" envisions a process where mothers not only experience physical safety but also emotional fulfillment throughout pregnancy and postpartum. Achieving this requires collaboration between healthcare professionals and families to create a supportive environment (Sandelowski, 2004). Actively engaging in fetal communication and establishing a comprehensive support system is expected to strengthen the bond between mother and child.

Additionally, fostering a culture where the entire family—including fathers and siblings—celebrates childbirth can significantly enhance the happiness of both mother and family members. Strengthened familial bonds provide emotional reassurance for mothers, positively influencing childbirth and parenting experiences. This holistic approach redefines childbirth, presenting it as a meaningful and shared family event.

By integrating the dual goals of health and happiness, this proposal introduces a new perspective to modern obstetrics. Childbirth with happiness as the goal transforms childbirth from a purely medical event into a celebration of life, deepening family ties and reaffirming the profound meaning of life itself.

11. THE IMPORTANCE OF HAPPINESS DURING THE PRENATAL PERIOD

Modern obstetrics and midwifery have made tremendous strides in improving maternal and neonatal health by focusing on physical well-being through scientific and evidence-based practices. However, the emotional and psychological dimensions of pregnancy, including "happiness," often remain overlooked (Verny, 1981). PME challenges this paradigm by emphasizing the equal importance of happiness and physical health during the prenatal period, proposing a holistic framework that integrates emotional, psychological, and physical well-being .

Happiness, in this context, is understood not as a fleeting emotion but as a complex and multidimensional construct influenced by several interconnected elements. These include:

Health: Physical and mental well-being as fundamental components of happiness (Linton, Dieppe, & Medina-Lara, 2016; Waldinger & Schulz, 2015).
Positive Relationships: Supportive and meaningful connections with family, friends, and society, which are essential for emotional stability (Linton et al., 2016; Waldinger & Schulz, 2010).
Economic Stability: A secure and stable living environment that fosters peace of mind and reduces stress (Linton et al., 2016).
Purpose and Achievement: The fulfillment derived from setting and achieving meaningful goals, which enhances life satisfaction (Ryff & Singer, 1998).
Self-Acceptance and Growth: Embracing oneself while striving for personal development, a critical aspect of psychological well-being (Ryff & Singer, 1998; Linton et al., 2016).
Resilience: The capacity to overcome adversity, which contributes to a sense of stability and satisfaction (Ryff & Singer, 1998).

These factors collectively shape a mother's overall happiness, highlighting its multidimensional nature. Furthermore, they exert a profound influence on the prenatal environment, creating conditions conducive to both maternal and fetal well-being.

Hormones play a critical role in shaping emotional states, with "happiness hormones" such as endorphins, serotonin, dopamine, and oxytocin fostering positive emotions and psychological equilibrium. In contrast, "stress hormones" like cortisol and adrenaline are associated with negative emotional states and physiological distress (Sapolsky, 2004). These hormones are dynamically regulated in response to environmental stimuli, forming the biochemical basis for emotional and psychological experiences.

During pregnancy, a mother's hormonal environment directly influences fetal development, affecting both physical growth and the long-term mental and emotional health of the child. Elevated maternal cortisol levels resulting from stress have been shown to disrupt the fetal hypothalamic-pituitary-adrenal (HPA) axis, increasing the risk of cardiovascular, metabolic, and psychiatric disorders in adulthood (Seckl & Holmes, 2009). Emotional and behavioral consequences for the child include heightened anxiety, stress-related behaviors, and difficulties in social adaptation.

PME highlights the importance of maternal well-being in creating a hormonal environment conducive to optimal fetal development. When mothers experience joy, contentment, and well-being, the balanced release of happiness hormones promotes healthy fetal growth and emotional resilience. This approach aligns with scientific findings while integrating spiritual perspectives, offering a holistic framework for maternal and fetal health.

For example, mothers who actively cultivate positive relationships, engage in mindfulness practices, and foster gratitude often report reduced stress levels during pregnancy (Field, 2008). Anecdotal evidence from practitioners of PME further suggests that babies born to mothers who prioritized happiness during pregnancy tend to exhibit calm and adaptable temperaments, contributing to a more fulfilling parenting experience.

In a world increasingly aware of the importance of mental health, understanding the relationship between maternal well-being and fetal development offers a pathway to more harmonious parenting and stronger family bonds. From the perspective of well-being and hormonal balance, the prenatal period is a critical time where minimizing maternal stress and fostering emotional openness are essential. Elevated stress levels, marked by the release of cortisol, can disrupt hormonal harmony, potentially affecting fetal development and long-term health. Therefore, techniques that alleviate maternal stress, promote relaxation, and encourage positive emotions are not only beneficial but necessary. By integrating science, spirituality, and lived experiences, PME has the potential to emphasize the profound impact of maternal happiness on both the mother and the child, offering an innovative and compassionate approach to nurturing life before birth.

12. THE FORMATION OF EMOTIONS BEGINNING IN THE FETAL PERIOD

The formation and regulation of emotions involve a complex interplay between the medulla oblongata and pons (brainstem), limbic system (especially the amygdala), and prefrontal cortex (Panksepp, 1998). According to Frontiers in Endocrinology (2022) and Springer (2019), prenatal and early postnatal environmental factors play a critical role in shaping neurodevelopmental outcomes. These functions are closely linked to the amygdala, a part of the limbic system responsible for processing emotions. The development and functionality of these brain structures can be significantly influenced by environmental factors during the fetal and infant stages (Meaney, 2001).

The brainstem, including the medulla oblongata and pons, is most sensitive to external influences during the mid-to-late fetal period (approximately weeks 10–30 of gestation) (Liley, 1969). During this critical phase, the primary structures of the brainstem rapidly develop, and its functions begin to activate. Both external and internal factors can profoundly affect this process:

- **External Influences**: Maternal stress, malnutrition, exposure to toxins, and infections.
- **Internal Factors**: Placental function, genetic predispositions, and maternal health conditions.

Together, these factors interact to shape the early neurological and emotional foundation of the fetus. Maternal stress during pregnancy, for example, exposes the fetus to elevated cortisol levels, which can alter the hypothalamic-pituitary-adrenal (HPA) axis and increase the risk of cardiovascular and emotional disorders later in life (Sapolsky, 2004).

Amygdala Development

The amygdala, part of the limbic system, responds to maternal stress and emotions through the HPA axis, playing a key role in regulating stress responses (Malcon et al., 2020). After birth, the amygdala develops rapidly and becomes central to emotional processing and social cognition between 6 months and 2 years of age. During this period, the fundamental structures for emotions such as anger and fear are established. Maternal emotional states during pregnancy significantly influence the child's emotional tendencies (Field, 2008).

Prefrontal Cortex Development

The prefrontal cortex, crucial for emotional regulation, begins forming around 20 weeks of gestation but remains underdeveloped during the neonatal stage (Giedd, 2004). Its maturation progresses significantly between ages 1 and 3, with full development continuing into the mid-20s. During this period, connections between the prefrontal cortex and the limbic system (including the amygdala) strengthen, gradually enhancing emotional regulation abilities (Davidson et al., 2003).

Implications for Emotional Health

From fetal to toddlerhood, the foundation for emotion formation is laid. After age 2, emotional regulation becomes the focus of development. Recognizing the importance of the fetal period in shaping emotions underscores the need for targeted interventions that support both the mother and the developing baby. Ensuring maternal well-being by creating a calm and relaxing environment is essential for fostering a positive emotional atmosphere for the fetus, as a supportive and stress-free setting can significantly influence the baby's emotional health (Verny, 1981). Additionally, encouraging mothers to engage in positive communication with their fetuses, such as talking to them, helps establish an early parent-child bond. This simple yet meaningful practice lays the foundation for emotional connections even before birth, nurturing a strong relationship that continues to develop after delivery (Chamberlain, 1998).

These measures can enhance self-regulation abilities and social skills, laying a robust foundation for future emotional health. Investing in the emotional development of children from the fetal period onward is an investment in the future. Early emotional support has implications for healthcare, education, and societal well-being. By integrating these insights into caregiving and education, families and communities can nurture emotionally stable and socially adaptable individuals.

13. EARLY HUMAN FORMATION AS THE KEY TO HAPPINESS

The Harvard Study of Adult Development, a landmark longitudinal study begun in 1938, explores factors influencing happiness and longevity. Its findings emphasize that the quality of human relationships—rather than wealth or fame—is the most significant determinant of happiness. Strong relationships contribute to mental stability, deepen social connections, and support physical health (Vaillant, 2012).

PME aligns with the importance of quality relationships by focusing on establishing parent-child bonds and social connections from the fetal period. This approach is based on the understanding that fetuses develop brain functions and respond to external stimuli even in utero (Chamberlain, 1998). Traditionally, science viewed the fetal brain as undeveloped and incapable of thought, a premise PME challenges .

By acknowledging the fetus as a sentient being with emotions and awareness, PME encourages active communication and emotional connections during pregnancy. This perspective fosters trust and love early, forming the basis for emotional stability and social competence after birth (Verny, 1981). For instance, talking to the fetus and observing its responses help parents cultivate a deep bond, promoting psychological health in both the parent and the child.

Conventional scientific approaches often overlook the significance of prenatal parent-child interactions. This oversight can delay trust and emotional connection after birth, potentially leading to emotional insecurity and isolation in children (Field, 2008). Differences in approaches during pregnancy can result in significant variations in parent-child relationships over time.

Recognizing the foundational role of human relationships in happiness highlights the importance of cultivating connections starting from the fetal period. Establishing trust, gratitude, and empathy with the fetus can lead to long-term benefits in emotional development and social skills. These principles extend beyond individual families, providing a framework for creating harmonious communities and a more interconnected society.

By emphasizing the development of early relationships, society can foster emotional stability and collaboration across various spheres—family, education, workplace, and community. Such an approach has the potential to enhance overall well-being, elevate societal happiness, and contribute to a more sustainable and compassionate future.

PME offers a pathway to this vision, underlining the critical role of early human connections in nurturing happiness and resilience for individuals, families, and society as a whole.

14. THE ROLE OF TRADITIONAL AND MODERN MIDWIFERY

Around the world, individuals provide childbirth support rooted in cultural and traditional practices rather than the scientific methods underpinning modern midwifery. These practitioners, often referred to as Traditional Midwives or Traditional Birth Attendants (TBAs), rely on generationally transmitted wisdom and experience rather than medical technology (Jordan, 1993). They play a vital role in offering emotional reassurance and treating childbirth as a cultural and social event within their communities (Davis-Floyd, 2003).

Traditional midwives provide comprehensive care, including prenatal encouragement, lifestyle guidance, labor support, and postpartum care. They integrate cultural practices such as prayers, rituals, and dietary recommendations to ensure not only the well-being of the mother and baby but also the harmony of the family and community (Hahn & Kleinman, 1983). By contrast, modern midwifery prioritizes safety through evidence-based practices and the use of medical technology, making it capable of addressing high-risk deliveries (WHO, 2016).

Rather than being oppositional, traditional and modern midwifery approaches can be complementary. Traditional midwifery emphasizes natural processes and cultural values, while modern midwifery focuses on risk management and safety.

Leveraging the strengths of both approaches based on situational needs can address diverse requirements effectively (Davis-Floyd, 2003). However, it is regrettable that the knowledge held by traditional midwives has been increasingly undervalued in modern contexts, often dismissed as unscientific (Jordan, 1993).

15. JAPAN'S TRADITIONAL MIDWIVES: THE "SANBA"

In Japan, traditional midwives, known as " " (Sanba), played a crucial role in supporting childbirth within communities during the Edo period (17th to 19th centuries) (Midwifery Today, n.d.). Sanba were not limited to medical assistance; they also provided spiritual reassurance and incorporated cultural rituals into childbirth practices. Their responsibilities extended from pregnancy to postpartum care, offering continuous support such as maternal encouragement, assistance during delivery, and health monitoring of mothers and newborns.

Sanba also viewed childbirth as a celebratory family and community event, facilitating cultural practices like preparing special postpartum meals for maternal recovery and conducting rituals for the newborn's health. They possessed extensive knowledge passed down through generations, including techniques for delivery positions, breathing methods, and dietary therapies to aid recovery.

With modernization, Sanba's roles were gradually taken over by modern midwives and physicians (Shirai,2020). However, as the importance of natural childbirth and emotional reassurance is being re-emphasized, efforts to integrate the wisdom and practices of Sanba into modern healthcare systems have gained traction (WHO, 2016). Far from being a relic of the past, Sanba traditions offer holistic perspectives on childbirth rooted in regional culture and values, contributing to richer and more diverse birthing experiences (Davis-Floyd, 2003).

16. THE CONTINUED IMPORTANCE OF TRADITIONAL MIDWIFERY IN MODERN TIMES

According to Shizuoka University (2017), traditional midwives in Japan were central figures in facilitating childbirth and mediating adoption, strengthening the social fabric of their communities.

Traditional midwifery has seen a resurgence in contemporary forms, including the role of doulas and traditional midwives. Doulas primarily focus on offering emotional and psychological support throughout pregnancy, childbirth, and postpartum, without performing medical procedures. Their role emphasizes guiding and supporting mothers and families, addressing emotional needs to make the childbirth experience positive and comforting (Wójcik-Brylska et al., 2023).

In Japan, the title for midwives has evolved from "sanba" to "josanpu," and eventually to "josanshi," reflecting changes in the status and scope of the midwifery profession (Shirai, 2020). According to Iimura (2015), midwives in Japan have historically played significant roles in childbirth and community care. While the professionalization of midwifery has elevated its role within modern medical systems, the community-based care and emotional support traditionally provided by sanba have diminished. With the loss of traditional practices such as specific birthing positions, postpartum recovery care, and rituals for safe childbirth, a gap has emerged in addressing the psychological and emotional aspects of childbirth.

Traditional elements of childbirth not only hold cultural significance but also contribute to the emotional stability and bonding of mothers and babies. For instance, region-specific birthing positions played a crucial role in reducing physical strain and facilitating natural delivery (Jordan, 1993). Additionally, postpartum care and rituals provided mothers with a sense of spiritual peace while also strengthening their connections with family and the community (Hahn & Kleinman, 1983). The erosion of these practices has isolated childbirth as a private event, reducing the psychological support mothers receive (Davis-Floyd, 2003).

Modern medicalized birthing environments prioritize physical safety, but this often comes at the expense of addressing the emotional needs of mothers. For example, fears and anxieties during childbirth may go unacknowledged (Field, 2008). Additionally, hospital policies can sometimes override maternal preferences, leaving mothers feeling disempowered. Furthermore, traumatic birth experiences may result in psychological distress, which can affect future pregnancies or childbirth (Takegata & Nakamura, 2014).

Traditional midwives and doulas address these gaps by focusing on emotional safety—ensuring mothers feel emotionally secure during and after childbirth. Emotional safety involves creating a supportive environment where mothers feel respected, valued, and at ease (Klaus & Kennell, 1993). This care not only enhances the mother's birthing experience but also strengthens the mother-child bond, fostering better long-term emotional health (Chamberlain, 1998).

By integrating traditional wisdom and cultural practices into modern midwifery, a more inclusive and human-centered approach to childbirth can emerge (Davis-Floyd, 2003). This integration not only preserves valuable cultural heritage by adapting it to contemporary needs but also addresses the emotional and psychological dimensions of childbirth. As a result, mothers can enjoy a more enriching and fulfilling birth experience. By combining the strengths of both traditional and modern midwifery, childbirth has the potential to become a safer, more holistic, and emotionally supportive experience for mothers, babies, and families, paving the way for a more compassionate future in maternal and newborn care.

17. PME AS A COMPLEMENT TO MODERN MIDWIFERY

Midwives are entrusted not only with ensuring maternal and neonatal health through medical expertise but also with fostering the bond between mother and child and providing emotional support (Verny, 1981). With the growing interest in prenatal memory research, the role of midwives is expanding. Prenatal memory explores the potential for fetuses to sense maternal emotions and environmental influences. Integrating this perspective into midwifery has the potential to deepen maternal-fetal relationships significantly (Gerland, J. 2022).

Research suggests that fetuses may establish emotional connections with their mothers during pregnancy, perceiving maternal emotions, voice, and affection (Chamberlain, 1998). By incorporating these insights, midwives can encourage mothers to recognize the fetus's presence and foster emotional bonding during pregnancy. This approach benefits both mother and child.

Midwives play a vital role in encouraging maternal-fetal communication by guiding mothers to engage in specific practices, such as talking to their unborn baby during quiet moments or responding to its movements with gentle touches or words of reassurance. These actions not only provide emotional comfort but also help mothers build a sense of connection and mentally prepare for the baby's arrival. Additionally, midwives facilitate emotional bonding through concrete physical interactions, such as teaching mothers to gently massage or cradle their belly in response to the baby's movements. These hands-on practices allow mothers to experience a deeper connection with their fetus, helping to reduce anxiety and cultivate a positive attitude toward childbirth and parenting.

PME allows midwives to introduce the perspective of respecting the fetus as an individual with emotions and awareness. By promoting this view, midwives enable mothers to strengthen their bonds with the fetus, enhancing attachment after birth (Verny, 1981). Such attachment supports the child's healthy emotional development and provides psychological fulfillment for the mother.

The bonds cultivated during pregnancy lay a strong foundation for postnatal relationships. Emotional connections established early have the potential to contribute to the child's social skills and emotional stability, while fostering trust and mutual understanding between parent and child. Midwives also serve as bridges, connecting medical safety with emotional well-being. By addressing maternal concerns through counseling and postnatal support, midwives can create a more comprehensive care experience (Davis-Floyd, 2003). By incorporating PME, midwives not only protect physical health but also support the next generation's emotional and developmental well-being. This holistic approach positions midwives as crucial agents in fostering both maternal and child happiness.

18. CHILDBIRTH AS A COLLABORATIVE TEAM EFFORT

Advancements in medical science have transformed childbirth into a specialized process. In Japan, where nearly all births occurred at home in 1950, this shifted to 99% of births taking place in facilities by 1975 (Shirai,2020). This transition often distanced childbirth from everyday life, making it feel like a "black box" experience. While some mothers now adopt birth plans or choose home births to reclaim a sense of agency, most continue to rely heavily on medical interventions. The COVID-19 pandemic further isolated childbirth, with many mothers giving birth without family support due to safety protocols. In such conditions, PME emerged as a valuable practice, enabling mothers to view the fetus as a companion and team member during labor. This perspective reframed childbirth, with mothers often describing their babies as calm and easy to care for, contributing to positive and less isolating birth experiences.

Research into the influence of consciousness on cellular functions, though limited, provides intriguing insights. Psychological states can impact cellular activity through mechanisms involving hormones, the immune system, and neural pathways (Sapolsky, 2004). For instance, meditation has been shown to influence cellular processes, and mental states such as stress or relaxation affect physiological responses (Davidson et al., 2003). Notably, research on athletes has demonstrated that focusing attention on specific muscles can increase blood flow and oxygen supply to those areas (Ranganathan et al., 2004). The author hypothesizes that pregnant women consciously directing their focus to organs like the uterus, placenta, and amniotic fluid could similarly enhance their function, potentially improving the childbirth process.

Practical applications of this theory have shown promise. Women with menstrual pain have reported significant relief by focusing on their uterus, which increases blood flow and reduces prostaglandin concentrations responsible for pain. Extending this concept to childbirth, PME encourages mothers to actively guide their body's natural processes, working in harmony with their fetus and biological systems. By framing childbirth as a "team process," where the mother and fetus collaborate toward a shared goal, this approach fosters a sense of connection and reduces maternal stress. Obstetricians, including Hedegaard et al. (1996) and Wadhwa et al. (2001), have observed that alleviating maternal stress leads to smoother labor progression, a key outcome supported by PME's emphasis on teamwork.

By recognizing the fetus as an active participant, PME shifts the mother's focus toward collaboration and empowers her to take an active role in the childbirth experience. This perspective not only promotes a smoother, more positive process but also marks an important step in reclaiming maternal autonomy from a traditionally hospital-centered, medically managed approach to childbirth. By encouraging mothers to embrace their role as active participants, PME transforms childbirth from a passive, medicalized experience into an empowering and deeply connected journey, fostering both emotional fulfillment and confidence.

19. BIDIRECTIONAL COMMUNICATION WITH THE FETUS

In Japan, the concept of communication between mother and fetus is often expressed through the term Ishin-Denshin ("heart-to-heart communication"), which embodies the cultural value of non-verbal interaction. Rooted in Japanese traditions, this idea aligns with beliefs in telepathic connections, similar to Western concepts like "Spirit Baby" or "Wonder Baby." While scientific evidence supporting such phenomena remains limited, Ishin-Denshin resonates deeply within Japanese culture, which places significant value on intuitive and emotional connections.

Building on this perspective, one method of maternal-fetal communication involves empathizing with and intuitively sensing the emotions or needs of the fetus, akin to a telepathic exchange. This practice encourages mothers to engage in a form of deep emotional resonance, fostering a sense of connection that transcends verbal communication. Although not scientifically validated, such approaches highlight the potential of shared empathy and awareness to strengthen the bond between mother and child, reflecting the broader cultural belief in the importance of Ishin-Denshin.

Telepathic communication, though not universally accepted in scientific circles, has been explored in various research endeavors. In the 1970s and 1980s, institutions such as Stanford Research Institute and Princeton University's PEAR lab investigated phenomena like remote viewing and consciousness-physical interactions (Targ & Puthoff, 1974; Jahn & Dunne, 1986). While these studies offered intriguing possibilities, their low reproducibility made practical applications challenging.

In Japan, similar explorations emerged, notably with Yumiko Tobitani's development of Quantum Speed Reading. This method reportedly enhanced cognitive and emotional development among children, sparking interpretations rooted in quantum mechanics, such as the observer effect (Tobitani, 2008). Although lacking definitive scientific validation, these findings highlight the potential for novel approaches to understanding human cognition and communication.

There are numerous cases where children, despite not being expected to remember events from their time in the womb, recount distinctive occurrences involving their parents before birth. Some children describe vivid memories of specific moments, such as their parents' actions or emotions during pregnancy. If such accounts are indeed factual, they may point to phenomena that cannot be fully explained by conventional scientific mechanisms. This suggests that it might also be possible for mothers to consciously convey positive information to their fetuses during pregnancy.

The potential benefits of fostering maternal-fetal communication are significant. Research indicates that emotional and psychological connections during pregnancy can positively impact postnatal bonding, parenting practices, and the child's development (Field, 2008). Encouraging mothers to engage in dialogue with their unborn child—whether through mindfulness, meditation, or simply speaking aloud—may enhance these bonds, contributing to healthier emotional foundations.

As the understanding of prenatal memory grows, societal acceptance of maternal-fetal communication could open new dimensions in parenting. For example, mothers who view their fetus as an aware and responsive being may experience reduced stress, increased emotional well-being, and stronger maternal instincts. These practices could also contribute to a broader cultural shift, promoting greater empathy and emotional connection within families and communities.

While scientific validation remains a challenge, the growing body of anecdotal evidence and cultural acceptance of maternal-fetal communication suggests promising avenues for further research. If safely and ethically embraced, these connections could enrich parenting and child development, fostering deeper relationships that benefit both mother and child. As science continues to explore the intersections of consciousness, emotion, and prenatal development, the potential for transforming early life experiences into a foundation for long-term well-being remains a compelling frontier.

This evolving perspective invites a reconsideration of how society views the prenatal period—not merely as a preparatory stage but as a formative time for nurturing the bonds that shape a child's future.

20. SOCIAL ACCEPTANCE AND SCIENTIFIC VALIDATION OF TAIKYO2.3

Validating Taikyo2.3 scientifically requires a collaborative, multi-disciplinary approach. This includes hypotheses such as the impact of maternal-fetal communication on reducing maternal stress and supporting fetal brain development (Verny, 1981; Chamberlain, 1998). Emerging technologies now enable sophisticated analyses of fetal physiological and neurological states. Techniques such as fMRI, MEG, and

1H-MRS can observe fetal brain activity and metabolic processes, while Electroencephalography (EEG) and Functional Near-Infrared Spectroscopy (fNIRS) provide real-time insights into neural development and brain oxygenation.

Additionally, Near-Infrared Spectroscopy (NIRS) and Fetal Magnetocardiography (FMCG) enable detailed assessments of fetal blood flow and cardiac activity, offering further opportunities to explore the physiological impact of maternal behaviors. Biomarkers like cortisol and oxytocin are crucial for quantifying the emotional and physiological connection between mother and fetus. Studies have shown that maternal cortisol levels can influence fetal development (Gitau et al., 2001), while oxytocin plays a significant role in fostering parent-infant bonding and emotional regulation (Feldman et al., 2007). Combining these tools creates a comprehensive framework to evaluate Taikyo2.3 scientifically.

Expanding research to include longitudinal studies tracking mother-child interactions from pregnancy through early childhood can illuminate the long-term implications of maternal-fetal communication (Gerland, 2022). These studies, paired with culturally sensitive practices like Taikyo and Ishin-Denshin, can align modern science with traditional values, fostering greater societal and academic acceptance.

To support the adoption of Taikyo2.3, findings must be disseminated through peer-reviewed journals and conferences. Practical applications, such as incorporating maternal-fetal communication into prenatal care, could produce measurable benefits, including reduced maternal stress and enhanced postnatal bonding (Sansone, 2019). Additionally, longitudinal and comprehensive studies are needed to evaluate the long-term impacts of Taikyo2.3 on mothers, children, and family dynamics. Such research would provide deeper insights into how maternal-fetal communication influences emotional well-being, developmental outcomes, and the overall harmony of family environments over time. These studies could further establish the enduring value of Taikyo2.3 as a transformative approach to prenatal care.

By combining interdisciplinary research, advanced technologies, and cultural perspectives, Taikyo2.3 has the potential to redefine the prenatal period as a formative stage for lifelong emotional and psychological well-being. Its integration of traditional wisdom with cutting-edge science can transform maternal-fetal relationships and enrich developmental experiences, creating a holistic framework for future generations.

21.THE PROCESS OF SCIENTIFICALLY VALIDATING TAIKYO 2.3

Establishing Taikyo2.3 (Prenatal Memory Education) as a scientifically validated concept requires a deeply interdisciplinary approach, as it spans multiple domains of expertise and calls for collaboration across diverse disciplines. This endeavor begins with defining clear and specific hypotheses that can serve as the foundation for empirical investigation. For example, researchers might hypothesize that maternal-fetal communication positively impacts the mother's mental health or that such interactions elicit measurable responses in the fetus's brain and physiological functions (Verny, 1981; Chamberlain, 1998; Sansone, 2019). These hypotheses are not only the starting points for rigorous scientific inquiry but also the stepping stones to building a robust framework for Taikyo2.3.

Given the complex and multifaceted nature of Taikyo2.3, it is essential to engage experts from neuroscience, obstetrics, psychology, developmental biology, and epigenetics. These fields provide complementary insights into key questions, such as how the emotional states of a pregnant mother might interact with fetal sensory and neurological development (Meaney & Szyf, 2005). For example, advanced imaging technologies like functional MRI (fMRI) and ultrasound can be used to observe how the fetal brain responds to stimuli such as maternal voice or meditative practices (DeCasper & Spence, 1986). Clinical trials focusing on the effects of intentional maternal-fetal communication can measure its impact on reducing maternal stress and strengthening postnatal bonding (Field, 2008). Furthermore, longitudinal studies that follow mothers and children from pregnancy through early childhood can illuminate the long-term developmental, emotional, and social implications of this communication (Gerland, 2022).

Interdisciplinary research is particularly critical in this field, as it lies at the intersection of biological, psychological, and cultural factors. For instance, epigenetic research can explore how maternal emotions and behaviors influence gene expression in the fetus, while psychological studies might examine how maternal-fetal communication shapes maternal instincts and attachment (Sapolsky, 2004; Meaney, 2001). These collaborative efforts are essential to unlocking the full potential of Taikyo2.3 as a scientifically credible framework.

In addition to empirical research, utilizing biomarkers like cortisol and oxytocin offers an objective way to measure the emotional and physiological connection between mother and fetus (Dawson et al., 1994). Wearable technology can further enhance these efforts by tracking maternal physiological changes during communication practices, providing additional layers of data to validate Taikyo2.3's effectiveness and reliability.

Cultural context is another key dimension of this interdisciplinary endeavor. The integration of Japanese cultural values such as Taikyo (prenatal education) and Ishin-Denshin (heart-to-heart communication) into Taikyo2.3 emphasizes its relevance and universality. Framing this concept within a cultural narrative that values emotional and intuitive connections can help bridge the gap between tradition and modern scientific understanding.

Finally, disseminating research findings through peer-reviewed journals and scientific conferences is essential to gaining recognition within the scientific community. Practical applications in maternity care, supported by real-world data, will further solidify Taikyo2.3's credibility and social acceptance (Chamberlain, 1998; Chamberlain, 2013; Sansone, 2019). By incorporating interdisciplinary insights and culturally informed practices, this approach can transition from a culturally inspired idea to a scientifically validated methodology with global implications.

Ultimately, Taikyo2.3 represents a field uniquely suited to interdisciplinary research, requiring the collective expertise of multiple domains to uncover its full potential. It offers the promise of transforming maternal-fetal relationships and enriching early developmental experiences, redefining the prenatal period as a foundational phase for lifelong emotional and psychological well-being. The collaboration of diverse specialists is not just beneficial but essential to advancing this visionary concept (Gerland, 2022).

22. A SIMPLE YET POWERFUL WAY TO STRENGTHEN FAMILY BONDS DURING PREGNANCY

One of the most effective practices discovered so far involves a simple yet meaningful act: having the expectant father place his hand on the mother's belly and engage in empathetic connection with the baby. This action not only fosters a sense of connection with the fetus but also creates a ripple effect of empathy between the parents. As attention shifts to the baby, the bond within the family strengthens, laying a foundation for deeper relationships after birth.

Mothers who have practiced this report feeling more supported and connected to their partners during pregnancy. After birth, babies born into such connected families often display remarkable behavior: they are more likely to meet their father's gaze with a smile and are less prone to cry inconsolably without clear reasons. This calm and positive interaction eases the emotional burden on mothers, giving them more confidence and emotional space to care for their child. As a result, the incidence of postpartum depression is significantly reduced, creating a healthier environment for both mother and baby (Meaney, 2001).

While this method has not yet been scientifically proven, the benefits observed by families who have tried it are compelling. The simplicity of this practice makes it accessible to anyone—no special tools or training are required. It emphasizes the importance of starting communication with the baby early, treating the fetus as a part of the family even before birth.

Sharing this practice with those who are pregnant or planning to conceive could have profound benefits. Encouraging expectant fathers to participate in such simple, empathetic actions strengthens their role in the pregnancy journey and fosters a sense of shared responsibility and connection. This, in turn, can lead to happier, healthier families and a more positive start to life for their child.

By promoting this easy-to-adopt habit, we can make a meaningful difference in the lives of parents and babies, even as we wait for scientific research to further explore and validate its effects.

CONCLUSION

This research demonstrates the potential of Prenatal Memory Education (PME) to foster self-awareness and well-being from the earliest stages of life. By encouraging empathetic communication with the fetus, PME strengthens parental bonds, reduces maternal stress, and creates a nurturing prenatal environment. These practices lay a foundation for lifelong psychological stability and a positive sense of self.

Scientific insights from neuroscience and epigenetics support the critical role of the prenatal environment in shaping emotional resilience and brain development. Evidence from 25 years of clinical observation suggests that children born into empathetic prenatal environments are more self-assured, socially connected, and altruistic.

While further research is needed to quantify these effects, PME's integration of traditional practices like Taikyo with modern science offers a holistic framework for redefining pregnancy as a transformative period for families. By promoting trust and emotional connection, PME has the potential to enhance the self-awareness and well-being of future generations.

REFERENCES

Barker, D. J. P. (1990). Fetal and infant origins of adult disease. *British Medical Journal, 301*(6761), 1111. DOI: 10.1136/bmj.301.6761.1111 PMID: 2252919

Barta, H., Jermendy, Á., Kovács, L., Schiever, N., Rudas, G., & Szabó, M. (2022). Predictive performance and metabolite dynamics of proton MR spectroscopy in neonatal hypoxic-ischemic encephalopathy. *Pediatric Research, 91*(3), 581–589. DOI: 10.1038/s41390-021-01626-z PMID: 34489532

Carman, E., & Carman, N. (2019). *Babies are cosmic: Signs of their secret intelligence*. Babies Are Cosmic.

Chamberlain, D. B. (1998). *The mind of your newborn baby*. North Atlantic Books.

Chamberlain, D. B. (2013). *Windows to the Womb: Revealing the Conscious Baby from Conception to Birth*. North Atlantic Books.

Clare, H. (2020). Spirit Baby: Communicate With Your Unborn Baby. Ease Your Birth. Authority Publishing. Kindle Edition.

Cutfield, W. S., Hofman, P. L., Mitchell, M., & Morison, I. M. (2007). Could epigenetics play a role in the developmental origins of health and disease? *Pediatric Research, 61*(5 Part 2), 68R–75R. DOI: 10.1203/pdr.0b013e318045764c PMID: 17413843

Daston, L., & Galison, P. (2010). *Objectivity*. Zone Books.

Davidson, R. J., Jackson, D. C., & Kalin, N. H. (2003). Emotion, plasticity, context, and regulation: Perspectives from affective neuroscience. *Psychological Bulletin, 129*(6), 890–913. DOI: 10.1037/0033-2909.126.6.890 PMID: 11107881

Davis-Floyd, R. (2003). *Birth as an American rite of passage*. University of California Press.

Dawson, G., Ashman, S. B., & Carver, L. J. (1994). The role of early experience in shaping behavioral and brain development and its implications for social policy. *Development and Psychopathology, 6*(4), 695–725. DOI: 10.1017/S0954579400004089 PMID: 11202040

Dawson, G., Hessl, D. A., & Frey, K. J. (1994). Effects of maternal behavior on infant stress physiology. *Developmental Psychology, 30*(6), 923–931.

DeCasper, A. J., & Spence, M. J. (1986). Prenatal maternal speech influences newborns' perception of speech sounds. *Infant Behavior and Development, 9*(2), 133–150. DOI: 10.1016/0163-6383(86)90025-1

Descartes, R. (1986). *Meditations on first philosophy* (Cottingham, J., Trans.). Cambridge University Press. (Original work published 1641)

Doi, M., Usui, N., & Shimada, S. (2022). Prenatal environment and neurodevelopmental disorders. *Frontiers in Endocrinology, 13*, 860110.

Feldman, R., Weller, A., Zagoory-Sharon, O., & Levine, A. (2007). Evidence for a neuroendocrinological foundation of human affiliation: Plasma oxytocin levels across pregnancy and the postpartum period predict mother-infant bonding. *Psychological Science, 18*(11), 965–970. DOI: 10.1111/j.1467-9280.2007.02010.x PMID: 17958710

Field, T. (2008). Pregnancy and labor alternative therapy research. *Alternative Therapies in Health and Medicine, 14*(5), 28–34. PMID: 18780582

Gao, W., Alcauter, S., Smith, J. K., Gilmore, J. H., & Lin, W. (2015). Development of human brain cortical network architecture during infancy. *Brain Structure & Function, 220*(2), 1173–1186. DOI: 10.1007/s00429-014-0710-3 PMID: 24469153

Gaskin, I. M. (2013). *Ina May's guide to childbirth* (Rev. ed.). Bantam Books.

Gerland, J. (2022). *Womb to Thrive: The Missing Keys to Heal Yourself, Your Family and the Planet*. Birthing The New Humanity.

Giedd, J. N. (2004). Structural magnetic resonance imaging of the adolescent brain. Annals of the New York Academy of Sciences, 102.0(1), 77–85.

Gitau, R., Fisk, N. M., Teixeira, J. M. A., Cameron, A., & Glover, V. (2001). Fetal hypothalamic-pituitary-adrenal stress responses to invasive procedures are independent of maternal responses. *Lancet, 357*(9251), 977–981. DOI: 10.1016/S0140-6736(00)04582-4 PMID: 11231985

Hahn, R. A., & Kleinman, A. (1983). Belief as pathogen, belief as medicine: "Voodoo death" and the "placebo phenomenon" in anthropological perspective. *Medical Anthropology Quarterly, 14*(4), 3–19. DOI: 10.1525/maq.1983.14.4.02a00030

Hallmayer, J.. (2011). Genetic and environmental influences on autism. *Archives of General Psychiatry, 68*(11), 1095–1102. DOI: 10.1001/archgenpsychiatry.2011.76 PMID: 21727249

Hedegaard, M., Henriksen, T. B., Secher, N. J., Hatch, M. C., & Sabroe, S. (1996). Do stressful life events affect duration of gestation and risk of preterm delivery? *Epidemiology (Cambridge, Mass.)*, *7*(4), 339–345. DOI: 10.1097/00001648-199607000-00001 PMID: 8793357

Heijmans, B. T., Tobi, E. W., Stein, A. D., Putter, H., Blauw, G. J., Susser, E. S., Slagboom, P. E., & Lumey, L. H. (2008). Persistent epigenetic differences associated with prenatal exposure to famine. *Proceedings of the National Academy of Sciences of the United States of America*, *105*(44), 17046–17049. DOI: 10.1073/pnas.0806560105 PMID: 18955703

Hume, D. (1739). *A Treatise of Human Nature*. Oxford University Press.

Ibuka, M. (1969). *Yochienn Deha Ososugiru* [Kindergarten is too late]. Kodansha.

Iimura, B. (2015). *History of midwifery in Japan*. Midwifery Today. Retrieved January 10, 2025, from https://www.midwiferytoday.com/mt-articles/history-of-midwifery-in-japan/

Ikegawa, A. (2005). Investigation by questionnaire regarding fetus/infant memory in the womb and/or at birth. Journal of Prenatal and Perinatal Psychology and Health (JOPPPAH), 20(2), 12.0–133.

Ikegawa, A. (2015). I remember, Mom: What can be understood from the womb. Tokyo journal of maternal health, 31(1), 8–12. [In Japanese].

Ikegawa, A. (2020). What is left behind? What is in the horizon? Quantum mechanical interpretation of prenatal memory. In Cárdenas, I. S., & Thorpe, M. (Eds.), *Change: Birthing & parenting at times of crisis* (pp. 199–248). Waterside Productions.

Ito, K. (2024). Prenatal memory therapy—Wonder Baby therapy: Dialogue with wonder baby. Pre- and Peri-natal Psychology Journal, 6(1), 72.

Jahn, R. G., & Dunne, B. J. (1986). *Margins of reality: The role of consciousness in the physical world*. Harcourt.

Jordan, B. (1993). Birth in four cultures: A cross-cultural investigation of childbirth in Yucatan, Holland, Sweden, and the United States. Waveland Press.

Kagan, J. (2004). *The psychological development of children*. Harvard University Press.

Klaus, M. H., & Kennell, J. H. (1976). *Maternal-infant bonding: The impact of early separation or loss on family development*. Mosby.

Klaus, M. H., & Kennell, J. H. (1993). *Mothering the mother: How a doula can help you have a shorter, easier, and healthier birth.* Perseus Publishing.

Lapehn, S., & Paquette, A. G. (2022). The placental epigenome as a molecular link between prenatal exposures and fetal health outcomes through the DOHaD hypothesis. *Current Environmental Health Reports, 9*(2), 155–166. DOI: 10.1007/s40572-022-00354-8 PMID: 35488174

Liley, A. W. (1969). The fetus as a personality. *The Australian and New Zealand Journal of Psychiatry, 3*(2), 57–63.

Linton, M. J., Dieppe, P., & Medina-Lara, A. (2016). Well-being is more than happiness and life satisfaction: A multidimensional analysis of 21 countries. *Health and Quality of Life Outcomes, 14*(166). Advance online publication. DOI: 10.1186/s12955-016-0530-0

Liu, D. (200 BCE). The Greater Dai's Book of Rites. Ancient Chinese text.

Liu, W., Zhang, L., Meng, T., Sun, H., & Gao, W. (2020). Functional connectivity development in the human fetal brain. *NeuroImage, 220*, 117090. DOI: 10.1016/j.neuroimage.2020.117090

Makichen, W. (2008). *Spirit Babies: How to Communicate with the Child You're Meant to Have.* Kindle Edition.

Malcon, L. M. C., Wearick-Silva, L. E., Zaparte, A., Orso, R., Luft, C., Tractenberg, S. G., Donadio, M. V. F., de Oliveira, J. R., & Grassi-Oliveira, R. (2020). Maternal separation induces long-term oxidative stress alterations and increases anxiety-like behavior of male Balb/cJ mice. *Experimental Brain Research, 238*(9), 2097–2.007. https://doi.org/DOI: 10.1007/s0022.0-020-05859-y

Meaney, M. J. (2001). Maternal care, gene expression, and the transmission of individual differences in stress reactivity across generations. *Annual Review of Neuroscience, 24*(1), 1161–1192. DOI: 10.1146/annurev.neuro.24.1.1161 PMID: 11520931

Meaney, M. J., & Szyf, M. (2005). Maternal care as a model for experienced-dependent chromatin plasticity? *Trends in Neurosciences, 28*(9), 456–463. DOI: 10.1016/j.tins.2005.07.006 PMID: 16054244

Midwifery Today. (n.d.). History of midwifery in Japan. Retrieved December 30, 2024, from

Ministry of Health. Labour and Welfare. (2020). Maternal and child health statistics in Japan. Government of Japan.

Nagel, T. (1974). What is it like to be a bat? *The Philosophical Review, 83*(4), 435–450. DOI: 10.2307/2183914

Ohkado, M., & Ikegawa, A. (2014). Children with life-between-life memories. *Journal of Scientific Exploration, 28*(3), 477–490.

Panksepp, J. (1998). *Affective neuroscience: The foundations of human and animal emotions*. Oxford University Press. DOI: 10.1093/oso/9780195096736.001.0001

Penrose, R. (1994). *Shadows of the mind: A search for the missing science of consciousness*. Oxford University Press.

Ranganathan, V. K.. (2004). Mental effort increases blood flow to muscles. *Journal of Applied Physiology, 97*(6), 2370–2380.

Reader, I. (2000). *Religious violence in contemporary Japan: The case of Aum Shinrikyo*. University of Hawai'i Press. DOI: 10.1515/9780824847135

Rose, J. (1991). Children recalling birth. Pre- and Peri-natal Psychology Journal, 6(1),91-104

Ryff, C. D., & Singer, B. (1998). The contours of positive human health. *Psychological Inquiry, 9*(1), 1–28. DOI: 10.1207/s15327965pli0901_1

Sandelowski, M. (2004). *Childbirth narratives: The cultural significance of birth stories*. Unknown Publisher.

Sansone, A. (2019). *Cultivating Mindfulness to Raise Children Who Thrive: Why Human Connection from Before Birth Matters*. Routledge.

Sapolsky, R. M. (2004). *Why Zebras Don't Get Ulcers: The Acclaimed Guide to Stress, Stress-Related Diseases, and Coping*. Holt Paperbacks.

Seckl, J. R., & Holmes, M. C. (2009). Prenatal stress, glucocorticoids, and the programming of adult disease. *Frontiers in Behavioral Neuroscience, 3*, 14. PMID: 19826624

Sharma, P., & Tucker, J. B. (2004). Cases of the reincarnation type with memories from the intermission between lives. *Journal of Near-Death Studies, 23*(2), 101–118.

Shichida, M. (1990). *Prenatal education and early childhood education*. Shichida Education Institute.

Shichida, M., & Tsunabuchi, Y. (1998). *The secret of birth trauma: Exploring the roots of personality through prenatal memory*. Diamond, Inc.

Shirai, C. (2020). Historical dynamism of childbirth in Japan: Medicalization and its normative politics, 1868–2017. *Technology and Culture, 61*(2), 515–545. DOI: 10.1353/tech.2020.0053 PMID: 33416778

Shizuoka University. Center for Research on Asia Faculty of Humanities & Social Sciences. (Year). *The social role of traditional midwives in Japan: Through the lens of mediating adoption.* Shizuoka University.

Springer. (2019). Prenatal and early postnatal influences on neurodevelopment. In *Advances in Brain Development Research* (pp. 85–100). Springer. DOI: 10.1007/978-3-030-25816-0_6

Taneichi, T. (2018). PF Theory and the multidimensional nature of human existence. *International Journal of Consciousness Studies, 14*(3), 101–120.

Targ, R., & Puthoff, H. E. (1974). Remote viewing and related phenomena. [Information transmission under conditions of sensory shielding.]. *Proceedings of the IEEE, 62*(6), 1081–1083.

Thomason, M. E., Scheinost, D., Manning, J. H., Grove, L. E., Hect, J. L., Marshall, N., & Ment, L. R. (2021). Weak functional connectivity in the human fetal brain prior to preterm birth. *Scientific Reports, 11*(1), 15621. DOI: 10.1038/s41598-021-95042-3 PMID: 34341418

Tobitani, Y. (2006). *Quantum speed-reading: Awakening your child's mind.* Hampton Roads Publishing.

Vaillant, G. E. (2012). *Triumphs of experience: The men of the Harvard Grant Study.* Belknap Press of Harvard University.

Verny, T. R. (2020). *The embodied mind: Understanding the mysteries of cellular memory, consciousness, and our bodies.* Pegasus Books.

Verny, (1981). The Secret Life of the Unborn Child. Dell Publishing.

Vlcek, J. (2017). *Tracking Consciousness Before Birth and Beyond.* FriesenPress.

Wadhwa, P. D., Culhane, J. F., Rauh, V., & Barve, S. S. (2001). Stress and preterm birth: Neuroendocrine, immune/inflammatory, and vascular mechanisms. *Maternal and Child Health Journal, 5*(2), 119–125. DOI: 10.1023/A:1011353216619 PMID: 11573837

Waldinger, R. J., & Schulz, M. S. (2010). What's love got to do with it? Social functioning, perceived health, and daily happiness in married octogenarians. *Psychology and Aging, 25*(2), 422–431. DOI: 10.1037/a0019087 PMID: 20545426

Wang, J. (2004). Prenatal influences: Historical perspectives and modern implications. [if available]. *The Journal of Maternal and Child Health*, *8*(3), 45–53. https://doi.org/10.xxxx/yyyy

Wójcik-Brylska, K., Pawlicka, P., Tataj-Puzyna, U., Szlendak, B., Węgrzynowska, M., Pięta, B., & Baranowska, B. (2023). Cooperation between midwives and doulas in the context of perinatal care: An integrative review of qualitative and quantitative studies. *Midwifery*, *126*, 103731. DOI: 10.1016/j.midw.2023.103731 PMID: 37321158

World Health Organization. (2016). *WHO recommendations on antenatal care for a positive pregnancy experience*. World Health Organization.

World Health Organization. (2016). *Standards for improving quality of maternal and newborn care in health facilities*. WHO.

World Health Organization. (2020). *Global maternal and perinatal mortality statistics*. WHO Publications.

Zhang, Z. (Ed.). (1983). *A Treasury of Mah_y_na S_tras: Selections from the Mah_ratnak_ta S_tra*. Penn State Press.

APPENDIX

Table 1. Comparative overview of maternal and fetal health approaches

Aspect	Prenatal Care	Prenatal Training	Taikyo
Primary Focus	Medical management and risk mitigation	Physical fitness and stress reduction	Emotional development and parent-child bonding
Conceptualization of Fetus	Developing biological entity	Supported indirectly via maternal stability	Sentient being with emotions and intentions
Methods	Medical oversight, diagnostics	Yoga, breathing exercises	Talking to fetus, music, meditation
Cultural Perspective	Universal	Regionally specific (e.g., yoga, cultural practices)	Unique to Japan, based on cultural values
Goals	Short-term: health and safety	Short-term: physical and mental preparation	Long-term: emotional stability, family harmony

Comparative Overview of Maternal and Fetal Health Approaches: Summarizes key distinctions among prenatal care, prenatal training, and Taikyo, highlighting their goals, methodologies, and conceptualization of the fetus.

Table 2. Key differences between Taikyo 1.1 and Taikyo 2.3

Aspect	Taikyo1.1	Taikyo2.3
Communication Type	Unidirectional	Bidirectional
Fetus Perception	Passive entity	Active participant with emotions and intentions
Participants	Primarily the mother	Mother, father, and fetus
Focus	External stimuli (e.g., music, calmness)	Mutual interaction and emotional connection
Objective	Fetal emotional development	Building familial bonds and mutual understanding
Symbolism of Name	".1" symbolizes one primary participant	".3" symbolizes a triadic relationship

Key Features and Differences between Taikyo1.1 and Taikyo2.3: Explores the evolution from traditional Taikyo practices to PME, emphasizing the bidirectional communication and inclusion of the entire family in prenatal bonding.

Chapter 3
Feeling (Remembering) the Connection With Invisible Things Is Necessary for the Future Evolution of Humanity

Shinichiro Sawano
Shin Sawano Photo Studio, Japan

ABSTRACT

Science has traditionally relied on hypotheses supported by precise statistics and evidence. However, this approach has limitations and often excludes phenomena beyond measurable logic. A new perspective is needed that goes beyond theory and speculation and embraces human sensitivity and intuition. This concept is consistent with Kansei Engineering, a field rooted in Japanese thought. The method presented here aims to guide individuals to a life aligned with the true essence of their mind, body and soul by emphasizing the innate sensitivity of human beings. It encourages people to recognize and feel the presence of phenomena that cannot be fully measured by current science, but that deeply impact harmony and interconnectedness. The integration of quantum theory and consciousness highlights this change and paves the way for the evolution and transformation of humanity.

DOI: 10.4018/979-8-3373-0360-4.ch003

INTRODUCTION

I am an artist, not a scientist. I am aware of the fact that the five senses that we humans originally possessed-taste, hearing, smell, sight, and touch-have been dulled by the abundance of knowledge that has accompanied the development of science and technology. I believe that if we can awaken the probably dormant sensors of the five senses and revive our senses, we can humbly realize that we are connected to nature and the universe, and that we are alive, including invisible beings, and lead a life that is uniquely our own. I am working on a method to revive this original sense. It is just an aggregation of subjective information.

However, if I quantify subjective sensations based on Kansei Engineering (Note 1), which originated in Japan as a technological field that explores the analysis, evaluation, and utilization of human sensitivity, a subjective response that is difficult to explain logically, using scientific methods, what I am practicing will be useful to society in new areas in the future, I believe that what I am practicing will be useful to society in new areas in the future.

I have come to realize that many people do not celebrate or truly enjoy their own lives. They live their lives for the purpose of gaining superiority over others, such as financial wealth and honor, out of fear of others' opinions and failure. Is this good or bad? It is not a question of whether it is good or bad, but rather a question of whether one's life is meaningful (was it enjoyable? Was it happy?) from the bottom of one's heart at the moment one's life is over.

How can a person regain his or her original way of life, a life that is truly radiant with joy from the soul? To live in such a state is to feel connected to the people around you, to nature, and to the universe, not theoretically, but from the bottom of your heart. People all over the world are becoming increasingly interested in and practicing Zen, meditation, and other forms of looking inward. However, based on Eastern thought, few people realize that their inner world creates the outer world, and that the inner and outer universes are connected and influence each other. Modern quantum theory, however, scientifically proves that the results of observation change according to the will of the observer. In other words, one's consciousness affects one's surroundings and changes the phenomena. I am very interested in the fact that cutting-edge quantum physics of our time has come closer to fundamental ideas such as Buddhism and Shintoism, and I research this every day alongside my artistic activities.

SECTION 1: BACKGROUND

In 1991 I came across what is said to be the world's largest wildflower garden in Namaqualand (note 2) in the Northern Cape region of South Africa.

The Northern Cape region is one of the least tourist-friendly areas of South Africa, and when I first visited in the early 1990s, it was a desolate area with a Mediterranean climate, rarely visited by tourists.

The area is said to be home to more than 3,500 species of wildflowers in the spring (see Figure 1,2,3 Session 101,203,103 Namaqualand). In the area where I usually stay, about 1,350 plant species have been recorded, a third of which are endangered species found nowhere else.

Because they are so densely populated, new varieties are created by mutation, and there is still no illustrated book that covers them all.

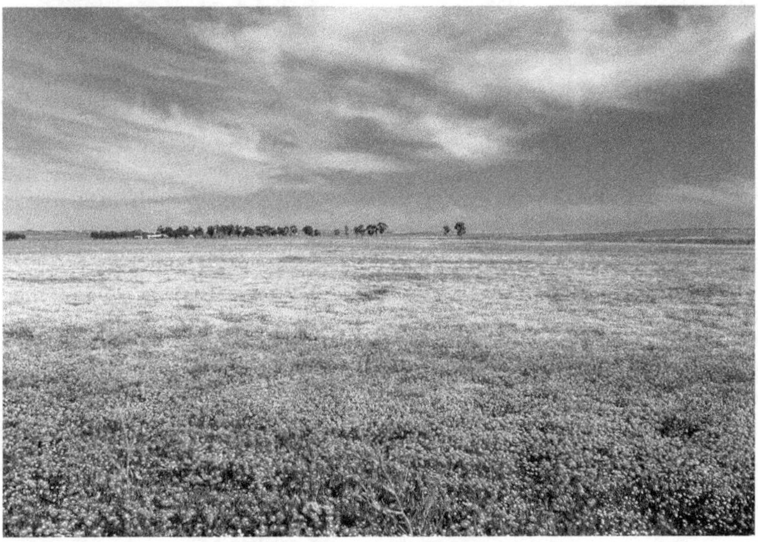

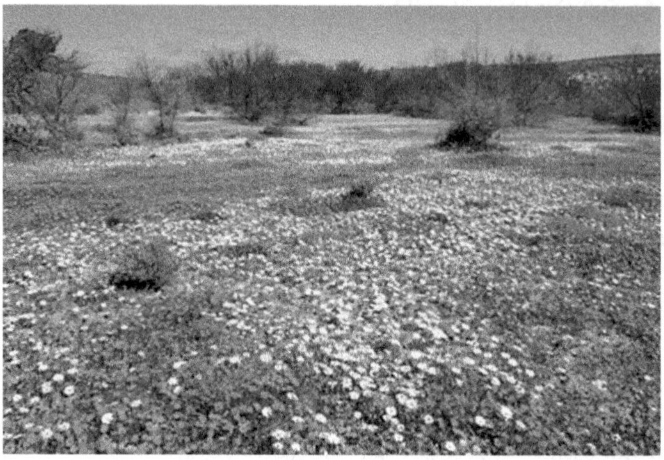

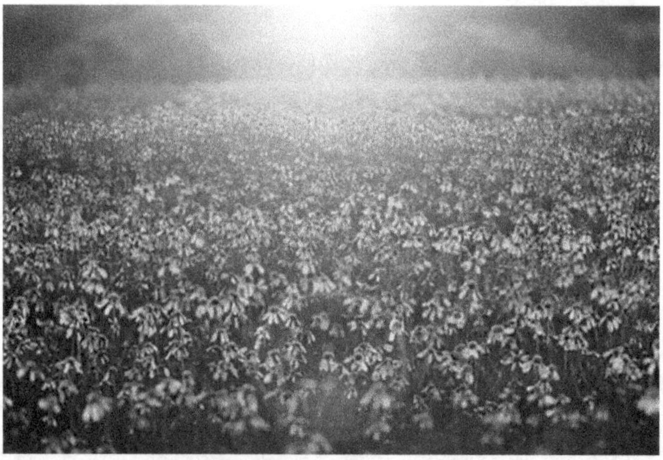

I was the first to introduce this place to Japan, and since 1997 I have made numerous appearances in the Japanese media and given lectures throughout the country.

Living in an environment where the seasons change abundantly, the Japanese people have a traditional culture of appreciating flowers. So many people have asked to visit this largest wildflower garden in the world.

I organized the first tour from Japan in 1998. Since then, I have organized a total of more than 30 tours until last year, 2024.

Since the first tour, I have always felt that the visitors are excited and energetic as if they were children again. When people visit this place, it is a fact that they are able to ground the negative thoughts and feelings of those who suffer from the stress of society and the city, and return their bodies and minds to their original healthy state. (see Figure 4 Session 104 Namaqualand)

At the peak of the flowering season, the carpets of flowers seem to glow like neon colors as they celebrate the brief spring in the rainy season to survive in the harsh, dry Mediterranean climate for most of the year. I was keenly aware that when people encounter this explosion of energy, they return to their original healthy state. (see Figure 5 Session 105 Namaqualand)

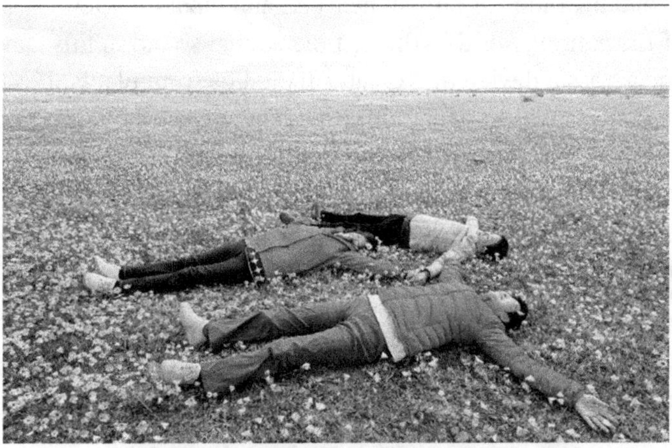

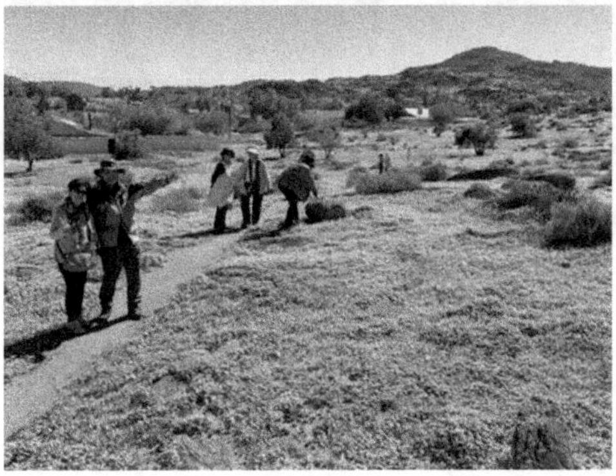

SECTION 2: REBIRTH OF NATURAL ENVIRONMENTAL MUSIC AND PLANT MUSIC

In the beginning, as a photographer, I visited South Africa every year, hoping to convey to Japan the energy that inspires people through photography. However, I had noticed that the natural world was full of melodies, not only the beautiful sight of flowers, but also the singing of wild birds and the sound of streams. Since my early days, I have been using high-resolution recording equipment capable of recording in an area beyond the range of human hearing, and binaural microphones to record the sounds of the natural world in three-dimensional sound in this flower garden.

I also came across a device that creates melodies from plants. I use it to record melodies extracted from plant matter on site and have workshop participants listen to them. It seems to have a relaxing effect, making people very sleepy when they listen to it. In the future, I would like to measure physical and psychological changes, such as brain waves and body temperature, with the help of medical professionals. (see Figure 6,7 Session201,202PlantMusic)

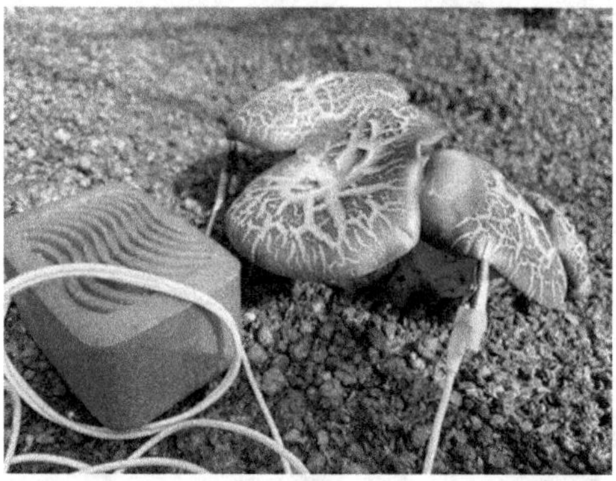

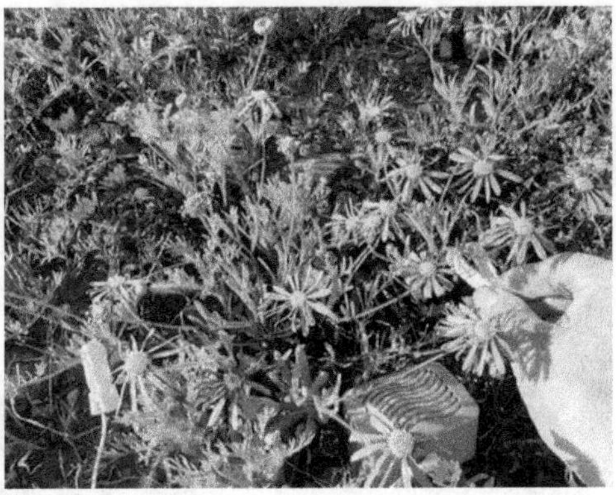

SECTION 3: FLOWER ESSENCES (FLOWER REMEDIES)

Another is flower essences (Note 3). Before my first visit to the flower gardens of South Africa, I came across batch flower remedies in Tokyo. I read a translated book, and without any discomfort, I intuited that plants have hidden abilities that cannot be scientifically analyzed. And it occurred to me that I could make this flower essence in Namaqualand, South Africa.

Using the Sun Method invented by Dr. Edward Batch, I began making flower essences in this pristine South African flower garden. The Sun Method is a technique in which flowers are picked in a glass vessel filled with water and floated on the surface of the vessel so that they are exposed to sunlight. Water is known to hold vibrational information. (Note 4)

However, as I mentioned earlier, there are many endangered species of plants in this area. Therefore, I put a few drops of the mineral water I brought with me into the petals of each flower, expose them to sunlight for a while, and gratefully suck out the water with a dropper. (see Figure 8 Session301FlowerEssence)

I have come up with a unique method of collecting water without picking the flowers and without damaging them, and I store the water with information about the flowers. (see Figure 9 Session302FlowerEssence)

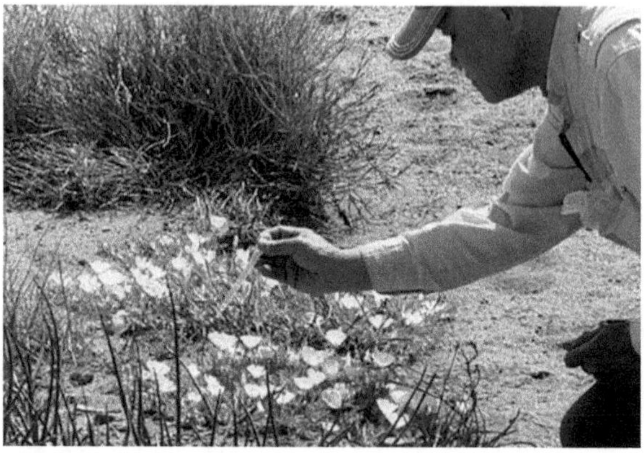

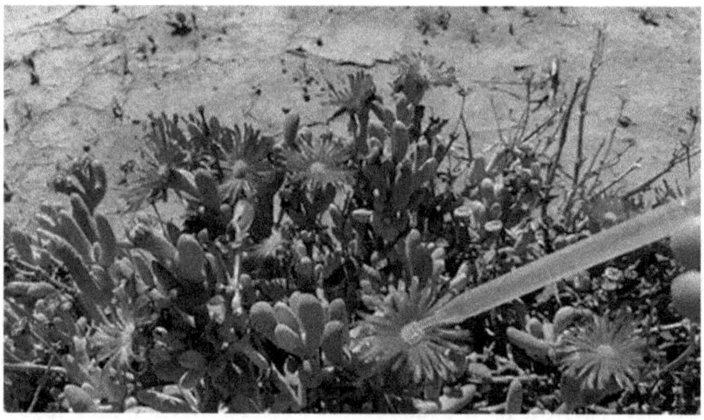

There are now as many as 5,000 or 10,000 different types of flower essences produced on five continents. The most common methods for choosing the right essence for you are pendulum, kinesiology, O-ring test, consultation with a flower essence specialist called a practitioner, or your own intuition.

SECTION 4: WORKSHOPS

My flower essence workshops are extremely unique and cannot be experienced anywhere else. It is a direct exposure to the light of the flower itself, the flower from which the flower essence is made, as well as a video recording of the flower essence itself. In other words, in the workshop, participants hold glass bottles containing only water for dilution and are directly exposed to the light of the flower garden as it is projected on a screen. In addition, the images of the subject were captured and recorded using a pinhole adapter attached to a camera without a lens. (see Figure 10,11,12 Session401,402,403PinholePhotography)

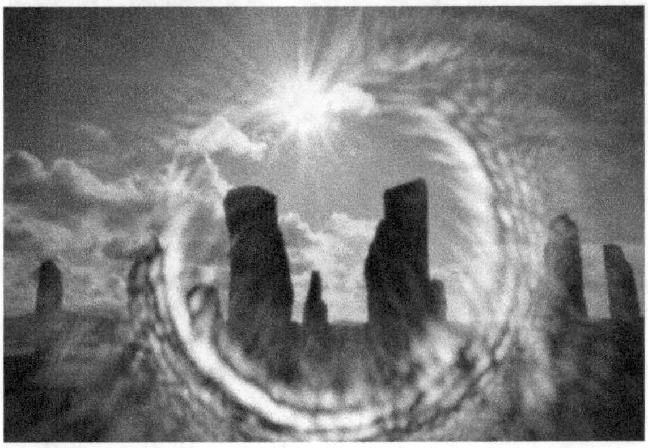

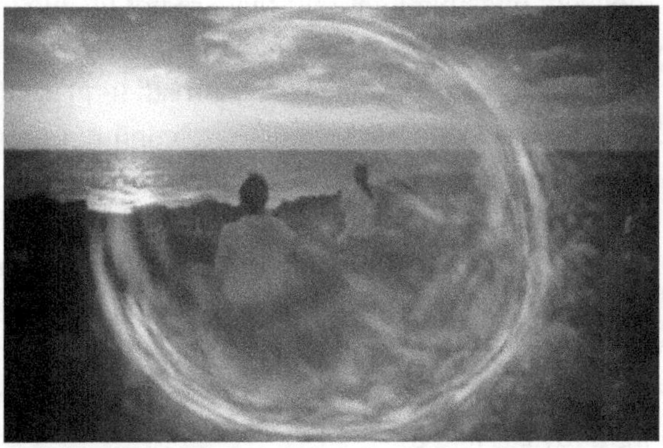

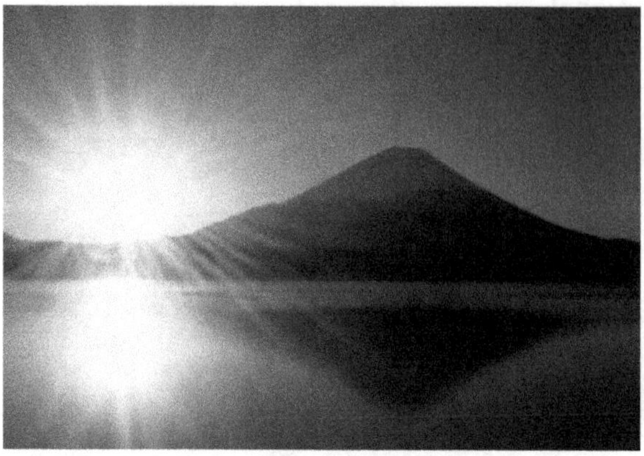

Digital image sensors are inherently sensitive to light in the ultraviolet and infrared regions other than visible light (Note 5), but if images are reproduced by capturing light in all sensitivity regions, they will be reproduced in colors that are different from the hues seen by humans. Therefore, in consideration of the color balance to be reproduced, invisible light rays that are not visible to the human eye are intentionally omitted by using lenses and internal filters. (General camera lenses, except for special applications, are designed to absorb all light except visible light).

I removed the lens and used a pinhole adapter to capture light in all the wavelength ranges that the image sensor can detect. (Note 6)

It is also known that skin absorbs colors in a certain range of wavelengths. (Note 7)

Therefore, knowing that human skin also absorbs light other than visible light, I dared to create a pinhole image with only a small hole to let light through.

The light is emitted by a video projector with a built-in state-of-the-art LED laser that bathes the participants in light; the LED video projector appears to contain a trace of invisible light rays. (Note 8)

With this setup, light other than visible light, including as much as possible, was absorbed through the skin rather than through the eyes (which were kept closed as direct eye contact is dangerous). It has been scientifically proven that sound is also absorbed through the skin in the form of vibrations. In particular, many people have experienced sound pressure and sound resonance not only with their ears, but also with their entire body when viewing fireworks or listening to a large percussion performance up close. (Note 9)

The bio-energy layer (bio-energy field) that extends outside the human body, also known as the aura, is round, spherical, and ideally shaped in newborns. As the child grows, the light of this sphere is often distorted or weakened by the influence of parents and social life.

The generally invisible layer of energy emanating from the physical body extends outward from the physical epidermis to the etheric, astral, and mental bodies.

Acupuncture works at the level of the physical body and the etheric layer immediately outside of it, while homeopathy works at the astral and mental body levels outside of it.

Flower essences have been shown to act on an even more subtle layer of energy, called the causal body, which is further removed from the physical body.

This is also described in the book "Vibrational Medicine" by Dr. Richard Gerber MD, an American Western physician. (Gerber, 2001) (Note 10)

I speculate that the comprehensive use of the various frequencies of vibration emitted by light, color, and sound can help restore balance to our natural ideal energy layer.

The following is an episode that led to this workshop approach. Around the year 2000, there was a friend of mine who had a kind of depression that kept him at home, unable to leave the house. One day he visited my studio and, with his permission, I exposed him to dozens of flower lights emitted from a video projector via my laptop for about 30 minutes. I heard from him about a month later. He told me that he had felt better since being exposed to the light, and that he had been able to keep his mind normal for several weeks without taking his doctor-prescribed medication. (see Figure 13,14,15 Session404,405,406workshops)

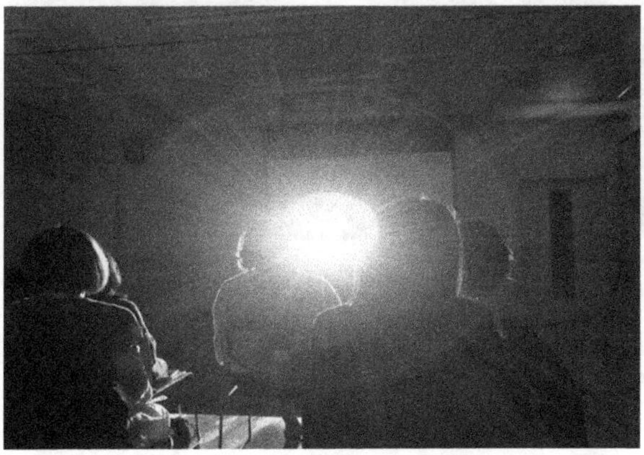

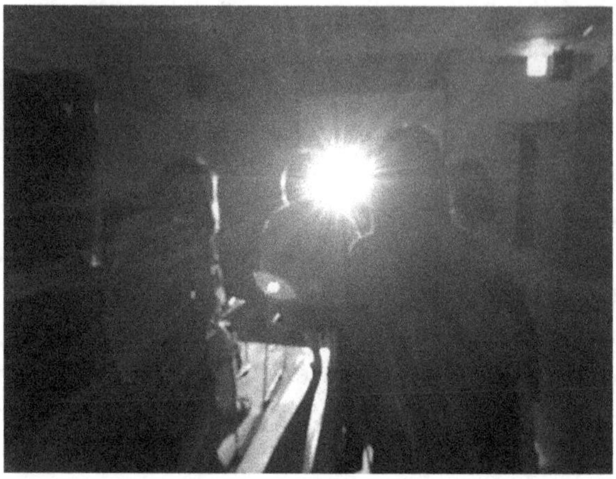

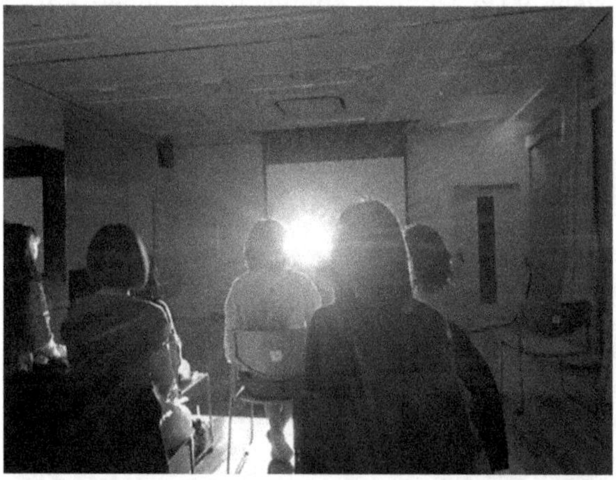

His feedback convinced me that even digital devices could convey information about the powerful flowers of nature.

Since then, I have created an immersive space during these flower essence sessions where people are exposed to light while listening to three-dimensional environmental sounds and plant music.

Currently, I have 30 types of flower essences in stock, mostly flower essences, but also other environmental essences such as full moon, stars, etc. Participants are exposed to each of these 30 types of light for 40 seconds, and I use a pendulum or O-ring test to determine which light and essence the participant is tuning into. (see Figure 16 Session407workshops)

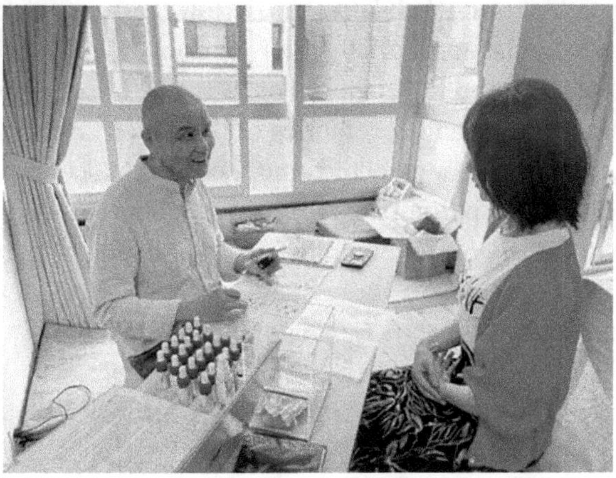

1) Experienced participants' impressions during the session:

Here are some of the participants' impressions immediately after being exposed to the specific light.
The energy is completely different from other essences:
Comments from experienced practitioners who use other specific brands of flower essences
I enjoy being in touch with my body and mind.
When I was exposed to light, I could smell certain lights. It was interesting to see how my body reacted to the light, feeling stronger, weaker, my hands felt hot, and so on.
I became very sleepy. But when it was over, I felt very comfortable and tired, which was strange.
I felt a cosmic expansion in my heart and a feeling of happiness and joy overflowing.
Depending on the light, my ears would feel vibrate and my hands would shake.
When I began to bathe in the Light, I felt very hot all over, but it was almost as if I was sleeping or meditating, but it was a time of slumber.
As I bathed in the light, I could feel my face beginning to feel mushy and bathed.
I was also born with color synesthesia. (Note 11)

To be more specific, even before I entered kindergarten, when I see a number, I think of a color. In other words, I was born with the sense that when I see or think of each number, I imagine a different color. The combination of each number and color has not changed from my childhood to the present. When I am conscious of it, the Japanese "Aiueo" and the ABC alphabet all bring up colors in my mind.

I apply this to each person when I customize flower essences for them, using my own intuition to advise the appropriate color for them. By appropriate, I mean to balance a person's energy and radiate more of their true bio-energy. For example, I recommend wearing clothes and accessories of that color, admiring flowers of the recommended color in their room, and eating foods of that color.

I have found that when participants follow my advice, when I see them again later, they are mysteriously positively transformed and radiant from the inside out.

2) Comments received by the experiencer after the session:

Here are some of the specific feelings, changes in their environment and impressions after the session.

"A healer attended my workshop and received a long feedback message the next morning. It is that she had a very realistic dream in the middle of the night. She woke up in the middle of the night with tears in her eyes, having had a very realistic vision of herself in a past life, in the Middle Ages, being hunted as a witch, escaping twice, but finally being executed the third time. She relalised that she was still attracted to her work as a healer, but something was holding her back, that she just couldn't cross the line, and the dream helped her understand why."

"I was able to follow my intuition and take a leap of faith on an issue that I had been unsure about."

"I felt so encouraged that I took the plunge, quit my job, got a new job and my relationships are better than before and my salary has improved."

"I was given advice on an unexpected color that I had never imagined, but when I took the plunge and started wearing it, my friends told me that I had become brighter. I, too, feel brighter and lighter these days."

In short, I believe that this workshop helps people to release the consciousness that they have unconsciously blocked. I have always believed that color is energy. However, I have found that a surprising number of women are indifferent to the colors they wear and look at. I explain that color has a great psychological effect on people and give them advice on how to live in a way that is unique to them, a way of living that their soul originally desires. (Note 12)

SECTION 5: SUMMARY AND ASPIRATIONS

By letting visitors experience a space that fully blends light, color, and sound with their whole bodies, I help revive their five dormant senses and awaken their intuitive or sixth sense, which can be described as animal-like and transcends the five senses.

In other words, I guide them to live their lives according to their conscience, their inner fit sensor.

How can I help people realize how much their lives can be brightened by feeling, rather than theorizing, that their inner and outer worlds are connected and influence each other? I believe that if people who have given up on having any impact on society can realize that they are connected and in resonance with nature and the universe, this will be the basis for a great harmony, a butterfly phenomenon, and this is what I am exploring every day as I improve this project.

From now on, with the cooperation of experts from various fields, I hope to apply Kansei engineering and advocate a new platform to the world by connecting existing science and invisible factors.

Note 1

Kansei engineering (Japanese: 感性工学 *kansei kougaku*, emotional or affective engineering) aims at the development or improvement of products and services by translating the customer's psychological feelings and needs into the domain of product design (i.e. parameters). It was founded by Mitsuo Nagamachi, professor emeritus of Hiroshima University (also former Dean of Hiroshima International University and CEO of International Kansei Design Institute). Kansei engineering parametrically links the customer's emotional responses (i.e. physical and psychological) to the properties and characteristics of a product or service. In consequence, products can be designed to bring forward the intended feeling. It has been adopted as one of the topics for professional development by the Royal Statistical Society. Product design has become increasingly complex as products contain more functions and have to meet increasing demands such as user-friendliness, manufacturability and ecological considerations. With a shortened product lifecycle, development costs are likely to increase. Since errors in the estimations of market trends can be very expensive, companies therefore perform benchmarking studies that compare with competitors on strategic, process, marketing, and product levels. However, success in a certain market segment not only requires knowledge about the competitors and the performance of competing products, but also about the impressions which a product leaves to the customer. The latter requirement becomes much more important as products and companies are becoming mature. Customers purchase products based on subjective terms such as brand image, reputation, design, impression etc.. A large number of manufacturers have started to consider such subjective properties and develop their products in a way that conveys the company image. A reliable instrument is therefore needed: an instrument which can predict the reception of a product on the market before the development costs become too large.

This demand has triggered the research dealing with the translation of the customer's subjective, hidden needs into concrete products. Research is done foremost in Asia, including Japan and Korea. In Europe, a network has been forged under the 6th EU framework. This network refers to the new research field as "emotional design" or "affective engineering". ("Kansei Engineering," n.d.)

Kansei Engineering Explained Simply

Kansei Engineering is a field of study that focuses on scientifically understanding how people feel comfort or beauty and applying that knowledge to product and service design.

For example, when someone says, "This car feels luxurious," or "I love how easy this appliance is to use," these impressions are based on their emotions and perceptions. Kansei Engineering gathers such feelings as data and uses them to improve designs.

Simple Examples

1. Car Design
    - When designing a car's interior, Kansei Engineering asks, "What colors and materials make the driver feel comfortable and secure?"
2. Smartphone Operation Sounds
    - It studies what kind of "click" sound when pressing a button makes people feel satisfied.
3. Drink Packaging
    - It examines how the shape and design of packaging can make a drink look more appealing or delicious.

How Does It Work?

Kansei Engineering uses methods such as:

- Conducting surveys to gather people's opinions.
- Measuring physical reactions like heart rate or brainwaves to observe how the body responds.
- Comparing impressions by slightly changing designs or shapes.

Why is it Impressive?

With Kansei Engineering, products aren't just functional—they're designed to feel good and bring joy to the user. It allows creators to design things that people find pleasant, exciting, or even emotionally touching.

What makes Kansei Engineering especially approachable for beginners is its focus on how people feel. It's not just about technology but about putting human emotions at the center of the design process. That's the true charm of Kansei Engineering!

Kansei Engineering: An Academic Explanation

Kansei Engineering is an interdisciplinary field that scientifically and technologically analyzes human sensitivity and sensory responses, applying these insights to the design and development of products and services. Originating in Japan, Kansei Engineering has become widely used in industries such as manufacturing and design. It integrates elements from psychology, cognitive science, statistics, design engineering, artificial intelligence, and other disciplines.

Basic Concepts

1. What is Kansei?

"Kansei" refers to a person's subjective senses, emotions, and impressions toward objects, environments, or information. For example, subjective reactions like "beautiful" or "comfortable" to specific colors, shapes, or sounds fall under Kansei. These responses are influenced by personal experience, culture, and context, making them highly complex.

2. Engineering Applications

Kansei Engineering quantifies subjective emotional responses and incorporates them into design and development processes. Examples include designing products that evoke a sense of "luxury" or creating soundscapes that users find "pleasant."

Research Process

Research in Kansei Engineering typically follows these steps:

1. Selection of Target
    - Identify the product, service, or object to be studied or developed.

2. Extraction of Kansei Elements
    - Define the elements related to users' Kansei, such as color, texture, sound, or shape.
3. Data Collection
    - Collect data through surveys, behavioral observation, or biological measurements (e.g., brainwaves, heart rate).
4. Analysis of Relationships Between Kansei and Design Elements
    - Analyze the relationship between Kansei (subjective evaluation) and design elements (product characteristics) using statistical methods like regression analysis or multivariate analysis.
5. Application to Design
    - Use the analysis results to design products or services that reflect user Kansei.

Applications

1. Automotive Industry
    - Designing interiors and control panels that convey "luxury" or "safety" to users.
2. Consumer Electronics
    - Creating button textures or operational sounds that feel "intuitive" and "comfortable."
3. Fashion
    - Selecting colors and materials that users perceive as "stylish" or "elegant."

Academic Background

Related Disciplines

- Psychology: Understanding perception and cognitive processes related to Kansei.
- Statistics: Analyzing and modeling Kansei data.
- Cognitive Science: Studying the relationship between Kansei and human cognitive processes.
- Engineering: Applying insights to product design and interface development.

Major Research Methods

- Quantitative Methods: Experimental data and statistical analysis.

- Qualitative Methods: User interviews and observations.
- Hybrid Methods: Combining qualitative and quantitative data for comprehensive analysis.

Significance and Challenges of Kansei Engineering

Significance
- Promotes user-centered design philosophy.
- Plays a critical role in differentiating products and services.
- Bridges technical factors and human sensory elements.

Challenges
- Kansei is subjective and varies greatly among individuals, making generalization difficult.
- It is heavily influenced by culture and era.
- Data collection and analysis require significant time and resources.

Kansei Engineering is a crucial academic field that harmonizes technological innovation with enhanced user experiences. Its continued development holds great promise for the future. (Source from ChatGPT)

Note 2

Namaqualand (Khoikhoi: "Nama-kwa" meaning Nama Khoi people's land) is an arid region of Namibia and South Africa, extending along the west coast over 1,000 km (600 mi) and covering a total area of 440,000 km^2 (170,000 sq mi). It is divided by the lower course of the Orange River into two portions – Little Namaqualand to the south and Great Namaqualand to the north.

Little Namaqualand is within the Namakwa District Municipality, forming part of Northern Cape Province, South Africa. It is geographically the largest district in the country, spanning over 26,836 km^2.[1] A typical municipality is Kamiesberg Local Municipality. The semidesert Succulent Karoo region experiences hot summers, sparse rainfall, and cold winters.[1]

Great Namaqualand, in the Karas Region of Namibia, is sparsely populated by the Namaqua, a Khoikhoi people who have traditionally inhabited the Namaqualand region.

The area's landscape ranges from an unexploited coastal strip in the west to semidesert areas in the north-east. Famed for its proximity to the Atlantic Ocean, its wild flowers during spring, its wealth of minerals, and cultural history, Namaqualand is a popular region for international and local tourists. The Namakwa coastline and the banks of the Orange River are popular for their hiking trails and off-roading routes.[1]

The beginning of the flower season varies from year to year, but usually occurs between August and October. The natural landscape is continually monitored with the first sign of spring and flower season being the arrival of Namakwa daisies. When purple vygies bloom, spring is coming to an end.[1]

The Namaqua National Park is situated west of the N7, one of South Africa's national roads. This conservation area is a great biodiversity hotspot, with the highest concentration of succulent plants of any of the world's arid regions. More than a thousand of its estimated 3500 floral species cannot be found anywhere else in the world.[2]

The Ai-Ais/Richtersveld Transfrontier Park, on the border of Namibia and South Africa, was known as the Richtersveld National Park in South Africa and the Ai-Ais Hot Springs Game Park in Namibia before the two parks were formally combined in August 2003.[1] What was once the Richtersveld National Park nurtures about 30% of South Africa's succulent species. (Source from https://en.wikipedia.org/wiki/Namaqualand)

Note 3

Flower essences are a type of natural therapy that captures the energy of specific flowers in liquid form, used to help balance emotions and the mind. They were developed in the 1930s by Dr. Edward Bach, known for Bach Flower Remedies, and are now used worldwide.

Features of Flower Essences

- Harnessing the energy of plants: They are made by immersing specific flowers in water and transferring their energy using sunlight or other methods.
- Contain no physical components: Unlike herbal medicine, flower essences do not contain the physical components of the flowers but are believed to carry their energy or vibrations.
- Work on emotional and mental levels: They are used to support issues like stress, anxiety, lack of confidence, or sadness.
- Chosen based on individual needs: The essences are selected according to the individual's emotional state or circumstances.

How to Use

Flower essences are typically used in the following ways:

1. Add a few drops to water or another drink and consume.

2. Place a few drops directly under the tongue.
3. Spray on the body or in a room.
4. Add a few drops to a bath.

Safety

Flower essences often contain alcohol as a preservative but are used in very small amounts, making them highly safe. They are considered a gentle therapy with almost no side effects and can be used for children and animals. ("Bach Flower Remedies," n.d.)

Bach flower remedies (BFRs) are solutions of brandy and water—the water containing extreme dilutions of flower material developed by Edward Bach, an English homeopath, in the 1930s. Bach claimed that the dew found on flower petals retains the supposed healing properties of that plant (Vohra, 2002). Systematic reviews of clinical trials of Bach flower solutions have found no efficacy beyond that of a placebo (Thaler et al., 2009; Ernst, 2002).

Description

The Bach flower remedy solutions, which contain a 50:50 mix of water and brandy, are called mother tincture (Weeks & Bullen, 1990). Stock remedies—the solutions sold in shops—are dilutions of mother tincture into other liquid. Most often the liquid used is alcohol, so that the alcohol level by volume in most stock Bach remedies is between 25 and 40% (Ernst, 2010). (50 to 80 proof). The solutions do not have a characteristic scent or taste of the plant because of dilution. The dilution process results in the statistical likelihood that little more than a single molecule may remain; it is claimed that the remedies contain "energetic" or "vibrational" nature of the flower and that this can be transmitted to the user placebo (Thaler et al., 2009). The solutions are described by some as vibrational medicines, (Cancer Research UK, 2013) which implies they rely on the pseudoscientific concept of water memory. They are often labeled as homeopathic because they are extremely diluted in water, but are not homeopathy as they do not follow other homeopathic ideas such as the law of similars.

Bach believed that illness was the result of a conflict between the purposes of the soul and the personality's actions and outlook. This internal war, according to Bach, leads to negative moods and to "energy blocking", thought to cause a lack of "harmony", thus leading to physical diseases (Graham, 1999; Wood, 2000).

Bach derived his solutions intuitively (Larimore & O'Mathúna, 2007) and based on his perceived psychic connections to the plants, rather than using research based on scientific methods (Robson, 2004, p 185) If Bach felt a negative emotion, he would hold his hand over different plants, and if one alleviated the emotion, he would ascribe the power to heal that emotional problem to that plant. He imagined that early-morning sunlight passing through dew-drops on flower petals transferred the healing power of the flower onto the water, (Barnard, 2004) so he would collect the dew drops from the plants and preserve the dew with an equal amount of brandy to produce a mother tincture which would be further diluted before use (Original Bachflower, 2020). Later, he found that the amount of dew he could collect was not sufficient, so he would suspend flowers in spring water and allow the sun's rays to pass through them (Barnard, 2004). If this was impractical because of lack of sunlight or other reasons, he wrote that the flowers may be boiled. The result of this process Bach termed the "mother tincture", which is then further diluted before sale or use.

Bach was satisfied with the method, because of its simplicity, and because it involved a process of combination of the four elements:

- The earth to nurture the plant
- the air from which it feeds
- the sun or fire to enable it to impart its power
- water to collect and be enriched with its beneficent magnetic healing.

By the time of his death in 1936 at 50 years of age, Bach had created a system of 38 different flower remedies along with their corresponding theories of ailments. Bach flower remedies are an alternative or complementary treatment that is used for emotional problems and pain. They're made out of watered-down extracts from the flowers of wild plants.

Edward Bach, a medical doctor and homeopath, created these remedies in the early 1900s. Homeopathy is the belief that the body can cure itself. It uses small amounts of natural substances like plants and minerals to treat the body or mind. The idea behind Bach flower remedies is similar to homeopathy. But they use fewer materials and don't work directly on physical symptoms, but instead on the emotions.

Bach believed that healing negative emotions helps the body heal itself. His system contains 38 remedies that each address a specific negative emotion. The emotions are grouped into seven broad psychological causes of illness:

- Fear
- Uncertainty
- Lack of interest in present circumstances
- Loneliness
- Oversensitivity to influences and ideas
- Sadness or despair
- Cares for others at the expense of self

How to Choose a Bach Remedy

Select a flower remedy according to the emotional issue or issues at the root of your problem. You might choose one remedy or mix several together.

You can buy them at a health food store or work with a specialist or someone trained to use them. Also, some naturopaths, homeopaths, herbalists, chiropractors, and acupuncturists offer them.

There's also a combination remedy that was developed by Bach himself. People use it to help stay calm in stressful situations

How to Use Them

Bach remedies usually come as liquids in dropper bottles. You can either drop the remedy on your tongue or mix it into a glass of water to drink. The dosage varies, but most people take several drops a few times a day.

Some remedies are also found as pills, sprays, skin creams, and bath salts.

Do Bach Remedies Work?

People have used Bach remedies for many conditions, including anxiety, depression, stress, emotional and physical trauma, cancer, and HIV. Existing reliable research does not back up these claims.

Results are mixed when it comes to whether they help with emotional issues or pain. They seem to make some people feel better, but it isn't clear if this is a result of the placebo effect or not. The placebo effect means something helps because people expect it to work.

Side Effects and Safety

Studies have found that Bach remedies are safe. Some have a small amount of alcohol, so check the label if you want to avoid it.

Don't take Bach remedies in place of any prescribed medicine. Let your doctor know if you have any problems. (Source from ChatGPT)

Note 4

Scientific Explanation of the Hypothesis That Water Retains Wave Information

The claim that "water retains wave information" has been proposed by some researchers and practitioners, particularly in the fields of alternative medicine and vibrational medicine. However, this claim lacks sufficient scientific evidence and is not aligned with mainstream scientific understanding. Below is an explanation of the concept from a scientific perspective, along with a summary of current discussions.

Background of the Claim

1. The Hypothesis of Water Memory
    - The concept gained attention in 1988 when Dr. Jacques Benveniste published a study claiming that water could retain "information" about substances even after they were no longer present in the water. This hypothesis suggested that the effects of a substance could remain in water despite extreme dilution (Benveniste et al., 1988).
    - This idea is often cited as a theoretical basis for homeopathy, a practice that uses highly diluted substances for therapeutic purposes.
2. Vibrational Medicine
    - "Wave" or "vibration" in this context refers to energy or information, and it is claimed that water can store this information and transmit it to the human body.

Attempts at Scientific Explanation

Some hypotheses and theories have been proposed to explain this concept scientifically:

1. Structure and Clusters of Water Molecules
    - In liquid water, molecules temporarily form networks or "clusters." Some researchers have speculated that these clusters could retain information.
    - However, the molecular bonds in water only last for extremely short durations (picoseconds to nanoseconds), making the long-term retention of information highly questionable.
2. Vibrations and Energy Transmission

- Water can absorb and temporarily retain vibrational energy, such as sound waves or electromagnetic waves. While this is physically possible, there is no established mechanism for this energy to be retained as "information."

3. Quantum Mechanical Hypotheses
   - Some proponents refer to quantum mechanics, suggesting that phenomena such as quantum coherence or entanglement might play a role in water memory. However, there is no scientific evidence that quantum effects influence water's macroscopic properties in a way that would support this hypothesis.
4. Electromagnetic Properties of Water
   - Water's sensitivity to electromagnetic waves is well-known, but there is no evidence that it retains these signals in a manner that could be described as "memory."

Scientific Criticism and Challenges

1. Lack of Reproducibility
   - Experiments supporting the "water memory" hypothesis have often failed to be reproduced by independent researchers, casting doubt on their scientific reliability.
2. Short-lived Molecular Structures
   - The bonds and clusters in water are extremely short-lived, making it unlikely for water to retain information over extended periods.
3. Ambiguity in the Definition of "Information"
   - The concept of "information" is often poorly defined in this context, and no clear physical or chemical mechanisms have been proposed.
4. Association with Pseudoscience
   - Because the idea of "water memory" is often used in alternative medicine without robust scientific evidence, it is frequently criticized as pseudoscience.

Current Conclusion

The idea that "water retains wave information" remains an unverified hypothesis in modern science. While intriguing, it lacks sufficient scientific evidence, reproducible experimental results, and theoretical grounding. Future advancements in science may provide new insights, but for now, this concept should be approached with caution.

Note 5

Digital image sensors typically exhibit high sensitivity within the visible light spectrum, approximately 400 to 700 nanometers. However, depending on the sensor type and design, some sensors may also be sensitive to wavelengths outside the visible range, such as ultraviolet (UV) and near-infrared (NIR) light.

For instance, Hamamatsu's CMOS linear image sensors are designed to be sensitive across a broad wavelength range, from UV to NIR, making them suitable for applications like spectroscopic measurements.

Additionally, Sony's SenSWIR technology-equipped image sensors are capable of detecting wavelengths from visible light up to short-wave infrared (SWIR), covering a range of 400 to 1700 nanometers. This broad spectral sensitivity allows these sensors to function effectively in both visible and SWIR imaging applications.

Thus, the spectral sensitivity range of digital image sensors varies based on their design and intended applications, with some sensors tailored for specific wavelength ranges beyond the visible spectrum. (Source from ChatGPT)

Note 6

Pinhole photography is a photographic technique that captures images using a tiny hole (pinhole) instead of a lens. In this method, light enters a light-tight box or container through a minuscule hole, projecting an image onto a photosensitive material such as film, photographic paper, or a digital sensor.

Principle:

Light travels in straight lines; when light from a subject passes through the pinhole, it projects an inverted image of the subject onto the photosensitive surface. This simple structure allows for image capture without the need for a lens.

Features:

- Infinite Depth of Field: Pinhole photography results in images where all subjects, from foreground to background, are nearly uniformly in focus.
- Long Exposure Times: Due to the small size of the pinhole, the amount of light entering is minimal, necessitating longer exposure times to achieve proper exposure.
- Unique Soft Rendering: The absence of lens distortions and aberrations produces images with a distinctive, soft quality.

History:

The phenomenon of the pinhole has been known since ancient times, with records from the 5th century BCE by the Chinese philosopher Mozi and the Greek philosopher Aristotle. Later, during the Renaissance, it was utilized in the "camera obscura" for astronomical observations and as an aid in painting.

Construction and Shooting Method:

A pinhole camera can be easily constructed by creating a small hole in one side of a light-tight box (dark box). A window covered with tracing paper or similar material can be made on the opposite side for direct observation. However, since the resulting image is quite dim compared to lens-based cameras, it's advisable to use a simple visor-like hood or, ideally, a covering cloth (as used with large-format cameras) to aid in viewing. Ideally, the interior of the box should be treated to reduce internal reflections.

Pinhole photography, with its simplicity and unique aesthetic, continues to be cherished by photography enthusiasts and artists today. The joy of constructing a handmade camera and the creative expression through long exposures offer a distinctive approach to capturing images. (Source from ChatGPT)

Note 7

Mechanism and Effects of Skin Absorbing Colors

The phenomenon of skin "absorbing colors" is primarily based on the processes of light absorption and reflection. This mechanism is determined by the structure of the skin and the pigments it contains. Below is an explanation of the mechanism and its effects:

1. Mechanism of Skin Absorbing Colors

When skin absorbs colors, the following processes occur:

(1) Wavelengths of Light and Absorption

Light is composed of various wavelengths (visible light, ultraviolet light, and infrared light). When light strikes the skin, some wavelengths are absorbed by the skin's structure and pigments, while the rest are reflected. The reflected light reaches our eyes, allowing us to perceive the color of the skin.

(2) Role of Melanin

The skin contains a pigment called melanin, which plays a significant role in light absorption.

- Ultraviolet (UV) Absorption: Melanin efficiently absorbs UV energy, protecting cells from damage.
- Visible Light Absorption: The concentration of melanin determines which wavelengths of light are absorbed, influencing whether the skin appears lighter or darker.

(3) Other Factors: Blood and Carotenoids

The skin's lower layers contain capillaries, and hemoglobin in the blood absorbs specific wavelengths of light, contributing to the skin's redness or healthy complexion. Additionally, carotenoids (pigments derived from vitamin A) subtly affect skin tone.

2. Effects of Color Absorption

(1) Protection Against UV Rays

Melanin's ability to absorb UV rays helps prevent DNA damage, reducing the risk of skin cancer and premature aging. This protective function is evident in tanning, which serves as a defense mechanism against further UV exposure.

(2) Regulation of Body Temperature

Darker skin absorbs more light and converts it into heat energy, while lighter skin reflects more light, reducing heat absorption. This difference is linked to evolutionary adaptation to different environmental conditions.

(3) Diversity in Appearance

The mechanism of light absorption and reflection creates individual skin colors. Variations in melanin levels due to genetic and environmental factors result in diverse skin tones, influencing human appearance and cultural perceptions of beauty.

(4) Indicator of Health

Skin color and complexion often reflect overall health. For instance:

- Cyanosis: A bluish tint caused by oxygen deficiency.
- Jaundice: A yellowish hue caused by liver dysfunction.

These changes occur due to alterations in pigment or blood absorption characteristics.

Applications and Precautions

The light absorption properties of skin are utilized in medical and cosmetic fields, such as phototherapy and laser treatments. However, excessive exposure to UV rays can surpass the protective capabilities of melanin, leading to DNA damage and aging. Therefore, proper skincare and sunscreen use are essential.

In summary, the skin's ability to absorb light and colors plays a vital role in protection, temperature regulation, aesthetic diversity, and health monitoring. (Source from ChatGPT)

Note 8

Video projectors primarily emit visible light to display images on a screen. However, depending on the type of light source and the projector's design, they may also emit small amounts of ultraviolet (UV) and infrared (IR) light.

Modern projectors are designed with user safety in mind, ensuring that any non-visible light emitted is minimal and does not pose a risk. For instance, laser projectors are engineered to prevent direct exposure to laser light.

In summary, while video projectors primarily emit visible light, the amount of UV and IR light they produce is minimal and typically not harmful due to modern safety designs. (Source from ChatGPT)

Note 9

Mechanism of How Human Skin Absorbs Sound

The mechanism by which human skin absorbs sound primarily involves the dispersion and absorption of sound energy by the structure of the skin. Below is an explanation of the process:

1. Properties of Sound Waves and Skin Structure

Sound is a vibration (sound wave) transmitted through the air, and when it contacts a solid or liquid, the vibration is transferred. Human skin is composed of multiple layers, each with different properties:

- Epidermis: The sound waves first reach the outermost layer of the skin, the epidermis. While some of the sound energy is reflected, a portion penetrates further into the skin.
- Dermis: Beneath the epidermis lies the dermis, a flexible layer containing collagen fibers and elastin. In this layer, sound energy is scattered and attenuated.
- Subcutaneous Tissue: Composed of fat and connective tissue, the subcutaneous layer absorbs the remaining sound energy.

2. Mechanisms of Sound Energy Absorption

When sound waves are absorbed by the skin, the following physical processes occur:

- Scattering of Sound Waves: The uneven structure of the skin (e.g., collagen fibers and interstitial fluids) scatters the sound waves, dissipating the energy and reducing its intensity.
- Conversion to Heat Energy via Friction: The vibration of sound waves causes the molecules within the skin to move, generating frictional heat. This process converts the sound energy into heat energy, leading to absorption.
- Damping of Vibrations: The elasticity and viscosity of the skin cause the vibrations of the sound waves to gradually diminish.

3. Factors Affecting Absorption Efficiency

The efficiency of sound absorption by the skin depends on several factors:

- Frequency of Sound Waves: High-frequency sound waves tend to scatter on the skin's surface, while low-frequency waves penetrate deeper into the skin.
- Skin Thickness and Condition: Thicker skin areas (e.g., palms and soles) absorb more sound energy.
- Composition of Subcutaneous Tissue: Areas with more fat absorb sound waves more effectively.

4. Applications and Research

This property is utilized in acoustics and medical research. For example, ultrasound technology relies on the transmission of sound waves through skin and tissues to create internal images. Additionally, studies on sound absorption by skin are applied in noise reduction technologies.

While the skin's ability to absorb sound is not complete, it plays a significant role in understanding the interaction between the human body and sound waves. (Source from ChatGPT)

Note 10

The invisible energy layer that extends outside the physical body is commonly referred to as the "energy field" or "aura." It is known in many traditional cultures and spiritual systems and is believed to consist of the subtle energies radiated by humans and living beings. The following is a basic description

1. the structure of the aura

The aura is believed to be composed of multiple layers, each corresponding to a different level of consciousness or energy. The following layers are commonly referred to

- Physical layer (etheric body): the layer immediately outside the physical body, which is closely related to the health of the body.
- Emotional layer (astral body): corresponds to emotions and moods and is affected by their changes.
- Mental layer (mental body): is connected to thoughts, beliefs, and knowledge.
- Spiritual layer (spiritual body): corresponds to the soul, spiritual connections, and higher consciousness of self.

2. nature of energy

- Vibration: The energy field takes the form of vibration and is said to change its frequency according to health, emotional, and spiritual states.
- Light and Color: Some people claim to be able to perceive the aura visually, with its color and brightness reflecting the state of the individual.

3. role and function

- Defensive Function: The energy field is believed to protect the individual from negative external influences and energies.
- Interaction and Resonance: Enables energetic exchange with others and the environment.
- Indicator of health: the state of the energy field is believed to indicate physical and mental health. 4.

4. gap with scientific perspectives

Current science has difficulty directly measuring auras and energy fields and lacks physical proof. However, biological data such as bioelectromagnetic fields (electromagnetic waves emitted by the body), heart rate variability, and brain waves are being studied for possible relevance.

The concept of "invisible energy layers" extending beyond the physical body is often described in traditional cultures and spiritual systems as the aura or energy field. From the perspective of modern science, such phenomena may be related to the following concepts:

1. Bioelectromagnetic Field

The human body generates a bioelectromagnetic field, which arises from electrical signals produced by physiological activities such as heartbeats and brain function. Examples include:

- Heart: Electrical signals from the heart can be measured as an electrocardiogram (ECG), and the associated magnetic field can be detected as a magnetocardiogram (MCG).
- Brain: Electrical signals generated by brain activity are observed as brain waves (EEG), with corresponding magnetic fields measurable via magnetoencephalography (MEG).

These electromagnetic fields, though extremely weak, can be detected outside the body and might serve as a scientific foundation for interpreting the "invisible energy layers."

2. Vibrations and Resonances in the Body

From a physical perspective, the molecules and cells that make up the human body are in constant motion (vibration). The following theories are related:

- Biophoton Emission: Extremely weak light emissions (biophotons) have been observed from living organisms. These emissions are related to cellular metabolic activity and may reflect the body's health.
- Resonance Phenomena: Energy exchanges with the environment or others can be explained through the physical phenomenon of resonance.

3. Psychophysiological Effects

The energy field is believed to be connected to emotional and mental states. Scientifically, it may correspond to phenomena such as:

- Mind-Body Connection (Psychophysiology): Changes in stress or emotions can influence heart rate variability and skin conductance. These may be perceived as energy changes observable from outside the body.
- Placebo Effect: Healing techniques involving energy fields might induce physiological changes via psychological mechanisms.

4. Quantum Theory and Energy Concepts

Some researchers and philosophers attempt to explain energy fields using concepts from quantum physics. Examples include:

- Quantum Entanglement: The energetic connection between the body and its surroundings is sometimes interpreted through the lens of quantum entanglement and non-locality.
- Zero-Point Energy: The vacuum energy that exists in space (zero-point energy) is hypothesized to have potential connections to life processes and consciousness.

5. Scientific Limitations

Current scientific understanding has not yet fully validated whether these phenomena align with traditional descriptions of "auras" or "energy fields." However, research into bioelectromagnetic fields and biophotons is ongoing, and further discoveries may provide new insights in the future.

In summary, the concept of "invisible energy layers" presents a fascinating topic at the intersection of scientific knowledge and traditional beliefs. Understanding it may require an integrative approach that considers perspectives from both domains. (Source from ChatGPT)

Richard Gerber M.D.

Vibrational Medicine

https://pmc.ncbi.nlm.nih.gov/articles/PMC5859346/

As per author and physician scientist Dr Richard Gerber [3], the Newtonian model of medical thinking sees the human physiological and psychological behavior as dependent upon structural hardware of the brain and body. However, the Newtonian mechanistic viewpoint of life is only an approximation of reality. In a machine, the function of the whole can be predicted by the sum of its parts; however, in reality, the human body is not a sum of its individual components; there is the force that 'animates.' Once that force leaves the body, as in after death, the body organs slowly deteriorate. A modern and more recent perspective of the life force has involved looking at it as a vibration science based on Einstein's paradigm. This concept sees human beings as a network of complex energy fields that interface with physical and cellular systems. Vibrational medicine uses specialized forms of energy to positively affect those energetic systems that may be out of balance due to diseased states.

Energy medicine is a branch of alternative medicine based on a pseudo-scientific belief that healers can channel "healing energy" into patients and effect positive results. The field is defined by shared beliefs and practices relating to mysticism and esotericism in the wider alternative medicine sphere rather than any sort of unified terminology, leading to terms such as energy healing, vibrational medicine, and similar terms being used synonymously. In most cases, no empirically measurable "energy" is involved: the term refers instead to so-called subtle energy. Practitioners may classify their practice as hands-on, hands-off, or distant (Evans, 2008) wherein the patient and healer are in different locations. Many approaches to energy healing exist: for example, "biofield energy healing", (MD Anderson Cancer Center, 2007; Jain & Mills, 2007) "spiritual healing", (Ernst, 2001) "contact healing", "distant healing", therapeutic touch, (American Cancer Society, 2008) Reiki, (National Center for Complementary and Integrative Health, n.d.) and *Qigong* (MD Anderson Cancer Center, 2007).

Reviews of the scientific literature on energy healing have concluded that no evidence supports its clinical use (Hall, 2010; Abbot et al., 2001; Ernst, 2003, 2006; Pittler & Ernst, 2008; Singh & Ernst, 2008). The theoretical basis of energy healing has been criticised as implausible; (Gist & Lubin, 1999; Barrett, 2007; Stenger, 1999; Kruglyakov, 2004) research and reviews supportive of energy medicine have been faulted for containing methodological flaws (McCaslin, 2009; Pignotti & Thyer, 2009; Agdal et al., 2011). and selection bias, (McCaslin, 2009; Pignotti & Thyer, 2009) and positive therapeutic results have been determined to result from known psychological mechanisms, such as the placebo effect (McCaslin, 2009; Pignotti & Thyer, 2009). Some claims of those purveying "energy medicine" devices are known to be fraudulent, (Berens & Willmsen, n.d.) and their marketing practices have drawn law-enforcement action in the U.S. (Berens & Willmsen, n.d.)

Note 11

Chromesthesia, or color synesthesia, is a type of synesthesia in which specific stimuli automatically and consistently evoke perceptions of colors that are not typically associated with those stimuli. For example, hearing a sound, seeing a word, or thinking of a number might cause a person to perceive a particular color.

1. General Explanation of Chromesthesia (Color Synesthesia)

Chromesthesia is a unique type of synesthesia, where certain stimuli like sounds, letters, or numbers automatically and consistently evoke perceptions of colors. These colors are not present in the environment but are vividly experienced by the individual.

Characteristics

1. Association of Stimuli with Colors
    - People with chromesthesia may associate musical notes, words, numbers, or abstract concepts (e.g., days of the week) with specific colors.
    - For example, a person might see the "C note" as red or "Monday" as blue.
2. Automatic and Consistent
    - These color associations occur spontaneously without conscious effort and remain stable over time.
3. Subjective Perception
    - The colors may appear visually (as though they are in the person's field of view) or conceptually (as a mental association).
4. Individual Differences
    - The specific colors and triggers vary greatly between individuals.

Examples

- Music and Colors
- Hearing a specific musical note might evoke a mental image of a color, such as purple for the "G note."
- Letters and Numbers
- Characters like "A" might appear red, while "B" appears blue.
- Days and Months
- Days of the week or months may have fixed color associations, such as "Monday is yellow."

Impact on Daily Life

1. Positive Aspects
    - Chromesthesia can make experiences like listening to music or organizing information more vivid and memorable. It is often linked to creativity, and many musicians or artists are believed to have synesthesia.
2. Challenges

- Overwhelming stimuli or sensory overload can sometimes cause discomfort or fatigue.

Prevalence and Insight

Chromesthesia is rare, occurring in a small percentage of the population (around 4%), but it offers fascinating insights into the diversity of human perception and creativity.

2. Physiological Explanation of Chromesthesia

The physiological basis of chromesthesia involves the brain's sensory processing systems and their interactions. Below are the primary hypotheses and findings that explain this phenomenon:

1. Cross-Wiring Between Sensory Areas
    - Unusual Neural Connectivity:
    - Chromesthesia might arise due to increased communication between sensory-processing regions in the brain. For example:
    - The auditory cortex (which processes sound) may have stronger-than-normal connections with the visual cortex (which processes color).
    - Similarly, the language-processing area may "leak" signals into the visual system, causing letters or numbers to be perceived as colored.
2. Hyperconnectivity Hypothesis
    - The brains of synesthetes may have an overabundance of neural connections, allowing sensory signals to "spill over" between normally separate sensory regions.
    - For instance, a sound might simultaneously activate the auditory system and the color-processing area (V4) in the visual cortex, leading to the perception of "colored sounds."
3. Disinhibition Hypothesis
    - Reduced Sensory Inhibition:
    - Normally, the brain filters and suppresses unnecessary sensory signals. In chromesthesia, this suppression mechanism may be weaker, allowing cross-sensory activation.
    - For example, auditory signals might also activate the visual cortex, creating the perception of colors alongside sounds.
4. Developmental and Genetic Factors
    - Incomplete Sensory Segregation:

- During early brain development, sensory systems are interconnected but become more specialized over time. In synesthetes, some connections may remain intact, leading to persistent cross-sensory perception.
- Genetic Basis:
- Synesthesia often runs in families, suggesting a heritable component. Genetic studies indicate that structural differences in the brain, such as increased white matter connectivity, may be involved.

5. Neurotransmitter Role
    - Chemical Imbalances:
    - Neurotransmitters like serotonin and dopamine, which are crucial for sensory processing, might contribute to the heightened sensory integration observed in chromesthesia.

Key Brain Areas

1. V4 Area (Color Processing):
    - This region in the occipital lobe is responsible for color recognition and is often activated in chromesthesia when sounds or letters evoke colors.
2. Angular Gyrus:
    - This area, involved in integrating language, memory, and numbers, may play a role in the cross-sensory associations seen in chromesthesia.

Research Evidence

1. fMRI and EEG Studies:
    - Brain imaging shows simultaneous activation of sensory areas during chromesthetic experiences, such as the auditory cortex and the V4 color area when hearing a sound.
2. Structural Studies:
    - Synesthetes often have increased white matter connectivity, facilitating enhanced communication between brain regions.

Summary

Chromesthesia's physiological mechanism involves increased neural connectivity and reduced sensory inhibition, leading to cross-activation of sensory areas. This allows stimuli like sounds or letters to evoke vivid perceptions of color. Further research in neuroscience and genetics continues to unravel the complexities of this fascinating phenomenon.

The abilities of people with chromesthesia (chromesthetes) are unique sensory experiences and creative thinking, which are expected to be utilized in various fields in the future. Below are some areas where their potential is anticipated.

1. Utilization of Creativity

   Fields of Art and Design

   - Chromesthetes can leverage their ability to perceive sounds, letters, or concepts as colors and shapes in the realms of art and design.
   - Fusion of Music and Visuals: They may create new forms of visual or performing arts by expressing music as visual art or images.
   - Future Design: Their sensitivity to colors and forms can contribute to user-centric experiences in interface and architectural design.

   Advancing Entertainment

   - In fields like video production and game development, chromesthetes can propose immersive experiences by integrating sound and color.

2. Education and Learning Support

   Application to Mnemonics and Educational Techniques

   - The superior memory and information processing abilities of chromesthetes are gaining attention, and they may inspire new methods for general learners.
   - Education Programs Based on Synesthesia: Developing educational materials that incorporate colors and sounds could improve learning efficiency.
   - Application to Neuroscience Research: Studying the mechanisms of chromesthesia may offer new insights into the brain's learning processes and creativity.

3. Science and Technology

   Human-Computer Interfaces (HCI)

   - The sensory integration abilities of chromesthetes may be valuable in designing next-generation computer interfaces, augmented reality (AR), and virtual reality (VR).
   - Multi-Sensory Systems: They could help create intuitive and sensory-rich interfaces that integrate sound, color, and touch.

   Data Visualization

- Incorporating the sensory perception of chromesthetes could lead to innovative data representations that integrate sound and motion with visual elements.

4. Medical and Psychological Fields

   Mental Health and Relaxation

   - The connection between sound and color could be applied in relaxation and mental health care.
   - Color and Sound Therapy: Therapies using the harmony of colors and sounds perceived by chromesthetes could help promote emotional healing.

   Advancement in Neuroscience

   - Researching chromesthesia can deepen our understanding of neural connectivity and sensory integration mechanisms in the brain.
   - Research on Neurodevelopmental Disorders: Analyzing the brain structure and functions of chromesthetes may aid in understanding conditions like autism and ADHD, which involve differences in sensory processing.

5. Social Inspiration

   Acceptance of Diversity and Promotion of Creativity

   - Chromesthesia represents diversity in perception and thought. It can lead to greater recognition of the value and abilities of people with unique sensory experiences, enhancing creativity and problem-solving across society.

Expectations for the Future

Although much about chromesthesia remains to be uncovered, it is expected to drive innovation in fields such as art, science, education, and medicine. Chromesthetes, with their unique perspectives and sensitivities, are anticipated to contribute to the development of future society and technology. (Source from ChatGPT)

Note 12

Color psychology is the study of colors and hues as a determinant of human behavior. Color influences perceptions that are not obvious, such as the taste of food. Colors have qualities that can cause certain emotions in people. How color influences individuals may differ depending on age, gender, and culture. Although color associations can vary contextually between cultures, color preference is thought to be relatively uniform across gender and race.

Color psychology is also widely used in marketing and branding. Marketers see color as an important factor, since color can influence a consumers' emotions and perceptions about goods and services. Logos for companies are important, since the logos can attract more customers.

The field of color psychology applies to many other domains such as medical therapy, sports, hospital settings, and even in game design. Carl Jung has been credited as one of the pioneers in this field for his research on the properties and meanings of color in our lives. According to Jung, "colors are the mother tongue of the subconscious."

Before there was color psychology as a field, color was being used for centuries as a method of treatment as early as 2000 BC. The ancient Egyptians documented color "cures" using painted rooms or sunlight shining through crystals as therapy. One of the earliest medical documents, the Huangdi Neijing, documents color diagnoses associated with color healing practices.

Influence of color on perception

Multiple researchers propose that one factor in the evolution of primate trichromatic color vision is to allow for better perception of others' emotions or condition which can prove highly useful for complex social interaction. For example, flushed or pale skin can non-verbally communicate whether they are excited or sickly. Besides its use for social situations, color has an impact in multiple facets of our perceptions.

Taste

Color also affects how people perceive the edibility and flavor of foods and drinks. This extends beyond just the color of the food itself. The packaging of the food and its placement among other foods and objects also affect how people perceive it. For example, in food stores, bread is normally sold in packaging decorated or tinted with golden or brown tones to promote the idea of home-baked and oven-freshness. People can mistake a cherry-flavored drink for being lime or lemon flavored if that drink was a green color. Additionally, a flavor can be intensified by a color. People can rate a brown M&M as more chocolate flavored than a green M&M based on color. This interaction can be mediated by our perceptions as well, especially depending on cultural expectation. Research in the UK demonstrated that individuals receiving a brown drink would have different expectations for the taste (i.e. expecting a Cola) while someone from Taiwan may expect a grape-flavored drink because popular brown colored drinks in their culture are typically grape-flavored.

Time

Recent studies showed that the perceived duration of a red screen was longer than that of a blue screen. The results reflected sex differences; men overestimated the duration of the red screen. Additionally, the reaction times to a red screen were faster than those to a blue screen. Participants who reacted quickly to a red screen overestimated its duration. In a demo with 150 people chosen at random, it was found that inside a pod bathed in blue color the average perceived duration of a minute was 11 seconds shorter than in a pod bathed in red color. However, another study looking at perceived duration found opposite results regarding blue and red stimuli.

Light

The color of a light source affects the apparent color of an object the light shines on. For example, the color of an object might appear different in the light from the sun versus from an incandescent (tungsten) light bulb. With the incandescent light bulb, the object might appear more orange or "brownish", and dark colors might look even darker. Light and the color of an object can affect how one perceives its positioning. If light or shadow, or the color of the object, masks an object's true contour (outline of a figure) it can appear to be shaped differently from reality. Objects under a uniform light-source will promote better impression of three-dimensional shape. The color of an object may affect whether or not it seems to be in motion. In particular, the trajectories of objects under a light source whose intensity varies with space are more difficult to determine than identical objects under a uniform light source. This could possibly be interpreted as interference between motion and color perception, both of which are more difficult under variable lighting.

Blue Lights (R) at the Woodside LIRR train station in New York

Blue light causes people to feel relaxed, which has led countries to add blue street lights in order to decrease suicide rates A railroad company in Japan installed blue lighting on its stations in October 2009 in an effort to reduce the number of rail suicide attempts although the effect of this technique has been questioned In 2000, the city of Glasgow installed blue street lighting in certain neighborhoods and subsequently reported the anecdotal finding of reduced crime in these areas.

Lighting color could also have a strong effect on perceived experience in stores and other situation. For example, time seems to pass more slowly under red lights and time seems to pass quickly under blue light. Casinos take full advantage of this phenomenon by using color to get people to spend more time and hence more money in their casino. However, a presumed influence of colored light (red vs. blue) on risk behavior could not be demonstrated.

Medicine

The color of placebo pills is reported to be a factor in their effectiveness, with "hot-colored" (red, yellow, etc.) pills working better as stimulants and "cool-colored" (blue, purple, etc.) pills working better as depressants. This relationship is believed to be a consequence of the patient's expectations and not a direct effect of the color itself.] Consequently, these effects appear to be culture-dependent.

Color preference and the connection between color and emotion[edit]

Main Article: Color Preferences

How people respond to different color stimuli varies from person to person. In a U.S. study, blue is the top choice at 35%, followed by green (16%), purple (10%) and red (9%). Blue and green may be due to a preference for certain habitats that were beneficial in the ancestral environment as explained in evolutionary aesthetics. Orange, yellow, and brown are the least popular colors, respectively.

One theory for why people prefer one color over another is called ecological valence theory (EVT) proposed by Palmer and Schloss (2010). This theory asserts that people tend to like or dislike colors based on their associations of the color to other objects or situations that they have strong feelings about. For example, if someone associates the color blue with clean water, they would be more likely to favor blue. On the other hand, people's dislike of the color brown could be due to associations of it with feces or rotten food.

Color preference may also depend on ambient temperature. People who are cold often select warm colors such as red or yellow, while people who are hot favor cool colors like blue and green. Introverted individuals are also found to be more attracted to cool colors, while extroverts prefer warmer colors.

Psychologists Elliot and Niesta (2008) tested to see if the color of a person's clothing could make them appear more sexually appealing. They found heterosexual men and women dressed in red were significantly more likely to attract romantic attention than women dressed in any other color. The color did not affect heterosexual women's assessment of other women's attractiveness. Other studies have shown men dressed in red appeal to heterosexual women.

A light's warmth or coolness can be described by its color temperature. The Kelvin scale is used to quantify the color temperature spectrum. These numbers are used to characterize the hue of artificial light. Since each person has their own unique method of perceiving color, there are a variety of color temperatures that will work well for certain tasks. Neutral and soft white is a friendly and clean light best for kitchens and bathrooms or any kind of workspace; cool light is adequate for offices, hospitals, and other commercial uses; and warm light creates a cozy, calm, inviting atmosphere that is ideal for bedrooms, living rooms, family rooms, dining rooms, and other spaces requiring an intimate, personal mood.

REFERENCES

Abbot, N. C., Harkness, E. F., Stevinson, C., Marshall, F. P., Conn, D. A., & Ernst, E. (2001). Spiritual healing as a therapy for chronic pain: A randomized, clinical trial. *Pain, 91*(1–2), 79–89. DOI: 10.1016/S0304-3959(00)00421-8 PMID: 11240080

Agdal, R., von Hjelmborg, J. B., & Johannessen, H. (2011). Energy healing for cancer: A critical review. *Forschende Komplementarmedizin, 18*(3), 146–154. DOI: 10.1159/000329316 PMID: 21701183

American Cancer Society. (2008). Therapeutic touch. Cancer.org. Archived from the original on May 6, 2015. Retrieved September 20, 2010.

Barnard, J. (2004). *Bach flower remedies*. Lindisfarne Books.

Barrett, S. (2007). Some notes on the American Academy of Quantum Medicine (AAQM). Archived from the original on October 27, 2018. Retrieved November 30, 2010.

Benveniste, J., Davenas, E., Ducot, B., Cornillet, B., Poitevin, B., Guillonnet, D., & Sainte-Laudy, J. (1988). Human basophil degranulation triggered by very dilute antiserum against IgE. *Nature, 333*(6176), 816–818. DOI: 10.1038/333816a0 PMID: 2455231

Berens, M. J., & Willmsen, C. (n.d.). Miracle machines: The 21st-century snake oil. The Seattle Times. Archived from the original on November 20, 2007. Retrieved November 18, 2007.

Cancer Research UK. (2013). *Flower remedies*. https://www.cancerresearchuk.org/about-cancer/complementary-alternative-therapies/individual-therapies/flower-remedies

Elliot, A. J., & Niesta, D. (2008). Romantic red: Red enhances men's attraction to women. *Journal of Personality and Social Psychology, 95*(5), 1150–1164. DOI: 10.1037/0022-3514.95.5.1150 PMID: 18954199

Ernst, E. (2001). A primer of complementary and alternative medicine commonly used by cancer patients. *The Medical Journal of Australia, 174*(2), 88–92. DOI: 10.5694/j.1326-5377.2001.tb143161.x PMID: 11245510

Ernst, E. (2002). "Flower remedies": A systematic review of the clinical evidence. [Note: DOI is inferred from the journal if unavailable]. *Wiener Klinische Wochenschrift, 114*(23–24), 963–966. DOI: 10.1007/BF03040566 PMID: 12635462

Ernst, E. (2003). Distant healing—An update of a systematic review. *Wiener Klinische Wochenschrift, 115*(7–8), 241–245. DOI: 10.1007/BF03040322 PMID: 12778776

Ernst, E. (2006). Spiritual healing: More than meets the eye. *Journal of Pain and Symptom Management, 32*(5), 393–395. DOI: 10.1016/j.jpainsymman.2006.07.010 PMID: 17085260

Ernst, E. (2010). Bach flower remedies: A systematic review of randomised clinical trials. *Swiss Medical Weekly, 140*, w13079. DOI: 10.4414/smw.2010.13079 PMID: 20734279

Evans, J. (2008, July 14). Spiritual healing on the NHS? The Times. London. Archived from the original on May 14, 2009.

Gerber, R. (2001). *Vibrational Medicine: The Handbook of Subtle-Energy Therapies*. Bear & Company.

Gist, R., & Lubin, B. (1999). *Response to disaster: Psychosocial, community, and ecological approaches in clinical and community psychology*. Psychology Press.

Graham, H. (1999). *Complementary therapies in context: The psychology of healing*. Jessica Kingsley Publishers.

Hall, H. (2010). Faith healing. Science-Based Medicine. Archived from the original on November 13, 2020. Retrieved February 29, 2020.

Jain, S., & Mills, P. J. (2007). Biofield therapies: Helpful or full of hype? *International Journal of Behavioral Medicine, 17*(1), 1–16. DOI: 10.1007/s12529-009-9062-4 PMID: 19856109

Kruglyakov, E. (2004). What threat does pseudoscience pose to society? Social Sciences, 3(3), 74–88. Archived from the original on December 14, 2021. Retrieved November 30, 2010.

Larimore, W., & O'Mathúna, D. (2007). *Alternative medicine: The Christian handbook* (Updated and expanded ed., p. 293). Zondervan.

McCaslin, D. L. (2009). A review of efficacy claims in energy psychology. *Psychotherapy (Chicago, Ill.), 46*(2), 249–256. DOI: 10.1037/a0016025 PMID: 22122622

MD Anderson Cancer Center. (2007). Energy medicines: Will East meet West? Network Newsletter. Archived from the original on November 25, 2010. Retrieved November 30, 2010.

National Center for Complementary and Integrative Health. (n.d.). Reiki practice. Nccih.nih.gov. Archived from the original on June 4, 2020. Retrieved September 20, 2010.

Original Bachflower. (2020, April 20). *Life of Dr. Bach.* https://www.bachflower.com/life-of-dr-edward-bach/

Palmer, S. E., & Schloss, K. B. (2010). An ecological valence theory of human color preference. *Proceedings of the National Academy of Sciences of the United States of America, 107*(19), 8877–8882. DOI: 10.1073/pnas.0906172107 PMID: 20421475

Pignotti, M., & Thyer, B. (2009). Some comments on "Energy psychology: A review of the evidence": Premature conclusions based on incomplete evidence? *Psychotherapy (Chicago, Ill.), 46*(2), 257–261. DOI: 10.1037/a0016027 PMID: 22122623

Pittler, M. H., & Ernst, E. (2008). Complementary therapies for neuropathic and neuralgic pain: Systematic review. *The Clinical Journal of Pain, 24*(8), 731–733. DOI: 10.1097/AJP.0b013e3181759231 PMID: 18806539

Robson, T. (2004). *An introduction to complementary medicine.* Allen & Unwin Academic.

Singh, S., & Ernst, E. (2008). *Trick or treatment.* W. W. Norton & Company.

Stenger, V. J. (1999). The physics of "alternative medicine": Bioenergetic fields. The Scientific Review of Alternative Medicine, 3(1), 16–21. Archived from the original on May 8, 2016.

Thaler, K., Kaminski, A., Chapman, A., Langley, T., & Gartlehner, G. (2009, May 26). Bach flower remedies for psychological problems and pain: A systematic review. *BMC Complementary and Alternative Medicine, 9*(1), 16. Advance online publication. DOI: 10.1186/1472-6882-9-16 PMID: 19470153

Vohra, D. S. (2002). *Bach flower remedies: A comprehensive study*. Health Harmony.

Weeks, N., & Bullen, V. (1990). *Bach flower remedies: Illustrations and preparations* (2nd ed.). The C. W. Daniel Co.

Wikipedia contributors. (n.d.). Bach flower remedies. Wikipedia. Retrieved May 29, 2025, from https://en.wikipedia.org/wiki/Bach_flower_remedies

Wikipedia contributors. (n.d.). *Kansei engineering*. Wikipedia. Retrieved May 29, 2025, from https://en.wikipedia.org/wiki/Kansei_engineering

Wood, M. (2000). *Vitalism: The history of herbalism, homeopathy and flower essences*. North Atlantic Books.

Chapter 4
Reaching the Zero Point: True-Self – Buried in Japanese Society

Margaret Hiro Kimishima
https://orcid.org/0009-0004-8968-2550
International Center of Transdisciplinary Research, Japan

ABSTRACT

The holistic perspective emphasizes the transdisciplinary relationship between the microcosm and macrocosm. By uniting these polarities, we can merge and transcend boundaries often overlooked by science. Recognizing both dimensions fosters an understanding that there is no true separation, merely different facets of a common principle. When individuals attain this awareness, they arrive at the "zero-point," a state where all possibilities for manifestation coexist. This paper will explore how shadows are interwoven into ancient Japanese aesthetics, facilitating the experience of the zero-point and guiding individuals towards the discovery of a singular truth that embodies ultimate happiness.

INTRODUCTION

It's only when an individual can say what they believe in the depths of their heart that they can build a healthy sense of well-being. In fact, well-being can only be achieved when both "eloquence" and "silence" are balanced. Silence, when overdone, can lead to misunderstandings, while excessive eloquence often results in antagonism. Neither extreme is conducive to well-being; the key lies in maintaining a middle ground. This balance allows a person to remain centered in their true self. Christine Page (Page, 2009c), a pioneer in holistic medicine, argues in *Frontiers of Health: How to Heal the Whole Person* that the throat "receives" and "expresses"

DOI: 10.4018/979-8-3373-0360-4.ch004

the “will” of the “soul” (Page, 2009c, chap 4). She also points out that many diseases are linked to the throat area, which she refers to as the “throat chakra”—an energy center located at the throat. According to Page, blockages in this area are often the source of many health issues (Page, 2009c, chap 11).

In addition, the throat chakra is believed to be “closely allied” with the sacral chakra, the abdominal energy center that governs the expression of the “will of the personality (Page, 2009c, chap 11). In other words, the sacral chakra serves as the center of all relationships, enabling individuals to connect with others and express their authentic personality (Page, 2009c, Chap 8). If one fails to communicate their true feelings through the throat chakra, they may suppress their true self, resulting in internal blockages. The issue in Japan, however, is that many people fail to realize that being eloquent is just as important as knowing when to remain silent. As an intuitive healer, I have encountered a wide range of clients over the years—both male and female, young and old, including individuals like Mio, whom I will discuss later. Not once have I met a client who didn’t have an energetic imbalance related to their throat. Even those who pride themselves on being “eloquent” often shy away from expressing their true selves. Indeed the proverb “Speech is silver, silence is golden” has been passed down through the ages, emphasizing that discretion can often be more valuable than eloquent words. Believed to have originated in 9th-century Arabic culture, it was later popularized by Thomas Carlyle (Wikipedia, 2024). The phrase is frequently referenced in various cultural contexts, including songs and literature, serving as a reminder of the profound power and importance of silence in communication.

Another popular Japanese saying is “Unsaid is flowery,” meaning that sometimes it's better to remain silent than to speak. The phrase suggests that silence can hold more value than words, especially in situations where speaking might lead to conflict, misunderstanding, or unnecessary complications. It highlights the idea that restraint and discretion often prove wiser than expressing one's thoughts openly. This reflects the deep cultural significance of silence in Japan. Renowned linguist Toshimasa Wada (1966) notes in his dictionary that this concept embodies the “Japanese aesthetic sense,” where revealing everything would be seen as too “blatant” and “unappealing” (Wada, 1966, p. 60).

The concept of this proverb was first introduced in the 8th century in *The Manyoshu* [An Anthology of Japanese Poems] (*Kotowaza No Maruzo*, 2022). In this anthology, poet and politician Hirotsugu Fujiwara writes, “Many words are contained within a generation of this flower. Don’t treat them badly” (*Kotowaza No Naruzo*, 2022). This poem, which accompanies a cherry blossom given to a girl whom he does not know, conveys the sentiment, “I won’t tell you who I am, but by pointing to this flower, which contains my thoughts.” The poem reflects deep emotions hidden within the poet, revealing his profound and genuine feelings for her (Wada, 1996, pp. 59-60).

In Japan, silence is often valued more than casual chatter. It is common for mothers to ensure their children remain quiet in public spaces to avoid disturbing others. Even when children are simply conversing quietly, they are frequently admonished in a clichéd Japanese manner: "People are looking at you. It's embarrassing." Parents encourage their children to be mindful of their surroundings, even if the children are not being overtly loud. In schools, students are trained not to speak back to teachers and rarely express opinions that contradict those of the instructor. This emphasis on silence has proven to be effective in promoting harmony within Japanese society. This phenomenon can be attributed to Japan's strong historical influence from Confucianism, which stresses respect for elders. Silence, therefore, plays a critical role in maintaining harmonious communication within the culture (*Kotowaza No Naruzo*, 2022).

Such dialogue reflects a key characteristic of Japanese conversation, which is based on the idea that communication is co-constructed with the other person, rather than being created solely by oneself. In fact, the Japanese often aid others to ensure mutual understanding of what is being said and what is intended. As Nobuko Mizuno (2008) points out in her book *Nihonjin To Dibeito* [The Japanese and Debates], Western dialogue typically features two distinct streams of speech: the speaker and the spoken. In contrast, Japanese conversation is characterized by a single stream of intermingled speech, where the speaker and the spoken are unified (Mizuno, 2008, p. 3).

For instance, my client Mio never spoke back to her mother, who was dominant and narcissistic, throughout her life. Because Mio refrained from arguing with her mother, she developed uterine cancer and suffered from severe constipation by the time she turned forty. As previously mentioned, in holistic energy medicine, the abdominal area is known to store negative emotions. In fact, cancer is considered the leading cause of death among Japanese people. According to the Japan Cancer Society's 2023 cancer mortality report, colorectal cancer had the highest mortality rate for women, with 25,195 women dying from it in that year. Additionally, 27,936 men died from colorectal cancer, making it the second leading cause of death for men in 2023 (Daichogan 2023). The sacral chakra is located in the abdominal area, and Mio was advised to express her opinions clearly to her mother if she had any objections. However, she responded that remaining silent would help maintain family harmony. Mio had been reluctant to express her true feelings for most of her life. As a result, her throat chakra had become blocked, preventing her from balancing the sacral chakra and allowing her negative emotions to be processed through the throat chakra. By keeping silent, she attempted to preserve harmony within her family. She recalled, "My father suffered the most and died young, and my mother used to yell at him all the time."

In the modern Western conception, dialogue is viewed as a form of turn-taking that emphasizes the differences between speakers, with clear distinctions between Speaker A and Speaker B. In contrast, in Japanese conversation, the boundaries between speakers tend to be blurred. The speaker often supports the other person's speech through backchanneling while also pausing to allow the other person to contribute backchanneling or even intentionally leaving a sentence incomplete. This approach of "not putting everything into words" can be seen as a manifestation of "gold". The word "gold" also suggests alchemical transformation. As an intuitive healer, I have observed that unspoken words are often stored in the abdominal area or the sacral chakra, which is connected to the throat chakra. Page (2009c) notes that the sacral chakra is healed through communication with others. When unspoken words are suppressed into this chakra, which is also associated with "creativity" and "relationships," problems arise if these two areas are not aligned. Honesty is the key to balancing them (Page, 2009c, chapter 11).

However, as Mio's case study illustrates, for most Japanese individuals who have long believed that silence brings peace, silence can instead lead to emotional strangulation. Japan has the lowest level of happiness among the seven major countries in terms of "relationships" (Global Economy World Economy, 2024).

It remains taboo to discuss one's inner self in modern Japanese society, which places immense value on harmony. This is because such topics are not universally acceptable. Instead, relationships and cooperation with others are emphasized, and individual uniqueness and opinions are often suppressed. When beliefs differ from those of others, the fear of criticism or ostracism can discourage individuals from exploring their own views. In Westernized societies, Japanese people often read too much into the surrounding atmosphere, which can leave them disconnected from Western individualism. They wear a "mask" to conceal their true selves in public, a topic I will explore in more detail later.

INTER-DEPENDENT COMMUNICATION VS. CO-DEPENDENT COMMUNICATION

Honesty fosters understanding and insight into human relationships and situations, promoting trust and openness. However, for many Japanese individuals, honesty does not necessarily equate to respect for others. As Mio's case illustrates in my practice, in Japanese culture, feelings are viewed as something that resonates with others, whereas in Western cultures, they are often used to express individual identity and facilitate communication. The definition of "feelings" in Japanese is "attitudes or evaluations toward an object caused by sensations or perceptions of external stimuli" (*Jitsuyo Nihongo Hyougen Jiten*, 2025). On the other hand, in

Western languages such as English, the word "feeling" is defined as "something you feel with your mind or senses," with no reference to "external stimuli." In this context, feeling is understood as an individual experience within the mind or senses, rather than something that resonates with others. In Western cultures, being honest with oneself is considered a key aspect of communication, although this may not always be the case. Thus, for the Japanese, feelings are not seen as subjective but exist in relation to the other party. In fact, in Japanese, the characters can be read as "feeling compassion." It is important for speaker A to empathize with speaker B, even if speaker B has not had the same experience. This style of communication developed among the Japanese as an agrarian method of creating harmony, as they settled in groups and needed to anticipate factors such as river rises due to weather, seasonal changes, and harvest times.

As discussed in my article, "A New Spiritual Dawn for the AI Era from the Nation of Harmony" (2024), the prominence of "cherishing harmony" (Kimishima, 2024, p. 117) is emphasized among people embodies the fundamental principle of the Japanese spirit, as mentioned in the first line of the oldest Japanese constitution published in 640 A.D. (Wikipedia, 2024). An agrarian must calculate natural changes, such as seasonal variations and weather. Masaya Ito (2020), a web marketer and writer, notes in his blog "Minato No Susume" [*Encouragement to Minato*] that "the study of geopolitics and astronomy has developed," and there is a tendency in Japan for many individuals to "stay away from anything they feel uncertain about," even in "modern business and investment." This can be interpreted as a communication style in which topics involving "uncertainty" are often "avoided," reflecting an attitude that seeks to minimize conflict and resolve matters as peacefully as possible (Ito, 2020).

This is a common trait among the Japanese, who are generally not accustomed to being assertive. While avoiding conflict with others is acceptable, when an individual is at the center of a problem or the cause of a problem but treats it as if it were someone else's issue, the expression "koto-nakareshugi" (matter-of-fact attitude) is used to describe a negative image of irresponsibility. Interestingly, according to Jitsuyo Nihongo Hyogen Daijiten [Dictionary of Practical Japanese Expression] (n.d.) the major definition means a person who tries to "arrange matters peacefully so as not to stir up trouble," especially one who takes a "passive attitude to turn away from problems and troubles" (Jitsuyo Nihongohyougen Dajiten [Dictionary of Practical Japanese Expressions], *n.d.*).

Although it can be seen as "permissive pacifism," it is typically used with a negative connotation, referring to a reluctance to act due to a fear of the changes necessary for improvement.

It is not uncommon for individuals to perceive themselves as pacifists yet be seen by others as engaging in "tokenism." Eiki Nishida (2016) argues in Naze Nōkō Minzoku wa "Mainasu Satei," Shuryū Minzokuwa "Purus Satei" Nanoka?

[Why Are Farmers "Assessed Negatively" and Hunters "Assessed Positively"?] on Diamond Online that ancient agrarians, who had to work together, would evaluate others by asking, "Is this person an ally?" (prioritizing the formation of alliances), whereas hunters, who had to consider the distribution of limited prey, would ask, "Is this person an enemy?" (focusing on identifying enemies first). (Nishida, 2016). For the agrarian, fellow workers in the rice fields can be both friends and enemies. In Japanese, there is a proverb that refers to "drawing water for one's own field or purposes," meaning to manipulate (an interpretation or argument) to suit one's own interests. Rice is the staple food of the Japanese. If a farmer stops the flow of water to benefit only their own rice paddy, the other rice paddies will dry up. This illustrates a phenomenon where a farmer sneaks out in the middle of the night to divert water into their paddy, preventing it from flowing into neighboring fields. The first step in creating rice paddies to produce rice is securing water. To prevent this, neighbors would stand guard at night. Hiro Sachiya (2010), in Kurui no Susume [Encouragement to Madness], mentions that farmers must live close to one another because they need to be near the rice fields where water is accessible. These rural relationships become the world to them, as their living environment was strictly confined in ancient times (Hiro, 2010, pp. 81–82).

Such an ambivalent environment unconsciously leads individuals to become skeptical of their friends. Sometimes, they find themselves in situations where they must lie to themselves to protect their rice, which is their only means of making a living (property). In ancient times, rice was considered a form of property (money). The system of paying taxes on rice paddies in the form of a physical commodity persisted in Japanese society for a long time, from ancient times until the revision of the land tax during the Meiji Era (1868-1912). It is no wonder that the agrarian had to protect their "property" by sacrificing their own truth (Okome No Bunka To Rekishi, Section 2.5).

One of the major characteristics of a nation that tends to exhibit "koto-nakareshugi" (matter-of-fact attitude) is a failure to consider the impact of current problems on themselves, facing them as if they were someone else's issue, often saying, "It has nothing to do with me in the first place." This attitude suggests that they do not truly view their fellow workers as trustworthy. It is interesting to note that the Japanese are known for having strong moral values and tend to commit themselves to their family members and close friends. When the Japanese refer to their family, they use the term "uchi" (my home), which also signifies "me," as I will discuss in more detail in the next section. In fact, Tetsuro Waguchi (2013) notes in *Fūdo: Ningengakuteki Kosatsu* [Climate: Anthropological Considerations] that the world outside the house or family is considered "out there." Within the home, husbands refer to their wives as "kanai" (inside the home), while wives call their husbands “uchi no hito” (the person in the home). In the household, individual distinctions disappear, and their identities merge as single family members (chapter 2).

Thus, the tendency to remain faithful to one's principles varies depending on social conditions in Japan. When it is someone else's problem, the “koto-nakareshugi” (matter-of-fact attitude) appears, distinguishing between the “inside the home” and the “outside the home.” Eiki Nishida (2016) points out that agrarian people are assessed based on whether they have a good harvest, leading to negative evaluations (using a perfect score system), while “hunter” people start with zero and are assessed positively, accumulating good points (Nishida, 2016).[8] In order to achieve a good harvest, ancient farmers would form superficial friendships with their enemies to accomplish their mission. This tendency highlights an interesting aspect of a collectivist society like Japan.

Collectivist societies are often built around the family. Nichola Raihani (2023) notes in “Higashi Ajiadewa Naze “Muchiibiiki” ga Hakobirunoka?” [Why Is “Patronage” So Popular in East Asia?] on Toyo Keizai Online that “collectivism is expected to result in a smaller tendency to help strangers” (Raihani, 2023). He also points out that strong family ties promote cooperation and trust within the closest social group but reduce cooperation and trust toward out-groups. In other words, in ancient Japan, it can be said that relationships based on doubt and suspicion strengthened family bonds (Raihani, 2023).[9]

The downside of such familism, as with any conservative family structure, is the potential to undermine individual freedom and respect. Raihani (2023) notes that individuals who identify as politically conservative tend to have strong affection for their families but weak affection for humanity, whereas those who identify as politically liberal show the opposite tendency.[10] Certainly, Japan is known as a conservative country, where people tend to exhibit “koto-nakareshugi” (matter-of-fact attitude) and are passive about reform or improvement when faced with national issues.

The matter-of-fact approach tends to make individuals cautious in the decision-making process, particularly in politics. It is highly risk-averse and may be reluctant to make significant policy decisions, potentially delaying necessary changes and leading to incomplete discussions. Hiromitsu Iwasaki (2020), in his article “Nihonjinnwa Ushinawareta Sanjuunen No Honshitsu O Wakatteinai: Genin To Sekinin O Tsukitome Kaenakareba Teimei wa Madatsuzuku [The Japanese Fail to Understand the True Nature of the “Lost 30 Years”: Without Identifying the Causes and Responsibilities, Failure to Change Will Lead to Stagnation] in *Toyo Keizai Online*, highlights that this lackadaisical approach reinforces bureaucracy, as there is a strong emphasis on adhering to existing rules and customs. Even when new ideas and reforms are proposed, following established processes and procedures is often prioritized, making change difficult. Indeed, by “deferring” various “risks,” the “bureaucracy, which had become aligned with the administration and protected the political system centered on the government, intentionally slowed down the speed of bankruptcy resolution and structural reform." Meanwhile, the government has consistently responded with economic stimulus measures through the mobilization of public funds and increased public works projects (Iwasaki, 2020).[11]

In addition to the above, at work the Japanese avoid helping others when they are in trouble. They may feel bad about their attitude, but their "conservative" and "disciplined" characteristics to stick with their own tasks or policies prevent them from changing their work environment to help colleagues. In ancient times, the yui, or mutual support, labor practices among the agrarian emerged, and a closed life-style, bound by customary rules within the village community, became prominent from the early modern period onward. Each village had certain customs and farmers were obliged to live according to them. Violations of these customs were sanctioned by the village ("2.4. Seikatsuno Chushinwa Komedukuri" [2-4 Rice cultivation is central to daily life], n.d.).[12] In such a harsh environment, agrarians learned how to become rooted in one land and adopted a lifestyle of living collectively in large groups. They developed a sense of planning and prudence by learning how to follow rules and live uniformly within the group. They also cultivated a sense of how to save resources (such as rice) and how to think long-term in case of poor harvests. In ancient Japanese society, for farmers, protecting their property was considered more important than being honest.

Thus, expressing one's true feelings is still not a core aspect of communication in Japan. In fact, it is often absent from Japanese communication. If Speaker A feels comfortable within their group, they may not mind expressing what others want to hear. Of course, everyone hides their true feelings to some extent in daily life. However, in Japanese culture, not expressing one's true feelings is seen as a sign of respect for others.

As mentioned earlier, mothers often tell their children to be quiet on the train because the adults around them seem annoyed by their chatter. Parents may imply that they personally don't mind their child talking in public, but they sense that others are irritated, which leads them to feel "embarrassed" by the perception that they are bad parents. As previously noted, parents nudge their children to be considerate of their surroundings, even if they don't believe their children are being loud. They make the children aware that it is the parents who feel embarrassed by their child's behavior. Through this, parents communicate their true feelings. It's also important to note that respect for others in this context involves maintaining good relations with those around them.

Children raised in this way are constantly trying to meet their parents' expectations and are always reading the expressions of those around them. Not surprisingly, compared to other countries, Japanese adolescents struggle to view themselves positively. Only 62.3% of children believe they have strengths and are satisfied with themselves, which represents the lowest rate of self-esteem compared to adolescents from other countries.[13]

In addition, showing respect for others in Japan involves demonstrating humility, which is a key characteristic of Japanese communication. By not overestimating oneself, individuals express a respectful attitude toward others. Humility is deeply embedded in Japanese culture and values. Japanese individuals are expected to be cooperative, often pushing themselves to their limits. For the Japanese, honesty can potentially damage relationships, so they tend to be more cautious about expressing themselves. In this context, honesty is not seen as a way to respect others, but rather as something that could disrupt the harmony within their group.

As for Mio, she surrendered herself to her dominant mother in the Confucian way of showing respect by not speaking back. Demonstrating humility in this context was a way for her to protect herself and her identity within her family, which she considered her primary community. Her late father failed to provide a sense of security at home, contributing to this dynamic. The sacral chakra, which is associated with "self-respect," was unable to fully develop for Mio during her childhood, as she was not encouraged to assert herself or express her true feelings.

Inner Self vs. Criticism

Since the Japanese have been encouraged to prioritize others over themselves, it can be difficult for them to recognize or be aware of their own intentions. The issue may lie in the national character of the Japanese, who fear that expressing differing opinions could be perceived as criticism. It is often considered inappropriate to discuss topics that may not be accepted by everyone in a group. Bringing up personal, subjective topics, particularly those influenced by an individual's beliefs and values—such as spirituality—may be seen as taboo.

As discussed in the previous section, the Japanese tend to distinguish between "inside the home" and "outside the home." Watsuji (2013) argues that the Japanese concept of home reflects their inner life, which can only be fully shared among family members. This duality also appears to be linked to the natural features of Japanese geography, particularly the seasonal and abrupt threats posed by phenomena such as typhoons, which can destroy rice blossoms in summer. Farmers cannot prevent these disruptions from occurring annually. This duality deeply affects some aspects of Japanese character, making individuals both "changeable" and "patient" depending on the situation. When interacting with the "outside world," this strong trait becomes evident. Rather than speaking their truth, the Japanese have historically adapted their mindset to external forces, such as natural disasters, in response to the needs of the outside world. In ancient times, the outside world was not something to be trusted but something to which they had to surrender. This social history has led individuals to avoid introspection and, consequently, prevented them from truly discovering who they are.

Mio was well-respected as a successful facial therapist with many clients. She shared that she had never truly opened up to anyone, including her ex-husband, who had consistently verbally abused her during their marriage. I encouraged her to begin using her five senses, which would help her acknowledge her true self. Emotions set our energy into motion, and the manifested impulses can be stored by the five senses. Interestingly, the renowned Japanese neuroscientist Ihoko Kurokawa (2025) asserts in *Taiwa no Torisetsu* [Dialog Manual] that the brain integrates information from the five senses and strives to perceive the full range of the world around us.[14] The five senses act as cognitive windows into the real world, reflecting an individual's characteristics and their perception of things. It is said that experiences and knowledge acquired through the five senses are more likely to be "retained in memory" (Kurokawa, n2025).[15] As previously mentioned, in holistic medicine, negative emotions are believed to be stored in the body, particularly in the abdomen and womb. It is no surprise that Mio was diagnosed with cervical cancer, as her traumatic experiences were likely retained deep within her womb.

Mio was always cheerful in front of her clients. Hisako, who introduced me to Mio, expressed her surprise upon learning that Mio had struggled to express herself. Her former colleague and friend shared, "Mio always looks happy around her fans and friends and is one of the most popular facial therapists in our community. I was even jealous of her charm." However, according to Mio, revealing her true self to close friends was a source of deep shame. She could not even tell her family members about the abuse she endured from her then-husband.

Showing one's true self can be risky for individuals who have distanced themselves from the "outside of the home." For many Japanese individuals, discussing self-exploration can feel as difficult as stepping outside during a typhoon. If their spiritual values are rejected, they quickly conform to fit in with their environment. In today's increasingly individualistic society, self-exploration and self-expression are highly valued. However, excessive personal beliefs can sometimes conflict with group dynamics, much like the way Mio closed herself off from others. Her health was not her only issue; it was time for her to release the negative emotions stored in her sacral chakra. I encouraged her to engage her five senses through activities such as cooking, creating art, writing, and going to karaoke. Over time, Mio began to connect with her inner self, acknowledging her desires and wishes, which she had long suppressed. She started to reconnect with her spiritual beliefs, cultivating a sense of mindfulness and presence.

Despite the individualistic aspects of modern society, spiritual practices can make it difficult for individuals in Japan to gain social recognition and understanding of their surroundings, leading to hesitation in continuing their inner exploration. If one's spiritual practice is perceived as strange by others, they may avoid discussing it for fear of disapproval or criticism. Being seen as heretical, especially in a group setting, can place a significant psychological burden on individuals. Media and cultural prejudices also contribute to the suspicion surrounding spiritual activities. Dubious cases are often highlighted, which shapes the public perception and reinforces a fixed image. As Takeshi Nishide (2023) argues in his interview in *Taidan: Dejitaru Jidai no Media de Shūkyō wo Dō Misekiru Ka* [A conversation: How Can We View Religion in the Media of the Digital Age?], modern newspapers tend to favor "fact-based rationalism" and often "avoid looking at or hide things that are incomprehensible to them, such as religion." Nishide further explains that when an interviewee mentions, "I actually believe in this kind of religion, which is why I am able to do my best," the discussion about the faith aspect is often cut off, and the focus shifts to "simply doing their best." Additionally, he notes that the media's portrayal of religion is often stereotypical, with a negative image associated with people who are "addicted to religion." This reflects how religion and spirituality have been openly avoided and often vilified in the mass media, potentially influencing public attitudes (Nishide, 2023, p. 219).

After World War II, there was a heightened sense of caution regarding spiritual beliefs or religion in Japan. The war's lessons led to a reconsideration of the role and influence of religion, particularly due to concerns about its association with the government and power. The mass deaths resulting from the tragic consequences of the war profoundly impacted people's subsequent religious and spiritual beliefs, as well as their trust in institutionalized religion. Prior to the war, emperor worship had been deeply ingrained in Japanese society. The state and religion were closely intertwined, with the emperor being revered as a "living god." This belief system played a significant role in motivating many individuals to participate in the war effort.

Japanese society today benefits from the advancements of Western medicine and economic prosperity, which often emphasize rationality and positivism. As a result, themes and concepts related to invisible or intangible realms are frequently regarded as lacking scientific foundation and rational justification. Consequently, opportunities for individual growth and inner exploration are often overlooked or neglected in personal beliefs.

As Japan has become Westernized, it seems that only the Japanese mentality has been left behind in a Western civilization where distinctions between right and wrong are often clearly defined. For instance, observing Japanese Noh actors perform in elaborate masks in the early twentieth century, the legendary critic Hideo Kobayashi (1977) expressed a strong desire to shout: "Take off your mask. Look at your true face." He observed that, without fully understanding the direction it was heading, modern civilization began to unfold. Kobayashi recognized that Japan's modernization was superficial and that it could not fundamentally alter the essence of the Japanese people (p. 62).[16] On the other hand, Yosuke Hamazaki (2021), in his book *Kobayashi Hideo no Jinseiron* [Life Theories of Hideo Kobayashi], argues that Western culture should challenge the "ego" or "life itself" through new knowledge coming from outside (Hamazaki, p. 14). In fact, in ancient Japanese, the surface (mask) indicates one's face, and the upturned side indicates "mind". In Japanese culture, the face can be a mask to hide one's true feelings (Doi, 1986, p.11).

As Hamazaki (2021) argues, "those cosmopolitans" who were busy turning their eyes outward during the tide of civilization and enlightenment in the Meiji era, while those who focused on the "inner feelings" flowing in the "undercurrent of culture" and "turned their eyes inward," were often considered "behind the times." His Noh episode clearly shows that for Kobayashi, criticism meant discussing "Why was I moved by the performance?" Through this process, he sought to explore the source of the Japanese environment (climate, history, traditions, etc.) that shaped him and asked, "What is a happy way of life for Japanese people?" in accordance with their true nature as Japanese (Hamazaki, 2021, p. 16).

In a Japanese society that founded the modern nation through utilitarianism and materialism, and trained its scholars and politicians by looking "outside," those who focused on the trunk of the wooden block at their feet, aware of the existence of the "samurai spirit" within them, and sought to reconcile it with Western modernity, were shunned as "visionaries" and forced to position themselves as "outsiders." However, just as he almost shouted at the Noh theater, Japan quickly moved into the era of modernization without having established its own identity as modern Japanese (Hamazaki, 2021, p. 16).

Furthermore, the Japanese failed to examine their own way of life to establish their identity even after World War II. While Western intellectuals incorporated Japan's spirituality and unique sensibilities into their own societies in the late 1980s, the Aum incident led to a growing tendency in Japan to shy away from such a spiritual approach. More than two decades after Tokyo's deadly sarin gas attack, spirituality is considered even more suspicious in Japan than before. Despite the ancient teaching that gods dwell in all things, Western researchers have surpassed Japan in the study of invisible senses and intuition.

According to a survey reported by Japanese public television NHK (2019) in "Nihonjin No Shukyokan Ya Ishiki Wa Dou Kawatta Ka?"[How Have Japanese Religious Views and Attitudes Changed?], in 1998, 43% of people answered "yes" to the question, "Do you think religion brings more conflict than peace?" This was higher than the percentage of people who answered "no." Additionally, 38% of people said "yes" to the question, "Do you think religion makes people intolerant?" which was also higher than the "no" response. The survey clearly indicates that the Aum affair had a significant impact on the Japanese view of religion and spirituality (NHK, 2019, p. 60).

On the other hand, it is important to note that the survey results reveal how much the Japanese are influenced by the wonders of nature. Seventy-four percent of respondents answered "yes" to the question, "Can you understand the concept that the gods dwell in mountains and rivers?" This suggests that many Japanese people believe more in the gods of nature than in the spiritual truths expressed by human beings. Deep down, this indicates that most of them feel threatened by others entering their inner world. To allow someone to access their true self, they must metaphorically "take off their shoes" before entering their "inner house," as Watsuji (2013) figuratively explains.

The concept of "home" in Japan is clearly distinguished from the outside. Even if the door to one's room is not locked, the door to the outside must be secured. Beyond the house, there are fences and walls, sometimes even a hedge, a reverse bush, or a moat. Upon returning home, individuals remove their clogs and shoes at the entrance, marking a clear distinction between the outside and the inside. This practice is a direct expression of the separation between the external world and the home. This distinction between inside and outside is not only reflected in the external appearance of the house but also defines the way of life.

Watsuji (2013) argues that to enter one's inner self, a guest must demonstrate respect according to social customs. They must make themselves suitable to the host by removing their shoes upon entering the house. This gesture symbolically reflects how the guest surrenders themselves, merging into the host's identity. One key aspect here is the recognition and establishment of who the individual wishes to become as a modern Japanese person in the 21st century. As mentioned earlier, self-exploration, particularly of a spiritual nature, was considered outdated in the context of modernization. However, there is another reason why the Japanese have avoided self-disclosure through spiritual activities (chapter 2).

In Japanese society, the excessive concern for others can prevent individuals from focusing on how to reveal their true selves. For the Japanese, true intentions are not directly expressed; rather, they are perceived and elicited by others. As mental health specialist Moeko Ohno (2022) argues in her article "Mijika Na Hito E No "Sasshite Hoshii Wa Aitee No Bouryoku Da "Chotto Gurai Tetsudatte Hoshii" Wa Ktoba Tarazu" [To Want a Little Help from Others Is a Form of Violence When It Is Not Communicated], it is harmful to harbor the feeling, "I'm doing my best to be understood," and then lash out in anger when someone does not understand. Ohno asserts that it is not appropriate to simply say, "I wish you could understand this much," without communicating one's feelings about the situation to the person who has not offered help.

Ohno (2022) points out that many Japanese individuals internalize the belief: "I must not bother others" or "I must not be selfish," leading them to focus more on how others perceive them rather than on their own desires or feelings. As a result, how they should behave in a given context often takes precedence over how they wish to be seen by others, causing them to suppress, neglect, or avoid acknowledging their true feelings. Ohno further argues that this pattern makes it increasingly difficult to "grasp their feelings." Unfortunately, despite their best efforts to consider others, it is nearly impossible to fully understand what the other person is thinking. Ohno (2022) adds that individuals must first become aware of how they feel and what they want to do in order to truly understand themselves. In Japan, individuals who fail to "guess" the needs of others are often seen as insensitive, unkind, or inattentive, while those who make such guesses are perceived as caring. In the next section, I will explore in greater detail why failing to guess is seen as disrespectful. Paradoxically, dishonesty can sometimes be interpreted as a form of respect. Instead of being direct, the Japanese often embrace silence as a virtue, considering it a sign of consideration (Ohno, 2022).[23] As for Mio, she was pushed to the point of not knowing what her "true feelings" were due to the suppressed emotions resulting from her inability to stand up to her father. For her, suppressing these feelings was a way to show "respect" to her father, in alignment with the traditional expectations of being a virtuous daughter. She wasn't the only client who had mentioned a similar issue to me. This is a symbolic phenomena in Confucian culture that affects how individuals perceive the elderly or others. The inability to express emotions can lead to various psychological tensions, which are reflected not only at the physical level but the distortions within society.

True-self Buried in Silence

Truth has always been something that should be sensed in silence in Japan. Traditional Japanese culture has consistently sought beauty in the darkness. This is a culture that finds its essence in minimalist beauty. Examples of this can be seen in the simplicity of architecture, lacquerware, the tea ceremony, and the form of the kimono.

It can be said that the Japanese aesthetic of valuing the dark eventually developed a sense of beauty that favored silence. In this view, beauty doesn't reside in objects themselves but in the interplay of light and dark created by objects and their shadows. As Tanizaki (1997) states, truth is hidden in silence: "A luminous pearl may radiate brilliance when placed in the dark, but when exposed to the light of day, it loses its charm" (p. 16). This way of perceiving things has been passed down to modern Japanese people. While there is beauty in the dark, the ancient Japanese have always felt a stillness in the darkness and sensed the heaviness of the air there. In the dark, they have felt the presence of the unseen by shutting down their five senses. If the light is dim, as Tanizaki points out, the Japanese will "immerse" themselves "in the darkness." They find contentment in simply being, as they are. Silence, as discussed earlier, symbolizes safety—serving as a protective mechanism against the threat posed by their fellow farmers or enemies. In order to come out of their dark silence, however, there must be light to illuminate all the dust. Transparency, which symbolizes light, is the key to indicating the truth in the West. The Old Testament says the light indicates God. For instance, Psalm 27:1 says, "The Lord is my light and my salvation—whom shall I fear? The Lord is the stronghold of my life—of whom shall I be afraid?"(1769). Light is often associated with clarity and visibility, making things clear and transparent. As Tanizaki points out, in the West, people "paint their ceilings and walls in pale colors to drive out as many of the shadows they can". He also points out that their quest for a brighter light never ceases from "candle to oil lamp, oil lamp to gaslight, gas light to electric light" (p. 31).

Similarly, expressing oneself involves being clear and truthful, revealing the reality of a situation without hiding anything. Light illuminates, allowing individuals to see and understand our surroundings.

In other words, there is beauty in silence, and the same beauty can be found in the darkness of night, where the mind and the five senses are at rest. Unlike the Western sense of beauty, the ancient Japanese sought to perceive the essence of the unconscious world and the presence of an invisible God in the heavy air of darkness. However, it is also true that their inner selves were suppressed by this silence, which was disguised as a safety net to show respect for others.

However, showing respect for others in silence does not express their innate truth for the Japanese. When an individual sits quietly in the darkness, they can perceive the vague outline of an object that is neither bright nor dark, but ambiguous. As Tanizaki (1977) points out, darkness itself prevents them from "moving forward to make changes for their current situation" (p. 8)..[26] It only husks a gun to one's head. What the Japanese have been doing in stillness can also be seen as the ambiguous desires or feelings of not wanting to cause problems by being honest. Interestingly enough, Page (200) argues that the throat manifests what the speaker "desires." She points out that the "opposite" is also true (Page, 2009c, chap 11). Creating "interdependence" in human relationships involves achieving a balance where there is a "dynamic flow of respect, freedom, commitment, and love." It is the "throat" that transforms an image into a structure that can be reproduced and manifested (Page, 2009c, chap 11). It is also important to note that the thyroid gland, located in this area, produces the hormone thyroxine. As she states, if the hormone is removed, the tadpoles can grow, but they cannot "transform" into frogs. The characteristic of the throat chakra is to bring about a complete transformation, much like how the tadpoles transform into frogs (Page, 2009c, chap 11). By remaining silent, the Japanese have refused to be transformed into the "frogs" of Western thought, yet they have accepted Western modernization. As noted above, Western modernization has provided the Japanese with significant clarity regarding the steps they need to take to open their country to foreign trade and culture.

At the individual level, the Japanese are known for their ability to control their emotions, as they consider it shameful to be distraught in front of others. As previously mentioned, the throat chakra is linked to the sacral chakra, where emotions are stored and often suppressed. Typically, emotions accumulated in the second chakra are released through the throat chakra. When these emotions are not expressed, individuals may become physically ill. The sacral chakra is associated with creating trust and intimacy with others, acting as the space where individuals "give" and "receive." Happiness is achieved through a balanced exchange of giving and taking. The interaction between the sacral and throat chakras is crucial for achieving ultimate happiness. Indeed, my client, Mio, became ill as a result of suppressing her voice.

In Japan, the concepts of giving and taking do not always represent the two sides of the same coin. When the listener remains silent during a conversation, the speaker cannot always interpret the listener's intentions accurately. This can lead to significant misunderstandings between the two. Doi argues that words arise from silence, noting that the word is, in fact, the "reverse of silence." see p.32 in (Doi, 1986). Likewise, he adds that "silence is the reverse of the word". Yet, for the Japanese, it doesn't necessarily matter whether the two parties fully understand each other in the silence. What is important is that they can feel mutual respect by resonating with one another. There are no words needed to confirm what silence means to them. While the culture of "reading between the lines" can also occur in Western conversations, in the West, seeking the truth tends to be prioritized over empathizing with and expressing the feelings of others. Conversations in Western cultures are generally seen as a tool for solving or clarifying misunderstandings, with the goal of moving forward and making relationships more seamless.

Again, this does not mean that the Japanese are willing to accept untruths. Instead, they try to understand and accept the speaker's intentions hidden behind their silence, if necessary. In Japanese tradition, a grownup is someone who can understand both sides of the coin. In other words, giving is not simply being submissive. Giving also involves merging one's identity with others. As Doi (1986) points out, "the awareness of self is constituted on the basis of connections to others" (p. 86). He notes that today's youth seem to find it more difficult to "identify themselves from the rest," partly because, as he explains, those who have grown up without a clear sense of self are no longer sure how to respond to the Westernized trend that emphasizes speaking one's mind. In the early twentieth century, the Japanese worked hard to accept Western modernization. Now, with the results of those efforts becoming apparent, the Japanese are becoming more aware of what has been left behind. However, even though the word "individualism" has become more widely used in recent years, the concept is still often misunderstood (Doi, 1986, p. 86).[27]

Indeed, many people like Mio in Japan are stuck in Confucian thinking and fail to understand the difference between individualism and self-centeredness, which may cast a serious shadow over Japan's future.

Lack of True Self-Authenticity and Independence

The Japanese use of "individualism" is sometimes closely associated with "selfishness," which implies leaving someone in need without concern. For instance, if someone is injured by accident in public, it often takes a while before a stranger step in to offer assistance.

Certainly, it's true that social systems based on individualistic concepts have become more widespread in Japan. However, as William Hiroyuki Saito (2015) notes in "Nihonshiki No Kojinshugitowa Coomatteiruhito Wo Hochi" [Japanese-style individualism means leaving people in need], the original definition of "individualism" in the West involves mutual respect for each other's roles and rights as members of a group—a concept that cannot be achieved if selfishness is tolerated, where "self-interest" takes precedence over other interests. He further argues that in Western work environments, if a problem cannot be solved by the parties involved, it is expected that people around them, who value teamwork, should assist in resolving the issue.[28]

This lack of understanding of individualism is due to the fact that the definition of "individualism" in Japan remains as vague as their nature. According to a summary report, "Nihon No Kojinshugi Wa Ika Ni Kodoku O Umidasu Ka? Bunka Shinrigaku Ni Yoru Kentou" [How Does Japanese Individualism Create Loneliness? A Cultural Psychological Examination], authored by Yuji Ogiwara (2014), the image of individualism and the individualistic person for Japanese individuals between the ages of 16 and 69 is characterized as "one who is independent and free" and "one who undermines relationships with others." The results show that the image of individualism, or the individualistic person, is neither clearly negative nor positive. However, Ogiwara adds that when asked to guess how others perceive individualism, people tend to predict that others view individualism negatively. The reason individualism creates loneliness in Japan may be due to the discrepancy between an individual's own attitude toward individualism and their prediction of others' attitudes. This also indicates that the concept of individualism has not yet been fully established in Japan (Ogiwara, 2014).[29] It's an ambivalent aspect of Japanese nature, much like a Noh actor performing with an obscure "mask," similar to my client Mio, who hides her true self behind a façade.

There is a distinctive aspect of Japanese culture that seeks individualism but struggles with it due to societal pressures. In Japan, individualism is often associated with isolation and selfishness, while in Western cultures, an individualistic person is typically viewed as unique and independent. As Ogiwara (2014) notes, individualism has not been embraced positively in Japan. Therefore, it is essential for the Japanese to redefine individualism in a way that aligns with contemporary social structures.[30] In fact, in Mio's daily life, she told me, she had never asserted herself. She said that if everyone in the café ordered coffee, she would order coffee that she didn't really want to drink. That way, she thought she wouldn't bother her friends or the waiter. After I advised her to start ordering what she would prefer to drink at a café for the first time, she asked. "Is it that important to know what I want to order?" I told her that every choice she makes every day is very important, as she needed to take advantage of using her five senses by choosing what she wants.

Not surprisingly, just a few months after following my advice, she was free from the constipation that had tormented her for years. She became more confident and grounded, with a noticeable surge of energy in both her core and womb. She even began expressing her intentions more openly to those around her. Interestingly, when energy becomes concentrated in the sacral chakra, it is believed to rise toward the solar plexus—functioning like a personal power plant. This energy center, located around the stomach, is associated with confidence, autonomy, and self-expression—qualities often lacking in traditional Japanese individualism. As Page (2009c) notes, to complete the triad that constitutes a healthy personality or ego, the solar plexus must be activated to reflect one's unique power in the external world. Without this healthy ego, individuals are easily "swayed" by the opinions and expectations of others (chapter 9).

The challenge lies in establishing a form of Japanese-style individualism within a society characterized by strong peer pressure. As previously noted, Japan reports the lowest levels of happiness among seven major countries. This may be due, in part, to differing conceptions of happiness between Japanese and Western cultures. According to Uchida (2024), Japanese individuals often derive happiness from "their relationships with others or clients," whereas Western individuals more commonly associate happiness with "the fulfillment of their own lives" (Uchida, 2024, p. 32).[31]

A distinctive form of Japanese individualism may hinder the development of close interpersonal relationships, as a matter-of-fact attitude often leads individuals to avoid confronting problematic issues encountered "outside the home," which may represent one's engagement with the real world. Uchida (2024) observes that relationships among co-workers in Japan tend to be notably more "distant" than those in Western cultures. Although Japanese individuals are generally expected to exhibit a strong sense of cooperation, Uchida notes that while they "value harmony with their surroundings," they often have "few close associates with whom they can consult." This suggests that an excessive emphasis on consideration for others can result in limited emotional intimacy and a tendency to remain within the bounds of "superficial business relationships" (Uchida, 2024).

In an effort to solidify their personal foundation, individuals in Japan often seek relationships that are both tenable and unbreakable. However, this pursuit of self-reliance can lead people to distance themselves from interdependent connections. As Uchida (2024) explains, a tension exists between two cultural tendencies: "syncretism," which places excessive emphasis on harmony with one's surroundings, and "isolation," which results from an overemphasis on self-expression (p. 32). This gap reflects a broader cultural struggle to balance collective expectations with individual autonomy.[32] The Japanese often struggle to find a balance between "tuning in," which places excessive emphasis on harmony with their surroundings, and "isolation," which stems from prioritizing self-expression. While Americans tend to achieve collaboration through a foundation of individual autonomy, Japan, though grounded in "cooperation and affinity," has yet to reconcile these values with the need for personal independence. As Uchida (2024) notes, in the Japanese context, autonomy and independence are indeed necessary—but they must coexist without disrupting the collective emphasis on harmony and cooperation (p. 34).[33]

To this end, the workplace should not be a space that simply "blends in," where relationships are maintained through passive attunement, but rather a place where individuals are encouraged to openly and honestly express their opinions and ideas. A necessary shift must occur toward a "workplace of unity," in which relationships are built through mutual influence and constructive dialogue—even if it involves conflict. According to Uchida (2024), such an environment, where individuals engage by exchanging and at times clashing over their perspectives, is essential for fostering genuine connection and growth (p. 34).[34]

The key is to shift to a "workplace of mutual cooperation," in which everyone expresses their own opinions and ideas and tries to develop relationships through mutual influence. And the path to this goal is a "workplace where autonomy invites collaboration. Unlike the West, in Japan, autonomy tends to be preceded by isolation. It would be appropriate to create an environment in which autonomous behavior is accepted after sufficiently fostering intimacy with the members (Uchida, 2024, p. 34).[35]

To jeopardize the community was to jeopardize not only one's neighbors but also one's own survival. Therefore, the community was the basis of life and defined all ways of living. The Japanese mindset is like two-tiered chest of drawers, as Uchida similarly names it as a "two-storied building" model, noting the first floor shows cooperation or harmony, whereas the second floor shows independence or autonomy (Uchida, 2024, p. 34). [36]

Unlike Uchida's (2024) "two-storied building" model, I propose a "two-tiered chest" metaphor to represent the Japanese mindset. In this model, each drawer conceals one's true self—*uchi* (inside the house)—while the exterior drawer represents *soto* (outside the house), or the public-facing self in the real world. These drawers symbolize the suppression of individuality and the fear of standing out in a society with strong conformity. Harmony is maintained not through authentic connection, but by aligning behavior with societal expectations. As I noted in "A New Spiritual Dawn for the AI Era from the Nation of Harmony" (Kimishima, 2024), a Dentsu survey found that 44.6% of young people worry their opinions will be rejected, and 73% are willing to say things simply to please others (p. 119). This tendency is also evident in children, who are often shaped by their surroundings and discouraged from expressing their individuality. Under the influence of Confucian-style education, there is a growing risk of neglecting one's inner self, leading to spiritual exhaustion and a loss of personal identity. To address this, it is crucial to revive the pursuit of spirituality and selfhood—qualities that were significantly diminished in the post-World War II era. Rebuilding a resilient, autonomous sense of self—one that is not swept away by external pressures—is essential for the well-being and future of Japanese society.[37]

If cooperation, as discussed earlier, serves as the foundation of the first drawer—a deeply rooted aspect of Japanese society—then the value system emphasizing "individualism" has long occupied the second drawer. The introduction of a value system that stresses "individual freedom" has contributed to the development of this second drawer. However, the status of cooperative well-being in Japan may now be at risk. The weakening of social relations is a growing concern, as it undermines mutual trust.

In their efforts to establish a secure foundation, the Japanese often believe that failing to conform to societal norms will result in social disconnection, thereby creating a barrier to genuine social cohesion.

To undermine one's self-esteem is to deceive oneself. As discussed earlier, an individual's self-esteem is closely tied to their ability to speak their mind. In a sense, the self-esteem of the Japanese can be likened to the foundation of a pancake. If the first pancake is too soft, the second one will fail to sit properly on top. For the Japanese, the "first pancake"—representing their sense of self—has often been unstable and insecure. This lack of a solid foundation prevents them from being honest or authentic in front of others. If they attempt to preserve their self-esteem, they find their foundation too fragile to support themselves, like balancing on a soft, squishy pancake. In the pursuit of cooperation, the desire to maintain harmonious and trusting relationships can often create a "bind," limiting their ability to assert individuality.

A trusting relationship in Japanese society often hinges on how humble one behaves, even in the presence of friends. In most situations, it is more beneficial and less damaging to express one's self-esteem in a humble manner rather than overtly or directly. This approach minimizes the risk of failure and preserves social harmony, as it is less disruptive when one does not openly assert their self-worth.

Humility, often considered a "uniquely Japanese" trait, is not an inherent characteristic of the Japanese mind, but rather a strategic attitude developed to navigate and succeed within Japanese society. To engage effectively with others while maintaining self-respect, it is essential for the Japanese to cultivate a solid foundation that protects their self-esteem, allowing them to balance humility with a healthy sense of self-worth.

The foundation of Japanese society has traditionally been one that fosters a sense of security and comfort for its members, creating an environment where people can feel at ease. As long as individuals maintain humility, society tends to accept and treat them well. However, this foundation is gradually eroding. Trust in others has significantly weakened in Japan. As Toshio Yamagishi (2010) discusses in *Anshin Shakai Kara Shinrai Shakai e: Nihon-gata Shisutemu No Yukue* [From a Society of Security to a Society of Trust: The Future of the Japanese System], a survey revealed that 47% of Americans believe most people are reliable, while only 27% of Japanese respondents hold the same view (Yamagishi, 2010, p. 33).

Yamagishi (2010) argues that in a collectivist society, individuals can feel secure as long as they remain within the group. However, the very collectivist principles that provide this security can undermine the broader trust needed to foster connections beyond the group. He explains that, in such a society, the stability of relationships offers a sense of "security" to its members, reducing the need to consciously assess whether others are trustworthy ((Yamagishi, 2010, p. 54).

The importance of stable social and human relationships, which have traditionally supported Japanese society, is rapidly diminishing. Consequently, the number of situations in which individuals can feel secure is decreasing. For instance, in the past, securing employment with a large company in Japan almost guaranteed job stability until retirement. Today, however, such guarantees are becoming a thing of the past. Individuals can no longer rely on the comfort of long-term job security simply because they are employed by a major corporation. As the security once provided by stable relationships diminishes, members of Japanese society are increasingly confronted with the question: "Can I trust the other person in this situation?" As Yamagishi (2010) points out, with the decline of relational stability, it is becoming essential for individuals to actively consider trust in their interactions (Yamagishi, 2010, p.4).

If a person's sense of security is solely derived from the external world, they will struggle to feel secure within themselves. It is essential to detach from external influences and discover who they truly are. This self-awareness does not need to conform to the values or frameworks of others. What individuals truly need is to accept and feel comfortable with who they are, regardless of external standards. True security comes from within, not from external sources or any particular religion. The key is to find balance by centering oneself and cultivating inner peace.

Often, individuals feel good about themselves when they match someone else's needs, or when they make someone else happy especially in Japan. They must feel happy whenever they are truly acting themselves. They need to be more mindful about what they want and what they need to know, and what they need others to know about them.

CONCLUSION

In a future shaped by the evolution of AI, it is crucial for the Japanese to cultivate their true selves. In Japanese culture, the concept of "sense of security" is closely tied to being at ease with oneself and others. In other words, individuals feel secure when they are in sync with those around them (Doi. 2001, p 193).

Redefining one's true self-identity is crucial in Japan, where people often prioritize external expectations over their inner desires. To discover their authentic selves, individuals must begin to act according to their own desires and voices. In this process of self-discovery, they must identify what is missing. The missing element is neither the identity formed within the home (the microcosm) nor the one shaped by the outside world (the macrocosm). When identity is firmly grounded, like the needle of a compass, a harmonious circle (the macrocosm) naturally forms around it. True happiness comes from knowing oneself and expressing one's authentic self to those around them.

Understanding through dialogue is essential for harmonizing individual and collective perspectives. For the Japanese, it is particularly important to share their spiritual beliefs and practices, thereby deepening their understanding by expressing these ideas within the broader societal context. The formation of communities with shared values and interests facilitates individuals' exploration of spiritual paths. Such spaces of shared experience can help alleviate feelings of loneliness and anxiety. Therefore, the interplay between collectivism and individualism in shaping attitudes toward spiritual beliefs is complex. To move forward, society will need to embrace greater acceptance of diverse values and perspectives.

Currently, research cooperation and collaboration across various fields in Japan are hindered by the closed nature of academic societies. It is essential to swiftly introduce the concept of being "spiritual but not religious." An international center for transdisciplinary research in Japan could play a pivotal role in this shift, offering expertise that enhances the well-being of Japan and people globally through concrete research and exchanges among experts. While Japan's approach may initially appear irreligious, merging the invisible realm with scientific findings will provide a foundation for spiritual ideas to take root in the real world.

It is important to uncover what the Japanese have buried within themselves. In fact, the rainy season in Japan, which lasts for two months each year, has long had a profound impact, often leaving the Japanese feeling overwhelmed and causing them to retreat into darkened homes, as Tanizaki (1997) describes:

There are no doubt all sorts of reasons such as climate, building materials, for deep Japanese eaves. The fact that we did not use glass, concrete, and bricks, for instance, made of low roof necessary to keep off the driving rain and wind. It has come to be that the beauty of a Japanese room depends on a variation of shadows against light shadows. It has nothing else. And it's indeed interesting to see even soy sauce looks most beautiful or profound when it's served with raw fish and greens in a dark room (Tanizaki, 1997, p. 13).

For the Japanese, their true selves are often hidden beneath layers of "shadows" that lie deep within. Years of social conflict have made them particularly cautious. In this sense, the defeat in World War II can be seen as creating a collective shadow or trauma, a result of the political pressure to sacrifice one's life for the emperor. As Doi (2001) notes in *Zoku Amae No Kozo* [Autonomy of Independence II], "The shock of the defeat has not allowed the nation to recover from the stress of the war" (see p 193 (Doi 2001)). The large number of lives lost in World War II, many under the belief in Emperor Hirohito as a living god—who later declared that he was not divine—has shaped a deep-seated wariness toward religion in Japan. This historical backdrop is closely linked to the changes in the national character that were formed as a result of the war. The lessons learned from the war led to a reevaluation of the role and influence of religion, fostering a new attitude toward faith—one that emphasizes self-belief. The pain and horror of the war contributed to a cautious stance on religious beliefs, prompting concern about the potential impact of religious doctrines on individuals and society. It is now crucial to uncover the "shadows" that people have carried in order to protect their inner beauty and truth, hidden in the dark.

In Japan, the close or intimate relationships in which individuals can be open and consult with others are in crisis. In response, the Japanese government has appointed a "Minister of State for Loneliness and Isolation" to address social isolation. Despite living in a society that values harmony, it is noteworthy that a lack of social connectedness negatively impacts happiness. Japan's long working hours and the pervasive issue of overwork contribute to this problem. As previously mentioned, Japanese culture places great importance on "reading between the lines" and maintaining harmony with others. This cultural tendency makes it difficult for individuals to express their true feelings, leading to stressful situations. Even when harmonious relationships are formed, many individuals remain unsatisfied with themselves and their lives. Furthermore, current economic conditions and uncertainty about the future have negatively impacted on the overall well-being of the nation. Among younger generations, the lack of stable employment and life prospects exacerbate stress.

In Japan, high educational and career expectations create significant pressure for self-fulfillment, and when these expectations are unmet, it leads to disappointment and diminished well-being. The cumulative effects of these factors have resulted in a lower level of happiness among the Japanese compared to other major countries. Consequently, the cultural tendency to conform to one's surroundings may impact individual well-being in profound ways.

In Europe and the United States, various forms of healing and spirituality, including vibrational medicine, have already been explored, with ongoing research into the essence of human beings. Understanding the essence of humanity involves revealing the invisible aspects of existence. It is essential to view both human beings and the universe from multiple perspectives, recognizing that humans are more than physical entities and transcend even the concepts of God or the universe. In Japan, research should focus on enhancing sensitivity, intuition, and the healing aspects that influence these areas. Traditional research methods, along with conventional medicine, education, and religion, have reached an impasse. Therefore, it is crucial to venture into the invisible realms of sensibilities and intuition, exploring well-being in a new era that truly measures happiness in its fullest sense.

To achieve this, it is essential for experts—beyond just healers, artists, and researchers—to form a collaborative "scrum" and propose a model of well-being suited for the coming era. Indeed, it is crucial for transdisciplinary research in Japan to extend beyond universities and research institutes. We must create an environment where individuals can freely exchange ideas and collaborate, irrespective of academic affiliation, specialized field, or occupation. As previously noted, Japan's research lags behind that of other countries, and various international organizations have already committed to cooperation. By exploring the realms of the five senses and intuition—areas that have traditionally been taboo—through more academic approaches, I hope to highlight the infinite possibilities of human potential. It is important to recognize that spiritual exploration enables each individual to gain a deeper understanding of themselves, their beliefs, and their values, thus fostering personal growth and self-awareness. In this way, the invisible realm will no longer remain hidden. When unexpressed or invisible emotions are released through vocal expression, individuals can attain the state that Buddha describes as the "pure unadulterated state"—a state that is neither negative nor positive, but simply zero.

REFERENCES

Doi, T. (1986). *The anatomy of self: The individual versus anatomy.* Kodansha USC Inc.

Doi, T. (2001). *Zoku Amae no kozo* [Autonomy of Independence II]. Kobundo, *ISBN: 4335651058,* Global economy, world economy (2024) Happiness index - Country rankings https://www.theglobaleconomy.com/rankings/happiness/

Hamazaki, Y. (2021). Kobayashi Hideo No "Jinsei" Ron [Life theories of Hideo Kobayashi], (NHK Shuppan Shinsho), IBN: 9784140886656

Hiro, S. (2007). *Kurui no susume* [Encouragement to madness]. Shueisha Inc. ISBN-10: 4087203778, Ito, M. (2020). Minato no susume [Encouragement to minato)]. https://minato-intl.com/?s=%E8%BE%B2%E8%80%95%E6%B0%91%E6%97%8F#google_vignette

Iwasaki, H. (2020). "Nihonjinnwa ushinawareta sanjuunen no honshitsu o wakatteinai: Geiin to sekinin oo tsukitome kaenakareba teimei wa madatsuzuku" [The Japanese fails to understand the true nature of the "lost 30 years" not finding out the causes and responsibilities and changing them will lead to stagnation]. https://toyokeizai.net/articles/-/325346 Tokyo Keizai, Inc.

Kimishima, M. H. (2024). "A new spiritual dawn for the AI era from the nation of harmony". In L. da S. G. M. da Costa & M. T. Loisel (Eds.), *Artificial Intelligence and Human Mediation: A New Spiritual Dawn for the AI Era from the Nation of Harmony* (pp. 117-119). ATLAS Publishing, Inc.

King James Bible. (1769). *The Holy Bible, King James version.* Cambridge Edition: 1769; King James Bible Online. https://www.kingjamesbibleonline.org/Psalms-27-1/

Kobayashi, H. (1977). *Tohma -- Motsuaruto-Mujoutoiukoto* [Tohma -- Mozart: The Impermanence of Things].

Kotowaza no naruzo [What's new for proverbs]. (2022). https://japanese-note.jp/iwanugahana/#index_id1

Kurokawawa, I. (2025). *Taiwa no torisetsu* [The Manual of Dialogue]. Kodansha.

Koekishadan hojin beikoku annteikyoukyukakuho shienkiko. (n.d.). Okome No Bunnka To Rekishi [Rice culture and history]. https://www.komenet.jp/bunkatorekishi/bunkatorekishi02/bunkatorekishi02_4

Mizuno, N. (2008). *Nijonjin to dibeito* [The Japanese and debates]. Miyachi, Y., Kai M. (Eds.), *Japanese linguistics.* Meijishoin, Inc.

Nakano, N. (2023). *Kanjō ni nagasarenai ressun* [Lessons on not being swayed by emotions]. President Inc.

NHK Broadcasting Culture Research Institute. (2019). *Nihonjin no shukyo teki ishiki ya koudou wa dou kawatta ka.* [NHK] https://www.bing.com/search?q=%E6%97%A5%E6%9C%AC%E4%BA%BA%E3%81%AE%E5%AE%97%E6%95%99%E8%A6%B3%E3%82%84%E6%84%8F%E8%AD%98%E3%81%AF%E3%81%A9%E3

Nikkei. (2015, April 6). "Nihon no kojinshugi wa ika ni kodoku o umidasu ka? Bunka shinrigaku ni yoru kentou" [How does Japanese individualism create loneliness? *Nikkei.* https://www.nikkei.com/article/DGXKZO85209440S5A400C1X12000/?msockid=3c749d55c913634810a78843c8166212%20Nikkei%20Asia

Nishida, E. (2016, September 13). "Naze noukouminzoku wa 'mainasu satei,' shuryuu minzokuwa 'purus satei' nanoka?" [Why are farmers 'assess negatively' and hunters 'assess positively'?]. Diamond Online. https://diamond.jp/articles/-/100036

Ogiwara, Y. (2014). "Nihon no kojinshugi wa ika ni kodoku o umidasu ka? Bunka shinrigaku ni your kentou" [How does Japanese individualism create loneliness? A cultural psychological examination] https://www.suntory.co.jp/sfnd/research/detail/2012_305.html

Ohno, M. (2022, January 24). Mijika na hito e no "sasshite hoshii wa aite e no bouryoku da "Chotto gurai tetsudatte hoshii wa kotoba tarazu". *Toyo Keizai Online.* https://toyokeizai.net/articles/-/503664

Page, C. (2009c). *Frontier of health: How to heal the whole person.* Random House.

Raihani, N. (2023, July 25). "Higashi ajiadewa naze 'muchiibiiki" ga hakobirunoka?" [Why is "patronage" so popular in East Asia?]. *Toyo Keizai Online.* https://toyokeizai.net/articles/- /678549?page=5

Tanizaki, J. (1997). *In praise of shadows* (kindle version). Leette's Island Books, Inc. XXXX

Uchida, Y. (2024). *Doucho kara ko o hiraku shakai e* [From harmony to an individualistic society]. Kokuyo Co., Ltd.

Wada, T. (1996). *Koji kotowaza meigen meiku jitsuyo* [Dictionary of Sayings, Proverbs, and Quotations for Practical Use]. Shufu To Seikatsu Sha. XXXX.

Wikipedia. (2024, August 27). *Junanajo kenpo [The Seventeen-article constitution].* Wikisource. https://ja.m.wikisource.org/wiki/%E5%8D%81%E4%B8%83%E6%9D%A1%E6%86%B2%E6%B3%9

Wikipedia. (2024b). *Speech is silver, silence is golden*. https://en.m.wikipedia.org/wiki/Speech_is_silver,_silence_is_golden

Yamagishi, T. (2010). *Anshin shakai kara shinrai shakai e: nihon-gata shisutemu no yukue* [From a society of security to a society of trust: The future of Japanese system]. CHUOKORONSHINSHA, INC.

Chapter 5
Zen and Mindfulness Practices to Increase Awareness of Inochi:
The Japanese Sense of Life as the Source of Ikigai

Mikio Shishido
https://orcid.org/0009-0009-2619-1515
International Center of Transdisciplinary Research, Japan

ABSTRACT

This chapter explores how sustainable well-being and a renewal of modern life can be achieved through an integrative understanding of ikigai, inochi, and Zen mindfulness. In today's society, rapid technological advancement, information overload, and a fading sense of purpose have heightened the need for self-awareness and well-being. Amidst this, the Japanese concept of ikigai has gained global attention. Commonly described as the intersection of what one loves, is good at, what the world needs, and what one can be paid for, in Japan ikigai often emphasizes purpose and service to others over monetary reward. At its core lies inochi—the Japanese view of life as interconnected with nature and society, rooted in the gratitude of living in the present moment. Zen and mindfulness practices help cultivate this awareness and promote mind-body harmony. Together, ikigai, inochi, and Zen mindfulness form a holistic framework that nurtures both personal fulfillment and social balance.

DOI: 10.4018/979-8-3373-0360-4.ch005

1. THE SEARCH FOR A JAPANESE SPIRITUALITY: AN ERA IN WHICH *IKIGAI* IS IN DEMAND

In today's society, the enhancement of self-awareness and well-being is becoming increasingly important. This is due to rapid technological evolution, increased stress caused by information overload, and a weakening of the individual's sense of purpose and purpose in life. Against this backdrop, *ikigai*, a traditional Japanese concept of "meaning of life" or "value of life," is attracting worldwide attention.

Ikigai is a concept that refers to the meaning of life or the purpose of life. Located at the intersection of one's passions, mission, vocation, and needs, *ikigai* brings a sense of purpose and satisfaction to one's daily life. Finding *ikigai* provides lasting motivation and happiness.

What is important in capturing one's *ikigai*? It is to feel the essence of life as life itself. This is where the Japanese view of *inochi*, a view of life that is at one with nature, becomes important.

In Japanese, *inochi* means "life itself". It is important to recognize the preciousness of life and the value of each moment, and to feel a sense of presence and vitality in our daily lives; becoming aware of *inochi* will increase our appreciation and awareness of the present moment and lead to a more fulfilling life. I would like to explain how Zen and mindfulness are effective in increasing the awareness of that *inochi*, which in turn increases self-awareness and well-being.

What is *ikigai* anyway? Why is it booming around the world? The main figures driving the worldwide boom in books about Japanese *ikigai* are Spanish authors Héctor García and Francesc Miralles, who have written a number of books on ikigai, including Ikigai: The Japanese Secret to a Long and Happy Life (García and Miralles, 2016).

Their book details the practical aspects of *ikigai* and its benefits by surveying Tokyo residents and longevity communities in Okinawa. Specifically, they used a simple framework to explain *ikigai* in terms of four elements: "what you love", "what you are good at", "what the world needs", and "what you can be paid for", providing a structure that anyone can understand and that has resonated with readers worldwide.

In fact, the Ohsaki Study conducted in Japan by the Tohoku University Department of Public Health (Ohsaki Study), which followed more than 40,000 middle-aged and older Japanese for about 7 years, showed that those who answered that they had no reason to live (*ikigai*) had a 1.5 times higher overall mortality rate than those who answered that they had a reason to live (*ikigai*). The risk was 1.6 times higher of death from cardiovascular disease. (Sone et al., 2008).

However, Garcia and Miralles' *Ikigai* framework has been criticized by Japanese researchers and cultural figures that this diagram is far from what Japanese people really feel. In fact, as a Japanese, I feel some discomfort. The most uncomfortable point is the "what you can be paid for" section. In Japanese culture, there are not many people who think of *ikigai* = earning a living, and I believe that many people feel *ikigai* in serving without asking for anything in return, as one of Japanese sensibilities.

In Japan, it is also said that work is called hata-raku, which means "to make things easier (*raku*) for the people around you (*hata*), as if to thank them for being a part of nature and for having already given you so much and kept you alive (*hata-raku*)" (Tasaka, 2011). " (Tasaka, 2011).

Gordon Mathews (1996) points out that the Japanese concept of *ikigai* is often found in more everyday, personal pleasures and relationships, as opposed to the Western framework that emphasizes external achievements such as professional accomplishment and monetary rewards. (Mathews, 1996).

Mieko Kamiya, a pioneer in the study of *ikigai* in Japan, in her book About the Meaning of Life (*Ikigai ni tsuite* in Japanese). argues that "through her work with leprosy patients, *ikigai* is deeply connected to 'service to others' and a sense of mission." She states that *ikigai* is "finding purpose and meaning in life," which leads to self-transcendent behavior and selfless service (without seeking anything in return)" (Kamiya Mieko, 1966).

One of the reasons why *ikigai* in Japan is different from that in the West is that in the West, influenced by the Christian worldview, the purpose of life tends to be strongly connected to "relationship with God" and "personal achievement" (Frankl, 1985), while in Japan, under the influence of Buddhism and Shintoism, human beings are seen as beings who live in relationship with nature and others (Frankl, 1985). In Japan, however, due to the influence of Buddhism and Shintoism, people are viewed as beings who live in relationship with nature and others, and *ikigai* has been nurtured as a value that is felt in social and relational connections rather than as an individual's internal satisfaction (Arai, 2001).

The Japanese concept of *ikigai* is not simply based on occupational achievement or reward, but is deeply rooted in meaning in daily life and in relationships with others. The background of this value system is particularly influenced by Zen Buddhism, one of the most important branches of Buddhism. In Zen, there is a spirit of "*sa-mu*," which concentrates on the "present moment (*sokkon sokusho*)" and regards everyday activities such as cleaning, cooking, and labor as practice in itself. This has been the foundation for cultivating a sensitivity to *ikigai* through the sense that "every action has meaning" (Suzuki, 1959).

In addition, Zen practice emphasizes values such as "no-self," "discriminating wisdom," and "oneness," and offers the perspective of viewing the self in relation to nature and others, rather than being bound by the ego. This resonates with the structure that *ikigai* is brought about not only by "joy of self" but also by "contribution to others and society" (Kumano, 2017).

It is then argued that the concept of *inochi* in Japanese Buddhism is not based on a self-contained existence, but rather on existence as part of cosmic life, and that this is the basis of *ikigai* in Japan (Arai, 2001). We would like to delve deeper into this background of Japanese *ikigai*, or *inochi*, which is the Japanese view of life.

An example of the English translation of the Japanese word "*inochi*" is "Our Lives" in the "Designing Future Society for Our Lives" theme for the 2025 Osaka Expo. The original Japanese word for "Our Lives" is "*inochi*," but in Japan, many people believe that "life" is not something that can be counted, but exists in a sense, in the place itself, in the connections.

In his article "Eastern Philosophy and Bioethics - A Response from Buddhist View of Life" (Haruhiko Masaki, 1992), Masaki explores the possibility of applying the Buddhist view of life to modern bioethics. In this article, through the concepts of *engi* and "no-self," which are fundamental tenets of Buddhism, the interdependence of inochi and emphasizes the non-fixity of the self. This presents a perspective that views life not as an individual possession, but in relation to others and the environment.

Beyond the mere existence of life as an individual, *inochi* emphasizes the harmonious presence of mind and body and a sense of oneness with nature. In his book "Japanese Spirituality" (Daisetsu Suzuki, 1972), D.T. Suzuki, who spread Zen culture throughout the world, describes spirituality as *daichisei* ("earthiness"), and it can be said that the Japanese way of feeling spirituality is to see life - *inochi* - as a unity with nature.

This concept is the foundation for deepening self-understanding and pursuing inner richness. In particular, Zen teachings and the practice of mindfulness have become widespread as an effective means of not only maintaining mental stability in today's busy lives, but also enhancing self-awareness based on a deep view of life.

Furthermore, the *inochi* view of life is deeply connected to the characteristics of Japanese culture, which values harmony with others and with nature. This fosters a perspective that takes into account the relationship with society and the environment when pursuing individual fulfillment of life. As a result, a sustainable and balanced way of life is promoted, not only for the well-being of the individual, but also for the harmony of the community as a whole.

In general, Japanese spirituality, based on *inochi*, is an essential element in the creation of *ikigai* in today's world, which demands increased self-awareness and well-being. Through the practice of Zen and mindfulness, individuals can pursue inner richness and build a harmonious life. This provides a clear path to a sustainable and fulfilling life.

I believe that there are four main elements of *ikigai* in terms of *inochi* as a Japanese spirituality.

--Recognition of the value of life: A deep understanding of *inochi* gives individuals the opportunity to reflect on their own existence and the meaning of life. This is the basis for self-awareness to find *ikigai*.
--Harmony with Nature: Feeling at one with nature enhances our sense of *ikigai*. Living in harmony with the rhythms of nature promotes stress reduction and mental stability, and helps us find our own purpose and joy.
--Connection to Community: *inochi* emphasizes holistic connections and relationships with others. By strengthening our ties to our communities and families, we find the relationships and social roles that are the source of *ikigai*.
--Spiritual Practices: Spiritual practices such as Zen and mindfulness deepen our understanding of *inochi* and assist in the creation of *ikigai*. Through these practices, focusing on the present moment and facing our inner selves helps us discover our true purpose in life.

As these elements suggest, the three elements of *ikigai*, *inochi*, and Zen/mindfulness, while independent concepts, are in fact deeply interdependent, mutually supportive, and resonate with each other. If *ikigai* is the energy of the mind that gives us a sense of purpose and motivation in life, then *inochi* is the sense of life as an underlying presence, and mindfulness is a way to establish both of these in our bodies as a daily practice.

In today's disconnected society, this chapter proposes that integrating these three concepts, rather than talking about them separately, is the path to a more essential and sustainable well-being. In other words, "awakening to *inochi* leads to a sense of *ikigai*, and walking mindfully along this path opens up an integrated view of life that transcends the divisions between inside and outside, self and others, nature and civilization.

2. *INOCHI:* THE JAPANESE SENSE OF LIFE

Inochi is a concept that represents the core view of life in Japanese spirituality. The word does not merely mean "Biological life" or "Existential life," but is deeply related to existence itself, the essence of life, and even the meaning and purpose of life. Below is a detailed explanation of how *inochi* shapes Japanese spirituality and is the source of *ikigai*.

Definition and Philosophical Background of *Inochi*

In Japanese, *inochi* means " existence itself," or " the essence of life," and is a broad concept that encompasses not only individual existence, but also oneness with nature and the universe. This view of life is rooted in the following philosophical background

The idea of *inochi* in Japan has been nurtured in a sense of coexistence with nature, a religious worldview, and a sensitivity that sees body and spirit as one. Arai (2001) argues that the introduction of Buddhism and its Japanization had a particularly significant impact on the formation of this conception of *inochi*.

Arai explains how the concept of *inochi* developed in a unique way in Japanese culture in relation to Buddhist thought as follows

1. Buddhist view of life and death and acceptance of samsara:

In Japanese Buddhism, life was not considered as an individual possession, but as an existence that arises and flows through causality and relationships. In particular, Mahayana Buddhism's concept of "emptiness" denies the materialization of individual *inochi* and creates an understanding that all beings exist together in connection.

2. Resonance with Nature:

The Japanese vernacular view of nature is also deeply rooted in the concept of *inochi*, which, according to Arai, is a Japanese interpretation of Buddhism that blends an animistic sense of spirituality and life not only in human life but also in all things in nature (plants, trees, mountains, and rivers).

3. Fusion of physicality and spirituality:

In Japanese Buddhism, the distinction between body and spirit, this world and the other world, is blurred, and *inochi* encompasses not only visible physical life but also life as an invisible spiritual existence. In this respect, it has a distinctly different structure from the biological and anthropocentric view of life of the Western modern era.

Despite this background, the Japanese view of life, *inochi*, is deeply rooted in Japanese culture and daily life and is expressed in the following aspects:

--Rhythm of Life: The rhythm of life, in tune with the natural changes of the seasons, reflects the Japanese value of respect for the cycles and changes of life. Seasonal events and festivals provide opportunities to celebrate the preciousness of life and harmony with nature.

--Harmony in Relationships: In Japanese society, harmony in groups and communities is more important than in individuals. Life has meaning in connection with others and is believed to be based on interdependence.

--Arts and Aesthetics: Traditional Japanese arts (tea ceremony, flower arrangement, calligraphy, etc.) express a sense of beauty that captures the transience of life and the beauty of the moment. Through these artistic activities, the profound value of life is experientially understood.

Within this *inochi* worldview, *ikigai* rooted in Japanese culture is created. As a life that captures *inochi*, *ikigai* exists as an expression of the "joy of living" or "purpose of life" and is the source of the sense of fulfillment and happiness felt by the individual.

Thus, *inochi* is more than just a life phenomenon; it is a comprehensive view of life that encompasses the dimensions of relationship, resonance, and spirituality, a concept deeply rooted in Japanese culture and spirituality. This sensitivity to *inochi* is nurtured through people's lives, art, and values, and leads to the creation of *ikigai*, a sense of personal meaning and significance of existence. This sense of living with *inochi* remains an important guiding principle in our search for a sustainable and harmonious way of life today.

A New Way of Perceiving *Inochi*

The way we perceive *inochi* overlaps with the worldview of the latest science, such as the theory of quantum mechanics, which has been revealed in the development of science, and we can see a new perspective on how *inochi* is perceived.

And it is said that the quantum world overlaps with the Zen ideas of "*mu-funbetsu* (non discrimination)" and "*mu-ni* (non-duality)" in Buddhism.

I would like to explore the world of Zen and the traditional Japanese view of life, *inochi*, which have influenced much of Japanese culture, and how these concepts interrelate and contribute to the reconstruction of self-awareness.

The term "nondiscrimination" refers to a state of cognition in which things are not perceived separately, i.e., there is no distinction between subject and object. In this state, there are no fixed ideas or categorizations based on sensation or thought, and it is possible to intuitively perceive pure existence itself. *mu-ni* expresses the non-duality of the whole being as one, without any division into two. This emphasizes the viewpoint that the subject (ego) and the object (world) are interdependent and not independent entities. The idea of nonduality suggests that all beings are interrelated and unified as one *inochi*.

The relationship between self and non-self from a Zen perspective provides an important perspective on self-awareness.

In Zen, "no-self" refers to the state in which there is no fixed "self" and all beings interact with each other. Through zazen and meditation, one transcends the distinction between self and non-self and experiences the sense that all is one. Understanding the relationship between self and non-self also allows individuals to break free from a self-centered perspective and view life and existence from a broader perspective!

Quantum mechanics is a theory that describes the behavior of matter and energy in the microscopic world and offers a different perspective from classical physics (Rosenblum & Kuttner, 2011). In quantum mechanics, nonlocal phenomena are observed in which particles affect each other instantaneously (Aspect, Dalibard, & Roger, 1982). This suggests that matter is not independent but interdependent. Also, in quantum mechanics, the observer and the object of observation are inseparable. The act of observation itself affects the state of the system, blurring the separation between subject and object (Wheeler & Zurek, 1983). Thus, the non-locality and observer effects of quantum mechanics resonate with the interdependence and unity in *inochi*. Self-awareness is deeply connected to physical phenomena and is the basis for understanding the interaction between self and the world, which is in response to the Zen view of the world.

Gaia Theory, proposed by Dr. James Lovelock, also views the entire earth as a single living system, in which living and nonliving organisms interact with each other to maintain the earth's environment. (James Lovelock, 2023) This theory resonates with the Japanese view of *inochi* and shows that each individual life exists as part of the entire global living system. This overlaps with the recognition that individual well-being is directly connected to the health of the planet, suggesting a new self-awareness. And this worldview of Gaia Theory, with its emphasis on sustainable ways of life and harmony with nature, raises environmental awareness as a source of *ikigai*. It suggests the possibility for individuals to find a deeper purpose in life by considering the health of the planet as a whole.

Other planetary health that microorganisms connect, advocated by Risa Kirimura, a Japanese physician and author of "Nurturing the 'Soil' of the Gut and Forest: Microorganisms Make People and the Environment Healthy" (Risa Kirimura, 2023), is the idea that the health of the entire planet and human health are closely related. Microbes are the key to this and play an important role in the earth's ecosystem and human health. Microbes, or intestinal bacteria, are vital to life in the human body and environment. Understanding the symbiotic relationship with microorganisms further deepens the Japanese view of *inochi*, and a healthy body and environment are the foundation for the creation of *ikigai*.

In particular, recent years have seen a focus on the gut-brain correlation, in which the gut microbiota has an impact on brain development, behavior, and mood, and gut microbes are involved in the production of neurotransmitters such as serotonin and GABA (gamma-amino acids), which influence stress response and behavior (2019. John F. Cryan and Timothy G. Dinan). In other words, gut conditioning leads to emotional stability and reduced depression/anxiety, which supports the foundation of *ikigai's* sensitivity = the ability to feel a sense of purpose in life.

The bacteria in the intestines are the "others" in our body, but they also support the "self" by establishing a symbiotic relationship. This awareness of the presence of others both inside and outside of the body creates an awareness that *inochi* is not one's own, but is an entity that resonates within the connection.

Understanding this relationship with microorganisms and maintaining a healthy microbial balance is directly related to improved self-awareness and well-being.

The Japanese view of *inochi* integrates these concepts in a comprehensive manner, offering individuals a new sense of self and the world as one, as well as a new way of firmly recognizing that physical and mental health are inextricably linked, helping to realize a fulfilling *ikigai*.

3. ZEN AND MINDFULNESS PRACTICES TO ENHANCE SELF-AWARENESS OF *INOCHI*, THE SOURCE OF *IKIGAI*

In today's Internet society, there is an overabundance of information, and search algorithms tend to give priority to information that is consistent with one's existing values. Furthermore, social networking sites tend to spread only "good information" that is easy to sympathize with, and a culture of transmitting and receiving information with concern for the eyes of others is spreading.

In such an environment, there is an increasing tendency to align one's values with those outside oneself, making it difficult to see what one really wants to do in life. Therefore, self-realization and finding one's purpose in life have become increasingly important themes for many people living today.

In addition, the rapid development of AI technology has led to an emphasis on efficiency and rationality, while at the same time, there is concern that the internal aspects of human nature, such as "life," subjectivity, and sensitivity, will be neglected. It is precisely in these times that we need to renew our focus on *inochi* as emphasized in the Eastern view of life, that is, the wholeness of life in its connection with others, nature, and the universe.

D. T. Suzuki taught that *inochi* and spirituality are not to be understood by the rational intellect, but to be embodied through mindlessness and intuitive awareness (Waddell, 2010). This is a fundamental value of human existence that AI cannot attain.

This chapter describes the role of Zen and mindfulness.

Zen Practice and the Look at Life

Zen, a branch of Buddhism, is a practice that aims for mental tranquility and enlightenment through zazen or meditation. Zen practice is a way of carefully living by adjusting the mind through zazen and daily life, focusing the consciousness on the present moment, and returning to what is truly important.

This is not simply to eliminate distractions, but to develop a freedom of mind to observe thoughts and feelings as they arise and to let them pass without being caught up in them. Through this process, one is freed from the attachment of the ego and opens the way to experience the true nature of the self and oneness with the universe.

Zen teachings do not seek truth in words or logic, but rather emphasize deep inquiry through physical sensation and inner experience. Through this practice, they help us to discern what is truly important to us and guide us toward a more harmonious way of life.

The Potential of Mindfulness in Today's World

Mindfulness is a concept originally derived from Buddhism, but in modern times it has transcended its religious background and expanded through scientific demonstration. Mindfulness is a state of mind that consciously focuses attention on the present moment and accepts experience as it is, without evaluation or judgment.

By focusing awareness on breath, bodily sensations, thoughts, and emotions, mindfulness increases awareness of the inner and outer world, reduces stress, promotes emotional stability, and deepens self-understanding. In fact, research has confirmed that mindfulness is effective in reducing stress hormones, improving concentration, and improving empathy (Tang, Hölzel, & Posner, 2015). It has also been applied in the treatment of depression and anxiety disorders (Wielgosz et al., 2019).

The practice of mindfulness calms the mind and facilitates listening to the inner voice and becoming aware of one's true desires and passions. This results in greater self-awareness and leads to the discovery of *ikigai* (Brown & Ryan, 2003).

As a Practice Connecting *Inochi* and *Ikigai*

As self-awareness deepens through mindfulness, *inochi*, the Japanese view of life, becomes recognized not as mere individual life, but as "existence itself" in connection with others and nature. By reaching such a state of being, people come to value harmony with nature and society and choose to live as one with self and others.

This perspective is deeply connected to Zen and mindfulness, and fosters an awareness that transcends the boundaries between self and others, self and nature. This broadened perspective is the foundation for the discovery and creation of *ikigai*.

With its gaze toward universal truths that transcend the self, Zen teaching reveals the meaning of one's own existence by moving away from a self-centered perspective and experiencing a sense of oneness with the whole. This sense of oneness is deeply related to the "contribution to others and society," which is at the heart of *ikigai*. Relationships with others are essential to the process of finding one's purpose in life, and Zen practice provides a solid foundation for the discovery of *ikigai*.

4. HOW TO PRACTICE ZEN AND MINDFULNESS TO IMPROVE WELL-BEING BY BECOMING AWARE OF *INOCHI* AND ENHANCING THE ABILITY TO PERCEIVE *IKIGAI*

Learn more about Zen and mindfulness practices that enhance your ability to experience *inochi* and connect with *ikigai* in order to improve your well-being (sense of well-being and health). Through these practices, you can deepen your self-understanding, balance your mind and body, and lay the foundation for a more fulfilling life.

(1) Feel Life Through Zazen

Procedure:

1. Choose a quiet place

   --Create an environment for zazen in a low-noise area.

2. Get the right posture

   --Sit on a cushion or chair and straighten your back.

   --Place both hands on your knees or in the shape of the Dharma Realm Teijin (right palm facing up, left hand facing up, overlapping, and lightly touching the tips of both thumbs together. The tips of both thumbs lightly touch each other.

3. Concentrate on your breathing

   --Focus on natural breathing and pay attention to your inhalations and exhalations.

--As if slowly and carefully receiving oxygen, a gift from the natural world, we inhale it and slowly and carefully exhale carbon dioxide, a gift that feeds the growth of plants in the natural world.

4. Getting a feeling of *inochi*

--Through breathing, we feel the rhythm of life and the presence of life.

5. Letting Go of Thoughts:.

--As thoughts come to mind, observe them without dismissing them, and then return your attention to your breath again.

Points:

--Regular practice will give you a deep sense of the value of life.

--Start with 5-10 minutes at first and gradually increase the time.

(2) Explore Ikigai Through Mindfulness Meditation

Procedure:

1. Relax in a quiet place:.

--Assume a relaxing position, such as sitting or lying down.

2. Concentrate on your breathing:.

--Breathe deeply and slowly, focusing on the rhythm of your breathing.

3. Observation of Emotions and Thoughts

--Observe without evaluating the emotions and thoughts that come to mind.

4. Explore thoughts related to *ikigai*

--Think about activities that you feel passionate about and find rewarding, and bring awareness to them.

5. Gratitude

--Feel a sense of gratitude for your present and surrounding environment.

Points:

--Use it as a time for self-exploration and help gain insight into *ikigai*.

--Regular practice leads to self-understanding and clarification of *ikigai*.

(3) Mindful Walking to Feel Inochi and Ikigai

Procedure:

1. Nature's Choice Walks:.

--Choose a place where you can experience nature, such as a park or forest.

2. Concentrate on walking

--Focus on the movement of the feet, the feeling of being grounded, and the rhythm of walking.

3. Observe the surrounding nature

--The movement of the leaves on the trees, the sound of birds, the feel of the wind, and other senses are used to feel the present environment.

4. Feeling the presence of life

--Realize our existence as part of nature and the connections between life.

5. Incorporate thoughts related to ikigai

--Think about your ideas and goals regarding what makes your life worth living.

Points:

--The natural environment during the walk will refresh your body and mind and promote a sense of *inochi*.

--Regular walking leads to ongoing mental stability and discovery of *ikigai*.

(4) Mindful Eating to Feel the Preciousness of Life

Procedure:

1. Take a deep breath before eating

--Take a few deep breaths and calm your mind before beginning to eat.

2. Observe your food

--Carefully observe the color, shape, and aroma of the food in front of you.

3. Eat carefully, one bite at a time

--Chew each bite more often and focus your attention on the texture and taste.

4. Feel the cycle of life

--Be aware that food is part of the life that sustains our bodies.

5. Gratitude

--Enjoy our meals while appreciating the people and nature that grew the food.

Points:

--By refraining from using cell phones during meals and concentrating on eating, we can deeply appreciate the preciousness of life.

--Mindful eating promotes healthy eating habits and satisfaction.

(5) Body Scan Meditation to Feel the Connection to Life

Procedure:

1. Relaxed posture

--Lie on your back or sit in a chair and relax.

2. Become aware of your breath

--Take several deep breaths to relax the mind and body.

3. Focus on each part of the body in turn: 1.

--Concentrate on each part of the body in turn, from the top of the head to the toes.

--Observe and relax the sensations and tensions felt in each part of the body.

4. Feel the connection of life

--Realize that your body is the vessel of life and that your whole body supports vital activities.

5. Feeling the whole body as one

--Finally, Feel the whole body as one cohesive whole and experience the oneness of life.

Points:

--Regular body scans deepen the connection between body and mind, and give us a stronger sense of the presence of life.

--It is effective when done before sleep or when stressed.

(6) Tips for Continuing Practice

--Make it a habit: Practicing Zen or mindfulness at a set time each day will make it easier to make it a habit. Find a time that works for you, for example, 5 minutes in the morning or 10 minutes before bedtime.

--Take it easy: Start with short periods of time and gradually increase the length of time. It is important to proceed at your own pace and not overdo it.

--Create the environment: Choose a quiet, relaxing place to create an environment in which you can concentrate on your practice. Scenting and music to create your own personal relaxation space can also be effective.

--Use guides: Use apps, guidebooks, and online videos to learn how to do it right. Guided practice is especially useful for beginners.

-Participate in a community: group practices and online communities make it easier to stay motivated. Working with others who share common goals makes it easier to keep going.

5. CONCLUSION

Throughout this chapter, we have explored the depths of Japanese spirituality based on three key concepts: *inochi*, *ikigai*, and Zen/mindfulness. Each of these concepts is important on its own, but it is the integration of these concepts that is of great significance for the reconstruction of human "self-awareness" and "well-being" in today's society.

First, we present the fundamental view of life that *inochi* is not an isolated existence of the self, but is kept alive in connection with nature, society, and others. This view of life, deeply rooted in the Zen and Buddhist teachings of "no-self" and "*engi*," brings awareness of existence in relationship, away from self-centered values.

This awareness of *inochi* brings a vivid sense of one's here-and-now and nurtures the foundation for a sense of being alive.

Ikigai is not just self-realization, but also a sense of giving to others without asking for anything in return, a sense of being fulfilled through empathy and resonance. In other words, true *ikigai* emerges from the awareness of the relationship of *inochi*.

Mindfulness is the bridge between awareness of *inochi* and insight into *ikigai*. The practice of mindfulness fosters the ability to observe and accept the "present moment" as it is, rather than being engulfed by the waves of thoughts and emotions. Through this process, we deepen our connection with our inner self and learn to listen to what is truly important, rather than being distracted by the noise of the outside world. Zen and Mindfulness are a proven technique and practical wisdom for experiencing *inochi* and discovering *ikigai*.

Furthermore, as discussed in this chapter, through the connection with the gut environment, symbiosis with microorganisms, the nondual worldview of quantum mechanics, and the Earth's entire life system (Gaia Theory), "*Inochi*," "*Ikigai*," and "Zen and Mindfulness" are no longer confined to the individual's inner world, but open up to the "connection between self and world" on a global and cosmic scale. The connection between the self and the world on a global and cosmic scale.

Thus, feeling "*Inochi*" and questioning "*Ikigai* " and walking that path through "Zen and Mindfulness" is a fundamental approach to not losing oneself and to regaining harmony with others and the world in this age of modern uncertainty.

The key to the revival of human dignity and spirituality in the future may lie in the practice of this trinity of "*Inochi* - *Ikigai* - Zen and Mindfulness". This is an irreplaceable gift that the wisdom nurtured in the climate and history of Japan can now deliver to the world.

REFERENCES

Arai, H. (2001). The concept of inochi (life) in Japanese Buddhism. In Keenan, J. P. (Ed.), *Japanese Buddhism and Ethics* (pp. 35–52). University of Hawai'i Press.

Aspect, A., Dalibard, J., & Roger, G. (1982). Experimental test of Bell's inequalities using time-varying analyzers. *Physical Review Letters*, *49*(25), 1804–1807. DOI: 10.1103/PhysRevLett.49.1804

Brown, K. W., & Ryan, R. M. (2003). The benefits of being present: Mindfulness and its role in psychological well-being. *Journal of Personality and Social Psychology*, *84*(4), 822–848. DOI: 10.1037/0022-3514.84.4.822 PMID: 12703651

Cryan, J. F., & Dinan, T. G. (2019). The microbiota-gut-brain axis. *Physiological Reviews*, *99*(4), 1877–2013. DOI: 10.1152/physrev.00018.2018 PMID: 31460832

Frankl, V. E. (1985). *Man's search for meaning*. Washington Square Press. (Original work published 1946)

García, H., & Miralles, F. (2016). *Ikigai: The Japanese secret to a long and happy life*. Penguin Books.

Kamiya, M. (1966). *Ikigai ni tsuite* [On the meaning of life]. Misuzu Shobo.

Kirimura, R. (2023). *Nurturing the "soil" of the intestines and forests: Microorganisms make healthy people and environment*. Kobunsha.

Kumano, H. (2017). Mindfulness, Buddhism, and the Japanese experience. mindfulness, 8(2), 295-300.

Lovelock, J. (2023). The Earth's life sphere (New ed.). Kosakusha.

Masaki, H. (1992). Oriental philosophy and bioethics: A response from the Buddhist view of life. *Journal of the Japan Society for Bioethics*, *3*, 48–52.

Mathews, G. (1996). *What makes life worth living? How Japanese and Americans make sense of their worlds*. University of California Press. DOI: 10.1525/9780520916470

Rosenblum, B., & Kuttner, F. (2011). *Quantum Enigma: Physics Encounters Consciousness* (2nd ed.). Oxford University Press.

Sone, T., Nakaya, N., Ohmori, K., Shimazu, T., Higashiguchi, M., Kakizaki, M., Fukudo, S., & Tsuji, I. (2008). Sense of life worth living (ikigai) and mortality in Japan: Ohsaki study. *Psychosomatic Medicine*, *70*(6), 709–715. DOI: 10.1097/PSY.0b013e31817e7e64 PMID: 18596247

Suzuki, D. T. (1959). *Zen and Japanese culture*. Princeton University Press.

Suzuki, D. T. (1972). *Japanese spirituality*. Iwanami Bunko.

Suzuki, D. T. (2010). *Japanese spirituality: A D.T. Suzuki reader* (Waddell, N., Ed.). University of California Press.

Tang, Y. Y., Hölzel, B. K., & Posner, M. I. (2015). The neuroscience of mindfulness meditation. *Nature Reviews. Neuroscience*, *16*(4), 213–225. DOI: 10.1038/nrn3916 PMID: 25783612

Tasaka, H. (2011). *How to live*. SB Creative.

Wheeler, J. A., & Zurek, W. H. (Eds.). (1983). *Quantum theory and measurement*. Princeton University Press. DOI: 10.1515/9781400854554

Wielgosz, J., Goldberg, S. B., Kral, T. R. A., Dunne, J. D., & Davidson, R. J. (2019). Mindfulness meditation and psychopathology. *Annual Review of Clinical Psychology*, *15*(1), 285–316. DOI: 10.1146/annurev-clinpsy-021815-093423 PMID: 30525995

Chapter 6
Mutual Nurturing:
Perspectives of the Law of Origin

Roberto Arturo Restrepo Arcila
https://orcid.org/0009-0005-6642-787X
Independent Researcher, Colombia

Oscar Eduardo Jordán
https://orcid.org/0009-0006-2702-5998
Kuska Cultural Center for Ancestral Wisdoms, Bolivia

ABSTRACT

The concept of "Mutual Nurturing" derived from the indigenous Law of Origin, emphasizing its significance in reshaping global education systems and fostering sustainable communities. Drawing on the ancient wisdom of American indigenous cultures, the study integrates perspectives on complex, transdisciplinary thinking advocated by modern initiatives like UNESCO's "Seven Necessary Knowledges for the Education of the Future." The Eagle's Vision metaphor is central to this discussion, illustrating the balance of context-awareness and precise action. The article examines the interplay of three "mind-souls"—body, reason, and emotion—and their role in achieving alignment and coherence in human experience. By revisiting ancestral philosophies and practices, the paper proposes a paradigm shift in education, public policy, and human behavior to restore harmony between humanity and the planet. The authors call for a transcultural dialogue and the reorientation of societal values towards mutual upbringing, enabling sustainable and equitable futures.

DOI: 10.4018/979-8-3373-0360-4.ch006

INTRODUCTION

Humanity is witnessing a crucial moment in the way the fabric of life can be affected at a planetary level. For centuries, our species has been concerned about the legacy it will leave to our successors, hence education has always been one of the most important principles of society. However, currently, we are faced with a reality that disdains the past and overestimates the future, prioritizing above all a Sustainable Development.

However, there is another paradigm of thought called the Law of Origin, coined by the indigenous peoples of the American continent—formerly called Abya Yala—and which has been shared continentally in a diachronic and synchronic way for more than 13,000 years. In common terms, the "operative part" of this vision is Mutual Parenting, a way of life, a being in the world in order to become fully human beings, not a being to be. A vision where the important thing is the way of making the path that weaves, forms and builds.

However, there is another paradigm of thought called the Law of Origin, coined by the indigenous peoples of the American continent—formerly called Abya Yala—and which has been shared continentally in a diachronic and synchronic way for more than 13,000 years. In common terms, the "operative part" of this vision is Mutual Parenting, a way of life, a being in the world in order to become fully human beings, not a being to be. A vision where the important thing is the way of making the path that weaves, forms and builds.

With the publication of "The seven complex lessons in education for the future" (Morin, 1999) the need to promote complex—transdisciplinary—thinking and define the human condition became evident, too become aware of the earthly identity and an ethic that allows us to guarantee a sustainable future —and present—; current generations —UNESCO postulated at the time— should have sufficient capacities to face the latent uncertainties in contemporary global daily life.

Solutions are needed that articulate formal and informal transdisciplinary knowledge on a global scale, as well as new models of public policies that are up to the multidimensional problems that nation-states must solve. The critical and open recovery of accumulated experience—successful and unsuccessful—must guide the design of effective solutions to the problems of human communities. The world requires immediate responses and the recovery of accumulated knowledge, through transcultural dialogue on a global scale; this is a priority on which the sustainability of this way of life that is our species depends. The production of knowledge must go beyond disciplinary areas based on new experiences of co-production of scientific knowledge in dialogue with ancient and current knowledge. Education systems must be reoriented towards achieving sustainable communities with the capacity to respond to uncertainties, which requires the creation of learning methodologies to sustain local ecosystems, as well as the development of self-learning and learning strategies that optimize the educational role of nearby environments—family and community[1] —in addition to granting new roles to formal education. This will be possible if we manage to establish a new model of societies/communities – oriented towards sustainable ecosystems – and of people (Multidimensional Subject/Multi-dimensional Citizenship).

The Experience of a *Chakaruna*[2 3]

I was walking in the Arizona desert in the company of a Navajo grandfather, understanding the landscape between the play of light and shadow that make up the "desert writing": at every moment, at every hour of the day, the imposing rock masses drew different images, depending on the intensity and direction of the sun's rays.

The Navajo wise man was trying to activate my "mind-souls" of the body and the heart in a person who, like me, had prioritized the "mind-soul" of reason, the head, motivated by my education system, with greater force in the Academy. He knew that my thoughts fluctuated between bewilderment and doubt, trying to keep my feelings and body language at bay. It was at that moment that his gaze caught a rising eagle. He caught my attention and asked me to follow it with my eyes, as it spiraled upwards towards the highest skies.

The old man explained to me that he might be able to help me understand the ancestral conception of the cosmos-world, like a fabric with its warp and weft.

— The eagle rises in a spiral because it opens up to the world of the day, to the life that manifests itself with the sun; it knows that it is time to experience light, action. Look at it as it rises and rises…

The eagle really rose to a very high point, where we could barely make it out as a diffuse shape in a bright blue sky.

— Now she is looking…looking for her food…she has a round and immense world to search.

I continued watching her while she made very wide circles in that almost infinite bright sky at that time of the morning. The old man spoke to me again:

— Stay still where you are and look at the horizon as far as you can.

Really, in that flat and open landscape, I could see very great distances to where the sky meets the curvature of the earth.

— Now go around, slowly, looking at everything, from near to far, from near to distant.

So I did, following a 360° circle, realizing, first, a landscape that I had only seen in pieces, now related, and the limitlessness of my peripheral vision.

— The eagle sees the same as you and beyond, but almost everything at the same time. It can see everything, looking for a rabbit or a fox to feed on.

At that moment the circle it traced in flight began to close in, becoming shorter.

— It has already discovered its food and now it is concentrating —the grandfather told me— it is looking at the terrain at the same time, where the little animal must go up and, therefore, walk more slowly; also the light, how it comes, so that it does not blind it when it comes down; the wind that can propel it or stop it; and the humidity that has to do with its flight. It looks at everything at once and calculates it so that its life journey is not a journey to death.

Suddenly the eagle seemed to shrink, turned into the tip of an arrow, and plunged into the void with increasing speed. It could have reached 200 km per hour. It descended rapidly and suddenly when I thought it would crash to the ground, it made an impossible turn, grabbed something with its claws, and ascended again; everything happened in seconds, instants of absolute precision.

— See? She launched herself into a journey to death which is, equally, a journey to the origin; if she makes a slight mistake she crashes and kills or injures herself; but if she does not take the prey, she loses all the energy of that flight, and her strength is diminished. That is why she must be very precise. From above, she sees at the same time the whole, the warp and weft of the fabric, the union of all its parts, and that is why she can calculate with precision; then she concentrates on the weft, on the detail, on the moment of space and time, and touches that fabric without damaging it and without damaging herself.

That is the vision we call that of the eagle, but it could be that of the quetzal or the condor; being able to see the whole—I thought of the term context—all the parts in relation, like a fabric; thus understanding the space-time in which we move; and in this way being able to touch the threads without ruining the fabric, leaving it healthy. It is woven between life and death.

I thought to myself about our education system, where we increasingly lose sight of the context, getting tangled up in the threads, leaving them so loose that the fabric falls apart, or so tight that it becomes uncertain, without a balanced use. At what point did we lose our true vision of this cosmos-world? Maybe when we became loose threads, individuals, who believe they can manage themselves and are only carried by the wind. (Field diary notes, 2024 [1975])

'Thinking'

The story of this Colombian *chakaruna* reminds us of the teachings of the Bolivian *jampiri*[4] Carlos Prado Mendoza, who in one of his spiritual sessions, sitting at the foot of a swing, told us: "nature is what teaches us, all knowledge is in it. Therefore, we must listen to nature, let it speak to you." We had a similar experience in the *kankurua*[5] of the villages of the Sierra Nevada de Santa Marta, when the *Mamo*[6] was 'thinking' the night when the four sacred fires of the four corners are lit around the central fire. The same thing happens when the zaila Gunadule, in his large community house, sings the songs that the assistant translates for us. All of them are thoughts from the Law of origin that our wise ones transmit to us so that we can act coherently in the world.

Our work experience has allowed us to connect with experts from peoples from Alaska to Patagonia, interweaving the Pacific with the Atlantic, in that cross and diagonals that is part of the order of the ancestral 'cosmos-world' In this way we arrived at the astonishing conclusion that all these peoples, diachronically and synchronically, for at least 20,000 years, shared and still share the same worldview, that is, a warp, which becomes more concrete in each cultural area (North America, Mesoamerica, Intermediate, Andean-Amazonian) through a procedure that many of these peoples call today "thinking," and which is projected in all that 'know-how' of mutual upbringing that is culture, the weaves of diversity that enrich the fabric of the world.

The important thing about experiencing this 'cosmos-world' fabric is that people can meet from the warp of worldview and thought, understand their common roots, be an extended family, *Ayllu* or *Calpulli*, feel a common origin and destiny, and respect and marvel at each other from the great web of the diversity of their cultural manifestations. Diversity in unity, as proposed by the *Whipala which* is the ancestral rainbow flag that continues to wave in the mountains and valleys of the Andes.

The second important aspect is the great coherence of the native peoples who have maintained the umbilical cord between warp and weft, ensuring that each cultural manifestation (territorial planning, urban planning, architecture, sacred objects, the different codices) is inextricably linked to thought and their worldview. It is because of them that today we can access, and we are doing so, the great original vision from those cultural manifestations that operate as true codices of their Law of Origin and vice versa.

A third aspect is the knowledge that the greater warp manifests itself as a Law of Origin that is inscribed in the three 'minds-souls' and operates as a navigation chart for this experience of full humanization, through naturalization and sacralization, in each "space-time" of the here and now, in this middle world that the Andean indigenous peoples call the *kay pacha*.[7]

This article attempts to explain both the three 'minds-souls' and the Law of Origin, the warp and weft, with its threads interwoven and shared by the different indigenous peoples, since the achievements obtained by them made possible some of our most desired current paradigms.

The Law of Origin, a Different Way of Explaining the 'World-Cosmos' and Human Experience

The Law of Origin, 'deep as the sea and simple as a ring' —named in a certain way by the poet Pablo Neruda (Benedetti, 2012)— is a summum of wisdom, simple and profound at the same time, which allowed us to achieve in the 'before' that we call the past some of our most precious paradigms, today increasingly far from being possible in this 'after' that comes behind and that we are unbalancing from the 'here' and the 'now'.

We can state the Law of Origin in two sentences, as a complementary duality, which according to sacred numerology, starts from 1 —unity— towards 3 —complementarity—. The first statement tells us that everything in this world is upbringing: 'I raise to be raised' that is, I am not a separate being nor the owner of the fabric of life, I am intertwined in that fabric like a thread or an embroidery, and therefore I raise myself, with the human community (*runa* in Quechua), with the community of nature (*sallqa*) and with the community of the sacred manifested in this plane (*waka*). This upbringing implies maintaining a constant dialogue, doing so in reciprocity, which allows for complementarity and completeness, respecting the free flow of life energies. The second statement is presented as an ethic and aesthetic of the upbringing process: 'how I raise I am raised' A Quechua scholar in Titicaca explained the following:

"It is simple, if I raise the earth (*ukku*), with love, cleanliness, respect, gentleness, just like that it raises me. The same with water (*unu*), fire (*nina*) and air (*wayra*). The same happens with my heart, with my bodies, with the family, the community, with the deepest nature and with the wakas. I do not know sir how we have forgotten to do it and that is why we all get sick at the same time."

In one of the many meetings held during the preparation of the books of the Trilogy of knowledge (Restrepo Arcila, 2002), held on Lake Titicaca with UNESCO, an Aymara scholar, after consulting with his Quechua peers and some Mesoamericans, took the floor and said:

When we are raised wisely, in *ayllu*, that is, among human communities, nature and the sacred, the result is the health of the entire fabric. That was the case before the invasion. But let us see now, in this time that passes like a straight line always progressing, but where there is no longer any upbringing: how is the health of the human people, do they respect each other or kill each other, do they eat well, do their body, heart and mind sing together, do they feel happy to live in this world and understand their path? And how is nature? Is it equally well or is it sick and depressed, almost without words? And our contact with the *illa tiqsi*, with the cosmos-world, with the fabric that embraces us, the sacred that you call, that fills the heart and enchants us, gives us happiness and security, communicates with the ancestors, and allows us to dialogue with the greatest and deepest in the heart of the stars and of this earth? Are they healthy? So, what happened to all this power and pride? What is all this knowledge for? (Field note, 2000)

According to the vision of the native peoples, we have chosen to live this human experience to become true human beings, relating to the 'cosmos-world' according to its Law of Origin, and understanding, between body, heart and mind, the mutual upbringing. We are raised with the human, nature and the sacred. And for this we must acquire the "eagle vision", how to understand, experience and respect the fabric of life between the three communities, weaving ourselves, in turn, with the *illa tiqsi*, the transcendent that is beyond our limited human vision. Understanding origin and destiny as a 'journey to the origin', the way of being in the world to be a true human being, impossible to achieve individually because it is a community process, of Ayllu. In this original worldview one is to be and one is not to be. For this reason, in the native languages the key to the sentence is the verb, not the subject. In our western world what matters most is the subject, because one is by the mere fact of existing in this human form. That is why we are based on a statement or a title, regardless of how we carry it out. The goals are more important than the way of making the journey, where the end justifies the means. We will see this in more detail in the concept of *Pacha*, the Andean 'space-time'.

The Three 'Soul-Minds'

In the ancestral worldview, particularly from the Andean *kamaska,* the greatest knower of this knowledge —which is still generically called shamanism—, the human being, must understand and learn to 'perceive-think-feel' from his three "soul-minds" or energy centers of knowledge of the 'cosmos-world'.

A first 'soul-mind' perhaps the most neglected by the prevailing Western thought, is the *nuna uchay*[8] in Quechua, *ihiyotl* in Nahuatl, located in the solar plexus, in relation to the liver, stomach and intestines, "soul-mind" of the body-form. This *nuna uchay* relates the human being essence-form or *kamaken* with the "cosmos-world" —*kamak*— through the senses: sight, hearing, smell, touch and taste, where the step from 2 to 3 is expressed with greater emphasis, that is, where the duality —two eyes, two nostrils, two ears, two hands, two oral cavities ordered by the tongue— from opposite becomes complementary, naturally. In this Andean and Mesoamerican thought, it is about perceiving by integrating the five senses as a unitary fabric, not in parts or separately as we do currently, thereby losing the context, the greater sensation, the integral relationship. This process of knowing the *nuna uchay* is also known as attention.

The second, *nuna sinchi*[9] in Quechua, *tonalli* in Nahuatl, is in the head, corresponds to our brain and its neural connections and is the "mind-soul" of reason, of thought as we know it. This process of knowledge is also known as intention.

The middle or third "mind-soul", *sunqu samay*[10] in Quechua, *teyolia* in Nahuatl, is in the *sunqu* or heart, it is the "mind-soul" of emotion-feeling, the coordinator of the true process of thinking with the body, mind and heart, a process known as intent. It is the "mind-soul" that remains after the person disincarnates, leaving their dense bodies and staying in their more subtle body, with the memory of the three "mind-souls" now deposited in the *sunqu samay* that accompanies this body through its transit from the end of this life to another life in a different dimension.

Nowadays, when the body's "mind-soul" tries to communicate something to us with its attention, we simply ignore it; this message touches the heart, which in its attempt guide us as a balanced response or action, which we also do not know; then we prioritize only the dictates of the cerebral "mind-soul" who, motivated by this absurd system of prevailing education and by the distorted and manipulated human communication, impels us to an inharmonious, unbalanced and unbalanced thought and reaction. The correct position must be, according to this ancestral vision, to align and interrelate attention, intention and intent to be able to respond adequately with our mutual upbringing to our relationship with the fabric of life in the 'cosmos-world'.

Between Creation and Upbringing, Defining the Basic Concepts

In a vision like ours, where the origin of everything that exists is linked to a form of creation from nothing, ancestral American thought is almost incomprehensible, as it does not link the origin to any process of creation, but rather to upbringing.

In no Andean language, and I would say ancestral American, does the term "nothing" appear (*manakaq* in Quechua means 'not yet to be') or the verb to create (something that comes out of "nothing"), only concepts like *kamay*, something new that emerges from an already existing energy, an upbringing. In Aymara the verb to form, to shape is *luraña*, which some mistakenly take to mean to create. The action of creating life is *uywaña* and creating as producing something is *achuyaña*. It was the intention of the Spanish chroniclers to give coherence to their forced process of evangelization and colonization, which led to misinterpretation of the basic concepts of origin and destiny of the ancestral worldview, managing to permeate leaders, scholars and entire communities.

There is a first great manifestation of the energy that is expressed in the "cosmos-world", in that liminal space-time between what we cannot perceive and what we can glimpse in the deeper and broader 'cosmos-world' (*ukhu* and *qawa*): the *illa tiqsi*: "*Illa*, Foundation, origin, beginning, cause. T*iqsi:* 'great Light', 'Primal Light, the foundation of light'. The ancestors said that everything originated from the *illa*, the energy from which the cosmos-world was formed (*kallpa, kamak*), expressing itself as a foundation in this form perceptible to us.

According to the chroniclers Blas Valera (1945), Guamán Poma de Ayala (1956) and Garcilaso de la Vega (2001 [1609]), the Andeans had the *Illa Tiqsi Wiraqucha* as their only deity, the solar light of the *Ti* (Sun) being its direct manifestation and for this reason they considered the Sun —*Ti*— to be the most sacred thing after the *Illa Tiqsi*. This deity embodies or manifests the *illa tiqsi*, and therefore forms, vitalizes, orders and gives movement to the "cosmos-world" in its different manifestations. This deity becomes complementary as *Pachakamak*: deity that animates, orders and gives form to the "cosmos-world", great bearer of the *kamak* in each "space-time" from the q*awa* to the *uku*, passing through the *hanan* and urin to the *kay*, all the *pachas* of manifestation. It seems that in the high Andes *Wiraqucha* was the predominant deity, while in the lower parts or yungas it was *Pachakamak*. From this conception two other essential terms are derived: *Tiqsi Kamay*, fundamental law, Law of Origin. And *Tiqsi Muyu Pacha*, world, universe in its visible and invisible expressions, from the *Qawa* to the *Uku*, at the point where they end up meeting.

The *Illa Tiqsi*, not perceptible by the 'mind-soul' of the body and its senses, but from the "mind-soul" of the heart, manifests itself as the first perceptible energy-form in the *kamak*: great vitalizing, organizing and forming energy of the Cosmos, poured from the *Illa Tiqsi*. This *kamak* permeates and expresses itself in the four levels of the world or living universe-form —*Kawsay Pacha*—: *Qawa Pacha*, the "space-time" beyond our capacity for perception, deep and wide; *Hanan Pacha*, the space-times that we can perceive as the World Above or celestial world, mainly during the day; *Kay Pacha* or middle world in which the three sister communities exist —*Runas, Sallqa, Wakas*—; the *Hurin Pacha* or Underworld, towards the interior of the Earth and the *Uku Pacha*, that deeper Underworld that manifests itself, above all, in the night sky. Each of the forces or energies that we find in the *Kay Pacha*, this middle world in which we exist as a human community, of nature and the perceptible sacred, manifestation of the duality-parity of the "cosmos-world", are considered expressions of *Illa Tiqsi* through the *Kamak* and receive a proper name and a particular form forming the wefts of the fabric when becoming *Kamaken*, each personalized and perceptible form.

Kamak is, therefore, one of the fundamental concepts of Andean spirituality and is derived from the verb *kama*[11], to animate, to give breath and the act of ordering. From there comes *kamay*, the breath, related to *sunqu*, the heart. The *kamaken* is, then, according to the definition given in the dictionary of Domingo de Santo Tomás (1951 [1560]): "Camaquenc, or camaynin, or *sunqu* anima por la qual viuimos". That is the anima of the heart that allows us life as a form. In a trial for idolatry between the Spanish inquisitors against the indigenous amautas, Duviols (2003) brings us this complement of the *kamaken*: "[…] he ordered the Indians to worship not God but his *Camaquenes Guacas* idols and malquis because these gave them clothing and food", from which it is deduced that the *kamaken* is each particular form that the energy of the sacred takes in this *kay pacha* or our middle world, and is distributed from the deity or the *waka*. From the same Duviols we take this other example:

"[…] that body was called Condortocas which was the malqui and camaquen of don Alomso Callampoma from where the said don Alomso and all the curacas his ancestors and other Indians of the Coto ayllo descended and that they all mochauan" (Duviols, 2003)

The concept then goes further, saying that this energy remains in the *malqui* or mummy of a person whose authority and dignity have earned him this treatment and whose connection with his community must remain. In other examples, they clarify that even sacred images have their own *kamaken*, that is, they carry that fundamental energy of all forms in this world. In the Huarochiri Manuscript, we find that the *kamaken* is every being "animated" by a protective god and a particular ancestor, that is, that his kamak is poured from the deity (in this case *Pachakamak*) and the founder of his lineage. (Duviols, 2016)

Kamaken is, as we have already explained, the *kamak* that animates and orders each living form of the five levels of the cosmos-world. This *kamak* penetrates the body-form from gestation to animate this new expression, personalizing itself, the part in the whole and the whole in the part. The same continues to occur in each birth and upbringing of the web of life. This implies that every form of life shares this spiritual essence and only differs in form and consciousness, opening the field to the interconnection and communication of the entire web of life.

An example of this is the dialogue of Inca Yupanqui with his father Inca Wiracocha; referring to the ordering deity of the cosmos-world, Inca Yupanqui says: "you are my father and you formed me and gave me being and the form of man" (de Betanzos, 1987)

Kamaken is a concept closely related to *kamachiy*, to command, to order from the *kamak*, energy of origin and ordering, and *chyi*, to flow in both directions. Something similar occurs with *kawsay*, to manifest life, to live, to exist, a concept that forms the *kawsachiy*, to sustain by ordering, to keep always flowing. Related to *kamaken, kawsaq* expresses that the being has vital energy, is alive because of this energy, complementing *kawsay*, which is the fact of living, existing.

Kamaken is the *kamak* personalized in a specific form within the communities —*runa-sallqa-waka*— that make up the fabric of life in the *kay pacha*; but it also inhabits the *hanan* and the *hurin pacha*, even forms that we do not perceive in the q*awa* and the *uku pacha*; everything that exists as a form carries that energy of the *kamak* because nothing exists without it, that is, everything carries that basic vital force. Therefore, communication between all beings in their various worlds and dimensions is made possible, because they are all part of the same world-form, with a common origin and destiny carried out through a Law of Origin that is Mutual Nurturing. The *kamaken* is made up of a complementary dual energy: *hucha* and *sami*. *Hucha* is a term related to *kama*, to animate; different sources indicate that it contains the possibility of becoming ill as it is a dense energy, necessary for the world-form, but that when accumulated in the being it limits it, for which reason it must be transformed into its complement, the more subtle energy called *sami*.

For this reason, in the ancestral vision of Abya Yala, there is talk of the double, that is, the *kamaken* or *nawal* that emerges into the world of form in pairs, complementary dualities, flowing at the same time between the human, the natural and the sacred manifested, called today by various Andean communities as the *huauqui* (brother of man) or *huaqui* (pair), which among the Incas had the character of an oracle. Duviols (2016) tells us how

> *"Manco Capac left his huauqui as an inheritance to his successors, but they had their own huauquis. Manco's successors would have had two huauquis then, at least until Pachacuti (Inga Yupangui). We know, in effect, that the personal huauqui of Sinchi Roca, the second Inca, was a stone fish called Huanachiri Amaru; that Lloque Yupanqui's was called Apa Mayta and that Pachakuti's was Inti Illapa, a large gold statue that represented thunder. Finally, it is well documented that each Inca was buried with his huauqui - and in fact, almost all*

of them were found next to the mummy - which implies that the successor had to choose another one".

This double initially inhabits the night sky, where the *Hanan-Qawa* and the *uku pacha*, the upper world and the underworld, meet. It is like an archetype of every form on a broader scale, of a community, not of a person, but of personal expression and communication towards behaviors that encompass the entire community. In the same Huarochirí document, the *kamak* is mentioned as the foundation of this double. Chroniclers such as Murúa (1987) and Polo de Ondegardo speak in their writings of all animals and birds having a 'similar' in the sky who was in charge of their procreation and multiplication (1965 [1603]). This 'double' is found, according to what has been compiled, in the stars; tradition speaks of every living being in the world of form having a celestial archetype, where the stars take the form of animals. Today we know that in archaeoastronomy and myths the planets are expressions of deities, the stars form animal archetypes and each terrestrial place referenced in the myth has its "double" in the celestial sphere (Santillana & von Dechend, 1969)

The Huarochiri manuscript (Taylor, 1987) calls the energy that allows the manifestation of these "doubles"—*kamak*—the same energy that animates the *wakas* as a manifestation of the sacred, a portal of communication with deities and ancestors. The same manuscript testifies that the people who understand and relate to this energy of the wakas or the "doubles" are the *kamaska*. Murúa says about this:

> *Los camasca...los quales eran como brujos, y tomaban la figura que querían, y yban por el aire en breuísimo tiempo mucho camino, y beían lo que pasaba: hablauan con el demonio, el qual les respondía en siertas piedras, o en otras cosas que ellos respetaban mucho. Estos serbían de adivinos, y referían lo que pasaba en lugares distantes y remotos, antes que se pudiese sauer o benir la nueua de lo que les preguntauan, y ansí en este Reino se an dicho alzamientos y motines y suzesos de batallas, en distancia de más de duçientas leguas y trecientas, el mismo día y tiempo, en que sucedían, o el siguiente, en que por curso natural era ymposible. (1987)*

Polo calls these healers *camasca* or *sunquyuc*. It is interesting to find here again the term *sunqu (shungu)*; it is the same word that, in the Lexicon of Saint Thomas (1951 [1560]), is transcribed as *sunqu* and that appears as a synonym of *camaquenc* and *camaynin*. Thus, *sonco* also designates the transmitted power and *soncoyoc* is the beneficiary of this transmission of power; *camaquenc (/kamaqi-n/ = /kama-q-NIn/)*, composed of *cama*, indicates the source of the vital force transmitted to someone while *camaynin (/kama-y -NIN)*, composed of *cama*, refers to the vital force that has been transmitted to him. This set of terms: *camaquenc*, *camaynin* and *sunqu* are translated by Saint Thomas as the "soul by which we live.'.

Today, *kamay* is the verb that indicates the act of animating, transmitting the vital force that allows the form and maintaining it in that order. In the world of form, the *kay pacha* in which we live, every form is animated to fulfill its origin-destiny, a being to be, and to carry out that experience of upbringing, then memory and knowledge that in the *runas* remains in the *sami* or soul mind of the heart, *nuna sunqu*. Garcilaso de la Vega (2001 [1609]) speaks of *kamak pacha (*in this case the same as *allpa kamak) as the* animating, organizing, feeding earth (potential and latent energy) while *allpa kamaska* is the already animated, fertilized, breeding earth. José María Arguedas (Mamani Macedo, 2019) is more complex in his definition of the llama's *kamak*: "it is like a llama's shadow, a double of this animal that walks through the center of the sky, because it is a darkness of the sky" alluding to the 'double' of the llama located in the dark cloud *—yana phuyu—* called *yamacñawin* or *yacana*, which appears in the greater mayu, the Milky Way, near the Southern Cross.

Then, in the process of formation, the deities, bearers of the *kamak*, do not perform an act of creation from nothing in the Christian style, but of animating, forming and ordering the world. And to do so, they personalize the kamak in kamaken, both at the level of the ayllus, community family among runas, sallqa and wakas, and at the personal level from the pakarinas. If we know how to read the chronicles, we will understand:

> *"... en Tiahuanaco el Hacedor empezó a hacer las gentes y naciones que en esta tierra hay, y haciendo de barro cada nación, pintándoles los trajes y vestidos que cada uno había de traer y tener; y los que habían de traer cabellos, con cabellos; y los que cortado, cortado el cabello; y que concluido, a cada nación dio la lengua que había de hablar, y los cantos que habían de cantar, y las simientes y comidas que habían de sembrar. Y acabado de pintar y hacer las dichas naciones y bulto de barro, dio ser y ánima a cada uno por sí, así a los hombres como a las mujeres; y les mandó se sumiesen debajo de tierra cada nación por sí; y que de allí cada nación fuese a salir a las partes y lugares que él les mandase; y así dicen que los unos salieron de cuevas, los otros de los cerros, y otros de fuentes, y otros de lagunas, y otros de pies de árboles, y otros desatinos de esta manera..." (de Molina, 1943 [1565])*

Likewise, the name of the major deity, *Pachakamak*, has been distorted by the early Quechua dictionaries and by the chroniclers, who were unable to understand the depth of the sacred language. Garcilaso de la Vega himself, who falls into these problems to justify the alleged 'civilization' of his Inca ancestors, nevertheless admits the great error when translating *Pachakamak*: "It is a name composed of *pacha*, which is world universe, and *Kamac*, present participle of the verb *cama*, which is to animate; which verb is deduced from the noun *kama*, which is anima: *Pachacamac* means he who gives anima to the world universe, and in all its own and entire meaning, it means he who does with the universe what the anima does with the body.

The visible plane, knowable by the senses of the body-form is called *ka*, its expression being *aka* (excrement), all fluid clearly perceptible by the mind-soul of the body. The invisible plane, not knowable by the senses, is *wa*, its expression being *awa* (warp). The great synthesis is *waka*, the sacred manifested on this plane, which brings together the two complementarities of the visible and invisible in an inclusive third plane, where everything is possible.

Another fundamental term in the Andean worldview is *Pacha*.

Pacha, understood as the 'space-time' in the "cosmos-world" of form, is everything that contains and sustains. The term is multi-meaningful and multi-dimensional; although the most used meanings are space and time as a complementary duality, it also encompasses place, world, time, and date. A more concrete way of seeing them. It represents two cosmo-telluric forces that interact and express what we know as life, the totality of the visible (pachamama) and the invisible (pachakamak). At the same time, it is pacha and pachakutik, complementary and cyclical duality of stable space-time and unstable, chaotic, transforming space-time, where both space-time and the levels of the world become 'upside down'. An example of a small-scale pachakutik is the transition from day to night, where space-time turns upside down and the uku pacha remains above, different from the hurin pacha which continues inside the allpamama.

Pachamama with her telluric force creates everything that exists in the 'cosmos-world', while the fertilizing principle of pachatata has its own pure cosmic energy invisible to the human eye. Thus, allpamama or Mother Earth emerges. Pachamama gives birth to a new pacha from time to time, a space-time cycle in the world of form.

Pacha as a cyclical and relative 'space-time'. The 'body-soul', the qualified kamaken between essence and form is expressed as an indissoluble unit within a specific space-time. A Quechua aphorism says: ñaupaqman puriy, qhepaman chayay, that is: 'Walk forward and then you will arrive back'. Time is cyclical and spiral in different rhythms that calendars allow, a consciousness of coiling and uncoiling with converging moments of here and now, similar, existential warps and wefts. By its nature, 'space-time' can be penetrated by the perception of the three minds-souls intertwined in a higher vision. It is the phenomenon of achinan, or the ability of the watuq (augurs) to know what happened in the visible before in the spiral and to approach the future, the after. The watuq are those living beings—men, animals or things—that can look forward and back with the lucidity of seers. Very different from our simple memory of past events and the fleetingness of the present. kashanmi is said in Quechua, manaraq chayamushaqtin (it exists, although it has not yet arrived).

For Andean man, *kallpa*, or universally manifested energy-force, is another constant of non-visible reality, complementary to all *kamaken*. It is innate to everything that exists and manifests itself in many ways. There is heat as a form of *kallpa*, either transmitted by the Sun and nesting in the entire fabric of life, protected within the Earth. Or the heat of fire, corporal heat and other forms of this *kallpa*. The seasons and climate depend on the way in which solar-terrestrial energy is distributed, as well as the existence of certain forms of life. Another form of energy is electricity coming from the *illapa*, which manifests itself in storms in the form of lightning (thunder and lightning). These are forms of *kallpa* that are not seen and are known only by their results.

There is a clear relationship between *kallpa*, *kapak* and *sinchi*, regarding energies that carry power, and are related to the powerful. *Kallpa*, as an energy-force, depends on the physical, emotional and mental effort of each *kamaken*, that is, a way of activating the *kamak* energy that each *kamaken* entails. It is this effort of the three minds-souls that allows the *kamaska*, the knower of the *kamak*, to obtain the "power" of acting and the know-how on the different planes of the cosmos-world.

Sinchi unites the quality of effort combined with courage and bravery and is therefore the "strength and courageous"; the strength and valor of the warrior in any of the three minds-soul in which it manifests itself.

Kallpa is used to indicate the power that comes from coherent effort and, above all, the power of the kamaska. Sinchi is the power associated with physical courage, and bravery. Kapak is the power that comes from know-how, from the coherence between what has been experienced, turned into wisdom and expressed as example and service, the authority, which allows the flow of prosperity.

The *kamaska* is the one who can perceive, let flow in himself and towards a being-form the powerful energy of the *kamak*. In the Huarochirí Manuscript, Taylor defines it as "the camasca, who received his "being and sustenance" from various sources, could increase the quality of his bed and become wide camasca (very lively), which allowed him to perform feats worthy of a shaman."

The *amautas* and *curacas* themselves maintained contact with the *kamaken* of their ancestors through the – bultos - or sacred objects, a form of the *kallpa*. There are, then, *kamaken* of the Q*awa-hanan pacha*, the *kay pacha* and the *Hurin-Uku Pacha*. The main ones are the solar bird-jaguar-serpent in their yellow-blue-red surroundings. Every *kamaken*, by having a specific form, carries the *kamak* or spirit of who it represents. It is not limited only to the sacred form, but rather it flows through it from the dimensions of the Q*awa* and the *uku*. Each *kamaken* responds to a specific space-time in the *kay pacha* but flows in the broader and more dimensional levels of the other levels, the *hanan* and the *urin*. It is through a specific ritual, depending on the sacred calendar that shows the space-time at the opening of the portals, when the wise men can, through these *kamaken*, communicate with their ancestors or with the deities that flow through the indicated *wakas*, the *kamaken* of the sacred. And according to the indications recorded by chroniclers and extirpators of idolatries, this communication was given from the soul that carries the *kamaken* to the *sami* or mind-soul of the receiver's *nuna sunqu*, when it is aligned with the *sinchi,* head reason and the *uchay*, mind of the body.

Even the wise men speak of how, if these sacred objects and bundles are destroyed with another intention, their *kamaken* remains available to establish communication with those who can do so in the appropriate space-time and ritual. When sacred objects such as fabrics or ceramics are intentionally broken, according to an established ancestral ritual, this *kamaken* is released to return to its source of *kamak*. Something similar to what happens to us when we pass through the Great Portal that communicates the space-times of what we call life and death, and we leave the two bodies and minds-souls - physical-etheric and rational mental -, passing its memory to the third body, mind-soul of the *nuna sunqu*, of the higher emotion-feeling, to continue our journey through the cosmos-world, in its different levels and dimensions.

That is why the knowledge of our Law of origin and the principles it entails is so important, to acquire the necessary experience of mutual upbringing that makes us true human beings. In this way, to the world that we arrive at to continue our path towards *illa tiqsi*, we will already be trained in that essential human step for our reunion with the Source.

CONCLUSION

The Role of the Amauta: Some Aspects Regarding Pre-Colonial Philosophy

The sources that must be looked at to find the vestiges of a pre-colonial philosophy are very dispersed because the great majority are not written. Oral memory is what has survived and is what has had to be cultivated to keep this vision of the world alive.

Some philosophical ideas are taken from literature, a discipline that has served as an umbrella to classify the production of all pre-colonial Andean knowledge.

The first vestiges of a true philosophical practice in American antiquity are found in the *Chavin, Nazca* and *Paracas* cultures. There we can say that the germ of a deep and complex philosophical practice is found.

What has been able to be collected regarding philosophical practices is based, among others, on the religious hymns compiled by Andrés de Pachacuti and Cristóbal de Molina, as well as the hymns of the *aukis* of *puquio*. In addition to data taken from F. de Montesinos (1642), Inca Garcilaso de la Vega and contemporary historians such as Josep M. Barnadas, Adolfo Cáceres and Jesús Lara among others.

Amawta [ay: wise; <?ama-uta: house of knowledge; <amayaña: to realize, to discover]

For D. de Santo Tomás he was the "curious, ingenious, wise or astute man"; for Ludovico Bertonio (Bertonio, 1612) "very wise, prudent", the Inqa Garcilaso usually defines them as philosophers; all this makes it difficult to ascribe the term to *Aymara* or *Quishwa*. In any case, the sources only manage to trace it in *Tawantinsuyu*, where they were the specialists who knew astronomy, chronology, weather forecasting, writing and preserving history (as a necessary part of the prediction of what can happen) and in all the activities that required the use of the calendar: conservation and interpretation, agricultural data, agronomy (as it appears in the agricultural laboratories of the *Inqa*) and everything related to worship (including the writing of prayers). The preservation of the information suggests the use of some Andean script or its equivalents (*qillqa* and *khipu*) (Barnadas, 2002).

The data from C. de Molina from Cuzco from the list of the *siq'i* of Cuzco (1943 [1565]) and from F. de Montesinos (Idem) suggest —despite the secret and esoteric nature of their knowledge— some direct contact with Spanish researchers. Although the sources do not identify them with the priests, they were at the top of the social hierarchy of the temples. In Montesinos' list it appears as the name or title of the kings of *Tiwanaku*.

Garcilaso de la Vega calls the *amautas* "men of good wit." "They philosophized subtle things and talked about these things in their republics," "they left nothing written because they were not literate," "their inventions died with their inventors," "they only discovered some principles traced in natural light," "they did achieve moral philosophy."

In *Ollantay*, the amauta[12], *Chay jamaut´a Willka Uma*, is mentioned in the personification of the wise old sorcerer *Willka Uma*, who with his mere presence is capable of instilling *mancharisqa*, fear, he is a *llayqata*[13] (*Chijnikunin chay llayqata*) and *watunña*[14]*(ñan watunña chaychu kaychu*), a witch and a sorcerer, who knows more things than other men —*Ñan yachanña iskay mit`a, "Tukuy imatan yachani qanña rikuy yuyawanki*"—.

The power of the amauta within the magical arts is extensible to everything, even to non-humans (*Ima qhenchas chaymi puma, Pay wan khuska purimusqan*). His power is so great even in the divinatory arts, being able to make omens (*Ancha llakita watujtin, Tukuy phutita watujtin*). In the time of the Incas he was an authority, (*Pay rimarin chay pachaqa*)

After defining these categories of the vision, thought, and culture of the original peoples of America, let us be convinced that their recovery is not only an attitude of respect towards our origins, but the possibility of having an essential tool to reorient the education system of the same peoples who inhabit the continent today, and of all the inhabitants of this world, in need of 're-enchanting' and 'reconnecting' as an integral part of the great fabric of life.

REFERENCES

Barnadas, J. (2002). *Diccionario Históríco de Bolivia*. Grupo de Estudios Históricos.

Benedetti, M. (2012). *Witness: The Selected Poems*. White Pine Press.

Bertonio, L. (1612). *Vocabulario de la lengua aymara*. Chucuito: Casa de la Compañia de Jesús por Francisco del Canto.

de Betanzos, J. (1987). *Suma y narración de los incas*. Ediciones Atlas.

de Molina, C. (1943). El Cuzqueño. In *R. Porres Barrenechea, Relación de las Fábulas y los Ritos de los Incas*. Editorial Miranda. (Original work published 1565)

de Montesinos, F. (1642). *Memorias Antiguas y Nuevas del Perú*. Biblioteca Nacional de España.

de Santo Tomás, D. (1951). *Lexicon, o Vocabulario de la lengua general del Peru*. Editado por Francisco Fernandez de Cordoua. (Original work published 1560)

Duviols, P. (2003). *Procesos y visitas de idolatrías. Cajatambo, siglo XVII: con documentos anexos*. Centro de Estudios Rurales Andinos "Bartolomé de las Casas".

Duviols, P. (2016). *Escritos de Historia Andina*. Instituto Francés de Estudios Andinos.

Garcilaso de la Vega, I. (2001). *Comentarios Reales que Tratan del Origen de los Incas, Reyes que fueron del Perú, de su Idolatría, Leyes y Gobierno en Paz y en Guerra*. Ediciones Catedra. (Original work published 1609)

Guamán Poma de Ayala, F. (1956). *La primera nueva crónica y buen gobierno*. Editorial Cultura.

Mamani Macedo, M. e. (2019). José María Arguedas: poeta quechua de la transformación. *Letras*, 110-137. Obtenido de http://www.scielo.org.pe/pdf/letras/v90n132/a05v90n132.pdf

Morin, E. (1999). *Seven complex lessons in education for the future*. UNESCO.

Murúa, M. d. (1987). *Historia Natural y Moral de las Indias*. Historia Viva. Crónicas de América.

Polo de Ondegardo y Zárate. J. (1965 [1603]). De las Huacas I Idolos. En J. Polo de Ondegardo y Zárate, *Relaciones de los ritos y fábulas de los incas* (pág. Cap 1). España: Biblioteca de Autores Españoles.

Restrepo Arcila, R. A. (2002). Sabiduría, Poder y Comprensión. América se repiensa desde sus origenes. Siglo del Hombre Editores: UNESCO.

Santillana, G., & von Dechend, H. (1969). *Hamlet's Mill: An Essay on Myth and the Frame of Time. Gambit*. Gambit.

Taylor, G. (1987). *Ritos y tradiciones de Huarochirí del siglo XVI*. Instituto Francés de Estudios Andinos.

Valera, B. (1945). *Las costumbres antiguas del Perú y La historia de los Incas*. Editado por Francisco A. Loayza.

ENDNOTES

1 There is a crucial difference between a society composed of autonomous individuals and a community, a fabric of human beings, nature and the sacred that act as a whole.

2 The term *chakaruna*, in the Quechua language, literally means "bridge man" and is used for those people who serve as a link between two different visions. They are the ones who create bonds of communication.

3 This subtitle corresponds to a field diary note of one of the authors whose original version is in Spanish and was made in contact with the indigenous spiritual wisekeepers of Abya Yala during his UNESCO position.

4 *Jampiri*, In Quechua, it refers to a herbalist who, by tradition, is dedicated to restoring balance and health to the body and spirit.

5 The term *Kankurua* refers to the ceremonial houses of the Ika, Kogi and Saha Indians of the Sierra Nevada de Santa Marta, Colombia.

6 *Mamo* is the name given to the wise man and spiritual leader of these indigenous Colombian peoples.

7 *Kay pacha*, literally means in Quechua "the land here", it is the conceptualization of the middle world

8 One could think of the combination of two terms: *nuna,* which means spirit, and *nunanchay*, which in Quechua means intellect, thought. It would be the intellect of the spirit.

9 In Quechua *sinchi* means strength.

10 The word *sunqo* in Quechua means heart, and *samay* also means time.

11 Also *Sama*, to encourage, to give breath.

12 Amauta is the philosopher, wiseman, the one who knows.

13 **layqay:***v.tr.* to bewitch; to bewitch; to enchant; **layqa**: s. sorcerer; witch; wizard; sorceress

14 **watuy:***s.* divination with coca leaves by Andean shamans; **watuy**: v.tr. to bewitch

Chapter 7
The Pakasqa Nuna Interface:
The Subconscious Neurophilosophy of the 'Unseen World' From the Law of Origin or First Law

Gabriel Peredo Albornoz
https://orcid.org/0009-0004-3847-249X
Universidad Santo Tomas, Chile

Carlos Prado Mendoza
https://orcid.org/0009-0003-8598-6656
Kuska Cultural Center for Ancestral Wisdoms, Bolivia

Luca D'Ascia
https://orcid.org/0009-0006-0713-4230
Scuola Normale Superior di Pisa, Italy

ABSTRACT

The study explores the intersection of neuroscience, neurophilosophy, and indigenous knowledge systems to address systematic and empirical evidence about the interface between visible and invisible - unseen world - phenomena by examining the Pakasqa Nuna (subconscious) at the ancestral medical practices, providing highlights in the integration of indigenous knowledge into contemporary biomedical and neurocognitive paradigms. Drawing on ethnomedicine practices, the paper proposes a consilient and trandisciplinary approach that bridges cultural and scientific perspectives. It emphasizes the health and wellness as rooted in the

DOI: 10.4018/979-8-3373-0360-4.ch007

interrelation of human, natural, and sacred communities. The study also critiques the limitations of reductionist views in neuroscience and psychiatry, advocating for the reconceptualization of mental health disorders. By exploring altered states of consciousness and their neurophenomenological impacts, the research offers new pathways for integrating spiritual dimensions into global health paradigms and science development.

INTRODUCTION

For many years the discussions and encounters of matter with consciousness have vexed most scientists and philosophers, Many dismiss the creation of reality by observation as having little significance outside the limited domain of the physics of microscopic entities; others, however, argue about the qualities of nature in terms of syntropy, space-time singularity, autopoiesis, dissipative structures, Gaia hypothesis, implicate order, fractal geometry, morphic resonance, synchronicity, syntergetics, neuronal holographic function, symbiogenesis, the memory of water, among others. All of them, at some level, have approached the constitutive matrices of the origin and order of life that the ancestral traditions of the world have shared synchronically and diachronically for more than 20,000 years. (Peredo Albornoz & Prado Mendoza, 2024) [The original version is in Spanish from authors]

In indigenous knowledge, there is no matter experience and consciousness activity without spirituality. A web of warps and wefts weave mutualistic relationships between living, nonliving and more than living organism, visible and invisible phenomena that inhabit to maintain harmony and health of all communities: human, sacred, and natural.

The principles and patterns of life interpretation of indigenous knowledge systems are contained in the Law of Origin, so named in territories of Abya Yala (Restrepo Arcila, 2008; Parra Witte, 2017; Rueda, 2022) or First Law in the indigenous peoples of Africa, Oceania, North America, Asia and Europe (Tanaka, 2000; Yunkaporta, 2019; Redvers, 2020; Grim, 2001; Muñóz González, 1998; Witt, 2006). Ancient cultures share a common core of conserving and strengthening life on the planet based on patterns and principles of nature. The understanding of health as general wellness or *Allinkay*, contains the principles of complementarity, interrelation, correspondence/analogy, and reciprocity for maintaining the rhythm and sequence of life. To treat the sacred or spiritual is to treat the vital energy in a way that illness indicates disharmony or stress in one of the parts of the whole: mind, body, or spirit, in the strict sense, and human community, natural or sacred, in the broad sense. From this framework, a consilient perspective available suggests that both points of view (scientific and cultural) about wellbeing:

(…) is possible only if the communities, which make up the living fabric as a whole, incorporate the sacred, spirituality, in and out of the equation; in this sense, the ancestral American wisdom, in its worldview, thought and culture, integrates the main quality of nature on the permanence of life: Tukuypaq or what is translated as the whole is summarized in the whole, the parts are the whole. As well as Morin's hologrammatic principle, Tukuypaq is a principle of the indigenous knowledge system that implies unity and singularity, with the substantial difference that the implication and translation of the system happen by mutual nurturing. This concept is substantially different from the self-organization of living systems because it considers that the energy/life link, called sahasrara, kumara, kallpa, ajayu, chi, or spirit for each different culture, can be stored even in organisms that do not necessarily possess or perform metabolic functions, have a brain or a nervous system. These conditions are referred to by the academic community as organisms or systems more than living ones, whose characteristic is that they comply with a principle of non-equivalent similarity. That is, organisms may be similar, but never equal in terms of structure, processes, and relationships, so that their contribution to everything fulfills functions with properties with implications in the configurations of life, mind, consciousness, and/or intelligence acquire broader dimensions but only if they are observed in complementarity (Peredo Albornoz & Prado Mendoza, 2024) [The original version is in Spanish from authors]

From this worldview, this paper seeks some guidelines to adjust the neurocognitive-biological-cultural model from Law of Origin and most particularly from the experience treatments reached at Kuska Cultural Center for Ancestral Wisdoms. We emphasize the importance of the P*akasqa nuna* (subconscious) to the understanding of the invisible or 'unseen world' and the possibilities of consilience between neuroscience and ethnomedicine from a neurophilosophy perspective.

STATE OF ART: GAPS AND VACUUMS

Many fundamental and widely applied concepts in neuroscience have a strong anthropological and to a lesser extent archaeological bias with a clear tendency to reduce the phenomena of Indigenous knowledge about human interaction with subtle energy (Sugano, Uchida, & Kuramoto, 1994) -and it is particularly subjective and personal characteristic-from Westernized 'shamanism' (Sun & Kim, 2024). There are two ways of looking at this problem. The first is from the social construction of science (Latour & Woolgar, 1986) and the second is from the scientific facts that contrast the conclusions of social science (Kuhn, 1970). It is important to clarify that what we are dealing with here is not to validate or invalidate the studies on shamanism but rather to make a counterbalance with the tools and advances of scientific knowledge to complement it with our Law of Origin.

Two of the main references, Winkelman (2000) and Eliade (1951), characterize the literature about shamanism from two positions: they propose this knowledge as an epistemology to face the problems of the world (Llamazares, 2011; Krippner, 2000; Cowan, 1999) and, on the other hand, as Yunkaporta state, that ancestral wisdom has been the object of a quasi-religion and a new age science (2024). As concepts, some authors characterize shamanism as: altered states of consciousness (Huels & al, 2021; Frecska, Hoppál, & Luna, 2016); symbolism and language (Hoppál, 2013; Walker, 2001); time and perception (Bogoras, 1925); embodiment and trance (Toriz & al, 2024; Qu, 2021); (Kolankaya-Bostanci, 2014) from the relationships established at the patient-healer level, from the interaction with 'sacred plants' (Schultes, Hoffman, & Ratsch, 2001) 'power animals' (Äikäs & Fonneland, 2012) or power objects (Schaefer, 2023), to bring about changes on the mental health and general well-being (Swanson, 2018) of a given person. The neurochemical and neurobiological processes that happen in conjunction with these elements, usually virtually boil down to the:

> *(...) altered states seem to involve a shift toward increased slow wave activity across the frontal lobes, coupled with increased dominance of limbic system activity (especially in the hippocampus, septum, and amygdala), and a shift toward parasympathetic dominance in the autonomic nervous system. Other common aspects of these states are said to include the synchronization of left and right frontal lobe EEG activity, along with a general shift toward right brain dominance. As the state deepens, there is a gradual decrease in frontal lobe activity followed by a similar decrease in limbic involvement, both of which seem to be associated with transcendent states of consciousness. Other neurological changes involve increases in certain neurochemicals, such as endogenous opiates, as well as blocking of the inhibitory effects of serotonin in the frontal lobes. The overall effect of this complex set of alterations is a broad integration of the various brain modules mentioned above. Winkelman cogently argues that this integrative organismic state is healthy for the client, and for widening circles of the community as well. (Krippner & Combs, 2002)*

From this point of view, studies of 'shamanism' are contextualized in a series of biases that are reduced to laboratory or field studies where behaviors and processes that do little to cover the realm of 'shamanic' power. For example, the extraction of the context and knowledge embodied in shamanism, regardless of where it comes from or is practiced, does not take care the mutualistic interactions with the ecosystem, mainly with the territories or sacred sites where most of the healings take place. On the other hand, shamanism it is not necessarily a concept related to ancestral medical practice in Abya Yala.

We believe that these issues have to do with a consequence of the reductionism that is inherent in any stage of maturity that occurs within science. Despite Indigenous knowledge has gained recognition in the environmental crisis context (Wall Kimmerer, 2020), has often been misinterpreted within decolonial frameworks, overlooking the importance of key concepts for science (social and cognitive), such as *kallpa* - spirit and vital energy - which are crucial for understanding ecosystem functions through mutualistic interactions and offering potential ways to prevent or mitigate the ongoing crisis.

Regarding this point of view, we found parallel concepts to "sacred," such as *illa* in Quechua. 'Plants as teachers' (Luna L. E., 1984), which are a very similar form of sacred plants mentioned below, are viewed as embodied spiritual entities. Even now neurobiology has confirmed that plants and fungi exhibit signs of cognition, consciousness, and communication, functioning like an underground nervous system (Mancuso, 2017; Whitman, 1975; Adamatzky, 2022; Money, 2021; Gardiner, 2012) or agency (Whitaker, Tamboli, Daly, & Lewy, 2024; Brenner & al, 2006; Bynum, 2022; Karban, 2008; Marder, Vattimo, & Zabala, 2013; Gibson & Brits, 2018; Fábregas-Tejeda, I., & Radick, 2025) . These scientific findings resonate with indigenous knowledge about the origin of life (Rueda & al, 2022), linking existence to cosmic and terrestrial ordering principles, and nurturing the anatomy of Mother Earth (Peredo Albornoz & Prado Mendoza, 2024). Forests and mountains are viewed as nerve endings, which connect *qawa* (the unseen world) with *ukhu* (the physical world) through *kallpa*, supporting a view of health that integrates human, natural, and sacred communities. On the human-sacred interactions the studies are commonly through the use of 'sacred plants' (Diaz, 2010; Shanon, 2003), but 'shamans' see the states of consciousness far as hallucinations or trance states of consciousness. They see it as a visit to realms where the sacred is *"Illa tiqsi"* or *"Illapa*, the lightning as ancestor," representing the fundamental and also invisible energy that gives and takes life (Luna & Amaringo, 1999; Restrepo Arcila, 2023).

Today, the 'invisible' is explored in modern biology through the study of morphic fields (Sheldrake, 2010) and the mycorrhizal network (Sheldrake M., 2023). Other "invisible" phenomena occur in what our indigenous knowledge finds as planetary nerve endings: mountains like the Great Tata Licancabur in the Atacama region (Glockner, 2004; Hubert, Baudry, & Saez, 2024) and forests (Dengel, Aeby, & Grace, 2009). Both are given by heightened cosmic ray activity.

From our cultural knowledge, to encourage this kind of exploration, concerning to the neurophenomenology of shamanism and following the steps of Varela (1996) about searching for additional pragmatism elements into neuroscience, perhaps have to start from what we call P*akasqa nuna (subconscious or the hidden spirit)* because in the light of the unseen world (Eddington, 1929) or spiritual world, there it happens most of the visible activity that is not registered by senses or by the classical physiological system model of the functioning of cognition and body.

Despite of science biases about shamanic practices, there is only a paper where most of the indigenous knowledge have been methodologically transducted (Ibañez, 1991) and is the most close related to what is the true image of what we are trying to show. The work of Trnka & Lorencova (2022), insights about similar concepts to consciousness. Extended reference were extracted.

In contrast to consciousness, the constructs of soul and spirit from the perspective of recent cognitive science are considered to be examples of supernatural, paranormal, or afterlife beliefs (…) Basic conceptualizations of consciousness varied widely across the studied indigenous cultures. Consciousness of an individual may be understood as a state of mind (e.g. San, Guajiro), faculty of mind (Kogi), subjectivity (Warlpiri), experience (e.g. Saami, Dene Tha, Oglala), kind of being (Blackfoot, Yuit, Kai), sensing (Yup´ik), living (Bakongo), as a kind of soul (e.g. Cherokee, Tungus, Ayoreao, Cashinahua), energy (Nahua), vital force (Tlingit), or capacity to respond to communicative signals (Araweté) (…) In a holistic sense, the consciousness is believed to be interconnected and shared with other humans, but also nonhumans (John, 2009). (…) consciousness is believed to be a kind of soul. For example, Cherokee people consider an individual's consciousness to be one of the souls that an individual owns (Kilpatrick, 1995). Four souls are distinguished by the Cherokee. The "soul of consciousness" denotes an individual's consciousness and is located in the head or throat. The remaining three souls are the "hepatic soul" located in the liver, the "visceral soul" located in the flesh and associated with blood, and the "osseous soul", which resides in the bones and is associated with sperm. The Cherokee model of consciousness considers an individual's consciousness to have the characteristics of a soul, which expects consciousness to be a spiritual essence of the human body.

Some indigenous cultures understand consciousness as an experience of the corporeal, real world. This is the case of Saami people, who distinguish two spheres of the world, the corporeal, or real world and the spiritual netherworld (Lehtola, 2002). Consciousness is closely related to all the experiences experienced in corporeal reality. However, the divide separating the spiritual netherworld from the corporeal, real world can be traversed when conscious experience is "transported" during a shaman's ecstatic practice.

Interestingly, conceptualizations of consciousness differ in the extent and diversity of the semantic space that relevant mental representations occupied in different indigenous cultures. Some of the concepts are highly polysemic. For example, the Nahua concept *teotl* includes many aspects, i.e. consciousness, but also an ever-flowing, ever-changing energy-in-motion, self-generating and self-conceiving sacred energy, power, or force, and a unified totality of all things (Maffie, 2008). In Cashinahua people, consciousness is identified with the concept of body soul, *yuda yuxin*, that, however, denotes also memory, thoughts, feelings, and individuality (McCallum, 1996). The Maasai concept of *oltau* at the same time denotes heart, mind, spirit, as well as soul (Westerlund, 2006). For Guna people, consciousness is a part of polysemic concept *burba* denoting soul, consciousness, the spiritual principle, shadow, reflection on water, echo, culture, essence, and way of being at the same time (Martínez Mauri, 2019). [The references are from the authors]

Even altered states of consciousness are added

> (…) some of the indigenous cultures understood altered states of consciousness as states with changed perception or imagination. Altered states are considered to be a different kind of "body knowing" (Cashinahua), ability to see spirits (Ndembu), personal visions (Blackfoot, Oglala), or hidden faculties of the mind enabling contact with the divine sphere, i.e. with the essence of being (Kogi). Second (…) are also understood as a different kind of being, e.g. as being outside one's own body, or as being possessed and detached from their one's vital force to search the cosmos for aid (Akawaio).

Third, are often explained as a kind of movement or travel, e.g. as moving into the magical sphere of ancestors' spirits (Bakongo). Saami people propose a kind of an ecstatic transport into the "other world" by traversing the divide separating the spiritual netherworld from the corporeal, real world (Lehtola, 2002). In Desana, altered states are understood as ecstatic flights, by which an individual is returned to the universe described symbolically as an immense womb. Inside this womb, an abstract cosmic brain charged with energies is believed to exist, and there, the individual becomes witness to cosmogonic episodes (Reichel-Dolmatoff, 1989). The metaphor of returning to an immense womb represents a symbolic return to a state before one's consciousness is born. From this perspective, altered states of consciousness are understood as a way of getting to the universal sphere of all-inclusive consciousness, which is represented by the immense womb. [The references are from the authors]

The same perspectives are integrated at Mind–Body and Soul-Body differentiation

In Nahua people, consciousness, mind, but as well as body and matter are considered to be of same quality, i.e. a kind of energy teotl denoting a unified totality of all things that is essentially becoming, changing, and in motion (Maffie, 2008). (…) Akan people believed that the soul is not connected with any bodily organ but is dispersed in every part of the human body as well as in body fluids (Akesson, 1965). Another pattern of soul-body differentiation can be found in Ata Tana 'Ai people (Lewis, 1988) who believe that self is created by a first layer, i.e. the body (ha lapen), which gives shape to the soul (rua lapen). Furthermore,

Tlingit people conceptualize a person to be composed of multiple layers. The incorporeal components of a person consist of two aspects, breath (x'aséikw), which is a person's life force, and a person's mind (toowú), the locus of thoughts and emotions. This incorporeal part of a person was believed to be enveloped by three layers, 1) the bones (sáagí) – the chief material component of the body and its inner essence, and the outer layers of 2) flesh (daadleeyí) and 3) skin (cháatwu). Very interestingly, Tlingit people do not even have a single term for a body as a whole (Kan, 2015). [The references are from the authors]

The same authors agree that concepts such as soul, spirit, and consciousness do not maintain stable semantic meanings over time, and this is because in indigenous knowledge every part comes the other but the same part at some point. In a previous work done (2024) *qawa* could take the form of *ukhu* depending on which cosmic or terrestrial order is located and what is talked about. At this point, the notion of 'unseen world' by René Dubos (1962) engages with indigenous knowledge. The complexity of the microbial world, offers a comprehensive view of how microorganisms interact with the environment and higher organisms like plants or sacred places, where human becomes *ukhu* of a more than living organism which is *Pachamama* Mother Earth and Space-Time at the same time.

Finally, additional consilience between science and cultural knowledge could be found.

other indigenous concepts of consciousness correspond less to recent scientific theories, for example, consciousness as being an energy, a vital force, or a kind of soul (but see recent discussions concerning the application of the free-energy principle to the hard problem of consciousness, e.g. Solms, 2019). (…) the conceptualization of altered states of consciousness by San people, also has its counterpart in scientific discourse. San people describe altered states as a kind of physical process that radically changes the state of matter. Similarly, Glicksohn (2001) compared the change of consciousness from a normal to altered state to be analogous to the change in physical state of water from liquid to steam or ice. This natural analogy of change of consciousness with physical processes mirrors the process called temporary symmetry restoration (Sundararajan & Fatemi, 2016) (…) Interestingly, some of the insights that emerged during the analysis of indigenous concepts may also suggest some broader implications. In Oglala and other Sioux groups, a fundamental force called the "Great Mystery" breathes the spirit into a human body at birth (DeMallie, 1987). After death, the spirit is believed to be transformed into a kind of non-local state that can be described as "being everywhere and pervading all nature". This idea is very similar to the concept of the "quantum sea", which originally emerged in physics (Puthoff, 2002) and was later also applied in anthropology (Trnka & Lorencova, 2016) and research of indigenous mythologies (Laughlin & Throop, 2001). The quantum sea is an all-pervasive energetic field including quantum vacuum energy that is a random, ambient fluctuating energy existing even in so-called empty space. This field is a single underlying substructure that is common for the entire universe and represents a primary source for the emergence of all material objects, as well as non-material processes (Puthoff, 2002; Trnka & Lorencova, 2016). The conceptual basis of the metaphor of the "quantum sea" is similar to the Sioux concept of the "Great Mystery". This example illustrates how conceptual development in science may reach similar conceptual meaning as indigenous knowledge. Of course, these similarities may be random results of parallel developments of thought in science and conceptual knowledge of some cultures. The parallel emergence of two similar conceptual meanings may be explained by the principle of equifinality (Pervin, 2001). This principle, coming from dynamic systems theory, suggests that the same endpoint can be reached through different routes. [The references are from the authors]

This linked knowledge suggests that the 'consilience' (Wilson, 1998) or transdisciplinary methodology (Nicolescu, 2010) from the indigenous knowledge framework is not only possible but urgent and even can be modelized. The key to managing planetary health is about integrating spirituality into the equation of life as the indigenous knowledge, enhancing our resilience against climate crises and pandemics. As Indigenous spiritual knowledge keepers teach: we must understand that together and not separated is the path to well-being (Kuska Cultural Center, 2024) (Wisekeepers, 2013). This is a time for the *chakaruna* (bridge people), time for the *Usqullu* embedded methodology, time to observe the Andean Cat (*Leopardus jacobita*) and to recover its ancient codex from the Atacama Desert (Villalobos, Sanderson, & Vergara, 2023).

BEYOND THE ARROW OF TIME. CONCEPTIONS IN THE EXPERIENCES WITH SACRED PLANTS AND IN THE REFLECTION OF CONTEMPORARY PHYSICS

Following the lines before, this section contribution is based is as we see about the visiting the unseen world that takes place in altered states of consciousness which exhibits a parallelism with the reflection of modern physics. This is not intended to confuse two epistemologies, the logical and the intuitive, but rather, respecting the specific contribution of each, to arrive at a fuller understanding of what sea quantum metaphor means from a various record testimony of people who have experience .

We will now clarify some points that are of great methodological relevance. In the set of experiences of alteres states of consciousness we find traditional contexts in which the entheogenic substance is delivered by a shaman belonging to an indigenous lineage and an increasing number of non-traditional contexts where the deliverer belongs to a hybrid culture and has appropriated indigenous elements from a requirement of enrichment of their "mestizo" or "western" culture, often with a scientific and/or therapeutic approach. It is obvious that there are clear differences between the two typologies: for example, indigenous societies were hierarchical, while hybrid groups tend to import elements ("We are all ancestors") into the entheogenic experience; and this element is framed in a strong subjectivization of the experience of expanded states of consciousness in hybrid contexts, as a result of which the attention to the individual subconscious replaces the listening to the spirits. However, we are convinced that these differences do not erase an underlying unity. If a westerner knows well the path of his own culture, he will intertwine in his experience the individual and the historical-mythological-collective in the same way as someone who belongs to a native people; he will observe with astonishment that some clearly metamorphic images and especially some reptiloid forms - for many Amazonian peoples taking ayahuasca, the entheogen that is most important for their cultural heritage, means looking at the world from the point of view of the serpent - bring him back to a jungle that perhaps he does not know in depth; He will even come to see, in its severe blackness of volcanic rock covered with thorns, those places of origin of the entheogen (the Wirakuta desert in the case of peyote) that he has never had the opportunity to visit in "real" life. We believe that this partial universality of experiences in the midst of a notable cultural difference has to do not so much with the biochemical modus operandi of the substance itself, which would be too generic a causal factor, as with a certain cognitive and psychological adaptogenic function of its prescribed use.

> *(...) the adaptogenic function that derives from the use of these psychoactive substances appears with sufficient clarity even when analyzing the exegesis that the natives themselves make of such consumption (...) That is to say, that the systemic order in which each subject is immersed - the mind and its cultural training - seems to receive a dynamic and renovating (neganotropic) orientation from the imagery generated by entheogens. For this, the subject must first enter into what we could call a controlled crisis, which allows to decompose the old order to verify its usefulness according to the new ends and resources envisioned, and thus keep the system in continuous movement, with life. (Fericgla, 1997) [The original version is in Spanish]*

The person, both 'shaman' and patient or non-indigenous, seeks through the intake of entheogens a better adaptation when making personal decisions, either by leaving behind concrete additions or by renewing his mental universe through a greater sense of connection - the living force of nature, the metamorphic "goddess" of which many Westerners educated outside of any religious dogma speak - that allows to relativize small and great personal sufferings (Badini, 2020). Taking this premise into account, it seems important to place the temporal perception in this adaptogenic context of the experience of entheogens: the time of everyday life, the time articulated in past, present and future, the time "divided into hours", as the existentialist poet Ingeborg Bachmann calls it, to have an intuition of the quantum "no time" and thus reach a better understanding of human time, the only one we really live, a limited but necessary perspective on the matter density experience.

We are now approaching the more specifically scientific part of this contribution where we will be guided by an Italian physicist who is not afraid of flat and informative exposition of concepts whose elaboration requires a very hard mathematical training: Carlo Rovelli. However, before arriving at this clarification it will be appropriate to clear the ground preliminarily of an objection raised by Fericgla himself. What kind of temporal alteration does the experience with entheogens really produce in us?

> *In any case, it is important to point out that under the effect of this entheogen neither the perception of time nor that of space is distorted. At most, it happens that during the two to three hours that the effect lasts, there are so many and so intense visions and/or experiences of endogenous origin that the subject is usually overwhelmed by it and has the sensation that time passes slower than usual. That is to say, there is a clear modification of the "experience of time" (the experience that each one has of time is related to the emotional content that tinges each moment of life), but there is no modification of the "temporal perception" (the experience that each one has of time is related to the emotional content that tinges each moment of life). (Fericgla, 1997) [The original version is in Spanish]*

This generalization, in our opinion rather hasty, contrasts with the evidence of the interviews with non-indigenous people who have participated in Ayahuasca ceremonies and who although they all begin with observations related to the "experience of time" -perhaps because it is the most accessible dimension to common sense-, "go up" to report an overcoming of the "Arrow of Time": from the past, anguishingly irrevocable, towards the future, supposedly open and anxiogenic because of this same openness. They "go up" to relate an overcoming of the "Arrow of time" as a condition of the adaptogenic and specifically therapeutic function of *illa.*

> *I would say that this happened to me twice, the two times that I took that were really transforming and that had a very different connection with time, because these two times are moments that I will not really call transcendental, but a very clear awareness of what was happening to me. It was like a visualization that put in mixture as past, present and future at the same time, like a certain key, it was as if at that point a certain knot, in my case in the reading that I make a certain psychological knot, a certain emotional knot or it could also be considered a spiritual knot, no, there is a certain point of jamming, a certain difficulty of resolution that in these points of jamming also that in the psychism*

itself are points that are outside of the temporal dimension so much that they are not resolved in linear time, they are things from the past that remain and things that you repeat and that... Therefore they are questions that are not in the time line of the daily action, but that base all your daily actions, a little bit more, and in these shots I really had even clarity, it is like a very big light, where there is a position from the outside, as if you look at the question where it comes from, where it is, where it goes, no, it is like an awareness, an instantaneous awareness of what is happening, and with this instantaneous awareness, this clarity that comes, this unblocking also produces lines that I would not say a direction of action, but lines of escape, no? Once you see this you can decide more clearly what lines of flight you are going to take, because even if the linearity apparently has a clear causality, in the point of view there are many causalities that are not in the consciousness, so this is already present in the daily life in a less conscious way. But in the taking of ayahuasca it is as if the consciousness of what is happening makes a splitting, a temporal splitting. You unfold yourself and this unfolding allows another position from where you start when you return from the process. That's why sometimes it can be so transforming, because as you have, you make a jump inside your own consciousness and you come out another, you don't come out another person but you come out another person, you come out another person with other perspectives of yourself and of what surrounds you. That it is possible, is what I am reflecting on now, it is possible that the cure, the healing that it produces comes perhaps from this unfolding of space/time that occurs in these moments where you can have experiences that occurred in another space and in another time and in some way also live space/time projections related to the experience (First Testimonial)

This testimony is interesting because it relates to a temporal experience that 'mental dialogism' in which Fericgla himself sees the active principle of the adaptogenic efficacy or *Illa* of Ayahuasca. The super-temporality of the algid moments of an "intake" acts, so to speak, as a homeopathic remedy for situations of psychological blockage which are also super-temporal insofar as they cage the neurotic subject in a coercion to repeat that hinders his adaptive evolution. But, at an even higher level of "controlled crisis", the super-temporality of entheogenic experiences exerts its therapeutic role above all by controlling the fear of death which is a consequence of the subject's immersion in linear time. As we shall see in more detail by approaching Rovelli's thought, the human experience of time is basically thermodynamic: the river of time coincides with the dispersion of heat that accompanies the work of a force; the second law of thermodynamics, which postulates the increase of entropy in the universe, is the only description of processes oriented in time admitted by physics. The old does not become young, hot things get cold. The physical wear and tear of the living organism, which day after day comes to place us in time, seems to deny the timeless giving of the superindividual life of nature - the *Pachamama (which means Mother Earth or Space-Time)* - is perceived instead in the sensory intensity of the expanded state of consciousness and which in Western philosophy Schopenhauer described as the "*Nunc stans*", the absolute presentiality of the universal preconscious will. However, symbolic death which is a simple psychological possibility in the context of ayahuasca, becomes an inevitable experience - according to the testimonies - before more powerful entheogens such as *Bufo alvarius*. After a deep darkness, this experience leads to a deep and luminous rebirth, as the womb narratives.

> *With the Bufo alvarius I can tell you that there I did experience death and the complete dissolution of everything, of everything: time, of space, of everything, but completely. As well as with the Ayahuasca, Wachuma, mushrooms and these types of substances there is always a space in which we leave space for the consciousness, that is, we do not completely turn off the rational part, we leave space for observation of what is happening, but with Bufo alvarius. It completely turns off this part and it is also the experience of living and being born as such. Everything disappears, everything, it is so difficult to explain, it breaks, everything breaks and suddenly you go to the light and you are light and a little bit the sensation of.... then when you take the Bufo there is a very strong fight because of course, you see that you are going to crash and you are going to die and the Ego has so much fear and so much resistance and you start a fight and it is something so strong that there is nothing as strong as that ... well the fight of pure and hard survival at some point, but there is a point when you cannot fight with and when you let go it is like the feeling of rising, you become part of the peak experience, that is, when you let go and let yourself go and it seems to me that it leaves a very transcendent sensation in this case, because that is what gives you life, the sexual aspect, the orgasm is what is in life and when we take the bufo and we die and we are born and really in this moment we die it is something so linked, it makes all the sense and it is also a very familiar sensation, like finding... as if all of a sudden you have been there, we have been dead, so we have been in the light and we have decided to reincarnate and we will die again and we will be there again and it is the cycle of life. So when you take the Bufo alvarius and you have this experience is that you no longer have doubts about anything, is that you already know, you know what it is, you have lived it, as if you could remember being dead and suddenly be born again, then, well, suddenly you find yourself in the light, everything is light, and you are part of the light and it is an absolute fullness. And from there, when you come back to yourself, the Bufo alvarius lasts about fifteen minutes, in fact I have a video that was made while I was on the trip, fifteen minutes, but, of course, the experience is eternal, that is eternal, there is no, there is no longer or shorter time, no, there*

is nothing like that, it is to be in the fullness and in the whole and you are part of it, but there is always the conscience, at least with the Bufo alvarius there is this conscience of I am, I am this, then when I opened my eyes and I came back to myself at the beginning my eyes opened and as I became conscious again of where I was, of who was with me, Michaela was with me, etc., but everything was white in my eyes, I could not see clearly, I saw everything white, it was all light and little by little the light went away and I was here again, it was like being born again, literally, being born again and understanding that we are here for something, we have a mission to do here, we have things to do here because if we would not be here, what are we doing here? We are working here and well, life here is finite, there are some physical laws that we have to weigh and, well, I remember that I came back to myself, I was looking at the grass, and then I looked at the tree tops and I started to cry and it was like the feeling of having died and being born again and the feeling that when I die, being dead is absolute peace, there is no need to be afraid of death because it really is peace. What happens is that if it is true that surrendering to death is something very strong because the Ego puts up a lot of resistance, but all the pain is caused by our Ego resistance, in reality if we were able to let ourselves flow through life as it is, we would not suffer, because we would understand that ... what I mean is that in the end all the pain we make ourselves. At least that is one of the teachings I had with it. (Second Testimonial)

In this striking testimony, different philosophical-religious traditions are mixed, from Buddhist detachment - which is also the renunciation of individual will, Schopenhauer's noluntas - to the Pythagorean-Platonic reincarnation, which is also a belief shared by some indigenous groups, especially by the indigenous populations of the region Mesoamerican Mayan cultures that conceive it as a reversibility of the "arrow of time" (the soul of the deceased, so to speak, "rejuvenates" until it is reincarnated) (Pitarch Ramón, 1996). However, beyond the complex syncretistic game that takes place when the context of the assumption of entheogens is not traditional indigenous but is framed in a situation of cultural hybridization, the central notion of a total time, without past, present and future, without directional arrow that heals the misalignments of the individual will is familiar to us if we look at the rivers of three banks of the Amazonian tradition. The river, symbol of time, has in mythology its "three-dimensional" moment: it is when it is not contained by its two banks only, which correspond to objective and instrumental time as a tool of scientific measurement which, as we shall see shortly, in the most recent developments of quantum theory has ended up disappearing from the equations that describe the fundamental structures of reality.

In the Amazonian cosmovision there is an antithesis between human time and the total time of nature. To delve into this antithesis we will choose as a guide the poet and novelist César Calvo, who intertwines ethnology and avant-garde literature in his disconcerting diary of travel and knowledge, “The three halves of Ino Moxo”. It is the “go on and further come on” of the Ayahuasca memories of an already unfolded protagonist, César Calvo, who is also his cousin César Soriano, who interacts with a series of increasingly ungraspable “sorcerers”, since each one of them is a mask, a mask of a “sorcerer”, because each one of them is the mask of another one who from deeper in the jungle (in the real and metaphorical sense) grants him his visionary powers, until he reaches the most powerful of all, the charismatic *amawaka* chief Ino Moxo, hero of the indigenous resistance against the rubber tappers' aggression. What the “sorcerer” Don Javier, supported by the sub-wisdom of Ino Moxo's alter ego, the chief campa Inganíteri, speaks about time deserves to be compared with the non-indigenous testimonies we have examined so far.

Back then, this time did not exist, the one that grows weary and lies down to rest like people do. It wasn't like it is now—fragmented. Today, only a few sorcerers, kaiziboreri, or smoking shamans, shirimpiáre, can manage to bring that time back, and no more than for one night, or two full nights at most. They summon it down from the air, gathering the scattered, orphaned remnants of that time and bringing them together through nights and nights of intense focus, after fasting for two or three weeks—days of eating only fire-roasted plantains, drinking only stream water, remembering, repeating, or inventing powerful prayers, magical songs, precise ícaros, and the most appropriate and powerful invocations.

That is how time returns, like a loving cloud of silvery pollen, and once again fills The House of the Calling. Master Ino Moxo is one of the rare shirimpiáre who possess the gift of persuading time to return to its original state, to fulfill its first purpose.

You must know that before, when Pachakamaite had not yet decided that Kaametza [the first woman] should be born, time did not serve to frame the cycle of the living. It was not its role to mark the transition from what lives to what dies and from what dies to what returns to life differently, eternally. No.

The first purpose of time was to create happiness, to prevent harm in life, in this world and in others beyond. If something or someone was occupied by evil and spread it, time would make that thing or person stop growing. It didn't kill them—no, because in the nature of that time, death did not exist. It would stop them, which was worse. At the same time, it would accelerate the greatness of what was great, nurturing the spirits Above. A young spirit would gain the wisdom of a thousand years.

Don't forget that time had three shores: it could go and return at the same time, while also remaining still, fixed, as landscapes moved around it. The landscapes were the ones that returned and advanced toward the sea.

That is why Master Ino Moxo, when he is under the cloud, after piecing together fragments of that time and bringing it down, infused with silvery breezes, nourishes his understanding with that ancient pollen. He multiplies the population of powers that live and work in his wisdom, fills his memory with the intelligence of thousands of lives, and strengthens his ability to see. (Calvo, 1995) [The original version is in Spanish]

Enrich this "mythology of time" with more details in another discourse by Don Javier, which points to a paradoxical and intrinsically contradictory conception of reality, akin to the "coincidence of opposites" in Western philosophy.

You will be granted the knowledge of truth, the deceitful face of truth, and timeless truth. You will see the three shores… The radiance and shadow of the blood of time, of time that is both one and all. What was true for yesterday will not be so for tomorrow. The same ancient time that brought us death also offered us the life to come. Hear me well: the air will become water, and the water will become air. Everything, absolutely everything, is reversed. Everything is always reversed. And the water, which is the air of the fish, will drown the wings of the Evil One. (Calvo, 1995)

It seems clear that this unfragmented time, which denies dualistic thought, carries a longing for renewal that a Westerner might rationalize in terms of individual psychological unblocking. However, for the Indigenous person, it is projected into objective configurations of a mythological nature, such as the enchanted being (the benign *Chullachaki*) who accompanies César Calvo to the village of Ino Moxo, a privileged place of initiation, and who not by coincidence appears as a child. But:

it is not a child, not the Chullachaki childhood of the Sorcerer of Sorcerers. It is timeless time—not this time that builds ruins and leads life to death, but the guide of death that lives. This child is the guide of lives that never die, the eternal creator of beauty and happiness. (Calvo, 1995)

The 'shaman' therefore heals by invoking an original, non-directional time. Something of the foundational utopia of the collective worldview and the fullness of mythological origins reverberates in individual healing. However, the direction of human time does exist and manifests as decline and diminishment. A loss of divinatory powers that also reminds us of the entropic dispersion of thermodynamics, but which should primarily be understood as a mythological transposition interpretation of specific circumstances in Indigenous origin narrative: diaspora, cultural uprooting, perception of threat due to the invasions of rubber tappers and settlers, expulsion from sacred places like the Gran Pajonal (an earthquake for the white people which is reinterpreted as the appearance of a Great Jaguar).

Because in this first then, day and night lived within a single one, there was no difference; by day it was, and by night it was the same time (...) And time passed in vain. It was there that time calmed down and divided, just like the Sacred River, the Urubamba, the Willkamayu of the Inkas of Cusco, father of the Ucayali and grandfather of the Amazon, who has no relatives. Time passed in vain, and no one responded to Narowé [the first man]. And Narowé knew the taste of tears (...) I have known, the air has provided me, that long before, all humans knew in advance, in the time without time, I have seen them. They looked at the future as one looks at what has already gone. With time, perhaps, or with their night, they began to lose these powers. Today, only a few can, generally children or shirimpiarés, sorcerers. As newborns, we all have such gifts, many more powers, but as we grow, we move backward, for whatever reason, and we lose them. Speaking, for example. (Calvo, 1995)

It would take us too far, within the scope of this contribution, to delve further into the specific context to which these words of Ino Moxo refer. It has become evident to us that in the Amazonian worldview, there is a direct relationship between the effectiveness of shamanic healing based on the use of entheogens and the evocation of a mythical time that is only possible through a change in the temporal perspective of the subject who takes the sacred potion. By questioning the arrow of time, this subject activates a set of "lost" neural connections, erased from an early age by education in instrumental rationality and its commands of discourse. Of course, there is a huge distance between the clear statements of ancestral wisdom – which, of course, become increasingly "unclear" as skepticism also progresses in the Indigenous world – and the vague perception of a temporal fracture that a Westerner may experience in the context of an "intake" of entheogens.

It seemed to me that I was climbing a spiral staircase, and from that moment onward, I found myself in an empty, dark space, where the plant continued telling me something, but it could not be visualized or heard. Instead, it was destined to remain inside, in a silence of the Self. And when the effect began to wear off, it seemed to me that that segment of my existence, of undetermined duration, did not fit in any way with the previous and subsequent phases of the "intake," which had been marked by the usual lucidity and clarity about "my" space-time location. (Third testimonial)

Despite this distance, there is a common element, which is perceiving everyday time as something constructed, not original and constitutive of reality itself. Going beyond this time is a mental experiment that can be beneficial. It is not a whim, but a cognitive necessity. Practical, fragmented time makes sense within a horizon of knowledge that relates it to something different, which does not negate it but assigns it a specific function, for us and not for the universe, and removes the illusion that it is reality. For the Amazonian worldview, as we already know, this "something different" is the river of three shores. But what about us Westerners, who insist on trivializing science into technology and time into linear progress, yet in reality, we know very well that the theory of our scientific knowledge operates on a completely different plane from our everyday certainties?

To answer this question, which is fundamental for situating expanded states of consciousness in a cognitive and adaptogenic dimension – the more we know that "there is also something else," the less we worry about the apparent limitations, which are not really limitations, of daily tasks – it will be necessary to take one more step in our intercultural conversation and invite the powerful Ino Moxo to hand the word over to the quantum physicist Carlo Rovelli.

This scientist from Verona, the Italian city where Dante Alighieri composed much of his *Divine Comedy*, is deeply convinced of the complementarity of knowledge, conceiving science as a dialectic of intuition and methodology. He does not hesitate to cite the Buddhist thinker Nagarjuna, who knew nothing of quantum energy or "non-commutative algebra," when presenting his fundamental thesis: reality is made of events, not things or substances, whether spiritual or material, that each take place in their own time, or better said, they are this time that is configured as a quantum field, not as an external and objective framework according to the Newtonian paradigm, and exist in their ever-changing relational context. Being-in-itself coincides with being-for-others.

None of the strata that time has lost (unity, direction, independence, present, continuity) calls into question the fact that the world is a network of events. One thing is time with its numerous determinations, and another is the simple fact that things do not "exist": they happen (...) For a long time, we have tried to understand the world in terms of some primary substance. Physics has perhaps pursued this primary substance more than any other discipline. But the more we study it, the less comprehensible the world appears in terms of something that "is"; instead, it seems much more understandable in terms of relationships between events (...) We understand the world in its becoming, not in its being. (Rovelli, 2018) [The original version is in Spanish]

The challenge is to continue thinking about reality as essentially dynamic – the metamorphic life of the jungle, which is updated in the imagery of ayahuasca, could be a good metaphor for this dimension – giving up a framework that, like Cartesian axes, assigns a priori meaning to any coordinate that may appear in the measurement-interaction process. What is imagined – imagined, as a sensory transposition of an enormously complex mathematical formalism – are rings of space-time (*Pachamama*) subject to a logic of probability like any quantum phenomenon since Heisenberg replaced the exact determination of the variables of a physical system with his "matrix" algebra that related tables of possible values. A microscopic dimension of which we can only have a highly abstract concept and/or a visionary intuition, which bears a strong resemblance to the "time without time" of expanded states of consciousness.

> *We cannot conceive of duration as continuous; we must imagine it as discontinuous: not as something capable of flowing uniformly, but as something that, in a certain sense, jumps, like a kangaroo, from one value to another (...) In the 12th century, the great philosopher Maimonides wrote: "Time is composed of atoms, that is, of many parts that can no longer be subdivided further because of their short duration" (Maimonides, Guide for the Perplexed, I, 73, 106a). (...) The physical substrate that determines duration and temporal intervals – the gravitational field – not only possesses a dynamics influenced by masses; it is also a quantum entity that has no determined values except when it interacts with something (...) Time is not unique: there is a different duration for each trajectory; it passes at different rates depending on the place and the speed. It has no orientation: the difference between past and future does not exist in the basic equations of the world, it is a contingent aspect that appears when we observe things, neglecting the details; from this blur, the past of the universe was in a strangely "peculiar" state. The notion of "present" does not work: in the vast universe, there is nothing we can reasonably call "present." The substrate that determines the durations of time is not an independent entity, distinct from the others that make up the world; it is an aspect of a dynamic field. It jumps, fluctuates, becomes concrete only when interacting, and is not defined below a minimal scale... What remains of time? (Rovelli, 2018) [The original version is in Spanish]*

What remains of time, according to Rovelli's hypothesis, is a "perspective" essential to the human biological being: a specific "blur" that, due to the impossibility of considering all the parameters of order, forces us to interpret thermodynamic phenomena as an increase in entropy. Once it is admitted that time is not a privileged, primitive variable, but a derived phenomenon, its emergence as a complex phenomenon can be explained from the first principle of thermodynamics (conservation of energy) as something that derives from the energy equilibrium state of a system that undergoes all possible microscopic (undetermined) configurations energetically equivalent. Not energy in time, but time in energy. The "river of time" would, in short, be a metaphor for an evolutionary adaptation: the movement from the past to the future and the irreversibility of processes that involve the dissipation of heat are nothing but the a priori form in which a given physical system, ours, shapes the information it has been storing (Manorea, 2004). Of course, we establish correlations with what is essential for our survival, just as any physical system has information about the other physical systems surrounding it (for example, the cell membrane of a marine bacterium reacts to the sugar levels in its environment, and this correlation is a basic form of information storage). The oriented time exists in us not in things. According to St. Augustine's intuition, while it does not exist for a "quantum" consciousness, purely hypothetical, which would imply the elimination of the specific "blur." As expressed by the protagonist of a science fiction novel by mathematician Alain Connes in terms that unmistakably evoke the experience of expanded states of consciousness.

> *I had the unheard-of fortune of experiencing a global perception of my being, not at a specific moment of its existence, but as a 'whole.' I was able to compare its finitude in space, against which no one rebels, with its finitude in time, which, on the other hand, scandalizes us so much." // Then, it will return to time: "I had the impression of losing all the infinite information provided by the quantum scene, and this loss was enough to irresistibly drag me into the river of time." The emotion that arises from this is an emotion of time: This emergence of time seemed to me a kind of intrusion, a source of mental confusion, of anguish, of fear, of dissociation. (Rovelli, 2018)*

Dissociation, that is bifurcation, which relativizes the 'sea quantum' feeling of belonging to nature, that subconscious memory of the amniotic waters that Freud spoke of, but which also gives us awareness of our non-autonomous existence, not as a supposedly self-sufficient form, but before that nature, before that quantum horizon that does not disappear entirely, but with its silence makes us perceive as authentic process the unfolding in time of our individual voice, just as in the cosmic background radiation, 300,000 years after the Big Bang, the tiny differences in temperature and pressure can be measured, which ultimately justify the existence of something. "A light of its own arose within us," says the poet, the same poet who had effectively translated, in a language that both the indigenous and the Western can share, the lesson of expanded states of consciousness.

> *What are we really? The movement of desire brought us into the world, the great membrane of love that unites the slightest of algae with the knots of the great galaxies, nothing exists on its own, nothing lives separated, we are a sacred mass interwoven by mystery, a step of light that transcends infinite time and space (Veramar, 2022) [The original version is in Spanish]*

The Parts of Human Being From Where to Access Into *Pakasqa Nuna: Quechua Experience*

In order to attend an adjustment to the neurocognitive-biological-cultural model from Law of Origin perspective, it is important to talk about DSM-5 from the *Tukuypaq* (Peredo Albornoz & Prado Mendoza, 2024) contributions to an integrative approach to epidemics or pandemics now that depression is one of the most long extended mental health problem around the world (Kupcova & al, 2023; Santomauro & al, 2021).

As it was exposed, relationality is one of the key factors from which cognition and behavorial schemes should be upgraded. Doing this will automatically reconceptualize concepts as health-illness, providing a wide range of analysis about how conserving life and harmony. Something very similar to Tukuypaq is the proposal of Bigaagarri Protocol. While the first emphasize on physical-spiritual harmonization on the relationships between matter-information-energy, mind-body-spirit and human-natural-sacred community, the second one provides a complementary vision about how the pathology comes from bias.

In the psychological orientation of these societies [western ones], there is a narrow visual focus and a dispositional bias in causal attribution that usually dominates cognition and behaviour (Varnum et al. 2010), which can present as collective pathologies such as racism and misogyny. (…) This orientation is part of what is termed field-independent cognition and behaviour (Murdoch 1988), which dissociates the mind and body of the thinker and doer from the field of interdependent relations in which they exist. From an Indigenous perspective informed by standpoint theory (Nakata 2007; Wilson 2008), this might be described as a pathology in which a person's ontology (what is real) becomes stifled by their relationally limited epistemology (what is true), which in turn affects their methodology (what is done), feeding back into an increasingly dissociative condition in their axiology (what is right). (Yunkaporta, Orcher, & Palmer, 2025) [The references are from the authors]

These approaches might provide some lights in analysing the DSM-5, particularly disorders of depression, trauma, stress, addictions and somatic which are most related with the subconscious activity according to our indigenous knowledge and experience applied in Kuska Cultural Center for Ancestral Wisdom treatments from the *Mancharisqa* treatment (Prado Mendoza, 2016).

From the perspective of the Andean worldview, the human being is divided into two parts: body (*ukhu*) and spirit (*nuna*). The five-dimensional dimension that we have defined according to the oral tradition of indigenous healers from our familial environment includes: *Jawa nuna* (open spirit, consciousness); *Pakasqa nuna* (hidden spirit, subconscious); *kallpa* (the soul, whose center, Chaupi, is the heart and lungs, and is related to life and thus to blood, bone marrow, water, milk, and fat, all of which generate strength and energy that sustain life): *pata ukhu* (the upper body), which is the head (*uma*) down to the neck; *ura ukhu* (the lower body), from the neck to the feet. Sunqu is the heart. *Ñuqtu* is the center of *Nuna*, the brain. Both are carriers of energy. *Ñuqtu* is divided into the female brain and male brain (*urqu ñuqtu, china ñuqtu*) and also into the right brain and left brain *(paña ñuqtu, lluqi ñuqtu*), which express themselves in different ways: The fundamental characteristic of both is that they have at their upper part the hole of life and death (*kawsay wañupta juskun*), which coincides with the fontanelle. In reality, however, we say that all people have three holes of life and death (the fontanelle of the head, the palms of the hands, and the soles of the feet), which is more of a metaphorical expression, so there is no need to wait to appreciate them, as they are merely vulnerable points that must be protected, for it is through them that the soul can escape.

Our ancestors understood these concepts as follows: *nuna* in Andean culture is *manchali, q'iwalu* (coward, easily scared). This human spiritual energy becomes disordered, lost, or easily recovered. People who lose or disorganize their soul or spirit also become physically ill, and it is not always possible to diagnose them using scientific methods. *Nuna* is part of the subtle energy generated in each individual from the mother's womb, and it does not disappear even with death, although it undergoes permanent transformations throughout life. Due to its behavior, *Jawa Nuna* is also known as *llankaq nuna* (active spirit) and *Pakasqa nuna* as *P'inqali Nuna* (fleeing spirit, timid spirit). When we perform mental health healings and severe disorders are present, we say they are located in P*akasqa Nuna,* and generally, it is only in these cases that sacred plants are applied in ritualized and carefully controlled ceremonies. For the treatment to yield better results, the healer must also take the medicine, so that the patient and the healer can communicate mentally even when they are at a distance (Bonilla, 2013). Two of the main ways to get access and reach the spirit recover at N*una* is thru nose (smells) and ears (sounds).

Most severe disorders are confused by psychiatric therapy with depression, whereas the context that enables this clinical picture is much broader. *Mancharisqa* comes from the word *manchariy*, which means fear, terror, panic, fright, surprise, shock, horror. *Mancharisqa* is the state of being scared, an effect produced in a person by strong impressions of some danger, fear of the unknown, which leads to a disturbance in the person to the point of affecting their physical health, or what is known as somatization, which is a multiple response of the neuropsychoimmuneendocrinological type (Saad, 2019; Adamczyk & al, 2015). It is essentially a spiritual imbalance, including the physical plane. It can occur at any age, culture, or society, and can happen at any time to anyone. It arises from the way in which we understand, are influenced by, and accept the interactions that exist between human beings, their environment, and their worldview. In any case, *Mancharisqa* is not just 'fear sickness'; this mental disorder that causes disharmony also refers to other mental states such as fear of the unknown, not knowing whether an illness will be easy or difficult to cure, the lack of information about which is the best path to choose to restore harmony, the insecurity of being able to face economic situations that the treatment will demand, or the debts that may exist. All these situations made *Mancharisqa* as different pathologie that is not contemplated on DSM-5.

CONCLUSION

A subconscious neurophilosophy of the 'unseen world' for treating the spiritual illness is possible to elucidate. The approach of the *Pakasqa nuna* as interface with the invisible phenomena provides a strong core foundation from which even DSM-5 could be observed and reconceptualized following the Law of Origin or the First Law Nations. We suggest that pathology come from bias, but we would develop this idea in further studies. This works explores about nature-sacred and sacred-human relationship and how this analysis brings new ideas into the neurocognitive-biological-cultural model. Still remains relationships between human-nature faraway from the classical functional perspective (medicinal plants and its benefits from the active principles) and a closer related to 'fractal communication' where the subconscious knowledge amplifies relationships with the plants spirit field. Yet, herbal teachings cannot be done outside of a shamanic interaction and guidance within a First Nation ancestral teaching context.

ACKNOWLEDGEMENTS

We are grateful for the wisdom of Mother Earth and the knowledge of our ancestors which allowed us to articulate the ideas that guide this work. We thanks to Prof. César Marín for reading and providing some suggestions for this work. We thank the institutions to which the authors are members of this work.

COMPETING INTERESTS

No conflict of interest is declared.

REFERENCES

Adamatzky, A. (2022). Fungal states of minds. *bioRxiv*, 1. DOI: 10.1101/2022.04.03.486900

Adamczyk, A. (2015). Neuropsychoimmunological mechanisms in the pathology of neurodegenerative diseases: From biomarkers to therapeutics. *The Days of Neurochemistry* (p.). Warsaw, Poland: Polish Academy of Sciences. doi:DOI: 10.5114/fn.2015.56554

Äikäs, T., & Fonneland, T. (2012). Animals in Saami shamanism: Power animals, symbols of art, and offerings. *Religions*, •••, 1–15. DOI: 10.3390/rel12040256

Badini, R. P. (2020). *Las dos mitades de Rafael Chanchari Pizuri. Testimonio critico shawi*. Editorial Horizonte.

Bogoras, W. (1925). Ideas of Space and Time in the Conception of Primitive Religion. *American Anthropologist*, *27*(2), 205–266. https://www.jstor.org/stable/661206. DOI: 10.1525/aa.1925.27.2.02a00010

Bonilla, E. (2013). Influencia mental a distancia sobre los organismos vivientes. *Investigacion Clinica*, •••, 427–454. https://www.redalyc.org/pdf/3729/372937694009.pdf PMID: 24502184

Brenner, E. D., Stahlberg, R., Mancuso, S., Vivanco, J., Baluška, F., & Van Volkenburgh, E. (2006). Plant neurobiology: An integrated view of plant signaling. *Trends in Plant Science*, *11*(8), 413–419. DOI: 10.1016/j.tplants.2006.06.009 PMID: 16843034

Bynum, H. (2022). Plant agency and planetary health. *Lancet*, *400*(10346), 90–91. https://www.thelancet.com/journals/lancet/article/PIIS0140-6736(22)01243-0/abstract. DOI: 10.1016/S0140-6736(22)01243-0

Calvo, C. (1995). *Las tres mitades de Ino Moxo y otros brujos de la Amazonía*. Grupo Editorial Peisa.

Cowan, T. (1999). *Shamanism as a Spiritual Practice for Daily Life*. The Crossing Press.

Dengel, S., Aeby, D., & Grace, J. (2009). A Relationship between Galactic Cosmic Radiation and Tree Rings. *The New Phytologist, 184*(3), 545–551. https://www.jstor.org/stable/27735807. DOI: 10.1111/j.1469-8137.2009.03026.x PMID: 19754637

Diaz, J. (2010). Sacred plants and visionary consciousness. *Phenomenology and the Cognitive Sciences, 9*(2), 159–170. https://philpapers.org/rec/DAZSPA-2. DOI: 10.1007/s11097-010-9157-z

Dubos, R. (1962). *The Unseen World.* Oxford University Press.

Eddington, A. S. (1929). *Science and the Unseen World.* USA: The Macmillan Company. Retrieved from https://ia801304.us.archive.org/0/items/scienceunseenwor00eddi/scienceunseenwor00eddi_bw.pdf

Eliade, M., (1951). *Shamanism: Archaic Techniques of Ecstasy.* Princeton University Press.

Fábregas-Tejeda, J. B. I., P. G., & Radick, G. (2025). *The Riddle of Organismal Agency. New Historical and Philosophical Reflections.* Routledge.

Fericgla, J. M. (1997). *Al trasluz de la Ayahuasca. Antropología cognitiva, oniromancia y conciencias alternativas.* La Liebre de Marzo.

Frecska, E., Hoppál, M., & Luna, L. (2016). Nonlocality and the Shamanic State of Consciousness. *NeuroQuantology : An Interdisciplinary Journal of Neuroscience and Quantum Physics, 14*(2), 155–165. DOI: 10.14704/nq.2016.14.2.934

Gardiner, J. (2012). Insights into plant consciousness from neuroscience, physics and mathematics: A role for. *Plant Signaling & Behavior, 7*(9), 1049–1055. https://pmc.ncbi.nlm.nih.gov/articles/PMC3489624/. DOI: 10.4161/psb.21325 PMID: 22899055

Gibson, P., & Brits, B. (2018). *Covert Plants, Vegatal Consciousness and Agency in an Anthropocentric World.* Brainstorm Books.

Glockner, J. (2004). Chamanismo en los volcanes. *Arqueología Mexicana,* •••, 40–47.

Grim, J. A. (2001). Indigenous traditions and ecology: the interbeing of cosmology and community. Cambridge, EEUU: Cambridge, Mass.: Distributed by Harvard Press for the Center for the Study of World Religions, Harvard Divinity School.

Hoppál, M. (2013). *Shamans and Symbols. Prehistory of Semiotics in Rock Art.* International Society for Shamanistic Research.

Hubert, G., Baudry, A., & Saez, A. (2024). Impact of Cosmic Rays on Radiation Exposures and Scientific Activities at the Atacama Large Millimeter/Submillimeter Array (ALMA) Sites. *Radiation Research, 202*(3), 523–540. DOI: 10.1667/RADE-24-00129.1 PMID: 39038818

Huels, E., Kim, H., Lee, U. C., Bel-Bahar, T., Colmenero, A. V., Nelson, A., Blain-Moraes, S., Mashour, G. A., & Harris, R. E. (2021). Neural Correlates of the Shamanic State of Consciousness. *Frontiers in Human Neuroscience, 15*, 610466. DOI: 10.3389/fnhum.2021.610466 PMID: 33815077

Ibañez, J. (1991). *El Regreso del Sujeto. La Investigación Social de Segundo Orden*. Editorial Amerinda.

Karban, R. (2008). Plant behaviour and communication. *Ecology Letters, 11*(7), 727–739. DOI: 10.1111/j.1461-0248.2008.01183.x PMID: 18400016

Kolankaya-Bostanci, N. (2014). The Evidence of Shamanism Rituals in Early Prehistoric Periods of Europe and Anatolia. *Colloquium Anatolicum*, 185-204. doi:https://dergipark.org.tr/tr/download/article-file/1715302

Krippner, S. (2000). The epistemology and technologies of shamanic states of consciousness. *Journal of Consciousness Studies, 7*, 11–12. https://philpapers.org/rec/KRITEA-3

Krippner, S., & Combs, A. (2002). The Neurophenomenology of Shamanism. An Essay Review. *Journal of Consciousness Studies*, •••, 77–82. https://philpapers.org/rec/KRISKA

Kuhn, T. S. (1970). *The structure of Scientific Revolutions*. The University of Chicago.

Kupcova, I., Danisovic, L., Klein, M., & Harsanyi, S. (2023). Effects of the COVID-19 pandemic on mental health, anxiety, and depression. *BMC Psychology, 108*(1), 108. Advance online publication. DOI: 10.1186/s40359-023-01130-5 PMID: 37041568

Kuska Cultural Center. f. A. (2024). *Talantaña Proposal for Planetary Harmony - Tiwanaku.* La Paz, Bolivia: Universidad Católica Boliviana. Retrieved from https://afgj.org/talantana-proposal-for-planetary-harmony-tiwanaku-bolivia

Latour, B., & Woolgar, S. (1986). *Laboratory Life. The Contruction of Scientific Facts*. Princeton University Press.

Llamazares, A. M. (2011). Injured West: The Healing Potential of Shamanism in the Modern World. *Journal of Consciousness and Transformation*, 67-104. Retrieved from https://ri.conicet.gov.ar/bitstream/handle/11336/28753/CONICET_Digital_Nro.6063bdfe-9243-4517-8147-5c45a3eece42_A.pdf?sequence=2&isAllowed=y

Luna, L. E. (1984). The concept of plants as teachers among four mestizo shamans of Iquitos, northeastern Peru. *Journal of Ethnopharmacology, 11*(2), 135–156. https://pubmed.ncbi.nlm.nih.gov/6492831/. DOI: 10.1016/0378-8741(84)90036-9 PMID: 6492831

Luna, L. E., & Amaringo, P. (1999). *Ayahuasca Visions: The Religious Iconography of a Peruvian Shaman—Unveiling the*. North Atlantic Books.

Mancuso, S. (2017). *El futuro es vegetal.* Giunti Editore S.p.A.

Manorea, A. (2004). Anticipation în the Context of Altered States of Consciousness. *Journal of Computing Anticipatory Systems*, 232-245. Retrieved from https://philarchive.org/rec/MANANT-2

Marder, M., Vattimo, G., & Zabala, S. (2013). *Plant-Thinking: A Philosophy of Vegetal Life*. Columbia University Press.

Money, N. (2021). Hyphal and mycelial consciousness: The concept of the fungal mind. *Fungal Biology, 257-259*(4), 257–259. Advance online publication. DOI: 10.1016/j.funbio.2021.02.001 PMID: 33766303

Muñóz González, Y. (1998). Ainu Moshir y Kamui Moshir. La cosmovisión religiosa del pueblo Ainu. *Estudios de Asia y Africa*, •••, 103–121. https://www.jstor.org/stable/40313265. DOI: 10.24201/eaa.v33i1.1490

Nicolescu, B. (2010). Methodology of Transdisciplinarity. Levels of Reality, Logic of the Included Middle and Complexity. *Transdisciplinary Journal of Engineering & Science, 1*(1), 19–38. http://www.basarab-nicolescu.ciret-transdisciplinarity.org/Docs_Notice/TJESNo_1_12_2010.pdf. DOI: 10.22545/2010/0009

Parra Witte, F. X. (2017). *Living the Law of Origin: The Cosmological, Ontological, Epistemological, and Ecological Framework of Kogi Environmental Politics.* Cambridge, USA: University of Cambridge. DOI: 10.17863/CAM.22047

Peredo Albornoz, G., & Prado Mendoza, C. (2024). El sistema Tukuypaq. Aportes de la medicina tradicional para el abordaje integral de epidemias o pandemias. *Revista de Investigación e Información en Salud, 19*(47), 94–108. DOI: 10.52428/20756208.v19i47.1218

Pitarch Ramón, P. (1996). *Ch'ulel. Una etnografía de las almas tseltales*. Fondo de Cultura Económica.

Prado Mendoza, C. (2016). *Mancharisqa no es depresión. Aporte etnomédico para la salud mental intercultural.* Cochabamba: Quipus. Retrieved from https://searchworks.stanford.edu/view/11879402

Qu, F. (2021). Embodiment of Ancestral Spirits, the Social Interface, and Ritual Ceremonies: Construction of the Shamanic Landscape among the Daur in North China. *Religions, 567*(8), 567. Advance online publication. DOI: 10.3390/rel12080567

Redvers, N. e., Poelina, A., Schultz, C., Kobei, D. M., Githaiga, C., Perdrisat, M., Prince, D., & Blondin, B. (2020). Indigenous Natural and First Law in Planetary Health. *Challenges, 11*(2), 29. DOI: 10.3390/challe11020029

Restrepo Arcila, R. A. (2008). *Cosmovisión y Pensamiento Americanos. Pueblos Originarios*. Inédito.

Restrepo Arcila, R. A. (2023). *La visión ancestral de la interrelación entre cultura y salud*. Unedited.

Rovelli, C. (2018). *El orden del tiempo*. Anagrama. Colección Argumentos.

Rueda, E. A. (2022). *Retornar al origen*. Montevideo, Uruguay: UNESCO-CLACSO. Retrieved from https://www.clacso.org/wp-content/uploads/2022/05/Retornar-al-origen.pdf

Rueda, E. A., & al, e. (2022). *Retornar al Origen. Narrativas ancestrales sobre humanidad, tiempo y mundo*. Montevideo: UNESCO-CLACSO.

Saad, M. D. (2019). Spirituality, Religiousness and Physical Health: Scientific Evidence. In Lucchetti, G. P. (Ed.), *Spirituality, Religiousness and Health. Religion, Spirituality and Health: A Social Scientific Approach (p.)*. Springer., DOI: 10.1007/978-3-030-21221-6_6

Santomauro, D. F., Herrera, A. M. M., Shadid, J., Zheng, P., Ashbaugh, C., Pigott, D. M., & Ferrari, A. J. (2021). Global prevalence and burden of depressive and anxiety disorders in 204 countries and territories in 2020 due to the COVID-19 pandemic. *Lancet, 398*(10312), 1700–1712.

Schultes, E., Hoffman, A., & Ratsch, C. (2001). *Plants of the Gods: Their Sacred, Healing and Hallucinogenic Powers*. Inner Traditions/Bear & Company.

Shanon, B. (2003). Altered States and the Study of Consciousness. The Case of Ayahuasca. *The Journal of Mind and Behavior*, 125-153. doi:https://www.jstor.org/stable/43853997

Sheldrake, M. (2023). *Entangled life*. Penguin Books.

Sheldrake, R. (2010). *La presencia del pasado: resonancia mórfica y hábitos de la naturaleza*. Kairós.

Sugano, H., Uchida, S., & Kuramoto, I. (1994). A new approach to the studies of subtle energies. *Subtle Energies, 5*(2), 143-166. Retrieved from https://journals.sfu.ca/seemj/index.php/seemj/article/view/182/147

Sun, H., & Kim, E. (2024). Archetype symbols and altered consciousness: A study of shamanic rituals in the context of Jungian psychology. *Frontiers in Psychology, 1379391*, 1379391. Advance online publication. DOI: 10.3389/fpsyg.2024.1379391 PMID: 38863671

Swanson, L. R. (2018). Unifying Theories of Psychedelic Drug Effects. *Front. Pharmaco, 9*(172), 0. DOI: 10.3389/fphar.2018.00172

Tanaka, S. (2000). *The Ainu of Tsugaru: the indigenous history and shamanism of northern Japan.* Point Grey, Canada: University of British Columbia. DOI: 10.14288/1.0076926

Toriz, H., Fagetti, A., Terán-Pérez, G., & Mercadillo, R. E. (2024). Neuroanthropology of shamanic trance: A case study with a ritual specialist from Mexico. *Frontiers in Psychology, 1325188*, 1325188. Advance online publication. DOI: 10.3389/fpsyg.2024.1325188 PMID: 38505362

Trnka, R., & Lorencova, R. (2022). Indigenous Concepts of Consciousness, Soul, and Spirit: A Cross-Cultural Perspective. *Journal of Consciousness Studies, 29*(1), 113–140. https://ssrn.com/abstract=4702526. DOI: 10.53765/20512201.29.1.113

Varela, F. (1996). Neurophenomenology. A Methodological Remedy for the Hard Problem. *Journal of Consciousness Studies*, •••, 330–349. https://unstable.nl/andreas/ai/langcog/part3/varela_npmrhp.pdf

Veramar, A. (2022). *Caballos que vienen del sueño*. Ediciones Veramar.

Villalobos, R., Sanderson, J., & Vergara, N. (2023). Largest known cat geoglyph in Chile identified as the Endangered Andean cat. *Oryx, 694-695*(6), 694–695. Advance online publication. DOI: 10.1017/S0030605323001151

Walker, M. (2001). The Language of Shamans and the Methaphysics of Language: Emerging Paradigms in Shamanic Studies. *Shaman*, 35-59. Retrieved from https://marilynwalkerproductions.com/wp-content/uploads/2019/10/language_of_shamans.pdf

Wall Kimmerer, R. (2020). *Braiding Sweetgrass. Indigenous Wisdom, Scientific Knowledge and the Teachings of Plants*. Penguin Books.

Whitaker, J. A., Tamboli, V., Daly, L., & Lewy, M. (2024). Plant Agency in the Guianas: Attraction, Assault, and Animacy. *Journal of Ethnobiology*, 347-359. doi:https://doi-org.pucdechile.idm.oclc.org/10.1177/02780771241277618

Whitman, J. (1975). *The pshych power of plants*. W.H. Allen & Co. Ltd.

Wilson, E. (1998). *Consilience. The Unity of Knowledge*. Random House.

Winkelman, M. (2000). *Shamanism. The Neural Ecology of Consciousness and Healing*. Praeger. DOI: 10.5040/9798216986232

Wisekeepers. (2013). *Declaración de Tezhúmake*. Colombia: UNESCO. Retrieved from https://3ffd5e52-dafa-446c-b353-5f1c24b5a836.filesusr.com/ugd/d666d5_dbf3291cd1ce4951ab8e42789de811c8.pdf

Witt, J. (2006). Nature in Asian Indigenous Traditions: A Survey Article. *Worldviews: Global Religions, Culture, and Ecology*, •••, 40–68. https://www.jstor.org/stable/43809322

Yunkaporta, T. (2019). *Sand Talk. How Indigenous Thinking can Save the World*. Text Publishing.

Yunkaporta, T. (2024). The Ancient Wisdom Grift: Mad Studies and Indigenous Methods applied to the problem of spiritual disinformation narratives. *International Mad Studies Journal*, 1-16. DOI: 10.58544/imsj.v2i1.8025

Yunkaporta, T., Orcher, P., & Palmer, V. J. (2025). Danger Is a Signal, Not a State: Bigaagarri—An Indigenous Protocol for Dancing Around Threats to Wellbeing. *Social Sciences (Basel, Switzerland)*, *27*(1), 27. Advance online publication. DOI: 10.3390/socsci14010027

Chapter 8

The Wisdom of the Senses of the Principles of Mother Earth: Notes From the Experience of the Degree Program in Pedagogy of Mother Earth

Abadio (Manibinigdinya) Green Stocel
https://orcid.org/0009-0007-3841-9682
Ministerio de Educación Nacional de Colombia, Colombia

ABSTRACT

This document is a profound and a systematization of indigenous knowledge and ceremonial practices centered on the teachings of the Gunadule people and their relationship with Mother Earth that turns into Bachelor's Program in Pedagogy of Mother Earth at the University of Antioquia which delves deeply into the spiritual and symbolic dimensions of human life, presenting the womb as a sacred space of origin and a living memory that informs the wisdom of all beings, offering a pedagogy that celebrates community, relationality, and the cyclical nature of existence. The document also emphasize its role in fostering ecological consciousness and spiritual resilience. This work contributes to broader discourses on education from first source of ancestral wisdom as vital pathways for addressing ecological and spiritual crises in the modern world. It invites readers to reconnect with their origins, embrace the principles of Mother Earth, and participate in collective healing through silence, sweet words, and good hearts

DOI: 10.4018/979-8-3373-0360-4.ch008

INTRODUCTION

To start, I must say that the program, was conceived as multiple stakeholder initiative based on the Indigenous Organization of Antioquia, the University of Antioquia through the Faculty of Education with the Diverse Research Group and the Indigenous Education Program, and the Indigenous communities of Antioquia, through their youth, women, and wise leaders, began to forge a path in 2005 where education is more directly linked to politics, and politics with education, in a common goal: "the defense of Mother Earth." The Bachelor's Degree in Mother Earth Pedagogy was created as a process to train and train us as teachers who are leaders of the people and, at the same time, as leaders with good pedagogy and a good heart.

Thru the years, the program has developed research lines. Some of these are the following (Antioquia, 2011):

Silence. Silence is a possibility to listen to ourselves and others. What we know as the "West" makes too much noise; academia is full of words, of truths. Silence as a pedagogical category invites us to look within, to know differently, and to recognize that through conscious silence, ancestral knowledge and peoples have survived. Silence is a permanent construction and is part of the way of knowing in the Bachelor's Degree in Pedagogy of Mother Earth.

Observation. Intentional observation, the gaze that recognizes, creates, and recreates life, people, education. It happens that we don't see each other often, we don't recognize our faces, nor the faces of our brothers and sisters, and this is how we lose our identity. Observing from the heart, from history, observing in order to walk.

Community. Communalism is an ancient practice of ancestral peoples, which we understand as a network of heterogeneous processes of exchange and social interaction between generations, within territories, where the re-creation and transmission of culture takes place. This promotes educational processes based on dialogue between students and communities based on their own realities and dynamics. The communitarian principle implies assuming a role as a political agent of transformation, with a value for history and for equitable intercultural construction. This principle challenges an individualistic view of the subject and cultures.

Decolonial. Postcolonial criticism and Latin American studies on the coloniality of knowledge, being, power, and nature resume discussions, contextualizing them within the framework of the relations of domination instituted during the long years of conquest and colonization of vast peoples and territories by Anglo-European metropolises, and whose ideological legacy is not easy to dismantle: the declaration and imposition of some knowledge as more advanced and legitimate, while other ways of inhabiting, thinking, and interpreting the world were usurped and delegitimized. Is a dialogue of knowledge with other peoples and cultures possible, within the framework of modern science, which considers itself a superior knowledge, and the mentality of progress and development? From the perspective of subordinate peoples (mestizos, indigenous peoples, Afro-Colombians, peasants, women), these discourses are merely different guises that perpetuate profound violence, not only territorial, political, and economic, but also epistemic, which makes a balanced dialogue of knowledge incompatible. That is why decolonialism is part of the transversal analysis of the entire process.

Dialogue of knowledge. The dialogue of knowledge and non-knowledge, or questions, as an exchange of knowledge and experiences in an exercise of "collective hermeneutics," where interaction re-contextualizes and re-signifies, enabling reflexivity and the configuration of meanings in processes, actions, knowledge, histories, and territorialities, expanding, in this case, not only the levels of understanding of the realities of communities, but also their theorization. The dialogue of knowledge provides us with intersubjective dialogic nuances to interact and discuss, that is, so that communities, students, teachers, and the organizations and institutions involved, both public and private, can listen to each other and build other possibilities of being, resolve difficulties, and find common ground for good living.

Weaving. Weaving with different materials and techniques has been one of the most enduring cultural expressions throughout human history. Cultures construct textiles as a form of their own language, to preserve memory, to express their thoughts, their material expression, to demonstrate the development and appropriation of environments, their ideas of beauty and their relationship with history, with individuals, family, politics, education, art, among others. In many cases and contexts, the materials change, as does what they communicate; however, their basic principle of interweaving through a warp, a weft, a shuttle, and an intention persists. The Bachelor's Degree in Mother Earth Pedagogy, in search of alternative possibilities different from the hegemonic ones regarding the way higher education curricula have been structured, proposes textiles as a metaphor for working with the diverse interweavings, commonalities, and differentials of its curriculum, with individuals, their histories, their communities, their cultures, their dreams, and possibilities. Weaving as a principle is understood as a permanent material practice and thought of cultures, which is built and recreated, reflects individual and collective participation, the intentionality for the useful and beautiful from the most complex collective and harmonious sense.

To date, the program is the only institutionalized Bachelor proposal on the continent authentically based on indigenous knowledge. However, there are similar curricula proposals in other documents such as Maya-Rose Simon & Hopi Martin (2023), Baltra-Ulloa & Kostecki (2024), Aghasaleh (2019), Mashford-Pringle, et al

(2019) and Smith-Gilman (2023). The common perspective on every contribution emphasizes on self-determined ways to early childhood education, in the last cases, university students in the first one. There are all thru indigenous nations experiences from Tasmania, Brazil, Canada, Turkey, Greece, US and Saudi Arabia.

METHODOLOGICAL BACKGROUND FOR THE BACHELOR PROGRAM IN LIGHT OF YESTERDAY, TODAY AND TOMORROW: WEAVING THE THOUGHT

In recent times, I have been weaving reflections on the meaning of transmitting the teachings of the Bachelor's Program in Pedagogy of Mother Earth. This has been done through healing ceremonies and dialogues with wisdom keepers of Mother Earth in Colombia and Abya Yala (America in the Gunadule language). I have also connected with plants through the ceremonies of my Gunadule people, where the grandmothers, the SOBIA mothers, have imparted the principles of Mother Earth: silence, listening, observing, weaving, sweet words, and a good heart . These teachings have been intertwined with the wisdom of Grandfather Yagé, who guided me along the pedagogical path to enrich our program with the principles of origin, disharmony, healing, and protection.

These teachings, which I have been weaving, are deeply tied to the challenging times humanity faces, particularly the current civilizational crisis. I have had the opportunity to reflect inwardly and connect with the ancestral territories of our peoples, where death looms constantly due to various capitalist-driven megaprojects. These projects ignore the diversity of health, education, worldviews, and spirituality. This disconnect became starkly evident during the pandemic, which exposed vulnerabilities in urban areas, rural villages, and within our communities. During this time, our elders and wise ones turned to the sacred plants' wisdom to help our millenary cultures persevere amidst other global cultures and peoples.

The pandemic's arrival in Colombia, and the world, highlighted the inefficiencies of our health systems under so-called democracies. These systems, rooted in profit rather than public welfare, failed to address the needs of their inhabitants. Public health responses to this crisis faltered because the foundation was not public but a business benefitting only a few.

During the pandemic, I took refuge in my 'womb home' where I had time to reflect spiritually on the journey we are undertaking through the Pedagogy of Mother Earth. In the silence of the nights, I conversed with myself, my history, and my people's history. I listened to the wisdom of my native language and felt the presence of grandmothers and grandfathers during the nightly fire ceremonies. These moments allowed me to revisit and feel the stories of my origins, weaving them with humanity's journey. I continued learning by listening to voices in the stillness of nights and dawns and recalling infinite conversations with my mentor, Grandfather Oloeligdiginya (Manuel Santacruz, an authority of my Ibgigundiwala community, Caimán Nuevo, Urabá, Antioquia). His wise words, along with the wisdom of other elders from various peoples who have contributed to my spiritual quest, guided me.

I felt the ancestral whispers emanating from the Gunadule language and remembered dialogues with Grandfather Yagé and the sacred grandmother plants during ceremonies held at my home in Caimán Nuevo, within the Ibgigundiwala Reserve, Gulf of Urabá, Antioquia. In this writing, I will focus on the principles of Mother Earth.

STORIES FROM THE WOMB

Silence revealed to me the meaning and awareness of time and the methodology rooted in the essence of the womb. It brought me greater clarity to nurture the pedagogy of Mother Earth and the meanings of life. The stories of the wombs, as great healers visible and invisible in the world, began to resonate deeply. I felt everything around me speaking to me, helping me understand the dimensions of the diverse conversations I've had. I came to recognize the importance of listening to the grandmothers and grandfathers—sparks of light who passed down their wisdom. These remarkable beings made it possible for me to soar, travel, and embrace my sisters, the stars, my grandmother Olowagli, and her seven siblings, the planets. In other words, the entire cosmos embraced me, guided me, and showed me how to live on this beautiful land, Mother Earth.

Through this woven writing, I wish to share with women, men, youth, children, and various collectives across the regions of this country, Abya Yala, and the world. Many are making an effort to seek balance and harmony for a good life on this beautiful Earth. I have found that the best way to perceive the spiritual path is to feel it, to connect with our womb stories—our origins. For years now, we have been weaving the experience of the Pedagogy of Mother Earth into academic life, resulting in substantial changes at the University of Antioquia.

From where I write and from my heart, I ask each of you who take the time to read this to journey with me along the trail of life born from our mothers' wombs. Most importantly, I invite all of you to join me in preserving the legacy of wisdom held within our mother languages.

The womb stories shared in this writing can be found in the memories of our grandmothers and grandfathers, in our families, in sacred plants, and in the ceremonies celebrated by diverse peoples to maintain the balance of their territories and humanity. These include rituals involving cacao, coca leaves, tobacco, joska,

Grandfather Yagé, Yopo, Peyote, the power of fire in Mayan ceremonies, temazcals, medicinal baths, dances, music, food, and more.

All these medicines guide us, weave us, and bring us back to the wombs of our mothers, grandmothers, great-grandmothers, and Mother Earth—the great womb of the Creator Mother, *Nanadummadi* (the Creator Mother who brought forth the cosmos and Mother Earth, along with the Creator Father). This journey allows us to return to our origin, to look directly into the essence of our being, and to rediscover our vitality through our connection to our great Mother Earth, leading us toward the fullness of healing.

This life journey reactivates the memory of all humanity, for we all come from the same womb—our first house of wisdom, our first territory. It was there that our ears, sense of smell, stomach, and heart received the cosmos's and nature's first lessons of wisdom. In this magical space, we wove and braided connections with all the beings of the cosmos and Mother Earth. It was where our parents, grandmothers, grandfathers, aunts, uncles, and Mother Earth taught us and communicated the transcendence of who we are, where we come from, why we are here, and our mission on this Mother Earth.

LIFE-WORD SIGNIFICATIONS: A PATH TO UNVEIL OUR MEMORY

For the Gunadule people, the womb is a portal that enabled our journey to these lands of our grandmothers and grandfathers, where we were chosen by our Great Mother and Great Father to come to these territories of Mother Earth. This has been humanity's story since life emerged in this beautiful existence millennia ago. The language of our ancestors is the Great Mother that explains our transcendence, the Great Grandmother who teaches and brings us closer to the mystery of life's meaning.

To clearly understand this message, I want to begin with the word <<pregnancy>> because it helps us better grasp the woven meaning of this word, filled with metaphor and poetry, which explains the meanings of life. The womb, in this context, enabled our journey to long memory, providing us with life's purpose in connection with the cosmos and Mother Earth.

In the Gunadule language, the word <<womb>> beautifully appears as an explanation. It portrays how the process of human gestation within the womb relates to the tree and the house of the Grandfather Sun: *sabbi ibedineggi.* This is what we will explore through the meanings of life and the wise resonance of words arising from our mother language.

Sabbi

means 'tree' and originates from two words:

Sabe + bi

Sabe: 'to love', 'to care for'. 'to protect'

Bi: an adverb meaning 'only' or 'solely'

Thus, the word *Sabbi* (tree) means to 'The tree that only knows how to love, care for, and protect'

And we continue with the following words to further complement the meaning of <<womb>>

Ibedineggi

Ibe: 'owner' but also refers to Grandfather Sun.

Di: a word that 'emphasizes' or 'points out'

Nega: 'house'

Gine: means 'in'

This gives us:

'The loving, caring and protective tree in Grandfather Sun's house'

Having this clarity about the meaning of the womb from the perspectives of life, it gives us the understanding that the tree represents the process of pregnancy, which takes place in the house of the grandfather sun, because the tree symbolizes love, protection, and wisdom. The womb, the space where pregnancy unfolds, is a place where we were nourished by the wisdom of ancestral memory and fed by the gifts of Mother Earth. It is a wonderful, magical place where we received various energies from the ancestors. The womb, the place of pregnancy, also relates to the house we inhabit, the House of Congress, where the entire community gathers to listen to songs, dances, rituals, and counsel, and it shares the same name, *IBE NEGA*, 'the house of the grandfather sun'. The house also represents the structure of self-governance, symbolizing the ancestral authorities who have safeguarded the territory, a process the Gunadule people have been weaving for centuries as part of their self-government.

In other words, pregnancy occurring in the womb is a tree-house, a space for life learning, where we were all formed with the wisdom of the plant grandmothers and grandfathers, and the spiritual grandmothers and grandfathers during the process of our germination.

This entire process of our gestation was meant to prepare us to give meaning to our existence on Mother Earth. It is an experience shared by all of humanity because all human beings come from the same place. The womb of a Japanese, Chinese, Russian, European, Maya, Êbera, Nasa, Iku, Wayúu, Dule, Kamentzá, Paisa, or Costeña woman is the same, woven from the same fabric. Therefore, we are all children of the same mother. We are all sisters and brothers on this planet.

Our umbilical cord was woven from the wombs of many mothers from my ancestors. There, our DNA, our memory, was lovingly stored for thousands of past generations. Within it lies the possibility of reaffirming who we are and becoming aware that we are perfect beings because we are the synthesis of the wisdom of the cosmos and Mother Earth. Each culture has connections to this story for healing, as the only true path to complete healing is returning to the womb. This is why each culture among the diverse peoples has recreated different ways to return to the womb, to find peace once again, and above all, to seek the wisdom of our peoples. And the Gunadule people, like all the peoples of the world, have their own healing practices. This is the message of life I want to share with you, a message I had the opportunity to hear, live, and feel in this experience.

Conversation with the Grandmother Plants, Sobia (weavers of beings in the womb)

In the month of January, eleven years ago (2014), I decided to undergo my healing, embracing the ancestral practices of my Gunadule people. The ceremony involved isolating myself for a month for my healing and receiving answers to the concerns I had been feeling since my experience in the Bachelor's Program in Pedagogy of Mother Earth, along with a firm conviction that I would drink from the wisdom of the grandmother plants, seeking both questions and answers.

The ceremony involves retreating for a month into a small space, where I was alone with various medicinal plants collected from the forest by a botanist. Before being placed into a small container filled with water, quartz, and medicinal stones, the elder botanist sang to the plants, giving them a mandate for my healing and learning. The cacao incense was present at all times during every moment of my healing. The plants were then placed in the container with the water for two days. This ceremony would be repeated every two days throughout the month, with the water and medicinal plants being changed every two days.

During that time, silence was the rule; I would not speak to anyone, except for an elder man or woman who would attend to my meals. These meals would be prepared without salt, spices, or meat—only small, smoked fish.

My experience during that month was one of spiritual healing, days filled with clarity and the wisdom of the grandmothers. Seventeen days into the ceremony, I began to feel desperate, longing to leave the space. Suddenly, I heard voices telling me to calm down and rest my head on the bed of my hammock. I obeyed, and they continued speaking. Suddenly, the three grandmothers appeared before me and immediately told me that we should talk about the origin of human life, my origin, and how my first threads were woven within my mother's womb. They had come to teach me and explain life in the womb. In this way, the grandmothers introduced themselves and said: 'We are *Sobbia'*.

I had never heard this name before, which is why it is important for me to understand its meaning.

Sobbia

Name of the spiritual grandmothers responsible for weaving the human being in the womb.

This name of the grandmothers comes from the following words

So+b(e)+b(i)+a

So: fire

Be: refers to the second person singular and also refers to the grandfather sun, and when combining the two words *SO* + *BE*, it means to weave, braid, create.

Bi = refers to the adverb 'only'

And by combining these words, we get the following:

'The grandmother weavers, braiders of life in a mother's womb'

After the introduction, they began to tell me and show me the process of fertilization of the seeds of my mother and father. It was the beginning of feeling and observing the process of my life, where I come from, my ancestry. I saw thousands of seeds from my father, and that only one of those seeds would enter to meet my mother's seed. What I witnessed next was a magical scene—I saw thousands of colors dancing in a spiral, forming various protective patterns, similar to those found in the designs of molas. There was no rush to move quickly; everything was slow, rhythmic, and filled with great beauty.

The *Sobbia* grandmothers told me that moving quickly does not mean reaching first. Instead, the seed that performs the best dance, with the most harmonious rhythm and colors like the rainbow, will be chosen by my mother's seed.

I saw when my father's seed, which was my being, united with my mother's seed, complementing each other. At that instant, a spark of fire was produced, continuing the spiral dance to extend the process of life in a woman's womb. The fire, with its heat, embraced the beginning of gestation. As the fire warmed, it facilitated the weaving of the different tissues, producing thousands of colors so the spiral movement could continue with more strength.

Slowly, at the center of the dance, a small drop appeared. The grandmothers questioned me, asking:

"What do you see?" I was in awe, unable to speak, silenced by the beauty of the spiral dance. One of the grandmothers gave me the answer: "What you see, what your eyes are witnessing at the center of the dance, is a marvelous being, reminding us of when life began in the cosmos and on Earth—the water. And when water appeared, so did the heat of the grandfather fire, and once again, the spiral dance continued, where the grandmothers and grandfathers danced in harmonious rhythm, producing thousands of colors in the garments of the ancestors (Sobbia Grandmothers, 2014)

As the dance progressed, the rhythm was filled with love. Gradually, at the center of the water, another marvelous being emerged from the shadow of the water—this time, it was blood, the liquid of life. The warmth of the spiral dance allowed life to emerge at the center, forming the heart.

From that magical place, the heart, the brain, lungs, bones, arteries, and liver were woven. It was the beginning of the heart's work—its beats weaving life—because in every pore of human skin, the heartbeat is present. The heart holds all the information of our being, just as the cosmos and Mother Earth do.

Likewise, the grandmothers told me that they wove the brain while observing and feeling the cosmos, meaning the brain is a reflection of the world above, the world of the ancestors where the grandmothers and grandfathers dwell—the world of the great house and the long memory.

These teachings from the Sobbia grandmothers reminded me of the stories left by wise elders, who taught that each organ in our body is a being, a community. The heart and brain are communities, and neither claims to be more important than the other. All are essential, all are interconnected, and whatever happens to one affects the entire organism, the entire being.

As Mother Giggardiryay and her brother Ibeorgun once said:

They used the pedagogy of the body as a unified whole, a single fabric to understand the importance of relationships—with my neighbor, with the community, with humanity, with Mother Earth, and with the cosmos. To explain this better, they gave an example: 'When a wasp stings a big toe, the other toe does not say, "I don't care." On the contrary, all parts of the body suffer—the body feels the pain and cries; the eyes shed tears of pain, the heart races, and the legs lose strength to walk. This means the entire body is connected, interrelated. If we understand this, it would help us grasp the importance of community: I feel the pain of what happens to each member of my community. Authorities should be like mothers and fathers to society. The same applies to our relationship with nature—her pain and joys should be my pain and joys.[1]

The heart was the first community to give the breath of life to our existence. The brain receives the heart's messages, not the other way around. The grandmothers wove our brains in the image and likeness of the cosmos.

The Womb as a Living Memory of Our Existence

From the womb, we learned to listen to our mothers—their songs, their worries, their dreams, and hopes. Everything we are today, our way of thinking, even our illnesses, is connected to the womb. Our DNA is inscribed in our umbilical cord.

When we are born, our umbilical cord is cut, separating us from our mothers. Many ancestral peoples hold rituals for planting the umbilical cord and placenta; many bury them in the earth, near the hearth, in the garden, or plant seeds of corn, coconut, and trees with the umbilical cord. This symbolizes that we are already part of the earth, our umbilical cord linked to Mother Earth, and we begin living within her womb.

We all come from a circular, cyclical, spiral world where the past is near—we can see it, feel it. Historical memory and the historical subject matter. Our history is our mark, our anchor, our center, our heart. The heart and reason are communities bound together, just as all organs are interconnected communities.

When we are born, the earth receives us. She too has the shape of a woman's womb. My Gunadule people call the Earth: *Nabba. Na* means totuma (vegetable vessel), and when repeated, *NANA* means mother. This suggests that our ancestors have long understood that the earth resembles the shape of a calabash or a pregnant woman's womb.

The womb of our mothers is circular-spiral, the earth is circular-spiral, the cosmos is circular-spiral, and other worlds are also spiral-circular.

From the womb, we learned to listen to our mothers, our grandmothers—their songs, their concerns, their desires, and hopes. Everything we are today, our ways of thinking, our illnesses, and our attitudes are woven into the wombs of our mothers, grandmothers, great-grandmothers, and great-great-grandmothers. Our DNA is a script written across every space of our being because blood flows everywhere, just like water flows through the body of Mother Earth.

To speak of our womb stories is to speak of our mothers' wombs, where our lives unfolded, full of stories of pain or joy. It was our first home, our first territory, our first learning space. Each fiber of our body was a source of strength and energy, where our placenta, umbilical cord, and navel protected us and embraced us with the love and tenderness of our mother and the creative grandmothers, *Sobbia.*

The Principles of the Senses of Mother Earth

From that thread of womb stories, I found that one of the paths to better explain the principles of Mother Earth was through the womb. I also took advantage of the time when humanity was within the womb of their homes, and I used this opportunity to better listen to the voices of my elders, in the mother languages, through the ceremonies of fire, accompanied by the sacred grandmother plants. I began to weave these principles together, keeping in mind the teachings I received from the grandmothers *SOBBIA*.

All the principles of Mother Earth are interconnected, like a large web, woven with love. Our bodies were woven in this way, like a great writing where the memory has been stored since we appeared in the memory of our great mother and great father. They wove our bodies to teach us about solidarity, community, fraternity, sorority, and communal work. From the body, we learn how to relate to others—feeling that 'the other is me'.

Silence, listening, observing, weaving, sweet words, and a good heart are principles that become very clear when we were in the wombs of our mothers. That is why, every time life is woven, these millennial stories from our cultures and our wisdom are remembered. And above all, we must ask ourselves: What are we doing in this world? What is our mission? What is our duty in this plane of human existence?

Principle of the Sense of Silence

All life begins in silence. All cultures of the world explain the creation of the Earth and the cosmos through beautiful words, and everything is woven harmoniously in relation to our lives, as life itself is the life of the cosmos and Mother Earth—our own weaving. Now, I want to recall how various peoples explain the beginning of life on Mother Earth:

> *Before creation, there were no humans, no plants, no animals... nothing manifested on the face of the Earth. Only the sea was suspended... There was nothing that had being... only the sea, the water which was calm, and so everything was in silence and darkness, as in a deep night." (Popol Vuh Maya-Toltec)*
>
> *The Mother existed when nothing existed. Nothing, nothing, just her. She is air, water, wisdom. She is the mother of the bubbling water, and the vapor that came from the depths was what, at one point, she gave birth to and became the Creator Father. This Mother existed before anything existed. She was the one who, silently, gave the first breath so that from that bubble, the Creator Father, Unámarai, was born. Through her, our Mother, the Only One, the creation began. (Creation Story, according to the vision and feeling of the Murui people)*
>
> *First there was the sea, everything was dark. There was no sun, no moon, no people, no animals, no plants. Only the sea was everywhere. The sea was the mother... and she would be the river, the lagoon, the stream, and the sea...*

Thus. First, there was only the Mother.(Creation Story of the Tayrona-Gágaba (Kogi) people)

In the beginning, everything was dark. A darkness so dense, as if two hands were pressing against one's eyes. There was no sun, no moon, the stars had not been born. Then Nanadummadi (Mother Creator) decided to create her daughter, the Earth, and Babadummadi (Father Creator) decided to create his daughter, the Earth. (Origin Story of Mother Earth from the vision and feeling of the Gunadule people)

Silence and darkness, as explained by the wise elders of our communities, mark the beginning of all life. This parallels our origin stories when everything began with the dance of the seeds of my mother and father in the womb. It was all silence and darkness; we saw nothing, absolutely nothing, only our ears, our stomach, our sense of smell perceived what was happening around our mother. Silence and darkness are stages of learning, of perceiving all the energies of our mother and our ancestors—places where the memory of our millennial cultures is present.

The placenta, the umbilical cord, and the navel remind us of the memory of our grandmothers, both the spiritual and earthly realms. The language itself is the same memory of a people that teaches us, points out the path, the knowledge, and the wisdom through the meanings of words, which I have called 'the meanings of life'. I wish to use these meanings of life and the meanings of the connections that held us connected to the outer world, such as the placenta, the umbilical cord, and the navel, all from the meanings of life.

Assu: The Placenta

It comes from the following words:

As(u)

It means 'sense of smell'

AS(u)(a)SU

It refers to the sense of smell twice.

The sense of smell is the tissue that bloomed quickly, and the tissues that enveloped our being. The tissue of the placenta is fragile, powerful, and fine, allowing us to perceive the outside world easily from within the womb. The placenta is the essential tissue that allowed my blossoming in the perception of the outside world. That is why, in my language, the verb to smell and to listen is the same word. For example, we say 'What a delicious sound', meaning 'What a delicious smell'. We could also say that the placenta is my guardian, my companion, my root, my origin, my memory.

To the umbilical cord, in the mother language, we say:

Simuduba

'The Bejuco (vine) of the Grandmother's Seat

The word S*I* refers to the state of being seated, and this sitting position is feminine because it is related to the puberty of girls. During the girl's first menstruation, she will sit, and the women of the community will come to cleanse her with the mother water for eight days of her learning. The word *MU* refers to the grandmother, as she, during these eight days, will oversee transmitting the wisdom of her people, the teachings of community life, the process of growing from girlhood to adulthood. The seat signifies the wisdom of the grandmother. The word *Duba* refers to the bejuco (vine) the umbilical cord, meaning that the umbilical cord not only represents the transmission of nourishment but also the path through which the wisdom of the ancestors arrives. However, when segmenting this thread, it brings other meanings such as: *Du* meaning cosmos, and *Ba(li)* meaning 'with'. The umbilical cord connects us, uniting the earth and the cosmos. The womb of my mother gave me the sweetness of my connection with the cosmos, where the grandmothers and grandfathers, and the mother earth reside, my territory as a space of learning. The placenta and the umbilical cord are tissues that made the passage of our lives in the womb of our mothers possible, and for this reason, in the Gunadule culture and in the other peoples of Abya Yala, they are planted in the place where the baby is born.

To the navel, we say:

SIMU

'The seat of the grandmother'

The navel represents the wisdom of our ancient cultures. Every wise elder in our communities has sat to learn from the teachers and masters of our communities. The navel is wisdom; that's why it is planted where the family's seeds are. In other words, the navel is buried, and on top of it, corn grains, cocoa seeds, or fruit trees are planted. In that moment, our navel connects us with Mother Earth, we are already part of her, we belong to her.

After explaining this, I begin to explain the principles of Mother Earth. The sense of silence is a privileged path of learning, because it allows us to have the capacity to perceive the meaning of everything around us; it is the highest state of learning. Silence is the category that enables greater learning from the wisdom of our people. In other words, we come from the wombs of our mothers with the ability to smell, feel, and experience the wisdom of our ancestors. So, what does the word silence mean in the native language of the Gunadule?

BOGGIGWA

Silence

It comes from the following words:

BO: Stillness, mist

GGI:

G(ine) Gi(ne)

'In the'

GWA:'Heart'

'The silence is in the heart of the mist'

Silence is mist, stillness, contemplation. It is the act of turning inward to understand the outside world. In other words, silence brings us back to our origin, to our womb; it is always a path to our healing. That's why many indigenous cultures of Abya Yala, in their ceremonies, always have the grandfather fire present, representing the beginning of life, warmth, and love.

The figure of mist symbolizes the closeness between the cosmos and the earth, as if they are conversing. It is a privileged time to regain strength and energy. This is how we are in the womb, a time of stillness, because silence and darkness are good companions for gaining wisdom. The womb is the space to listen to the voices of the grandmothers and grandfathers. In this sense, all cultures of many indigenous peoples learn through silence, listening to songs and words. In my experience, to approach the wisdom of my people, my teacher Manuel Santacruz listened to me in silence for a year before imparting his wisdom. He wanted to hear me, my journey, my memories, my mistakes, my family's story, and only then did he begin to share the stories. I heard from the silence the ancient stories of my people. That's why, in general, teachings are given at night, in darkness, to remember our first lessons, which were in the womb, in darkness, and in silence.

Principle of the Sense of Listening

In order to listen from the heart, we must be in silence. That is, I must be empty to be filled by the other. And precisely in the womb of our mothers, we developed this sense of listening more fully, as we were in silence and darkness. Only our ears, sense of smell, and stomach were attentive, perceiving, because the grandmothers were preparing us fully to listen to the wisdom of the world, of the earth, and of the cosmos.

Now, let us listen to the grandmother language of the Gunadule, the meaning of the word <<Listen>>:

IDDOGE

Listen

I: Feeling of emptyness

D(O)DO: Play, girl, boy

G(U)E: 'to become'

'To empty, to become a girl/boy'

The womb, my first home, my first territory, was my first space of listening, learning, and above all, feeling the energy of my mother, father, family, and society. Everything I learned in that time became my light, my guide, my path in this vast and long journey in the bosom of Mother Earth.

With great clarity, the Gunadule people challenge us on this principle, as it refers to two important aspects: play and being a child. I find this essential because play is the best way to learn, and being a child is the best stage of life for wisdom because their lives are in a process of rapidly absorbing knowledge. These two figures offered by the Gunadule language give us strength to affirm that listening is a privileged stage of learning from others. And to learn from others, I must feel empty, and through listening to others, I will be filled. The joy of having listened to the other will arise in me, and the knowledge and feelings of the other will become my pride, my wisdom, and above all, our healing; they heal, and I heal.

Listening is the best way to learn from others and from myself; in this sense, the principle of silence is connected because we cannot listen to others without silence. I cannot listen only from my own point of view; I must be like the child who is always available to listen, to learn. Today, politicians, leaders, and educators are not listening because they think and feel that they already possess the truth, that they know more than others. There is no sense of emptiness. The truth is that one is nothing without the other, that we are complementary beings, that we learn from one another. This is why play is a pedagogy of learning through play, and feeling like a child is a form of learning through tenderness.

Principle of the Sense of Observation

Observing does not mean seeing with the eye, just as listening is not only from the ear; rather, all the principles we have outlined so far occur from the heart, that is, from the senses. This is because in the womb of our mothers, we developed these principles, which allow us to sense and listen to our own bodies, as well as to Mother Nature and the cosmos that also reside within us. Our grandmother language, Gunadule, gives us enough clarity in the meaning of the principle of observation:

DAGGE

Observe

DA(DA): Grandpa, refers to the Grandpa Sun

G(UE)G(U)E: 'To become, to become

' To become, To become Grandpa Sun'

Everything we have learned from our language, from our body, is related to Mother Earth and the cosmos. For this reason, in the Gunadule language, the singularity of being does not appear, but rather the collective, the reciprocity. Therefore, the principle of observing is linked to the grandfather Ibelele (Sun), who observes all of us—trees, plants, animals, insects, large and small fish. Not only does he observe all living beings on Mother Earth, but also the entire galaxy, the cosmos. It is the principle that we human beings are endowed with the privilege of feeling in observation, which is why we can observe beyond what our eyes can see because we possess the energy of grandfather Sun. In the Gunadule language, all these principles are contained to give meaning to our existence, to the heart of being. In every sound, in every word, the grandmothers and grandfathers are present. For example, in the Gunadule language, when referring to personal pronouns: I, you, she, or he, it is clear that it refers to the individual, but in the Gunadule language, it has other perceptions:

ANI:

'I'. First person singular pronoun

A: Refers to a person who is not present.

NI: Moon

The first person singular refers to the Moon, and it is our grandfather, the father of the Sun and all the planets. For the Gunadule people, the Moon is the grandfather, the Sun is his son. The Earth is the mother of all planets and stars, meaning that the stars are the daughters of the Moon. This is why we can affirm the importance of the Moon in human life, as it guides our path and life. Therefore, the phases of the Moon are related to the life of the Earth.

BE: 'You'. Second person singular pronoun

The second person singular has a direct connection with the grandfather Sun. In the Gunadule language, we say *IBE* which means precipice, creating a feeling of emptiness when one looks into the abyss. We all have energy, sometimes strong, sometimes soft, but we can affect others. In the context we are discussing, the second person singular in Dulegaya refers to the grandfather *Dada Olowaibibbilele* or *Ibelele* (Sun). So, when I say 'you' then I am recalling the grandfather Sun.

WE: 'He' or 'She'. Third person singular pronoun

The third person singular has a direct relationship with Mother Earth. It is a story related to the tale of the eight brothers, who are the planets, and it is the story of our origin.

In this sense, if we interpret silence, listening, and observing, they are closely related to the personal pronouns we are referring to because they concern the origin of our people. The grandparents, the Moon and the Sun, are far from us, but at the same time, they are close because they are within us. We are cosmos, we are earth, which is why personal pronouns refer to ourselves, to the Moon, the Sun, and Mother Earth—they are us.

Principle of the Sense of Weaving

In the Gunadule language, to refer to weaving, we have two words: *sobe* and *magge*. *Sobe* is used when building a house, as mentioned earlier. It refers to the political and organizational governance of the Gunadule people. That is, for the

Gunadule, it refers to community governance, and it is linked to the weaving of the house. In other words, governance is a weave to govern the Gunadule community.

The weaving of the house begins by placing the main posts in the center, and they must be strong, resistant to termites, the force of the wind, the rain, and able to last for 20, 30, or even 40 years. This construction weave represents the community authorities, whom we call *SAGLAMALA*—they are the central posts. But they cannot resist alone; they need other posts for support. That is why next to the main posts are smaller posts, which we call *ARGALA*. These are tied with a special vine called *sargi*, a strong jungle vine. These are weavings where the large and small posts are interwoven, making them strong and resistant. But these large and small posts cannot govern alone; they need others, which is the Indigenous guard, *sowalibedi*.

Similarly, the word *sobe* is also related to the womb because the process of gestation is also a weaving. Our entire body is a weave, and water recreates, transforms, creates, and weaves. Similarly, we can speak of Grandfather Fire as the great sage who was present at the creation of Mother Earth in the great mother's womb. Our Creators, *Nanadumadi* and *Babadummadi*, recreated their bodies to weave the life of their daughter, *Nabgwana* (Mother Earth). The fire wove inside the womb of the mother. Fire transforms, it is love, it burns, and light appears. Mother Earth is fire within, in her bones, her muscles; in other words, Mother Earth is fire, water, wind, and medicinal plants.

Now let's explain the other word that also refers to weaving, which is the word *magge*. This word means to paint, and the word painting means protection. When a woman *dule* (weaves) the *mola*, using different colored fabrics and creating geometric or non-geometric figures, she is weaving, protecting, and painting. Similarly, when we paint our faces with *achiote*, we obtain the color red, and when we paint with *jagua*, we obtain the color black. These paintings represent protection for our lives when we enter the forest or jungle because there live various beings that could harm us physically or spiritually.

In the same way, we could say that when a woman *dule* (weaves) her *molas*, she recreates according to her sense. That is why no *mola* is the same; they are all different because they align with nature. There are *molas* that refer to the corals of the sea, to the vertebrae of each tree leaf, to the flight of the eagle, the path of the tapir, the snakes, and the mountains. In other words, when a woman *dule* (weaves), she connects with the world around her, and she also thinks about the protection of the people who will wear that art of the *mola*.

The Sense of the Word 'Sweet' and the Sense of the 'Good Heart'

All the principles of Mother Earth are interconnected, and even more so when we talk about these two principles. As we were weaving these principles, I began to delve deeper into the sense of Mother Earth, and each time I found that they are wonderful weavings, because these principles are in my body, they are everywhere, and this is precisely what we find in pedagogy, to explain life, as defined by the wise people in the Bachelor's Program in Pedagogy of Mother Earth: "The pedagogy of Mother Earth is a pedagogy to learn the stories and accompany dreams."

And precisely this is what all the ancestral peoples of the world agree on: that our origin is in the cosmos, Earth is a step to return to the origin. But the difference lies in that some cultures say they come from water, that they come from the serpent, that their ancestor is the whale, that they come from the rainbow, but all are related to nature. It is extremely important, and I believe we must continue delving into this topic.

In Gunadule culture, when one is asked how much knowledge they have learned, what is being asked is: How many fires from the bones of the mother do you know? Knowledge is from the fire of the mother's bones, it is the great wisdom that is woven into every pore of our skin because Earth is my life. I am within her womb, constantly transforming, gestating until my death, and after death, we will continue weaving until we reach the realm where our great mother and father are. If we understand this lovingly and in balance, we approach the sense of the sweet word and the good heart, because this is precisely what will unite us to understand these principles: the heart. In the Gunadule language, this is very clear because to the word sweet, we say:

Gwabin ossigwa: 'The tongue has the smell of pineapple'. In Dulegaya, we say the tongue *Gwabin*, which comes from two words: *gwa*, referring to the heart and *binnni*, meaning to move or turn. The word for tongue refers to the heart that moves and turns, meaning the tongue is the voice of the heart. In this sense, the tongue can heal. This is why in Gunadule culture, there are various therapeutic songs, which are beautiful and metaphorical.

Ossigwa: 'It is the heart of the pineapple'. The word <<Sweet>> comes from the smell of the pineapple, and once again, the heart appears in reference to the scent. If we combine these words, we get the sense of the good heart, meaning the sweet word refers to the sweetness, the flavor of the pineapple. This is how the word should be understood; it is healing. And our encounter with the sweetness, with the flavor of the word, begins from the womb of our mothers, because the grandfather, the grandmother, sang stories of the plants, the community, and the heart of the words was present in my gestation process in my mother's womb. This is why the program in the Bachelor's Degree in Pedagogy of Mother Earth, when referring to the <<Sweet>> word and the 'good heart', along with the other principles we previously mentioned, weaves, intertwines, and unites as a whole.

Now we can understand that the sweet word comes from the depth of the wisdom of my people, which turns into poetry, becomes metaphor. In this sense, we cannot speak in just any way about what we have lived; it is something extraordinary. This is why we must speak to women, nature, and Mother Earth from the sweet word, from the good heart.

Gwage nuedi: 'Good Heart' comes from the following words: '*Gwage*', which refers to the heart, and it in turn comes from two words: Gwa, meaning center or essence, and the word *G(u)e*, meaning 'being being'. That is, when we say the word 'good heart' it means 'being being essence, center'. In other words, the heart is the center of our existence.

In this sense, all of us who are involved in the pedagogy of Mother Earth cannot have just any heart, but must have a good heart, because it is about healing. When we talk about healing, we refer to the care of the life of Mother Earth, and for this, therapeutic songs must be present: songs for cacao, for spicy chili, for basil, for healing plants, for birth and death, for the spirits of the grandmothers and grandfathers. All of this must be through beautiful words.

Here, the researcher of Mother Earth cannot be just anyone because it involves all the ethics of respect, of valuing things from the heart, from the sense of things, not just from the rationality that we have been taught until now. It is time to return to the thought of corazonar (thinking with the heart). We must feel the research from the depth of my being and my community.

I believe that this is not only our task as students in the Bachelor's Program of Mother Earth but for all academics, for all human beings because the heart of Mother Earth is speaking to us, it is calling us. If we do not listen to her, we are heading straight to death, to chaos.

The world needs to listen, we need to listen to each other in silence to observe, to weave from the sweet word and the good heart, the events of history. This would allow the sense of our existence to be linked, connected with the cosmos and the earth, allowing us to dance with grandfather *Ibelele* (the Sun).

CONCLUSION

These principles of Mother Earth are connected to spirituality, and each people has their way of relating to their surroundings. Each people has their grandmothers and grandfathers who weave with the spirits of their ancestors. Each people has been recreating for thousands of years through their ceremonies, dances, songs, foods, and Mother Earth has entrusted us with the delegation of her principles, as a path to continue recreating the meaning of life, a meaning that we lost with rationality, which caused us to lose the sense of human existence.

For this reason, the Bachelor's Degree in Pedagogy of Mother Earth will continue inviting us to return to the womb, to return to our origins, to stay connected with all cosmic beings and all beings of Mother Earth, since we were conceived by the energy of our mother and father. We are special beings who were created with multiple energies, capable of perceiving what is happening in the cosmos and in every pore of the skin of our Mother Earth.

The only person who is permanently caring for the life of the community, for all beings on earth, is a woman. She is the mother of all living beings. The Earth is also a mother, who loves us all equally. If we recreate the many language spoken in Abya Yala we would realize that as we evoke the words, we would begin to understand and reveal the face of our ancestors and the meaning of things and life, thus better understanding the meaning of good living for our future generations, since everything depends on us, the survival of our habitat.

I use this methodology of learning our mother tongue from the meanings of words as a pedagogical contribution so that new generations have greater arguments to continue resisting from their own perspective, and thus prevent us from being co-opted by neoliberal policies that do not prioritize collective interests, but rather specific interests for the well-being of their class. This linguistic tool becomes powerful for the defense of our culture and our territories. In other words, we find greater arguments to defend our Mother Nature against large development megaprojects, which have seen large mining deposits in our territories and thus threaten us daily. This contribution is essential, since the Spanish language, for centuries, has been doing its work of diminishing the flavor and importance of the wisdom of our grandfathers and grandmothers when they pass on their words. The Pedagogy of Mother is even a path to start learning how to interact with nature composed by living organisms and more than living organisms.

REFERENCES

Aghasaleh, R. (2019). *Children and Mother Nature. Storytelling for a Glocalized Environmental Pedagogy*. Brill Hes & De Graaf. DOI: 10.1163/9789004399822

Antioquia, U. d. (2011). *Licenciatura en Pedagogía de la Madre Tierra*. Obtenido de Líneas de formación o investigación: https://www.udea.edu.co/wps/portal/udea/web/inicio/unidades-academicas/educacion/oferta-pregrado/licenciatura-pedagogia-madre-tierra/!ut/p/z1/3ZRLc5swFIX_ClmwxBJv6M51mATbcYyfMZuOkK4xHZAIxqbtr69wunGa2Olk2JQNkubc7zCXo4ti9IRiTo5ZSupMcJLL_SZ2vk0iO9CNAR7jeejgK

Baltra-Ulloa, J., & Kostecki, T. (2024). Engaging care for Mother Earth as central pedagogy for sustainable and regenerative Social Work. En M. Kumar, S. Pattanayak, & N. Belford, *The Layered Landscape of Higher Education. Capturing Curriculum, Diversity, and Cultures of Learning in Australia* (pág. 11). London, UK: Taylor & Francis Group. DOI: 10.4324/9781032715544-16

Green Stocel, A. (2011). *Anmala Gaya Burba: Isbeyobi Daglele Nana Nabgwana Bendaggegala. Significado de Vida; Espejo de Nuestra Memoria en Defensa de la Madre Tierra*. Universidad de Antioquia.

Mashford-Pringle, A.; Stewart, S. L.; et al. (2019). Akiikaa (it is the land): exploring land-based experiences with university students in Ontario. Global Health Promotion. 64-72. DOIi:DOI: 10.1177/1757975919828722

Simon, M.-R., & Martin, H. (2023). Mother Earth as Emergent Curriculum. En P. Trifonas, & J. S., *Handbook of Curriculum Theory and Research* (págs. 4 - 11). Ontario, Canada: Springer Nature Switzerland. DOI: 10.1007/978-3-030-82976-6_43-1

Smith-Gilman, S. (2023). *Mother Earth's Way. A beginning resource guide for early childhoods educators*. McGill. Obtenido de., https://www.mcgill.ca/walkingalongside/files/walkingalongside/wa_sheryl_fnl_draft_vocabbeg-1.pdf

ENDNOTES

1 Some ideas for the presentation at the education forum – Basic Principles for Self-Education and Life- a lecture by the author at the National Meeting of the Ministry of Education (MEN), Colombia.

Section 2
Practices and Pedagogies for Personal and Collective Growth

Chapter 9
Integrating Mindfulness Into Parenting and Education:
A Pathway to Child Wellbeing and Emotional Resilience

Richi Simon
https://orcid.org/0000-0003-4961-2609
IGNOU, India

Hannah John
https://orcid.org/0009-0004-2654-9066
Madras School of Social Work, India

Shumayela Hasan
The Bal Bhawan School, India

ABSTRACT

The chapter explores the integration of mindfulness into parenting and education as a transformative approach to addressing child anxiety and fostering emotional resilience. The analysis highlights the role of mindfulness in mitigating the challenges faced by children and adolescents, particularly in the post-COVID-19 era, where stressors have amplified mental health concerns. Grounded in cultural sensitivity, the chapter examines the interplay of parenting styles, educational practices, and sociocultural influences, advocating for mindful parenting and classroom strategies that enhance self-awareness, emotional balance, and adaptive coping mechanisms. Through a synthesis of theoretical insights and practical applications, it emphasizes mindfulness as a culturally adaptable tool for nurturing children's well-being

DOI: 10.4018/979-8-3373-0360-4.ch009

and resilience in a rapidly evolving global society. This holistic approach not only addresses the immediate symptoms of anxiety but also promotes long-term psychological stability, making a case for integrating mindfulness into broader child development frameworks.

INTRODUCTION

Anxiety in children, characterized by physiological responses like muscle tension and rapid breathing, is an adaptive reaction to perceived threats. This emotion is influenced by a range of factors, including parental styles and cultural expectations, which shape a child's interpretation of threat and coping mechanisms. Emerging research suggests mindfulness is a viable tool for managing childhood anxiety. By integrating mindfulness into parenting and everyday practices, children can learn to approach their feelings with curiosity rather than fear, potentially mitigating the impact of anxious thoughts and fostering resilience.

Anxiety, an emotion associated with apprehension and somatic symptoms of tension whereby individuals expect misfortune, danger or even catastrophe. This perception of threat is addressed by the body in the form of tension in muscles, fast breathing and rapid heartbeats. Anxiety, a future oriented, long acting response focused on diffusing threat (*APA Dictionary of Psychology*, n.d.). APA also associates anxiety with recurring intrusive thoughts. Response normally takes the form of "flight or fight" (Felman, 2020).

Wittchen et al. (2011) found that anxiety is more common than any mental illness in Europe among those in the age bracket of 14 to 65 years. Further, women suffer two to three times more than men. IHME (2019) indicates anxiety disorder as the most widespread of all mental disorders, i.e., 31% of the 13% of the global population having mental disorders are victims of anxiety disorder, the next in line is depressive disorders comprising 28.9%. WHO (2022) also indicate that rates of already common conditions such as depression and anxiety went up by more than 25% in the first year of the pandemic. There are several factors associated with anxiety which are discussed in the sections below.

Anxiety and Age

Anxiety is found across people of all age groups. However, research studies indicate that anxiety disorders mostly begin in childhood with separation anxiety marked in 23% of preschool or school goers (Beesdo, 2010). Also, WHO (2022) quotes "Our infancy and childhood set the tone for the rest of our lives." Anxiety disorders onsets during childhood, adolescence, or early adulthood. A peak is reached in middle age, this may decrease with older age (Bandelow & Michaelis, 2015). It is further found that the median age for anxiety is 11 years (Kessler, Berglund, Demler, Jin, Merikangas, & Walters, 2005).

Parenting significantly influences childhood anxiety. Research has shown that authoritarian and neglectful parenting styles are often linked to higher anxiety, whereas authoritative parenting—with its balance of warmth and control—promotes emotional security. Introducing mindfulness within parenting practices offers an additional layer of support, as it teaches both parents and children to acknowledge emotions without immediately reacting. This mindfulness-based approach enables children to view their anxiety with a balanced perspective, ultimately reducing the power of their anxieties over time.

Parenting is complex and often described with a key focus on normal variations in parenting emphasizing the issues of control (Baumrind, 1991). Maccoby & Martin (1983) discussed two elements of parenting as parental responsiveness and behavioural control and proposed a typology of 4 parenting styles depicted in Figure 1-

Figure 1. Parenting Style Typology (Maccoby & Martin, 1983)

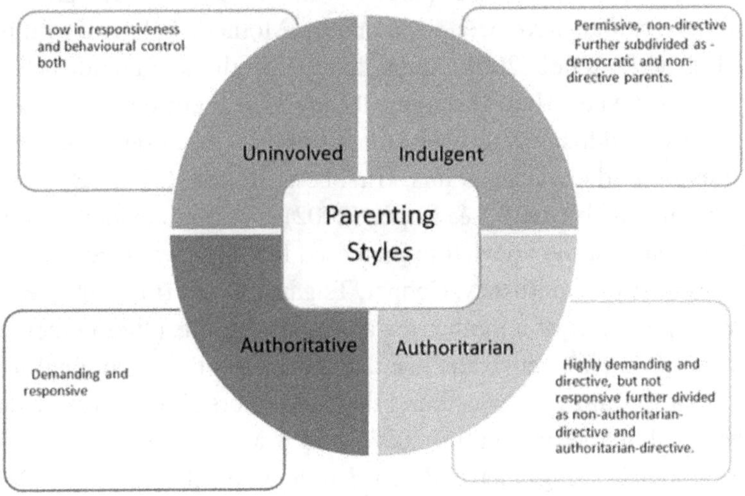

Barber (1996) added another dimension – Psychological control, i.e., those attempts to control emotional and psychological development of the child prompted by acts of guilt induction, shaming, withdrawal of love etc.

Anxiety disorders are often characterised by complex interaction of environmental factors and multiple genetic variants at chromosomal loci (Gottschalk & Domschke, 2016). Bandura (1997) suggested that interactions between parents and adolescents can affect the well-being of young ones. Also, interpersonal factors play a key role in elevating anxiety sensitivity (Taylor, Jang, Stewart, & Stein, 2008).

Grüner, Muris, & Merckelbach (1999) also found that child anxiety resulted from both maternal and paternal rejection. Van, Tillfors, & Trost. (2018) noted the difference in causative factors resulting in social anxiety across gender. While for girls it was higher parental worry, for boys it was high parental over control.

Exploring the factors leading to anxiety in children the top down studies have indicated that children of the adults who had suffered from anxiety disorders are more prone to anxiety disorders (Barrett, Dadds, & Rapee, 1996) and also the bottom up studies also show that the parents of children with anxiety disorders have increased prevalence of anxiety themselves (Cooper, Fearn, Willetts, Seabrook, & Parkinson, 2006). Child anxiety and depression were significantly related to parent anxiety symptoms. (Burstein, Ginsburg, & Tein, 2010; Biederman et al., 1991; Turner, Beidel, & Costello, 1987). Children of parents with anxiety disorders had higher mean levels of all types of symptomatology relative to children of parents with no psychiatric diagnosis. Burstein et al., (2010) also suggest that children of parents with both anxiety and externalizing problems are more likely to develop anxiety themselves than children of parents with only anxiety problems.

Further, most studies have been done on how Mother's behavior results in anxiety, like, Hudson & Rapee (2001) found that the Mothers of anxious children are more controlling and negative. The atypical caregivers themselves have been found to have an unresolved history of mourning or trauma – emotional, physical or sexual or are traumatized (Zeanah, Danis, Hirshberg, Benoit, Miller, & Scott, 1999). With the experiments by Gerull & Rapee (2002) it became evident that mother's fearful expression to some toys led to increased fear and avoidance in off springs towards the same toys. De Rosnay, Cooper, Tsigaras, & Murray (2006) established that anxious expressions of a mother towards a stranger resulted in increased fear and avoidance in infants and further, reduction in positive emotional tone upon advancement of a stranger. It was found that if Mothers show intrusive control or ridicule their children (Rubin et al., 2002), and if Mothers exhibited anxiety and less interest in social settings then children also show social withdrawal (De Rosnay, Harris, & Pons, 2008). It was further found that higher level of maternal control can increase anxiety particularly when the children are given to being fearful (Thirlwall & Cresswell, 2010).

Though mainly such studies are done on Mothers, research study by Cooper et al. (2006) found that fathers of anxious children have increased lifetime history of anxiety themselves. Merikangas, Avenevoli, Dierker, & Grillon (1999) found that the presence of anxiety disorder among both the parents double the chance of their offspring to have anxiety disorder. Parents with SAD are likely to implement over controlling behaviours (Ballash, Leyfer, Buckley, & Woodruff Borden, 2006). Field,

Lawson, & Banerjee (2008) found that children's avoidant behaviour and fears are influenced by the information they receive.

Further, the parent and child factors also affect internalization (Brumariu & Kerns, 2010) and externalizing of the problems (Gross, Shaw, & Moilanen, 2008). Barrett et al. (1996) found that discussion with parents and their interpretations and response shape the level of anxiety in children which further effects their planning. They proposed 'FEAR' effect: Family Enhancement of Aggressive or Avoidant Responses. These results were consistent among fathers and mothers. Study done by Platt, Williams, & Ginsburg (2016) indicated that stressful life events and anxiety symptoms were mediated by the levels of parenting stress, parental anxious rearing, and dysfunctional parent child interaction.

Thus, research studies point that parenting can trigger anxiety and affect anxiety levels in children and plays a crucial role in the development of a child.

Erozkan (2012) found that there is a significant relationship between anxiety sensitivity and parenting styles. Further, overprotective and authoritarian parenting styles affect child's interpretations of events as threatening (Chorpita & Barlow, 1998). Mannuzza, Klein, Moulton, Scarfone, Malloy, Vosburg, & Klein (2002) found that perceived parental pressure correlated positively with trait anxiety and with anxiety sensitivity. Parental over involvement (Hudson & Rapee, 2001), lack of bestowing autonomy (Moore, Whaley, & Sigman, 2004), intrusive control (Wood, 2006) are all forms of parental control. Moreover, parents' excessive regulation makes the child believe that the world is dangerous (Hudson & Rapee, 2004). Wood (2006) found that intrusiveness may result in Separation Anxiety Disorder (SAD).

The case study by Siddaway, Wood, & Cartwright Hatton (2014) bridges theory and practice by providing a practice evidence explaining the interplay between child anxiety theory and evidence. The study also emphasizes upon the role of parents in CBT for treatment of child anxiety.

A diathesis-stress model helps understand the factors resulting in anxiety among children. It is depicted in Figure 2.

Figure 2. Diathesis Stress Model of Child Anxiety

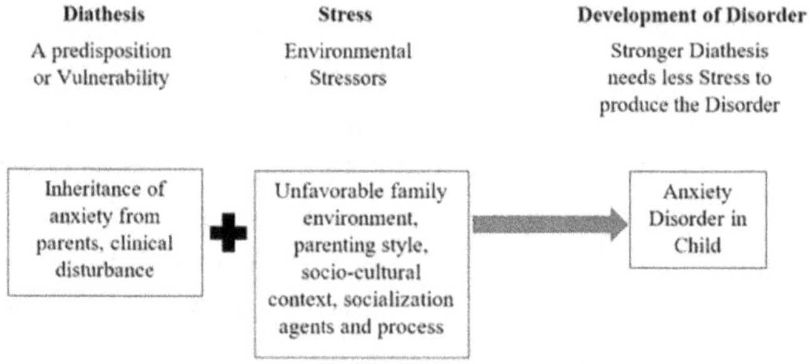

Effect of Mindfulness on Emotional Resilience

According to Connor and Davidson (2003), resilience is "the personal qualities that enable others to thrive in the face of adversity." The resilience model proposed identifies key protective factors, including self-efficacy and adaptability, which align closely with mindfulness practices. The ability of a person to cope with hardship, whether it comes from inside or beyond, is referred to as resilience (Zsido et al., 2022). Bogaerts et al. (2021) describe resilience as the capacity to adapt adaptably, stay afloat, or even develop in the face of stress or hardship. By intentionally focusing on the present moment without passing judgment, one can attain mindfulness, a state of elevated awareness (Marenus et al., 2021). Mindful exercise is exercise that integrates physical exertion with kinesthesia (Mitchell, 2021). Mindfulness practitioners seem to be better able to regulate negative thoughts and feelings, as well as to take in and learn from their experiences without passing judgment (Sünbül & Güneri, 2019).

According to Shapiro et al. (2006), "attention," "intention," and "attitude" are three axioms of mindfulness that emphasize the attitudinal orientation in consciousness. Integrating mindfulness can strengthen these protective factors, enabling children to regulate emotions and cope effectively with challenges. Twelve characteristics of "meditative mindfulness" were identified by Shapiro and Schwartz, including patience, trust, gentleness, generosity, empathy, appreciation, openness, non-striving, acceptance, and loving-kindness (Shapiro & Schwartz, 2000).

In their study, Niazi & Niazi (2011) investigate Mindfulness Based Stress Reduction (MBSR) therapy as a meditation technique. Originally created for stress management, MBSR therapy is currently being used to treat a number of illnesses, including cancer, diabetes mellitus, depression, anxiety, chronic pain, hypertension, skin, and immune disorders. Patients with chronic diseases benefit from MBSR, which also helps them manage a wide range of clinical issues. Jain (2024) discovered that among young individuals, mindfulness, resilience, and quality of life were significantly positively correlated. In particular, people who reported feeling more aware tended to be more resilient and to think that their quality of life was higher.

According to the findings of Philippe et al. (2021) mindfulness practice increased the practitioners' initial level of resilience, indicating that mindfulness meditation may be used as a coping mechanism after a potentially stressful situation. Also, Holas and Jankowski (2013) found that attentive individuals are more likely to use the link between awareness and meta-awareness to track their cognitive processes. These individuals can perceive their feelings, ideas, and experiences more clearly.

Parenting and Mindfulness

If parenting affects anxiety in children, the question arises - what factors affect parenting? Harmon & Brim (1980) pointed that there are 4 factors that affect parenting viz. 1. Generic Cultural Factors 2. Individual Factors 3. Interpersonal Factors and 4. The Setting. Another researcher, Belsky (1984) proposed 3 determinants of parenting as – 1. Personal psychological resources of parents (which are further shaped by developmental history of the parent), 2. Characteristic features of child (goodness of fit between parent and child), and 3. Contextual sources of stress and support (like marital relationship, employment, social network).

Culture shapes the way anxiety is perceived and expressed, influencing both parenting styles and children's responses. In many non-Western cultures, authoritative parenting may be associated with respect and obedience, yet integrating mindfulness can introduce flexibility, allowing children to process emotions healthily within culturally appropriate boundaries. When mindfulness practices are adapted to respect cultural values, they can offer children tools to navigate cultural expectations without succumbing to anxiety. This culturally sensitive mindfulness approach respects traditions while promoting emotional resilience.

In the words of Marsella, "Culture refers to the shared learned behavior which is transmitted from one generation to another for purposes of individual and societal growth, adjustment, and adaptation; culture is represented externally as artifacts, roles and institutions, and it is represented internally as values, beliefs, attitudes, epistemology, consciousness, and biological functioning" (Marsella, 1988). Researchers have argued that the observed ethnic differences in the association of parenting style and child outcomes may be due to the differences in the social context, parenting practices, or the cultural meaning of specific dimensions of parenting style (Chao, 1994; Darling & Steinberg, 1993). Cultural beliefs and values about parenting can affect how anxiety is expressed in children. In Western cultures, authoritarian parenting that restricts autonomy is linked to clinical anxiety, whereas in non-western cultures, it is not. This indicates that different cultural ideologies shape the way anxiety is perceived and experienced (Wood, McLeod, Sigman, Hwang, & Chu, 2003). Chorpita, Brown, Barlow (2016) evaluated structural models and investigated the relation of perceived control and attribution to family environment, negative affect, and clinical disturbance. The study depicted the mediating role of cognitive dimensions between family environment and clinical anxiety and mood disturbance. The family environment is certainly build within the cultural framework as culture shapes one's belief system and parents act upon them while treating their young ones (Ochs, 1988). Culture is believed to impact psycho social dimensions and the manner in which they interact to produce risk for or protection from the emergence and maintenance of anxiety problems (Kirmayer, 2001). Culture shapes parents and parenting (Bornstein, 2014). Interestingly, parenting and culture reciprocate, parenting embeds culture and meaning in itself. Also, culture is inherited through parenting (Bornstein & Sameroff, 2009; Bornstein, 2012). Moreover, Bernstein (2013) pointed that the different perceived parenting styles bring different outcomes across different cultures. Culture, the set of distinct patterns of beliefs and behaviours is shared by a group of people for the purpose of regulation and control. Hofmann & Hinton (2014) established Ethnopsychology/Ethnophysiology (the mental and bodily processes) and contextual factors (norms and rules including the individualistic/collectivist disposition) as factors leading to anxiety. Economic and social disadvantages further increase the risk of anxiety. People living in the countries with a vast gap between the rich and poor and where social polarization persist also have greater risk to anxiety (WHO, 2022).

It must be noted that the concept of mindful parenting has existed since 1997. The study by Wong et al. (2017) investigated whether children's social and personal decision-making is predicted by attentive parenting. After adjusting for confounders, more sharing was strongly predicted by more attentive parenting from mothers. For all of the individual decision-making indicators, there was no discernible major effect of mindful parenting by mothers. The results indicate that children's social decision-making is supported by mindful parenting. One promising strategy that encourages emotion management in both parents and kids is mindful parenting (Duncan et al, 2009). The way parents connect with their children is influenced by their own emotional regulation skills, and differences in this capacity are influenced by a number of cognitive, social, physiological, and neurobiological variables (Morris et al., 2007). According to Rutherford et al. (2015), parents who are unable to set an example of effective control through their conduct and parenting techniques help their kids struggle with emotion regulation, which may have a negative effect on their development inadvertently. Duncan et al. (2009) expanded the mindful parenting model by incorporating mindfulness principles into parent-child relationships. The model includes five dimensions: listening attentively, accepting self and child, emotional awareness, self-regulation, and compassion. These dimensions improve parenting behavior, leading to more positive, supportive relationships. A natural everyday practice, dispositional mindfulness has been associated with better mental health symptoms and better emotion control (Fogarty et al., 2013; Bravo et al., 2018).

With the given backdrop, the objectives of the study are –

1. To examine the interplay between culture, parenting styles, and child anxiety, with a focus on understanding how these factors influence children's emotional well-being.
2. To explore the impact of different parenting styles on children's perception and expression of anxiety.
3. To investigate the role of cultural influences, communication patterns, and coping mechanisms in shaping children's anxiety levels within diverse cultural contexts.
4. To assess the effectiveness of support systems in mitigating child anxiety and promoting emotional well-being.
5. To identify potential areas for improvement in parenting approaches and support systems to reduce child anxiety and foster a healthier parent-child relationship.

Hypotheses:

1. Children raised in authoritative parenting environments characterized by balanced rules, open communication, and support will exhibit lower levels of anxiety compared to those raised in authoritarian, neglectful, or overprotective environments.
2. Cultural norms and gender roles will significantly influence the perception and expression of anxiety in children, with variations observed across different cultural contexts.
3. Effective coping mechanisms, such as engaging in hobbies, practicing mindfulness, and participating in physical activities, will be associated with lower levels of anxiety in children.
4. Support systems, including friends, teachers, and counselors, will play a crucial role in mitigating child anxiety and promoting emotional well-being.
5. Parental involvement in education and the establishment of clear guidelines, warmth, and understanding will positively impact children's anxiety levels and emotional well-being.

RESEARCH METHODOLOGY

The study is qualitative in nature. The study employs data triangulation, combining information from clients and parents in each case, alongside literature reviews and scrutiny of 30 distinct cases selected from the Sanskar Valley School, Bhopal, to enhance credibility and ensure robustness. The participants were selected using purposive and volunteering sampling, thus, only those children who had the problem of anxiety and who along with their parents consented to be a part of the study were selected as participants. Research ethics were followed, oral consent was sought from the participants and only those who were willing to be a part of the study were included in the study. The participants were made aware of the study's objectives and confidentiality was maintained. The participants were debriefed about the study and were allowed to withdraw from the study within a time period of two weeks from their interview. Need based counselling services were also assured.

The study also utilizes comprehensive literature reviews and adheres to well-established anxiety disorder definitions from organizations such as the APA and WHO, reinforcing the validity of its findings. Additionally, the study employs a grounded theory approach to develop a theory regarding child anxiety and its relationship with parenting styles, cultural influences, communication patterns, and coping mechanisms. This methodology amalgamates existing knowledge, strengthening the overall validity of the research findings. Wordclouds were used to analyse the interviews.

The participants were from The Sanskar Valley School, Bhopal as the school demonstrates a daily practice of mindfulness.

About The Sanskar Valley School

Sanskaar Valley School is a non-profit co-educational, day boarding-cum-residential institution established by the Sharda Devi Charitable Trust. Located on a 40-acre campus, the school offers 2.5 lac square feet of built-up area and focuses on nurturing individuals towards excellence in a happy, value-based, and progressive learning community.

Mindfulness Sessions at The Sanskar Valley School

The Sanskaar Valley School in Bhopal integrates mindfulness into its curriculum, addressing rising stress and anxiety among students. Tailored 15–20-minute sessions incorporate practices like guided breathing, body scan meditation, yoga, and visualization to enhance relaxation, emotional balance, and self-awareness. Reflective journaling encourages introspection in older students. These culturally sensitive sessions blend universal mindfulness techniques with Indian traditions, ensuring relevance and effectiveness. Students report improved focus, reduced anxiety, and enhanced emotional resilience, while teachers and parents observe better behavior and coping skills. The program demonstrates the school's commitment to fostering holistic development and emotional well-being in its students.

The demographic profile for both anxious children from The Sanskar Valley School and their parents is presented in Table 1.

Table 1. Demographic Profile

Children			Parents		
Criteria	**Description**	**Frequency**	**Criteria**	**Description**	**Frequency**
Age	7-10 years	6	Gender	Male	15
	10-13 years	9		Female	15
	13-16 years	15	Economic Class	Upper Class	5
Gender	Male	15		Middle Class	15
	Female	15		Low Class	10
Assessed level of anxiety	Mild	12	Employment status	Self-employed	5
	Moderate	8		Public sector	8
	Severe	9		Private sector	7

Table 2. Tools used for the study

Interview Schedule administered to the anxious children	**Interview Schedule administered to the parents of anxious children**
1. Demographic Information: a. Age: b. Gender: c. Grade/Year in School: 2. Parenting Style Perception: 3. Parental Involvement: 4. Cultural Influences: 5. Anxiety Perception: 6. Parent Child Communication: 7. Impact of Parenting on Anxiety: 8. Expression of Anxiety: 9. Support Systems: 10. Coping Mechanisms: 11. Suggestions for Improvement: 12. Additional Comments or Insights:	1. Background Information: a. Parent's Name: b. Child's Name and Age: c. Family Background: 2. Exploration of Child's Anxiety: a. Signs or Symptoms: b. Duration of Symptoms: c. Professional Help: 3. Parenting Style and Practices: a. Parenting Style: b. Influence on Child's Anxiety: c. Handling Anxiety: 4. Cultural Influences on Parenting and Anxiety: a. Influence of Cultural Beliefs: b. Cultural Factors in Anxiety: c. Navigating Cultural Differences: 5. Communication Patterns and Coping Mechanisms: a. Communication about Anxiety: b. Coping Mechanisms: c. Supporting Expression: 6. Impact of Parental Involvement and Support Systems: a. Involvement: b. Support Systems: c. Changes in Anxiety: 7. Suggestions for Improvement and Parenting Approaches: a. Improvement Areas: b. Effective Strategies: c. Building a Healthier Relationship:

Table 2 details the interview schedule administered to anxious children and the parents of anxious children enrolled in The Sanskar Valley School. The schedule mostly had open ended questions. While there were twelve questions in the schedule, with one question having three parts administered to the children, the schedule administered to the parents of the anxious children had seven questions, with each question having three parts.

DATA ANALYSIS

Figure 3. Word cloud depicting the central themes of childrens' transcripts

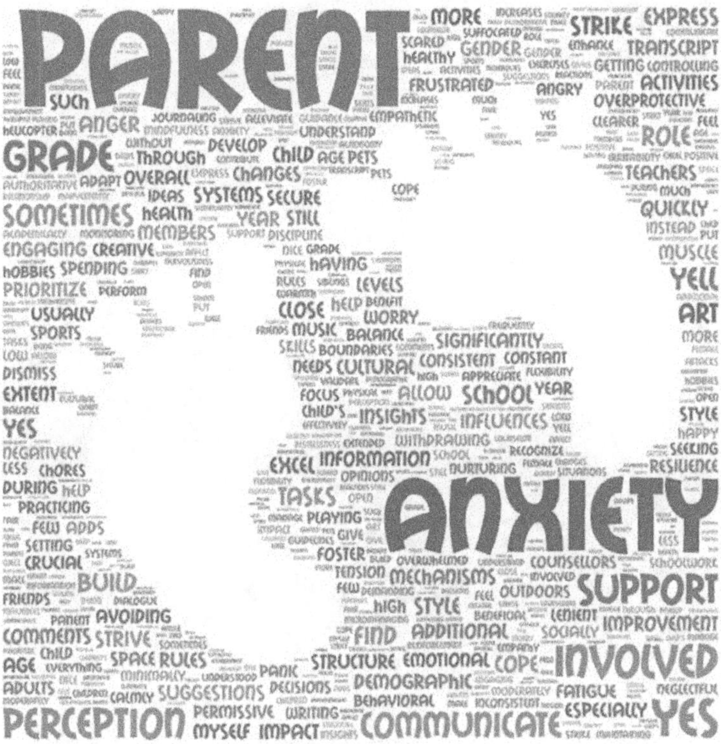

Figure 3 depicts the central ideas in the transcripts of children. "Anxiety", "grades", "parenting", "parents", "communication", "perception" and "support" are the central ideas as discussed by the children with anxiety clearly depicting the family micro-environment and areas of improvements for addressing anxiety.

Figure 4. Word cloud depicting the central themes of parents' transcripts

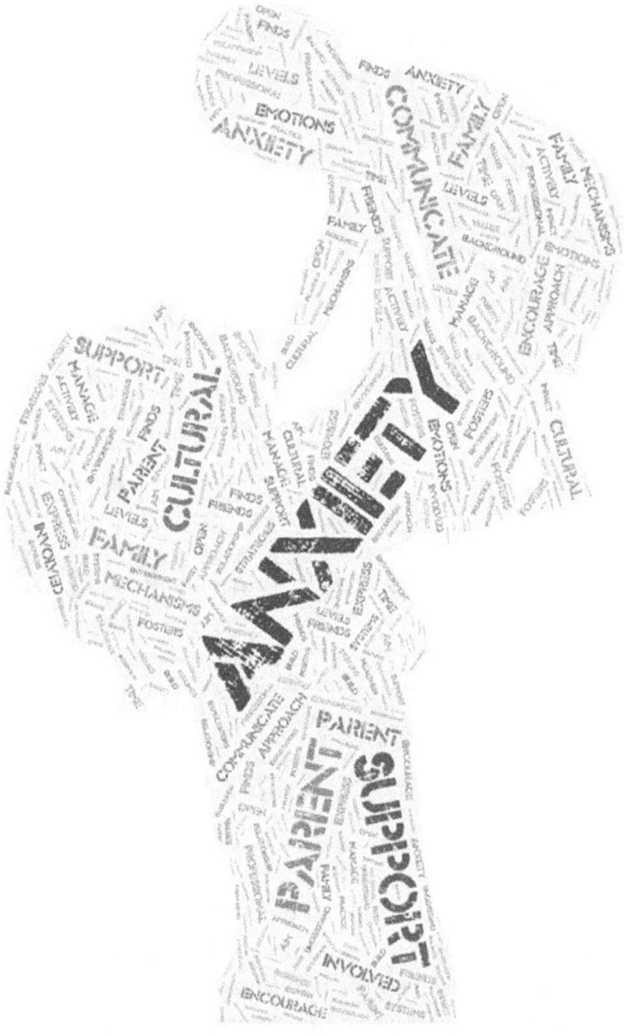

Figure 4 presents the central themes in the transcripts of parents. Words like "emotional", "parenting", "activities", "feelings", "communication", "support", "individual", "concerns" and "changes" represent the central themes.

Further word clouds were generated on the text queries of anxiety, support, parenting and culture.

Upon analysing the transcripts of both parents and children, the word cloud depicted in Figure 5 was constructed. The word cloud projects the central theme as "anxiety", further major themes are "support", "cultural", "communication", "parenting", "family" . Thus, it is clear that anxiety is related to culture, parenting, communication, support and family. Family environment and communication patters rely on culture and parenting style.

Figure 5. Word cloud depicting the overlapping central themes of both parents and children

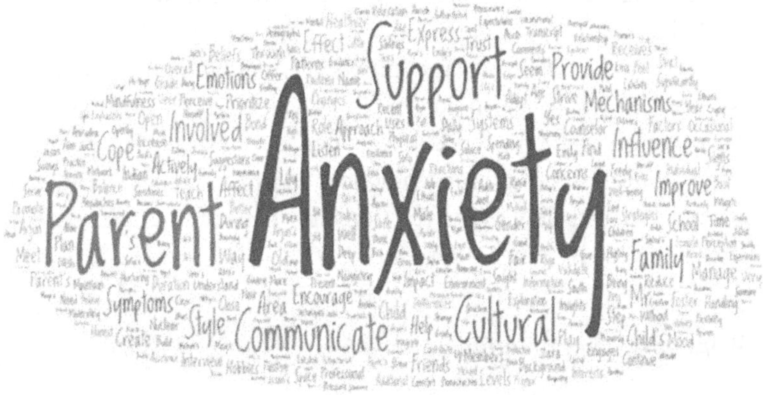

Figure 6. Word cloud on anxiety

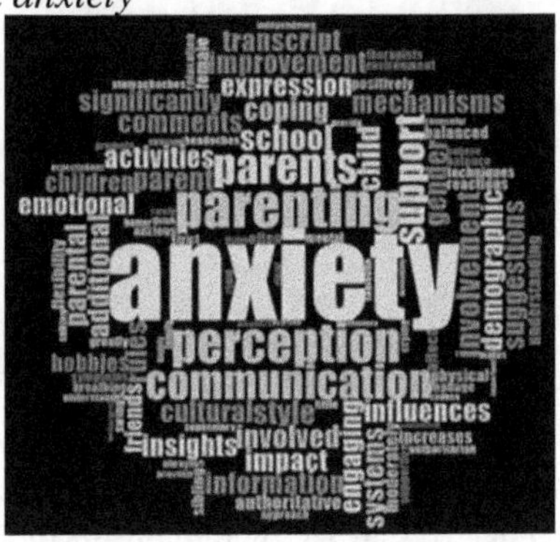

The word cloud in figure 6 visually represents key term – "anxiety" from the transcripts. The central focus is "anxiety," surrounded by terms like "parenting" and "perception," highlighting their roles in linking parenting practices to children's anxiety. This underscores the need to explore how various factors contribute to children's anxiety.

The word cloud also reveals different parenting styles and their effects on anxiety. Words such as "authoritative," "strict," "involved," and "support" suggest how different parenting approaches may impact anxiety, possibly reflecting cultural differences. Terms like "cultural," "style," and "gender" show that cultural norms and gender roles are crucial in understanding anxiety in children, affecting how parenting practices influence emotional health. Additionally, "communication" stands out, emphasizing its role in parent-child interactions and cultural norms influencing anxiety. Words like "coping," "mechanisms," "support," and "activities" point to coping strategies in various cultural contexts. The inclusion of "stomachaches," "headaches," and "symptoms" indicates the physical signs of anxiety and their cultural interpretations. The presence of "gender" suggests examining how gender intersects with cultural and parenting practices to affect anxiety. The word cloud thus offers a concise overview of the relationships between culture, parenting, and children's emotional well-being.

Figure 7. Word cloud on Parenting

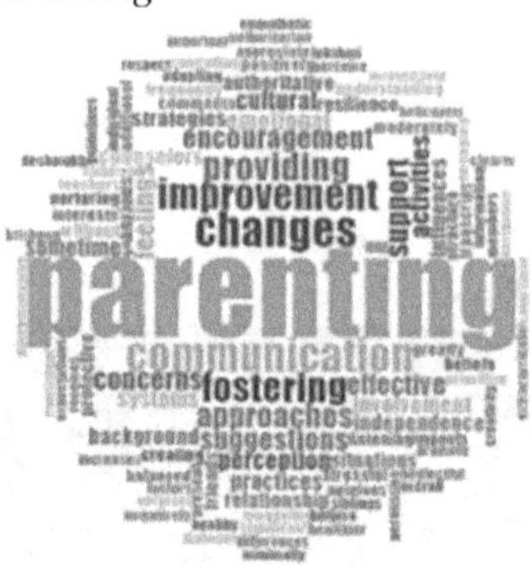

The "Parenting" word cloud in figure 7 reveals the complexities and stresses parents face in managing their responsibilities. Key words like "children," "stress," "support," "work," "home," and "education" illustrate the multifaceted nature of parental roles. Parents discuss the stress of balancing work and family life, highlighting the need for robust support systems. The term "education" points to the critical role parents play in their children's learning and development, indicating that educational support is a significant aspect of parenting. The emphasis on "home" reflects the dual function of the household as both a workplace and a nurturing environment for children.

The "Culture" word cloud depicted in figure 8, underscores the influence of cultural norms and traditions on family dynamics and gender roles. Words like "culture," "traditions," "gender roles," "patriarchy," "family," and "community" suggest that cultural expectations significantly shape the experiences of families. The focus on "gender roles" and "patriarchy" highlights the structural barriers women face, which can affect family dynamics and individual well-being. The presence of "family" and "community" emphasizes the importance of these social units in providing support and navigating everyday challenges, illustrating the deep-rooted impact of cultural context on family life.

Figure 8. Word cloud on Culture

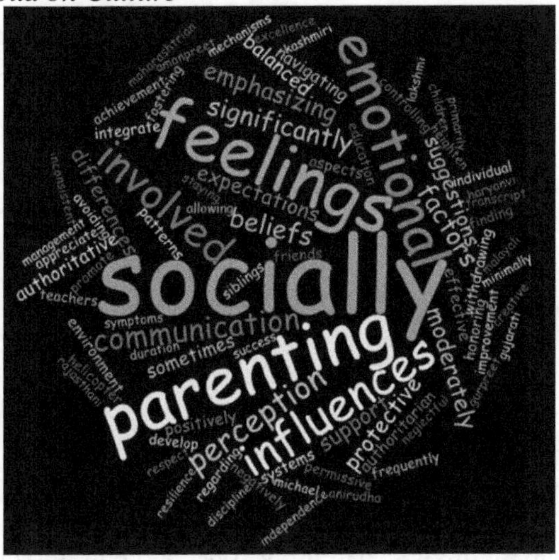

The "Anxiety in Children" and "Parenting" word clouds both highlight significant stress and anxiety, indicating a mutual influence where the well-being of parents and children is closely linked. Educational challenges are prominent in both children's and parents' experiences, underscoring the importance of academic support. The cultural word cloud connects these experiences to broader cultural norms and gender roles, suggesting that traditional expectations and patriarchy exacerbate stress and responsibilities within families. This holistic view illustrates that addressing these interconnected issues requires an approach that considers emotional support, educational assistance, and cultural context.

Also, thematic analysis was carried on the interview transcripts to understand the major themes emerging during the interviews. The results are depicted in figure 9.

Figure 9. Thematic map

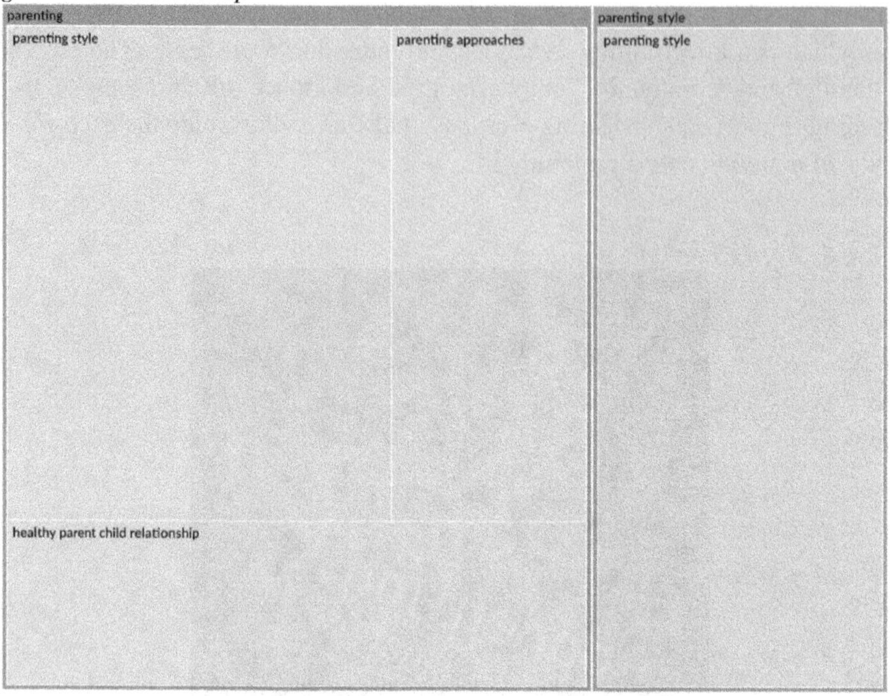

The thematic map highlights "parenting style" as central to effective parenting, emphasizing how authoritative, authoritarian, permissive, or uninvolved styles impact child development. Parenting approaches—methods like positive reinforcement, discipline, and communication—are also key, aiding in managing behavior and promoting growth. A healthy parent-child relationship, characterized by trust, respect, and support, is essential for children's social and emotional well-being. The analysis shows a strong link between parenting style, approaches, and relationship quality, as parenting style influences the methods used, impacting the parent-child bond. Overall, nurturing relationships and effective approaches are crucial for children's holistic development.

Grounded Theory

Based on the data collected open, axial and selective codes were generated using the data gathered from the interviews. Interviews were carried on until saturation was reached (Strauss & Corbin, 1997). They are presented in Table 3.

Table 3. Coding

Open Codes	Axial Codes	Selective Codes
Parenting styles: Authoritative, Permissive, Neglectful, Overprotective	Parenting Styles and Anxiety Perception: Authoritative and Overprotective styles are specifically linked to anxiety.	The impact of parenting styles, cultural influences, and communication patterns on child anxiety and their coping mechanisms.
Cultural influences: Norms, values, expectations	Cultural Influences and Parenting Behaviors: Norms, values, and expectations shape parenting behaviors.	
Communication patterns: Open, supportive, non-verbal	Communication Patterns and Anxiety Management: Effective communication (open, supportive, non-verbal) and ineffective communication.	
Coping mechanisms: Cognitive strategies, emotional strategies, behavioral strategies	Coping Mechanisms for Child Anxiety: Cognitive strategies (positive self-talk, problem-solving, cognitive restructuring, mindfulness) Emotional strategies (deep breathing, relaxation techniques, expressive writing) Behavioral strategies (exposure therapy, systematic desensitization, reward systems)	

Using the codes, a mind map is presented in Figure 10.

Figure 10. Mind map

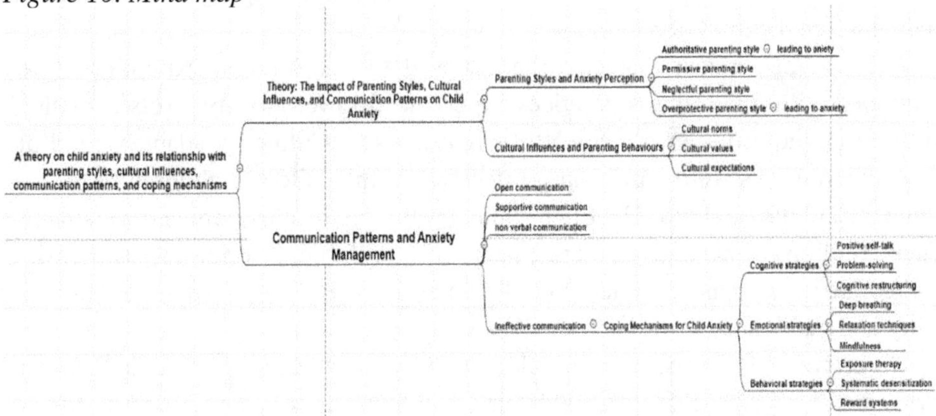

The mind map presents a theory on child anxiety, exploring how parenting styles, cultural factors, communication, and coping strategies shape anxiety levels. Authoritative and overprotective parenting can increase anxiety, while permissive and neglectful styles influence stress management. Cultural norms affect parenting practices, which can either alleviate or heighten anxiety, especially in societies with high academic and social expectations. Effective communication, allowing children to express emotions openly, reduces anxiety, while poor communication worsens it. Coping mechanisms—like mindfulness, relaxation, problem-solving, and reward systems—play a crucial role in helping children manage anxiety, fostering a supportive environment for emotional resilience.

Major Findings

Objective 1: To examine the interplay between culture, parenting styles, and child anxiety, with a focus on understanding how these factors influence children's emotional well-being.

The findings reveal that children exposed to authoritative parenting styles combined with mindfulness practices experienced lower anxiety levels compared to those in authoritarian or neglectful environments. Culturally adapted mindfulness interventions were particularly effective, as they allowed children to remain connected to their cultural identities while developing healthy coping mechanisms. These findings emphasize the importance of mindfulness in not only addressing immediate symptoms of anxiety but also in establishing long-term emotional stability and resilience.

Objective 2: To explore the impact of different parenting styles on children's perception and expression of anxiety.

The findings reveal that children exposed to authoritative parenting styles combined with mindfulness practices experienced lower anxiety levels compared to those in authoritarian or neglectful environments. Culturally adapted mindfulness interventions were particularly effective, as they allowed children to remain connected to their cultural identities while developing healthy coping mechanisms. These findings emphasize the importance of mindfulness in not only addressing immediate symptoms of anxiety but also in establishing long-term emotional stability and resilience.

Objective 3: To investigate the role of cultural influences, communication patterns, and coping mechanisms in shaping children's anxiety levels within diverse cultural contexts.

The findings reveal that children exposed to authoritative parenting styles combined with mindfulness practices experienced lower anxiety levels compared to those in authoritarian or neglectful environments. Culturally adapted mindfulness interventions were particularly effective, as they allowed children to remain connected to their cultural identities while developing healthy coping mechanisms. These findings emphasize the importance of mindfulness in not only addressing immediate symptoms of anxiety but also in establishing long-term emotional stability and resilience.

Objective 4: To assess the effectiveness of support systems in mitigating child anxiety and promoting emotional well-being.

The findings reveal that children exposed to authoritative parenting styles combined with mindfulness practices experienced lower anxiety levels compared to those in authoritarian or neglectful environments. Culturally adapted mindfulness interventions were particularly effective, as they allowed children to remain connected to their cultural identities while developing healthy coping mechanisms. These findings emphasize the importance of mindfulness in not only addressing immediate symptoms of anxiety but also in establishing long-term emotional stability and resilience.

Objective 5: To identify potential areas for improvement in parenting approaches and support systems to reduce child anxiety and foster a healthier parent-child relationship.

The findings reveal that children exposed to authoritative parenting styles combined with mindfulness practices experienced lower anxiety levels compared to those in authoritarian or neglectful environments. Culturally adapted mindfulness interventions were particularly effective, as they allowed children to remain connected to their cultural identities while developing healthy coping mechanisms. These findings emphasize the importance of mindfulness in not only addressing immediate symptoms of anxiety but also in establishing long-term emotional stability and resilience.

Based on the information provided, the document discusses the interplay between culture, parenting styles, and child anxiety, emphasizing the influence of parenting styles and cultural factors on children's anxiety levels. It also highlights the impact of authoritarian and overprotective parenting styles on children's susceptibility to anxiety and the mediating role of culture in shaping parenting and influencing the expression of anxiety in children. The study underscores the need for balanced and authoritative parenting approaches to reduce anxiety and promote healthier emotional development in children.

Hypotheses-Wise Findings

Hypothesis 1: Children raised in authoritative parenting environments characterized by balanced rules, open communication, and support will exhibit lower levels of anxiety compared to those raised in authoritarian, neglectful, or overprotective environments.

The findings reveal that children exposed to authoritative parenting styles combined with mindfulness practices experienced lower anxiety levels compared to those in authoritarian or neglectful environments. Culturally adapted mindfulness interventions were particularly effective, as they allowed children to remain connected to their cultural identities while developing healthy coping mechanisms. These findings emphasize the importance of mindfulness in not only addressing immediate symptoms of anxiety but also in establishing long-term emotional stability and resilience.

Hypothesis 2: Cultural norms and gender roles will significantly influence the perception and expression of anxiety in children, with variations observed across different cultural contexts.

The findings reveal that children exposed to authoritative parenting styles combined with mindfulness practices experienced lower anxiety levels compared to those in authoritarian or neglectful environments. Culturally adapted mindfulness interventions were particularly effective, as they allowed children to remain connected to their cultural identities while developing healthy coping mechanisms. These findings emphasize the importance of mindfulness in not only addressing immediate symptoms of anxiety but also in establishing long-term emotional stability and resilience.

Hypothesis 3: Effective coping mechanisms, such as engaging in hobbies, practicing mindfulness, and participating in physical activities, will be associated with lower levels of anxiety in children.

The findings reveal that children exposed to authoritative parenting styles combined with mindfulness practices experienced lower anxiety levels compared to those in authoritarian or neglectful environments. Culturally adapted mindfulness interventions were particularly effective, as they allowed children to remain connected to their cultural identities while developing healthy coping mechanisms. These findings emphasize the importance of mindfulness in not only addressing immediate symptoms of anxiety but also in establishing long-term emotional stability and resilience.

Hypothesis 4: Support systems, including friends, teachers, and counselors, will play a crucial role in mitigating child anxiety and promoting emotional well-being.

The findings reveal that children exposed to authoritative parenting styles combined with mindfulness practices experienced lower anxiety levels compared to those in authoritarian or neglectful environments. Culturally adapted mindfulness interventions were particularly effective, as they allowed children to remain connected to their cultural identities while developing healthy coping mechanisms. These findings emphasize the importance of mindfulness in not only addressing immediate symptoms of anxiety but also in establishing long-term emotional stability and resilience.

Hypothesis 5: Parental involvement in education and the establishment of clear guidelines, warmth, and understanding will positively impact children's anxiety levels and emotional well-being.

The findings reveal that children exposed to authoritative parenting styles combined with mindfulness practices experienced lower anxiety levels compared to those in authoritarian or neglectful environments. Culturally adapted mindfulness interventions were particularly effective, as they allowed children to remain connected to their cultural identities while developing healthy coping mechanisms. These findings emphasize the importance of mindfulness in not only addressing immediate symptoms of anxiety but also in establishing long-term emotional stability and resilience.

Cultural Sensitivity in Mindfulness Practices: Adapting to Global Perspectives

Mindfulness based interventions facilitate a means to connect with the cultural and social identity (Li et al., 2024). Kabat-Zinn (2003) emphasizes that while mindfulness has universal benefits, its Western adaptation often disregards its spiritual and cultural origins. Addressing cultural sensitivity is essential to respect its roots and ensure its ethical application in diverse cultural contexts. Integrating indigenous perspectives into mindfulness practices enhances inclusivity and avoids cultural appropriation. Singh et al. (2021) highlight that mindfulness programs in Asian societies resonate more when incorporating native philosophies like Confucianism or Hinduism. These adaptations not only preserve cultural authenticity but also increase the efficacy of mindfulness interventions. The globalization of mindfulness has led to ethical dilemmas surrounding cultural appropriation. Hyland (2015) critiques the commercialization of mindfulness in Western markets, which often strips the practice of its original cultural and ethical dimensions. Ethical mindfulness practice demands acknowledgment of its Buddhist heritage while fostering intercultural understanding and respect. Wong (2018) explores how culturally adapted mindfulness programs in educational settings enhance students' emotional regulation and social skills. Tailoring these programs to reflect the diverse backgrounds of learners ensures inclusivity and relevance. Wilson (2019) suggests that mindfulness practitioners can learn from indigenous practices of holistic well-being, which align with mindfulness principles but are grounded in unique cultural contexts. Such integration fosters mutual respect and learning between traditions. Mindfulness practices can support cultural identity when adapted appropriately. According to Kim et al. (2022), culturally sensitive mindfulness interventions empower marginalized groups by validating their cultural heritage within therapeutic settings. Many studies have shown that regular meditation practice, even for a short period, can lead to positive results such as reduced stress, improved focus or mindfulness, and improved health, as evidenced by the growing acceptance of meditation as a mainstream practice (Chiesa, Calati, & Serretti, 2011; van den Hurk et al., 2010).

Victor (1992) identified five cultural characteristics: emphasis on written word, adherence to law, governance of interpersonal behavior, agreements based on personal promises, and agreements based on written word or contract. Low-context cultures emphasize written word, rigid adherence to law, flexible governance of interpersonal behaviors, and binding agreements based on personal promises or contracts.

Educational Settings as Platforms for Mindfulness-Based Learning

Educational institutions hold the unique potential to shape children's mental health and emotional resilience. As centers of learning and development, schools provide an optimal platform for introducing mindfulness practices that not only enhance academic performance but also equip children with essential life skills. Mindfulness programs in schools—ranging from structured breathing exercises to guided meditation and reflective journaling—have been shown to improve emotional regulation, attention, and empathy in students.

The Role of Educators: Teachers play a pivotal role in implementing mindfulness in classrooms. Training programs for educators can empower them to model mindfulness practices, creating an empathetic and inclusive environment for students. Mindfulness instruction equips educators with the tools to manage classroom stress and foster a culture of calm and focus.

Integration with Social-Emotional Learning (SEL): Mindfulness aligns seamlessly with SEL frameworks, which emphasize skills like self-awareness, emotional regulation, and effective communication. By embedding mindfulness into SEL curricula, schools can enhance students' ability to navigate social interactions and cope with challenges effectively.

Practical Implementation

Strategies for incorporating mindfulness in schools include:

- Daily mindfulness moments: Brief sessions of focused breathing or silent reflection integrated into the school day.
- Mindful movement exercises: Activities such as yoga or tai chi to improve body awareness and stress reduction.
- Mindfulness corners: Designated classroom spaces for relaxation and grounding practices.

By embracing mindfulness, schools can become catalysts for nurturing resilience and emotional intelligence, creating a supportive foundation for students to thrive academically and personally.

The Future of Mindfulness in Child Wellbeing: Opportunities and Challenges

The evolving landscape of mental health and education presents a fertile ground for the integration of mindfulness. However, scaling mindfulness practices for widespread adoption involves navigating opportunities and addressing significant challenges.

Opportunities

- Advancements in Research: Ongoing studies continue to highlight the cognitive, emotional, and physiological benefits of mindfulness for children. Future research could explore long-term impacts, including its influence on academic achievements, interpersonal relationships, and mental health outcomes.
- Policy Integration: Governments and educational bodies have the opportunity to adopt mindfulness as part of public health and educational policies. National-level initiatives can allocate resources for mindfulness training and implementation across schools and community centers.
- Technology and Accessibility: Digital platforms and mobile apps offer scalable solutions for mindfulness practice. Tools such as guided meditations, reminders, and interactive exercises can bring mindfulness to underserved populations, bridging gaps in accessibility.
- Collaborative Networks: Partnerships among educators, psychologists, policymakers, and technology developers can create interdisciplinary frameworks for delivering mindfulness programs effectively.

Challenges

- Cultural Sensitivity: Implementing mindfulness in diverse cultural settings requires thoughtful adaptation. Practices must respect local traditions, beliefs, and societal norms to ensure acceptance and relevance.
- Training and Resources: Effective mindfulness instruction necessitates extensive teacher and parent training, as well as access to quality resources. Funding and logistical support remain critical barriers in resource-constrained environments.
- Sustainability and Consistency: Integrating mindfulness into daily routines without overwhelming educators or caregivers requires strategic planning. Ensuring that mindfulness practices are sustainable over time is a significant challenge.

LIMITATIONS, SCOPE, AND IMPLICATIONS

The study is limited by its small sample size, as only 30 cases were examined due to time constraints. Participants were drawn from a single school in India that practices daily mindfulness, focusing on children experiencing anxiety and their parents who volunteered for the study. The primary data collection is restricted to Indian culture, and findings predominantly reflect authoritarian parenting styles, which may result from this cultural focus. While the literature review broadened the context and supported the findings, the geographic and cultural limitations suggest that further research across diverse settings is necessary to enhance generalizability.

This research investigates the integration of mindfulness practices into parenting and educational settings, emphasizing their potential to mitigate child anxiety and foster emotional resilience. It examines theoretical foundations, empirical evidence, and practical applications, exploring the relationship between cultural norms, parenting styles, and mindfulness-based interventions. The study evaluates schools as critical platforms for mindfulness practices, highlighting strategies like guided meditations, reflective journaling, and mindfulness-based stress reduction (MBSR) programs. These practices are analyzed for their impact on emotional regulation, academic performance, and social skills in children.

Cultural sensitivity forms a core aspect of the study, focusing on how mindfulness can be adapted to align with diverse cultural values and ethical considerations. Although the primary data reflects the Indian context, the research incorporates global insights to identify universal principles of mindfulness, making the findings relevant beyond India.

The study provides actionable insights for parents, educators, and policymakers. For parents, it emphasizes the value of mindful parenting—characterized by empathy, emotional awareness, and self-regulation—in reducing anxiety and nurturing emotional resilience in children. For educators, it outlines strategies to incorporate mindfulness into classroom environments, including daily mindfulness sessions, reflective practices, and mindfulness corners. Schools are positioned as key environments for promoting mental well-being and enhancing social-emotional learning (SEL).

On a broader level, the findings underscore the importance of culturally sensitive mindfulness interventions. Policymakers and mental health practitioners can use these insights to design programs that respect cultural contexts while addressing the universal issue of child anxiety. Integrating mindfulness into education and public health policies has the potential to scale its benefits, making the practice more accessible and inclusive.

The study lays a solid foundation for future research. Expanding the scope to include diverse cultural and socio-economic contexts will improve the generalizability of findings. Additionally, training parents and educators to implement mindfulness practices effectively is crucial for ensuring the sustainability of these interventions. With further development, mindfulness can become a vital tool in fostering emotional resilience and reducing anxiety in children worldwide.

DISCUSSIONS

The study's limitations are noteworthy and impact the generalizability and depth of its findings. Firstly, its exclusive focus on India limits the applicability of results to diverse cultural settings, where distinct parenting styles and societal norms may influence the interplay between culture, parenting, and child anxiety differently. The reliance on a small sample size of only 30 cases raises concerns about representativeness within the broader population, and potential selection biases may have affected external validity. The study's concentration on authoritarian parenting styles restricts insights into the broader impact of different parenting approaches on child anxiety. It also overlooks various potential contributors to child anxiety, such as genetic predispositions, environmental stressors, and peer influences. The study inadequately accounts for the cultural diversity within India, potentially oversimplifying the complex interplay between culture, parenting, and child anxiety. The lack of explicit consideration of temporal changes in parenting styles and cultural dynamics may hinder understanding of their evolving interactions. The assumption of direct parental influence on child anxiety without exploring other factors oversimplifies the intricate web of influences on children's emotional well-being. Lastly, the overemphasis on maternal influences neglects the potential significant role of paternal influences in shaping child anxiety. To enhance understanding, future research should address these limitations through diverse samples, a comprehensive exploration of contributing factors, and a nuanced consideration of both maternal and paternal influences.

The study illustrates that integrating mindfulness into parenting and educational practices offers a practical, culturally adaptable strategy for managing childhood anxiety. Mindfulness provides children with tools to address their emotions constructively, fostering an inner resilience that complements the guidance provided by authoritative parenting. Future research should expand on the role of mindfulness across diverse cultural contexts, refining techniques that respect cultural values while promoting well-being. This approach underscores a promising path for reducing anxiety and enhancing emotional health in children globally. Mental health exists on a complex continuum with experiences ranging from an optimal state of well-being to debilitating states of great suffering and emotional pain. With an understanding that out of 8 people every 1 lives in a mental health condition (WHO, 2022), it makes it utmost important to understand mental health and develop ways and means to address them. Anxiety, a complex emotion, involves apprehension and physiological responses like muscle tension and fast breathing. It's prevalent across ages, peaking in middle age, and has diverse disorders categorized by APA and WHO. Parenting significantly influences childhood anxiety; maternal and paternal behaviors impact children's anxiety levels. Parenting styles, including authoritarian and overprotective approaches, affect susceptibility. Cultural factors also shape parenting and impact anxiety expression in children. Culture mediates and moderates parenting anxiety relationships. Understanding these connections can guide interventions for anxious children. Further research is necessary to explore the intricate interplay between parenting, culture, and child anxiety for effective prevention and treatment.

CONCLUSION

Integrating mindfulness into parenting and educational practices offers a transformative approach to addressing child anxiety, fostering emotional resilience, and promoting long-term psychological well-being. The findings highlight the significance of authoritative parenting styles and culturally sensitive mindfulness practices in reducing anxiety among children. By incorporating mindfulness strategies tailored to diverse cultural contexts, parents and educators can bridge traditional values with modern therapeutic approaches, ensuring inclusivity and effectiveness.

This study underscores the interconnected roles of parenting, culture, and educational systems in shaping a child's emotional health. Authoritative parenting, when combined with mindfulness, fosters a balanced environment that supports children in navigating their anxieties while remaining connected to their cultural identities. In educational settings, mindfulness practices not only enhance academic performance but also cultivate emotional intelligence and social adaptability, creating resilient learners capable of managing stress and uncertainty.

Challenges remain in adapting mindfulness practices to diverse cultural and socio-economic settings. Future research should aim to explore broader applications of mindfulness across varied cultural landscapes, ensuring sustainable implementation through training, resources, and policy integration. Addressing these barriers will allow mindfulness to serve as a universal tool for enhancing child well-being and building emotionally resilient societies.

By prioritizing mindful parenting and education, stakeholders can create a nurturing foundation for children, empowering them to navigate the complexities of a rapidly evolving global environment with confidence, compassion, and resilience.

REFERENCES

Ainsworth, M. D. S. (1989). Attachments beyond infancy. *The American Psychologist, 44*(4), 709–716. DOI: 10.1037/0003-066X.44.4.709 PMID: 2729745

APA Dictionary of Psychology. (n.d.). Anxiety. https://dictionary.apa.org/diathesis-stress-model

Ballash, N., Leyfer, O., Buckley, A. F., & Woodruff-Borden, J. (2006). Parental control in the etiology of anxiety. *Clinical Child and Family Psychology Review, 9*(2), 113–133. DOI: 10.1007/s10567-006-0007-z PMID: 17089199

Bandelow, B., & Michaelis, S. (2015). Epidemiology of anxiety disorders in the 21st century. *Dialogues in Clinical Neuroscience, 17*(3), 327–335. DOI: 10.31887/DCNS.2015.17.3/bbandelow PMID: 26487813

Barber, B. K. (1996). Parental psychological control: Revisiting a neglected construct. *Child Development, 67*(6), 3296. DOI: 10.2307/1131780 PMID: 9071782

Barrett, P. M., Dadds, M. R., & Rapee, R. M. (1996). Family treatment of childhood anxiety: A controlled trial. *Journal of Consulting and Clinical Psychology, 64*(2), 333–342. DOI: 10.1037/0022-006X.64.2.333 PMID: 8871418

Baumrind, D. (1991). The influence of parenting style on adolescent competence and substance use. *The Journal of Early Adolescence, 11*(1), 56–95. DOI: 10.1177/0272431691111004

Beesdo, K., Pine, D. S., Lieb, R., & Wittchen, H. U. (2010). Incidence and risk patterns of anxiety and depressive disorders and categorization of generalized anxiety disorder. *Archives of General Psychiatry, 67*(1), 47–57. DOI: 10.1001/archgenpsychiatry.2009.177 PMID: 20048222

Belsky, J. (1984). The determinants of parenting: A process model. *Child Development, 55*(1), 83–96. DOI: 10.2307/1129836 PMID: 6705636

Bernstein, D. A. (2013). *Essentials of Psychology*. Cengage Learning.

Biederman, J., Petty, C., Hirshfeld-Becker, D. R., Henin, A., Faraone, S. V., Dang, D., & Rosenbaum, J. F. (2006). A controlled longitudinal 5-year follow-up study of children at high and low risk for panic disorder and major depression. *Psychological Medicine, 36*(8), 1141–1152. DOI: 10.1017/S0033291706007781 PMID: 16700966

Bogaerts, S., van Woerkom, M., Erbaş, Y., De Caluwé, E., Garofalo, C., Frowijn, I., Jeandarme, I., Masthoff, E., & Janković, M. (2021). Associations Between Resilience, Psychological Well-Being, Work-Related Stress and Covid-19 Fear in Forensic Healthcare Workers Using a Network Analysis. *Frontiers in Psychiatry*, *12*, 678895. DOI: 10.3389/fpsyt.2021.678895 PMID: 34177662

Bornstein, M. H. (2009). Toward a model of culture↔parent↔child transactions. In Sameroff, A. (Ed.), *The transactional model of development: How children and contexts shape each other* (pp. 139–161). American Psychological Association., DOI: 10.1037/11877-008

Bornstein, M. H. (2012). Cultural approaches to parenting. *Parenting, Science and Practice*, *12*(2-3), 212–221. DOI: 10.1080/15295192.2012.683359 PMID: 22962544

Bornstein, M. H., & Cote, L. R. (2014). Immigration and acculturation. In Bornstein, M. H., & Cote, L. R. (Eds.), *Handbook of Cultural Developmental Science* (pp. 543–564). Psychology Press. DOI: 10.4324/9780203805497

Bravo, A. J., Pearson, M. R., & Kelley, M. L. (2018). Mindfulness and Psychological Health Outcomes: A Latent Profile Analysis among Military Personnel and College Students. *Mindfulness*, *9*(1), 258–270. DOI: 10.1007/s12671-017-0771-5 PMID: 29430258

Brody, G. H., & Ge, X. (2001). Linking parenting processes and self-regulation to psychological functioning and alcohol use during early adolescence. *Journal of Family Psychology*, *15*(1), 82–94. DOI: 10.1037/0893-3200.15.1.82 PMID: 11322087

Burstein, M., Ginsburg, G. S., & Tein, J. Y. (2010). Parental anxiety and child symptomatology: An examination of additive and interactive effects of parent psychopathology. *Journal of Abnormal Child Psychology*, *38*(7), 897–909. DOI: 10.1007/s10802-010-9415-0 PMID: 20432062

Chao, R. K. (1994). Beyond parental control and authoritarian parenting style: Understanding Chinese parenting through the cultural notion of training. *Child Development*, *65*(4), 1111–1119. DOI: 10.2307/1131308 PMID: 7956468

Chiesa, A., Calati, R., & Serretti, A. (2011). Does mindfulness training improve cognitive abilities? A systematic review of neuropsychological findings. *Clinical Psychology Review*, *31*(3), 449–464. DOI: 10.1016/j.cpr.2010.11.003 PMID: 21183265

Chorpita, B. F., & Barlow, D. H. (1998). The development of anxiety: The role of control in the early environment. *Psychological Bulletin*, *124*(1), 3–21. https://psycnet.apa.org/doi/10.1037/0033-2909.124.1.3. DOI: 10.1037/0033-2909.124.1.3 PMID: 9670819

Chorpita, B. F., Brown, T. A., & Barlow, D. H. (2016). Perceived control as a mediator of family environment in etiological models of childhood anxiety. *Behavior Therapy*, *47*(5), 622–632. DOI: 10.1016/j.beth.2016.08.008 PMID: 27816075

Connor, K. M., & Davidson, J. R. (2003). Development of a new resilience scale: The Connor-Davidson Resilience Scale (CD-RISC). *Depression and Anxiety*, *18*(2), 76–82. DOI: 10.1002/da.10113 PMID: 12964174

Cooper, P. J., Fearn, V., Willetts, L., Seabrook, H., & Parkinson, M. (2006). Affective disorder in the parents of a clinic sample of children with anxiety disorders. *Journal of Affective Disorders*, *93*(1-3), 205–212. DOI: 10.1016/j.jad.2006.03.017 PMID: 16675030

Darling, N., & Steinberg, L. (1993). Parenting style as context: An integrative model. *Psychological Bulletin*, *113*(3), 487–496. DOI: 10.1037/0033-2909.113.3.487

Dattani, S. (2021, August 20) Mental Health. *Our World in Data*. https://ourworldindata.org/mental-health

De Rosnay, M., Cooper, P. J., Tsigaras, N., & Murray, L. (2006). Transmission of social anxiety from mother to infant: An experimental study using a social referencing paradigm. *Behaviour Research and Therapy*, *44*(8), 1165–1175. DOI: 10.1016/j.brat.2005.09.003 PMID: 16288978

De Rosnay, M., Harris, P. L., & Pons, F. (2008). Emotion understanding and developmental psychopathology in young children. In Fonagy, P., & Goodyer, I. (Eds.), *Social Cognition and Developmental Psychopathology*. Oxford University Press., DOI: 10.1093/med/9780198569183.003.0012

Duncan, L. G., Coatsworth, J. D., & Greenberg, M. T. (2009). A model of mindful parenting: Implications for parent-child relationships and prevention research. *Clinical Child and Family Psychology Review*, *12*(3), 255–270. DOI: 10.1007/s10567-009-0046-3 PMID: 19412664

Erozkan, A. (2012). Examination of relationship between anxiety sensitivity and parenting styles in adolescents. *Educational Sciences: Theory & Practice*, *12*(1), 52–57. https://files.eric.ed.gov/fulltext/EJ978432.pdf

Felman, A. (2020, January 11). What to know about anxiety. *Medical News Today*. https://www.medicalnewstoday.com/articles/323454#what-is-anxiety

Field, A. P., Lawson, J., & Banerjee, R. (2008). The verbal threat information pathway to fear in children: The longitudinal effects on fear cognitions and the immediate effects on avoidance behavior. *Journal of Abnormal Psychology*, *117*(1), 214–224. DOI: 10.1037/0021-843X.117.1.214 PMID: 18266499

Fogarty, F. A., Lu, L. M., Sollers, J. J.III, Krivoschekov, S. G., Booth, R. J., & Consedine, N. S. (2015). Why it pays to be mindful: Trait mindfulness predicts physiological recovery from emotional stress and greater differentiation among negative emotions. *Mindfulness*, *6*(2), 175–185. DOI: 10.1007/s12671-013-0242-6

Gerull, F. C., & Rapee, R. M. (2002). Mother knows best: Effects of maternal modelling on the acquisition of fear and avoidance behaviour in toddlers. *Behaviour Research and Therapy*, *40*(3), 279–287. https://psycnet.apa.org/doi/10.1016/S0005-7967(01)00013-4. DOI: 10.1016/S0005-7967(01)00013-4 PMID: 11863238

Gross, H. E., Shaw, D. S., & Moilanen, K. L. (2008). Reciprocal associations between boys' externalizing problems and mothers' depressive symptoms. *Journal of Abnormal Child Psychology*, *36*(5), 693–709. DOI: 10.1007/s10802-008-9224-x PMID: 18288602

Grüner, K., Muris, P., & Merckelbach, H. (1999). The relationship between anxious rearing behaviours and anxiety disorders symptomatology in normal children. *Journal of Behavior Therapy and Experimental Psychiatry*, *30*(1), 27–35. DOI: 10.1016/S0005-7916(99)00004-X PMID: 10365863

Hofmann, S. G., & Hinton, D. E. (2014). Cross-cultural aspects of anxiety disorders. *Current Psychiatry Reports*, *16*(6), 450. DOI: 10.1007/s11920-014-0450-3 PMID: 24744049

Holas, P., & Jankowski, T. (2013). A cognitive perspective on mindfulness. *International Journal of Psychology*, *48*(3), 232–243. DOI: 10.1080/00207594.2012.658056 PMID: 22506609

Hudson, J. L., & Rapee, R. M. (2001). Parent-child interactions and anxiety disorders: An observational study. *Behaviour Research and Therapy*, *39*(12), 1411–1427. DOI: 10.1016/S0005-7967(00)00107-8 PMID: 11758699

Hudson, J. L., & Rapee, R. M. (2004). From anxious temperament to disorder: An etiological model of generalized anxiety disorder. In Heimberg, R. G., Turk, C. L., & Mennin, D. S. (Eds.), *Generalized Anxiety Disorder: Advances in Research and Practice* (pp. 51–74). Guilford Press.

Hyland, T. (2015). Mindfulness in education: Can schools make students better people? *Educational Studies*, *41*(1-2), 34–50. DOI: 10.1080/03055698.2014.1002387

IHME. (2019) Global Burden of Disease Study 2019 (GBD 2019) Data Resources. http://ghdx.healthdata.org/gbd-results-tool?params=gbd-api-2019-permalink/5066-348dc958b095cb6ceb4bfd9c3e07

Jain, S. (2024). Impact of Mindfulness on Resilience and Quality of Life among Young Adults. *International Journal of Indian Psychology, 12*(2). Advance online publication. DOI: 10.25215/1202.322

Kabat-Zinn, J. (2003). Mindfulness-based interventions in context: Past, present, and future. *Clinical Psychology : a Publication of the Division of Clinical Psychology of the American Psychological Association, 10*(2), 144–156. DOI: 10.1093/clipsy.bpg016

Kessler, R. C., Berglund, P., Demler, O., Jin, R., Merikangas, K. R., & Walters, E. E. (2005). Lifetime prevalence and age of onset distributions of DSM-IV disorders in the National Comorbidity Survey Replication. *Archives of General Psychiatry, 62*(6), 593–602. DOI: 10.1001/archpsyc.62.6.593 PMID: 15939837

Kim, S. H., Kang, E., & Choi, H. (2022). Culturally responsive mindfulness: Addressing mental health disparities among marginalized populations. *Journal of Counseling Psychology, 69*(3), 210–220. DOI: 10.1037/cou0000598

Kirmayer, L. J. (2001). Cultural variations in the clinical presentation of depression and anxiety: Implications for diagnosis and treatment. *The Journal of Clinical Psychiatry, 62*, 22–28. PMID: 11434415

Li, W. W., McIntyre, R., Reid, C., & Chao, M. (2024). A Systematic Review on the state of the Art of Culturally Adapted Mindfulness-Based Interventions for First Nations Peoples: Cultural Adaptation, Effectiveness, and Feasibility. *Mindfulness, 15*(9), 2147–2172. DOI: 10.1007/s12671-024-02440-4

Maccoby, E. E., & Martin, J. A. (1983). Socialization in the Context of the Family: Parent-Child Interaction. In Mussen, P. H., & Hetherington, E. M. (Eds.), Handbook of Child Psychology: Vol. 4. *Socialization, Personality, and Social Development* (pp. 1–101). Wiley.

Mannuzza, S., Klein, R. G., Moulton, J. L., Scarfone, N., Malloy, P., Vosburg, S. K., & Klein, D. F. (2002). Anxiety sensitivity among children of parents with anxiety disorders: A controlled high risk study. *Journal of Anxiety Disorders, 16*(2), 135–148. DOI: 10.1016/S0887-6185(01)00095-0 PMID: 12194540

Marenus, M. W., Murray, A., Friedman, K., Sanowski, J., Ottensoser, H., Cahuas, A., Kumaravel, V., & Chen, W. (2021). Feasibility and Effectiveness of the Web-Based WeActive and WeMindful Interventions on Physical Activity and Psychological Well-Being. *BioMed Research International, 8400241*(1), 8400241. Advance online publication. DOI: 10.1155/2021/8400241 PMID: 34660800

Marsella, A. J. (1988). Cross-cultural research on severe mental disorders: Issues and findings. *Acta Psychiatrica Scandinavica, 78*(S344), 7–22. DOI: 10.1111/j.1600-0447.1988.tb08998.x PMID: 3067531

Merikangas, K. R., Avenevoli, S., Dierker, L., & Grillon, C. (1999). Vulnerability factors among children at risk for anxiety disorders. *Biological Psychiatry, 46*(11), 1523–1535. DOI: 10.1016/S0006-3223(99)00172-9 PMID: 10599480

Millon, T. (2006). Biography. http://www.millon.net/content/tm_bio.htm

Mitchell, A. E. P. (2021). Resilience and mindfulness in nurse training on an undergraduate curriculum. *Perspectives in Psychiatric Care, 57*(3), 1474–1481. DOI: 10.1111/ppc.12714 PMID: 33355935

Moore, P. S., Whaley, S. E., & Sigman, M. (2004). Interactions between mothers and children: Impacts of maternal and child anxiety. *Journal of Abnormal Psychology, 113*(3), 471–476. DOI: 10.1037/0021-843X.113.3.471 PMID: 15311992

Morris, A. S., Silk, J. S., Steinberg, L., Myers, S. S., & Robinson, L. R. (2007). The Role of the Family Context in the Development of Emotion Regulation. *Social Development, 16*(2), 361–388. DOI: 10.1111/j.1467-9507.2007.00389.x PMID: 19756175

Niazi, A., & Niazi, S. (2011). Mindfulness-based stress reduction: A non-pharmacological approach for chronic illnesses. *North American Journal of Medical Sciences, 3*(1), 20. DOI: 10.4297/najms.2011.320 PMID: 22540058

Ochs, E. (1988). *Culture and Language Development: Language Acquisition and Language Socialization in a Samoan Village*. CUP Archive.

Philippe, R. A., Schwab, L., & Biasutti, M. (2021). Effects of physical activity and mindfulness on resilience and depression during the first wave of COVID-19 pandemic. *Frontiers in Psychology, 12*, 700742. Advance online publication. DOI: 10.3389/fpsyg.2021.700742 PMID: 34393936

Platt, R., Williams, S. R., & Ginsburg, G. S. (2016). Stressful life events and child anxiety: Examining parent and child mediators. *Child Psychiatry and Human Development, 47*(1), 23–34. DOI: 10.1007/s10578-015-0540-4 PMID: 25772523

Rapee, R. M., & Spence, S. H. (2004). The etiology of social phobia: Empirical evidence and an initial model. *Clinical Psychology Review, 24*(7), 737–767. DOI: 10.1016/j.cpr.2004.06.004 PMID: 15501555

Rubin, K. H., Burgess, K. B., & Hastings, P. D. (2002). Stability and social behavioral consequences of toddlers' inhibited temperament and parenting behaviors. *Child Development*, *73*(2), 483–495. DOI: 10.1111/1467-8624.00419 PMID: 11949904

Rutherford, H. J., Wallace, N. S., Laurent, H. K., & Mayes, L. C. (2015). Emotion Regulation in Parenthood. *Developmental review: DR, 36*, 1–14. https://doi.org/ DOI: 10.1016/j.dr.2014.12.008

Shapiro, S. L., Carlson, L. E., Astin, J. A., & Freedman, B. (2006). Mechanisms of mindfulness. *Journal of Clinical Psychology*, *62*(3), 373–386. DOI: 10.1002/jclp.20237 PMID: 16385481

Shapiro, S. L., & Schwartz, G. E. (2000). The role of Intention in Self-Regulation. In *Elsevier eBooks* (pp. 253–273). https://doi.org/DOI: 10.1016/B978-012109890-2/50037-8

Siddaway, A. P., Wood, A. M., & Cartwright-Hatton, S. (2014). Involving parents in cognitive behavioral therapy for child anxiety problems. *Clinical Case Studies*, *13*(4), 322–335. DOI: 10.1177/1534650113510398

Singh, R., Patel, K., & Mehta, J. (2021). Eastern philosophies in mindfulness-based interventions: Bridging the gap. *Asian Journal of Psychology*, *26*(3), 241–256. DOI: 10.1037/ajo0000258

SingleCare. (2022) Anxiety statistics 2022. https://www.singlecare.com/blog/news/anxiety-statistics/

Strauss, A. L., & Corbin, J. M. (1997). Grounded Theory in Practice. *Sage (Atlanta, Ga.)*.

Sünbül, Z. A., & Güneri, O. Y. (2019). The relationship between mindfulness and resilience: The mediating role of self-compassion and emotion regulation in a sample of underprivileged Turkish adolescents. *Personality and Individual Differences*, *139*, 337–342. DOI: 10.1016/j.paid.2018.12.009

Taylor, S., Jang, K. L., Stewart, S. H., & Stein, M. B. (2008). Etiology of the dimensions of anxiety sensitivity: A behavioral genetic analysis. *Journal of Anxiety Disorders*, *22*(5), 899–914. DOI: 10.1016/j.janxdis.2007.09.005 PMID: 18029140

Thirlwall, K., & Creswell, C. (2010). The impact of maternal control on children's anxious cognitions, behaviours, and affect: An experimental study. *Behaviour Research and Therapy*, *48*(10), 1041–1046. DOI: 10.1016/j.brat.2010.05.030 PMID: 20594546

Turner, S. M., Beidel, D. C., & Costello, A. (1987). Psychopathology in the offspring of anxiety disorders patients. *Journal of Consulting and Clinical Psychology*, *55*(2), 229–235. DOI: 10.1037/0022-006X.55.2.229 PMID: 3571678

van den Hurk, P. A. M., Giommi, F., Gielen, S. C., Speckens, A. E. M., & Barendregt, H. P. (2010). Greater efficiency in attentional processing related to mindfulness meditation. *Quarterly Journal of Experimental Psychology*, *63*(6), 1168–1180. DOI: 10.1080/17470210903249365 PMID: 20509209

Van Zalk, N., Tillfors, M., & Trost, K. (2018). Mothers' and fathers' worry and over control: One step closer to understanding early adolescent social anxiety. *Child Psychiatry and Human Development*, *49*(6), 917–927. DOI: 10.1007/s10578-018-0807-7 PMID: 29730770

Victor, D. A. (1992). *International Business Communication*. HarperCollins Publishers, Inc.

WHO. (2022) *World Mental Health Report: Transforming Mental Health for All*. https://apps.who.int/iris/rest/bitstreams/1433523/retrieve

WHO. (2022, February) *ICD-11 for Mortality and Morbidity Statistics*. https://icd.who.int/browse11/l-m/en#/http://id.who.int/icd/entity/1336943699

WHO. (2022, March 2) COVID-19 pandemic triggers 25% increase in prevalence of anxiety and depression worldwide. https://www.who.int/news/item/02-03-2022-covid-19-pandemic-triggers-25-increase-in-prevalence-of-anxiety-and-depression-worldwide

Wilson, P. (2019). Indigenous traditions and mindfulness: Pathways to intercultural synergy. *Indigenous Mental Health Review*, *8*(2), 65–80. DOI: 10.1111/imhr.2019.08

Wittchen, H. U., Jacobi, F., Rehm, J., Gustavsson, A., Svensson, M., Jönsson, B., Olesen, J., Allgulander, C., Alonso, J., Faravelli, C., Fratiglioni, L., Jennum, P., Lieb, R., Maercker, A., van Os, J., Preisig, M., Salvador-Carulla, L., Simon, R., & Steinhausen, H. C. (2011). The size and burden of mental disorders and other disorders of the brain in Europe 2010. *European Neuropsychopharmacology*, *21*(9), 655–679. DOI: 10.1016/j.euroneuro.2011.07.018 PMID: 21896369

Wong, K. (2018). Mindfulness in multicultural classrooms: Adapting practices for inclusivity. *Journal of Educational Psychology*, *110*(1), 1–12. DOI: 10.1037/edu0000207 PMID: 30739953

Wong, K., Hicks, L. M., Seuntjens, T. G., Trentacosta, C. J., Hendriksen, T. H. G., Zeelenberg, M., & van den Heuvel, M. I. (2019). The Role of Mindful Parenting in Individual and Social Decision-Making in Children. *Frontiers in Psychology, 10*, 550. DOI: 10.3389/fpsyg.2019.00550 PMID: 30949094

Wood, J. J. (2006). Parental intrusiveness and children's separation anxiety in a clinical sample. *Child Psychiatry and Human Development*, *37*(1), 73–87. DOI: 10.1007/s10578-006-0021-x PMID: 16932853

Wood, J. J., McLeod, B. D., Sigman, M., Hwang, W., & Chu, B. C. (2003). Parenting and childhood anxiety: Theory, empirical findings, and future directions. *Journal of Child Psychology and Psychiatry, and Allied Disciplines*, *44*(1), 134–151. DOI: 10.1111/1469-7610.00106 PMID: 12553416

Zeanah, C. H., Danis, B., Hirshberg, L., Benoit, D., Miller, D., & Scott, H. S. (1999). Disorganized attachment associated with partner violence: A research note. *Infant Mental Health Journal*, *20*(1), 77–86. DOI: 10.1002/(SICI)1097-0355(199921)20:1<77::AID-IMHJ6>3.0.CO;2-S

Zsido, A. N., Arato, N., Inhof, O., Matuz-Budai, T., Stecina, D. T., & Labadi, B. (2022). Psychological well-being, risk factors, and coping strategies with social isolation and new challenges in times of adversity caused by the COVID-19 pandemic. *Acta Psychologica*, *225*, 103538. DOI: 10.1016/j.actpsy.2022.103538 PMID: 35219042

Chapter 10
Mindfulness and Self-Recovery:
A Consideration of an Integrative Approach to Recovery From Long-Term Social Withdrawal

Masaya Fujimura
https://orcid.org/0009-0008-2815-4841
International Center of Transdisciplinary Research, Japan

ABSTRACT

This study analyzed the author's own recovery process from a decade of social withdrawal from the perspective of mindfulness, wellbeing, and a holistic approach. In particular, it focused on the internal transformation and gradual process of social participation that occurred as a result of a change in outlook on life and death at the age of 39, and explored the recovery mechanism. The analysis revealed that mindfulness practice enabled the individual to distance himself from anxiety about the past and future, that the five elements of the PERMA theory developed while influencing each other, and that the integration of physical, mental, and social approaches promoted comprehensive recovery. These results indicate that a combination of internal awareness and gradual social participation is effective for recovery from long-term withdrawal, and present the possibility of a new support approach.

DOI: 10.4018/979-8-3373-0360-4.ch010

I INTRODUCTION

Hikikomori, especially among adults over 30, has become a significant issue in Japan, involving complex factors like self-denial, cognitive and emotional decline, and isolation, making recovery difficult. The challenges faced highlight the inadequacy of current support mechanisms and the need for improved intervention models (Nakajima, 2023).

This study analyzes the recovery of a Japanese man, named Ma from ten years of hikikomori, using established theoretical frameworks to provide new insights and improve support for hikikomori individuals. While hikikomori has various typologies (Kawakita, n.d.), the study focuses on cases of profound despair and persistent suicidal ideation, where individuals are trapped in a psychological dilemma, leading to prolonged withdrawal. The study seeks to clarify how such a state forms, the internal changes that facilitate recovery, and how these processes can be understood.

This study focuses on a specific type of hikikomori, offering insights for individuals facing low self-esteem, depression, or suicidal ideation. The findings contribute to broader discussions on psychological resilience and recovery. Driven by Ma's personal experience, the study reevaluates recovery, emphasizing a pivotal realization at age 39: "If I die, even if misunderstood, my words will never reach others again." This insight shifted Ma from passive resignation to proactive recovery.

This transformative moment led Ma to pursue recovery through three theoretical frameworks: Mindfulness, Wellbeing, and a Holistic Approach. Organizing the process within these models provides a universal understanding of recovery from hikikomori, contributing to more effective support strategies for related psychological challenges.

This chapter presents a comprehensive framework for hikikomori recovery using Mindfulness, Wellbeing, and Holistic Approaches. It emphasizes the importance of internal awareness and gradual social participation in recovery. These approaches work together to support long-term recovery, particularly in cases of prolonged social withdrawal. The study aims to guide more effective interventions for hikikomori individuals.

The findings aim to establish a new theoretical foundation for recovery support and offer practical insights for developing interdisciplinary systems. This research seeks to advance future intervention strategies and support frameworks for individuals experiencing prolonged social isolation.

Research Background: The Social Challenge of Hikikomori and the Elucidation of the Recovery Process

Hikikomori has become a significant social issue in Japan, particularly affecting adults over 30 who experience prolonged social withdrawal. These cases involve self-negation, cognitive and emotional decline, and increasing isolation, creating a complex state that complicates recovery (Nakajima 2023).

Recovery from chronic hikikomori requires an integrative approach addressing physical, psychological, and social aspects. Key elements include transforming negative cognitive patterns and promoting gradual social participation (Kato, 2019). However, research on recovery mechanisms for long-term hikikomori, especially in adults over 30, remains limited. The lack of detailed analysis and empirical validation of approaches like Mindfulness, Wellbeing, and Holistic practices underscores a significant gap, which must be addressed for more effective, evidence-based support frameworks.

Despite the complexity of hikikomori, empirical research on recovery mechanisms for long-term cases, particularly in adults over 30, is limited. The lack of analysis from those who have recovered, along with limited validation of support methods like Mindfulness, Wellbeing, and Holistic practices, highlights a significant gap. Addressing this gap is crucial for advancing the field and developing effective, evidence-based support systems.

This study focuses on two key components: the existential shift in perspective on life and death, and gradual social reintegration. It emphasizes the critical role of these elements in recovery, providing both theoretical and practical insights for supporting those with prolonged hikikomori.

The research clarifies recovery mechanisms and proposes practical methods for social reintegration. The findings suggest that recovery is most effective when multiple approaches work together. Combining internal awareness (mindfulness and existential transformation) with gradual social participation is essential. This study aims to contribute to better support models for long-term hikikomori by examining how these elements interact.

Research Objective: Elucidating the Recovery Process Through an Integrated Approach of Mindfulness, Wellbeing, and Holistic Frameworks

This study analyzes recovery from ten years of hikikomori using three frameworks: Mindfulness, Wellbeing, and Holistic Approaches. It explores how these frameworks interact to support sustainable recovery.

First, the study examines mindfulness, focusing on how present-moment awareness reduces past regrets and future anxieties, aiding social reintegration. It also explores mindfulness's role in emotional regulation, self-acceptance, and resilience, contributing to gradual recovery.

Second, the study applies the PERMA model of wellbeing to explore how elements like Positive Emotion, Engagement, Relationships, Meaning, and Achievement foster growth, aiming to inform long-term recovery strategies for hikikomori.

Third, the study investigates the synergistic effects of combining physical, mental, and social approaches, such as martial arts, mindfulness, and communication. It aims to understand how these elements reinforce each other and support recovery.

The research will demonstrate the effectiveness of this integrative approach, identifying key factors for sustainable recovery and informing interventions and policies for hikikomori support.

Significance of the Study: Empirical Elucidation of the Recovery Process and Its Societal Applications

This study provides value from three perspectives. First, it offers an empirical analysis of recovery from hikikomori, focusing on individual experiences. Using Mindfulness, Wellbeing, and Holistic Approaches, it clarifies recovery mechanisms and explores how internal change and external support interact, highlighting personal growth and social reintegration. Second, the study contributes to intervention strategies by showing a phased approach to social reintegration, from online to face-to-face interactions, integrating physical, mental, and social support. It demonstrates the effectiveness of gradual participation. Third, the study shows that recovery is possible even for individuals over 30, highlighting Ma's journey of existential transformation and social engagement.

These insights offer practical guidance for developing interventions and support frameworks for hikikomori recovery, contributing to better intervention strategies.

II PATHWAY TO SELF-RECOVERY: AN EMPIRICAL EXAMINATION OF REINTEGRATION FROM SOCIAL WITHDRAWAL TO SOCIETAL INTEGRATION

Background Leading to Social Withdrawal and the Catalyst for Societal Retreat

Ma's strict upbringing, including corporal punishment and emotional reactions, suppressed emotional expression and influenced cognitive and emotional development. This led to emotional suppression, negative thoughts, and hindered social skills, fostering avoidance and withdrawal. Addressing these familial impacts emphasizes the need for interventions targeting emotional and relational factors, with a focus on systemic approaches alongside individual therapy.

Family Environment and the Suppression of Self-Expression

A significant episode occurred when Ma, pretending to be ill because he did not want to go to school, was forcibly taken to school in his pajamas without being asked about his true feelings. This caused him humiliation and increased his fear of his father, which restricted emotional expression.

This experience fostered a need for external validation, with academic performance becoming his sole measure of self-worth. These maladaptive patterns, rooted in emotional suppression, played a crucial role in his social withdrawal.

The findings suggest that early familial experiences, including coercive control, contributed to Ma's withdrawal. Effective interventions should address both individual cognitive patterns and broader familial dynamics.

Changes in Family Dynamics and Their Impact

After Ma's parents' divorce, he lived with his father and two younger brothers, creating psychological distance between him and his siblings. As the eldest son, he faced strict discipline from his father, with high academic expectations. His brothers received more lenient treatment, creating unequal familial roles.

This imbalance reinforced Ma's sense of isolation and internalized maladaptive cognitive patterns. His self-worth became heavily tied to meeting external standards, leading to a constant pressure to conform.

Ma's reliance on external validation for self-worth hindered the development of a stable self-concept and contributed to ongoing psychological distress, leading to social withdrawal. Effective interventions should focus on rebuilding self-worth through internal validation, addressing these familial dynamics.

The Progression of Social Maladaptation

During middle and high school, Ma struggled with expressing emotions, leading to heightened sensitivity and hyper-vigilance. This hindered genuine engagement with others and fostered a maladaptive coping mechanism of excessive self-restraint to maintain superficial harmony. However, this strategy caused chronic tension and stress, worsening Ma's sense of inadequacy.

The suppression of the authentic self-eroded self-esteem and reinforced negative cognitive patterns. Emotional suppression led to superficial stability, but deepened internal dissatisfaction, reflecting social anxiety and maladaptive perfectionism. Ma's transition to university worsened these struggles. Despite financial success, he developed a gambling addiction, leading to severe financial instability and using it as a maladaptive coping mechanism to relieve distress.

Gambling provided temporary relief from emotional pain but reflected broader issues of impaired impulse control and dysfunctional coping. The resulting financial strain worsened Ma's distress, perpetuating a cycle of avoidance and self-denigration. The reliance on gambling highlights maladaptive coping in response to emotional and cognitive dysregulation. Combined with social anxiety and cognitive suppression, these factors led to a decline in psychological well-being, contributing to prolonged isolation.

The Immediate Catalyst for Social Withdrawal

After the Great Hanshin-Awaji Earthquake, Ma moved to Yokohama and worked as a mobile phone salesperson at 27. The job caused psychological distress due to emotional labor and the need for superficial relationships. This led to anxiety, a desire to avoid social contact, and, after a year, an abrupt severing of ties with the workplace, starting nearly a decade of social withdrawal.

Initiation and Early Phase of Hikikomori

At 27, Ma worked at an electronics store but struggled with authentic self-expression, leading to prolonged stress. Eventually, he severed all social ties by disappearing from work.

After a brief period of vagrancy, he returned home and entered a prolonged state of social withdrawal by 28, marking the start of his hikikomori condition and initiating a decade of reclusiveness.

Lifestyle Patterns and Social Isolation

During the early phase of hikikomori, Ma used separate entrances to avoid his father and only procured food when his father was absent. This minimalistic lifestyle was a deliberate means of social isolation, helping him evade interactions and maintain psychological detachment.

Progression of Psychiatric Symptoms

Throughout the hikikomori period, Ma attempted social reintegration, consulting healthcare providers and receiving a major depressive disorder diagnosis. In the later stages, symptoms worsened, leading to significant psychological decline. The last four years were marked by anhedonia, psychomotor retardation, and a lack of motivation, rendering Ma unable to perform basic daily tasks. He described this period as feeling like a "living corpse," reflecting a severe decline in cognitive and functional capacity.

Conflict with Suicidal Ideation

Each time Ma experienced intermittent periods of hikikomori, Ma faced persistent suicidal thoughts and made several attempts. Despite writing numerous suicide notes, frustration remained as he struggled to express his true emotions. A critical realization emerged: "If I choose death, even if others misunderstand me, my words will never reach them." This insight marked a pivotal turning point, reshaping Ma's path toward recovery.

Manifestations of Social Disconnection

The disconnection from society manifested itself through a recurrent and cyclical pattern, as evidenced by the following dynamics:

Attempts at Social Reintegration and Failures

Individuals who withdraw often experience guilt (Employment Continuity Navigation 2024). Ma made ten reintegration attempts, driven by guilt toward his father, but each failure worsened his suicidal thoughts. Contemplating death, he feared his words and actions would be lost forever, making misunderstandings irreversible. This conflict deepened his despair.

Limited Social Interaction Through SNS

At 38, during his withdrawal, Ma used SNS to create a virtual identity, offering minimal connection to society. This became his only way to engage, providing temporary escape. After reintegration, he continued online, forming a supportive relationship with an older woman, which helped with self-expression and emotional relief.

Turning Point and Process of Social Reintegration

The most critical turning point in the recovery was a shift in Ma's perception of life and death. After ten years of withdrawal and suicide attempts, this realization at age 39 accelerated his recovery. This section explores the process of social reintegration that began with this breakthrough.

Fundamental Transformation in Perception of Life and Death

At 39, Ma had a pivotal realization: "If I die, my words will never reach others." This shift from passivity to a resolve to live marked a critical turning point, redirecting Ma's path toward recovery and reintegration.

Gradual Approach to Social Reintegration/Initial Stage: Initiation of Internet-Based Business

Ma's first step toward reintegration involved engaging in internet-based business activities, minimizing direct contact to reduce anxiety. The internet served as an effective medium for reducing barriers associated with social anxiety (Organisation for Economic Co-operation and Development [OECD], 2025).

Intermediate Stage: Experience in a Venture Company

Drawing on the skills he had developed through years of self-directed learning, Ma eventually secured a position at a venture company operating in the online business sector. This new role marked a significant step forward in his journey, offering him a structured environment where he could apply his abilities and begin to reconnect with the world beyond his home.

As he settled into his job, the nature of his work gradually brought more opportunities for face-to-face communication. These interactions, while promising, also introduced new challenges. Ma found himself overly preoccupied with how others perceived him, often consumed by worry over interpersonal dynamics. Social engagements, though essential for his reintegration, left him mentally and physically drained. Even expressing his thoughts and feelings openly proved difficult, as lingering inhibitions from his years of withdrawal surfaced in moments that required vulnerability.

Despite these hurdles, Ma continued to navigate this unfamiliar terrain with resilience, slowly adapting to the demands of social and professional life. Each challenge became part of the broader process of reclaiming his place in society.

Establishment of Financial Independence:

As Ma immersed himself in his work at the venture company, his efforts began to bear fruit—not only professionally, but personally. Over time, he achieved financial independence, a milestone that marked a significant turning point in his journey. No longer reliant on his parents, Ma experienced a profound sense of liberation. This newfound autonomy played a crucial role in restoring his self-esteem, allowing him to see himself as capable and self-reliant.

With economic stability came something even deeper: the formation of a renewed social identity. Through his business activities and ability to sustain himself, Ma began to redefine how he related to others—not as someone in need of support, but as a contributing member of society. This shift brought a quiet but powerful confidence, reinforcing his sense of purpose and place in the world.

Social Development Beyond the Late Forties

In his late forties, Ma actively engaged in society through speech clubs and marriage events. In his fifties, he married a confident woman he met at a social gathering, further advancing his reintegration and personal growth.

Current Social Activities

After marriage, Ma became deeply involved in social activities, organizing home parties and participating in community events. Communication is now central to his life, as he continues to grow through learning and social engagement.

Reconstruction of Communication Skills

The enhancement of communication skills following social reintegration was characterized by a gradual, phased approach. This developmental process began with online interactions and progressively evolved into direct, face-to-face interpersonal communication.

Initial Efforts

In the early stages of reintegration, Ma engaged in online business to limit direct contact. Initially focused on self-learning, he later attended business seminars, interacting with like-minded individuals. Shared objectives made interactions natural, allowing him to gradually deepen social engagement and rebuild communication skills.

Experience at a Shared Office Space

Ma's time in a shared office space with entrepreneurs marked a pivotal turning point. Initially, he only responded to others, but over time, he began initiating conversations, significantly improving his social and communication skills.

English Speech Club Activities

Thanks to an introduction from the former president of a foreign-affiliated logistics company, Ma joined Toastmasters—a global organization dedicated to developing public speaking and leadership skills. Ma began attending meetings twice a month, a routine he maintained for eight years. This consistent, structured environment became a vital space for personal development, offering Ma the opportunity to practice and refine his interpersonal communication in a supportive setting.

At Toastmasters, Ma found a safe space to express himself, gradually building confidence as he stood before others and shared his thoughts. His speech skills improved step by step, guided by thoughtful feedback from fellow members. The meetings were more than just exercises in public speaking—they became a gateway to deeper social interaction.

After each session, informal gatherings allowed Ma to connect with others in a relaxed atmosphere, further sharpening his communication abilities. Over time, these experiences transformed his relationship with social engagement. Participating in speech contests, where he earned awards, became not just a measure of progress, but a celebration of his journey—from isolation to confident self-expression.

Practice of Humor Communication

Ma's participation in humor communication workshops over a span of more than seven years marked a profound turning point in his ability to build and maintain meaningful relationships. Attending bi-monthly classes, he immersed himself in a unique environment where laughter, expression, and connection came together as powerful tools for personal growth.

Through these sessions, Ma significantly enhanced his communication skills. He became a more attentive listener, learning to observe subtle reactions in others and ask thoughtful, timely questions. Ma speaking style evolved as well—he developed a sense of rhythm in his delivery, using voice modulation, facial expressions, and body movement to convey his messages with greater clarity and impact.

The workshops also brought about deep psychological transformation. As his confidence grew, Ma found himself able to speak more openly, even about the most personal chapters of his life, including his hikikomori experience. Smiling became more frequent, not just as a performance tool, but as a genuine reflection of his renewed outlook. Ma learned to approach conversations cheerfully, embracing the art of uplifting communication.

Beyond technique, Ma cultivated a multifaceted way of seeing the world. He developed an open-minded attitude, eager to engage with new experiences and perspectives. Perhaps most importantly, he nurtured resilience—adopting a mindset that prioritized enjoyment and connection over the fear of failure. Through humor and human connection, Ma rediscovered the joy of being present with others, and with himself.

III ENCOUNTER AND PRACTICE OF MINDFULNESS

Encounter with Mindfulness

In 2015, Ma discovered mindfulness through Masaaki Yoshida's blog.[1] and his book *Introduction to Mindfulness*[2]. This led to serious practice, with a CD offering practical guidance. A key moment came with *Search Inside Yourself* (Chade-Meng Tan, 2016, May 25), which highlighted mindfulness' effectiveness in business settings like Google's programs. Mindfulness helped Ma overcome self-doubt and anxiety, offering a new perspective on self-reflection and techniques to distance from past regrets and future anxieties.[3]

Methods of Practice and Application to Daily Life

The practice of mindfulness began with fundamental meditation techniques and gradually expanded to encompass various aspects of daily life. The following section outlines the specific methods of practice and their developmental progression.

Fundamental Meditation Practice

Ma began with short, breathing-focused meditations lasting 5-15 minutes, redirecting attention to the breath to enhance present-moment awareness. A one-minute pre-work meditation proved particularly effective for mental resetting and focus (Tan et al, 2012). Currently, Ma practices guided meditation with a therapist every morning, incorporating mindfulness into his daily routine.

Practice in the Workplace

In the midst of his busy work life, Ma began incorporating mindfulness into his daily routine—a quiet, personal practice that brought clarity and calm to his day. Each morning, before diving into his tasks, he would take a few moments for a brief meditation, grounding himself before the demands of the day unfolded.

During lunch breaks, he blended mindfulness meditation with short naps, creating a restorative pause that helped him recharge both mentally and physically. Throughout the day, he maintained a gentle awareness of his breathing, using it as an anchor whenever stress or distraction crept in.

These small but intentional habits made a significant difference. Ma found that his concentration sharpened during the often-drowsy afternoon hours, and his overall stress levels gradually diminished. Mindfulness became not just a tool for focus, but a quiet ally in his journey toward balance and well-being in the workplace.

Practice in Daily Life

Ma's mindfulness practice gradually extended beyond the workplace, weaving itself into the fabric of his everyday life. During his daily commutes, he transformed routine walking into a meditative exercise. With each step, he brought focused attention to the soles of his feet, silently repeating "right, left, right, left" in rhythm with his movement—a grounding technique that brought calm and clarity before entering the bustle of the day.

Meals became another opportunity for presence. Through mindful eating, Ma began to slow down, paying close attention to the flavors, textures, and sensations of each bite. Rather than rushing through his meals, he savored them, treating eating as a rich sensory experience rather than a mere necessity. (The Nutrition Source, 2024)

At concerts and events, he practiced sustained concentration, allowing himself to become fully immersed in a single sound, image, or moment. This heightened presence deepened his appreciation and enjoyment of cultural experiences.

Even in conversation, mindfulness played a role. Ma trained himself to truly listen—setting aside distractions and tuning in completely to the person in front of him. With undivided attention, he not only improved the quality of his relationships but also enriched his own sense of connection and understanding.

These daily practices became quiet anchors, nurturing a sense of balance, attentiveness, and joy in Ma's evolving life.

Changes Resulting from Practice

The continuous practice of mindfulness brought about significant changes in both psychological well-being and interpersonal relationships.

Psychological Changes

As Ma deepened his mindfulness practice, subtle but profound psychological shifts began to take root in his life. One of the most noticeable changes was in his ability to concentrate. Where once his mind constantly darted from thought to thought, he gradually developed the capacity to focus with clarity and intention. This newfound attentiveness became particularly evident in his professional and academic pursuits, where sustained focus on immediate tasks became not only possible but natural (Goleman, 2019).

Alongside improved concentration came greater emotional stability. The emotional turbulence that had once weighed him down began to ease. Depressive states, which in the past could linger for days or even weeks, now lifted more quickly. He found himself recovering from emotional lows with a resilience that had previously felt out of reach (Stromberg, 2015).

Ma also developed a healthier relationship with loss and failure. Rather than clinging to past disappointments, he learned to acknowledge them and move forward with a constructive mindset. His attachment to what once was began to loosen, replaced by a capacity to meet challenges with acceptance and a quiet inner strength (Christina et al., 2012).

Perhaps most notably, Ma experienced relief from anxiety. By turning to deep breathing and focused attention during moments of stress, particularly in social situations, he was able to calm his nerves and ease the tension that once made interactions feel overwhelming (Luo et al., 2025). Mindfulness didn't erase life's difficulties, but it gave Ma the tools to face them with steadiness, presence, and grace.

Changes in Interpersonal Relationships

As Ma continued to grow, notable qualitative improvements emerged in his interpersonal relationships. A key development was his increased capacity for self-disclosure. He became more willing to acknowledge his own weaknesses and mistakes, which allowed him to communicate with greater sincerity and authenticity (Ketay et al., 2022). This openness marked a shift away from guarded interactions toward deeper, more meaningful exchanges.

Alongside this, Ma cultivated a new attitude toward apologizing. Rather than deflecting blame or making excuses, he learned to admit his faults directly and humbly. This shift led to healthier, more constructive relationships rooted in accountability and mutual respect (Ketay et al., 2022).

These changes contributed to a general deepening of his connections with others. His interactions began to feel more genuine, as he developed a heightened ability to understand others' emotions and perspectives. This empathic insight enriched his relationships and helped him form more enduring bonds (Suttie, 2022).

Additionally, Ma's listening skills improved significantly. He learned to fully concentrate on what others were saying, resisting the urge to interrupt or mentally prepare responses. This level of attentiveness led to more effective and meaningful communication, strengthening both personal and professional interactions (Beloborodova, 2023).

Changes in Daily Life

Ma also experienced tangible improvements in his daily life, reflecting the far-reaching impact of his mindfulness practice. One of the most noticeable changes was in his sleep quality. Where he had once struggled with only 4 to 5 hours of rest, Ma began regularly sleeping 6 to 7 hours per night. This shift brought not just longer sleep, but deeper, more restorative rest, which significantly improved his overall well-being (Alvarado-García et al., 2025).

His increased energy translated into a more active lifestyle. Ma found himself not only able to engage in multiple activities throughout the day but also more willing to embrace new opportunities. Whether participating in community events, hobbies, or physical movement, he approached life with renewed vitality (Pacheco et al., 2024).

Importantly, this new rhythm of life came with stabilized energy levels. Rather than experiencing highs and crashes throughout the day, Ma was able to maintain a steady, sustainable pace. This consistency enhanced his ability to navigate daily tasks with greater ease and satisfaction.

Together, these changes demonstrated that mindfulness was more than just a mental exercise. It had become a holistic practice that enriched many dimensions of his everyday life—from sleep and energy to active engagement—contributing to a more balanced and fulfilling lifestyle.

Relationship with Medical Support

The practice of mindfulness was an independent effort undertaken by Ma in parallel with existing medical support.

Combined Effects with Pharmacotherapy

To support his ongoing recovery, Ma adopted a dual approach by integrating mindfulness practice with pharmacotherapy, particularly during periods of depressive episodes. This combination proved especially effective in managing mild depressive states. The synergy between the two methods often accelerated recovery, suggesting that mindfulness could enhance the therapeutic effects of medication.

However, the benefits of this integrated approach were more limited during severe depressive episodes. In such cases, even the combination of mindfulness and pharmacological treatment did not always yield immediate improvements, highlighting the complexity of treating deeper psychological conditions and the potential need for more intensive or alternative interventions.

Despite these limitations, the long-term preventive effects of mindfulness became increasingly evident. As Ma maintained a consistent mindfulness routine, he was gradually able to adjust the dosage of his medication under professional guidance. This suggested not only improved self-regulation but also the potential for reducing medication dependency through sustained mindfulness practice.

Relationship with the Treatment Process

Ma's relationship with his primary physician was largely centered around conventional care, consisting of regular symptom monitoring and medication adjustments. While Ma shared that he had been practicing mindfulness, the physician offered no specific advice or direction regarding this aspect of his self-care.

Instead, Ma pursued mindfulness on his own initiative, integrating it into his recovery process without formal medical endorsement. Over time, the effectiveness of this practice became evident through Ma's personal experience. Rather than being a structured part of his clinical treatment, mindfulness emerged as an experiential and self-directed approach that complemented the medical care he received.

Approaches to Overcoming Challenges

Ma encountered several practical challenges in maintaining a regular mindfulness practice, but he addressed them with thoughtful strategies that prioritized sustainability over perfection. One of the key turning points was his conscious release from perfectionism. Instead of criticizing himself for missed sessions or perceived shortcomings, Ma cultivated a more accepting mindset—one that allowed space for imperfection without falling into self-denial. He learned to shift his attention away from what hadn't been done and toward the value of his ongoing efforts.

He also adopted a flexible and adaptable approach to practice. Rather than confining mindfulness to formal sessions, Ma began integrating it naturally into his everyday life. He experimented with brief exercises, such as one-minute meditations, and discovered moments for mindful attention even during routine activities like commuting or eating. This made practice more accessible and less burdensome, especially during busy or emotionally demanding periods.

Ma's approach was deliberately gradual. He focused on building confidence through small, achievable successes, which in turn sustained his motivation. Even brief, consistent sessions were seen as meaningful progress. Over time, he gradually expanded both the length and frequency of his practice, allowing mindfulness to take root more deeply in his daily rhythm.

By releasing rigid expectations and embracing a flexible, steady path, Ma was able to weave mindfulness into his life in a way that was both realistic and enduring. It was this deliberate integration into daily routines that became the cornerstone of his consistent growth and well-being.

IV ANALYSIS FROM THE PERSPECTIVE OF WELL-BEING

This section analyzes recovery using the PERMA model: Positive Emotion, Engagement, Relationships, Meaning, and Accomplishment. It explores how successful experiences in each element advanced Ma's recovery, providing a comprehensive analysis of the process.

Cultivation of Positive Emotion

The first critical turning point in the self-recovery process was the positive emotional experience derived from the relationship with an older woman met through social networking sites. Particularly, the unconditional acceptance and wholly affirming interactions within this relationship played a pivotal role in facilitating recovery.

Accumulation of Positive Experiences

The cultivation of positive emotions in Ma's life was facilitated by several key factors. One of the most significant was the continuous exposure to non-judgmental experiences. Unlike his past interpersonal relationships, Ma found himself in a safe psychological space where he could engage in self-disclosure without fear of judgment. This newfound freedom allowed for deeper emotional expression and growth.

In addition to this, positive feedback played a crucial role in Ma's development. As he began to receive accepting and encouraging responses to his self-disclosures, his confidence in his ability to express himself grew. This reinforcement helped him embrace vulnerability and further opened the door for meaningful communication.

Finally, social success experiences contributed to Ma's increasing sense of confidence in social participation. Activities like dining out and engaging in karaoke not only provided enjoyable moments but also served as stepping stones toward deeper social involvement. These experiences enabled him to feel more comfortable and capable in face-to-face interactions, solidifying his reintegration into social life.

Reconstruction of Self-Esteem

The self-esteem that had been eroded by years of social withdrawal gradually recovered through a series of transformative processes. One key aspect was Ma's gradual self-disclosure within safe and supportive relationships. By opening up progressively in environments characterized by psychological safety, he began to regain a sense of trust and acceptance, which was essential for rebuilding his self-esteem (Harvey, 2021).

Another significant factor was Ma's practice of social skills in accepting environments. Engaging with others in spaces where acceptance was consistently offered allowed him to refine his interpersonal abilities and gain confidence in his social interactions (Winarsunu et al., 2023). This ongoing engagement provided opportunities for growth without the fear of rejection.

Additionally, the accumulation of small successes played an instrumental role in the recovery of Ma's self-esteem. Achieving minor successes in various aspects of his life, however small they seemed, served as positive reinforcement, helping to restore his confidence (Ishida, 2024).

Engagement (Immersion in Activities)

A significant turning point in the recovery process was Ma's deep engagement in online business. This activity possessed characteristics that facilitated a gradual reintegration into society from the state of social withdrawal.

Characteristics of the Activity

The effectiveness of Ma's approach to online business can be attributed to several key factors that aligned well with his personal needs and preferences. First, the minimization of direct contact with others was crucial. During times when Ma experienced intense anxiety about face-to-face communication, the online business environment allowed him to continue working without the added stress of interpersonal interactions.

Additionally, the ability to learn and practice at his own pace played a significant role in his success. With no fixed time constraints or locations to worry about, Ma could acquire knowledge and skills as he saw fit, making the learning process self-directed and flexible.

Lastly, the visibility of tangible results greatly contributed to Ma's sense of accomplishment. The ability to see concrete outcomes, particularly in numerical form, provided clear evidence of his progress, which served as a powerful motivator and affirmed his efforts. This combination of reduced social pressure, autonomy in learning, and measurable success helped Ma thrive in his online business endeavors.

Experience of Flow State

During the process of self-learning web-related knowledge, Ma experienced several distinctive features of the flow state, which contributed to his deep engagement and motivation. One of the most notable aspects was the loss of the sense of time. As he immersed himself in learning, Ma entered a state of intense concentration where the passage of time seemed to fade away, allowing him to focus fully on the task at hand.

The learning process also provided an appropriate challenge level. Ma had the freedom to adjust the difficulty of the material to his own pace, which kept him engaged and continuously motivated to tackle new challenges. This personalized approach enabled him to maintain a steady rhythm in his learning journey, ensuring that he was always moving forward.

Furthermore, Ma benefited from immediate feedback within the learning environment. The direct confirmation of his progress not only reinforced his understanding but also fueled his motivation, helping him to stay on track and continuously improve. This combination of time loss, tailored challenges, and instant feedback created an optimal learning experience, enabling Ma to advance in his self-directed web education.

Developmental Effects of the Activity

This period marked a pivotal turning point in Ma's life, shifting him away from a pattern of aimless time-spending toward a more intentional and purpose-driven way of living. As he began to engage more meaningfully with his surroundings, his motivation to learn surged—fueled by a genuine curiosity and a desire to grow. With each new skill acquired and challenge overcome, Ma's sense of self-efficacy deepened, allowing him to recognize his own potential and take pride in his progress. Alongside this inner transformation, he also began to restructure his daily routine, filling his time with activities that carried personal meaning and direction. Through this evolution, Ma laid the foundation for a life guided by purpose, learning, and self-belief.

Relationships (Reconstruction of Interpersonal Connections)

The reconstruction of interpersonal relationships was carried out gradually, with experiences gained at each stage serving as steppingstones for progression to subsequent stages.

Gradual Development Process

The process of developing social relationships unfolded gradually, beginning in the digital realm. At first, interactions were limited to social networking sites, where Ma could safely experiment with self-expression. By constructing a virtual self, Ma created a protective buffer that allowed them to engage in social contact while maintaining a sense of security. This early stage provided a low-risk environment to practice self-disclosure and test the waters of social connection.

As confidence grew, the next stage was marked by the deepening of trust with a particular, reliable figure—an older woman who offered consistent, nonjudgmental support. Through this nurturing relationship, Ma began to rebuild self-esteem, feeling genuinely accepted for who he was. Encouraged by this experience, online interactions gradually gave way to real-life engagements, such as meeting for meals or enjoying karaoke together—steps that strengthened the connection and bridged the virtual and physical worlds.

In the final stage, the focus shifted toward building relationships in a business context. Operating within the more structured and less socially demanding setting of a shared office space, Ma maintained minimal interpersonal contact while becoming more familiar with the professional environment. Participation in business seminars offered opportunities to enhance social skills and connect with others who shared similar aspirations,

Active Social Participation

From his late forties onward, Ma took intentional steps to broaden his interpersonal relationships, embracing new opportunities for connection and personal development. He became a regular participant in speech clubs, where he not only practiced communication but also formed lasting relationships with others who shared his interest in self-improvement. At the same time, Ma actively engaged in marriage-oriented activities, seeking deeper companionship and emotional fulfillment. This journey ultimately led Ma to meet a partner with strong self-esteem and a supportive spirit—someone whose presence reinforced his own recovery and growth. Together, their relationship became a source of mutual strength, marking a new chapter of connection, confidence, and renewal in Ma's life.

Current Social Activities

After getting married, Ma began to engage more actively in social life, gradually expanding his circle of interaction and deepening his connection with others. Hosting home parties became a way to bring people together in a warm, welcoming environment, turning his residence into a hub of shared laughter and conversation. His voluntary involvement in community activities further strengthened these bonds, allowing him to contribute meaningfully to the neighborhood while building trust and camaraderie. At the same time, Ma remained committed to personal growth, continuously learning and exploring the art of communication as a central life theme.

Meaning (Rediscovery of Life's Purpose)

The rediscovery of life's meaning deepened through three distinct stages. This process evolved beyond mere survival instincts, becoming a journey toward uncovering a deeper sense of personal significance and purpose.

Reaffirmation of the Meaning of Survival

The critical turning point was the realization that self-expression ends with death. The insight, "If I die, even if misunderstood, my words will never reach them," shifted Ma from passive survival to actively seeking deeper meaning in life.

Acquisition of Social Roles

The journey toward acquiring meaningful social roles unfolded through a combination of personal initiative and community engagement. Gaining economic independence through online business played a foundational role, allowing Ma to establish a clear social identity rooted in self-sufficiency and purpose. This sense of identity was further strengthened by active involvement in speech club activities, which served as a platform to refine social skills and gain confidence in public interaction. As these abilities grew, so did the desire to give back—leading to participation in community activities where the individual could contribute meaningfully to others. Through these interconnected experiences, a fuller social role took shape—one defined not only by personal achievement but also by a commitment to connection and contribution.

Recognition of Existential Value Through Relationships

The recognition of existential value gradually emerged through meaningful interactions with others, reshaping Ma's sense of purpose. At the heart of this transformation was the deepening relationship with a spouse—a partnership grounded in mutual understanding and unwavering support. Beyond the intimacy of the home, involvement in community activities opened new pathways for social connection, fostering a sense of belonging and shared humanity. Through these experiences, communication became more than a skill—it evolved into a lifelong pursuit, a central theme in the ongoing journey of personal growth. As these relationships deepened and communication flourished, The meaning of Ma's life expanded beyond the boundaries of personal survival, finding richness and fulfillment in the shared space between self and others.

Accomplishment (Sense of Achievement in Social Activities)

The sense of achievement in social activities was attained through a gradual, step-by-step process. Successful experiences at each stage enabled Ma to take on new challenges and progress to subsequent stages of growth.

Achievement of Financial Independence

Achieving success in online business marked a major turning point, symbolizing both personal and professional growth. By establishing a stable and independent source of income, Ma not only gained financial security but also took a meaningful step toward self-reliance. This newfound economic independence allowed for a gradual liberation from parental support, reinforcing a sense of autonomy and adult identity. Alongside these achievements, real-world business activities became a training ground for acquiring and applying practical skills—turning each challenge into a learning opportunity and each success into a building block for future ventures.

Improvement of Interpersonal Skills

Communication abilities were gradually enhanced through a mix of structured practice and natural social interaction. Regular participation in speech club activities provided consistent opportunities to engage in public speaking and refine interpersonal skills in a supportive environment. These experiences were complemented by real-world application, as communication techniques were tested and honed in professional business settings. Over time, Ma also learned to incorporate humor into conversations, using it as a subtle but powerful tool to ease tension and create more comfortable, engaging interactions. Perhaps most naturally, communication grew through informal lunch gatherings after karate training sessions—unassuming moments that offered rich, low-pressure chances to practice conversational flow and social nuance.

Personal Life Achievements

In his fifties, Ma stepped into a new chapter of life marked by personal growth and renewed purpose. He met and married a partner whose strong sense of self deeply inspired him, and together they built a stable and supportive family life. It was also during this time that Ma took on a bold new challenge—beginning karate training at the age of 50. What started as a personal endeavor soon became a powerful journey of continuous improvement, both physically and mentally.

With each practice and promotion examination, Ma experienced not only technical advancement but also a profound sense of fulfillment. The discipline and dedication required by karate helped him cultivate inner strength and resilience, leading to noticeable mental growth. Through these experiences, Ma gradually shaped a new social identity—one grounded in self-assurance, commitment, and the joy of lifelong learning.

Achievement of Social Integration

Following his marriage, Ma began to engage more actively in social life, embracing new opportunities to connect with others. He regularly hosted home parties, turning his residence into a welcoming space for friends and neighbors. His involvement extended beyond the home as he voluntarily participated in various community activities, building bridges and nurturing a sense of belonging.

Throughout this period, Ma made communication a central focus—continually learning, refining, and practicing the art of meaningful interaction. These efforts not only reflected his personal growth but also marked a significant step toward deeper social integration. Each successful experience reinforced his belief in his own abilities, fueling a cycle of motivation and confidence that empowered him to take on new challenges.

His steady progress in karate mirrored this journey. With every advancement, he not only honed his technical skills but also experienced mental and emotional growth. This discipline became a powerful medium for connecting with others, deepening social ties while enriching his sense of purpose and identity.

V EFFECTS OF THE HOLISTIC APPROACH

This section examines the holistic recovery approach, focusing on physical, mental, and social aspects. It highlights how karate, mindfulness, and social participation complemented each other to foster recovery, emphasizing their therapeutic significance.

Transformation Through Physical Approach

The recovery of physical functions diminished by long-term social withdrawal was significantly enhanced through core strengthening achieved by practicing karate, which Ma began at the age of 50. This new challenge not only contributed to the improvement of physical capabilities but also exerted positive ripple effects on mental aspects (Moore 2019).

Physical Transformation Through Karate

Practicing kata, the fundamental movements of karate, had a series of significant effects on Ma's physical and mental well-being. Through consistent practice, he strengthened his core muscles, which not only improved his physical fitness but also enhanced his overall body awareness. This increased awareness allowed him to develop a deeper connection with his movements, fostering better control and precision.

In addition to physical benefits, Ma mastered the coordination of his movements with breathing techniques, a key aspect of karate that brought both technical improvement and mental clarity. This integration of breath and motion further amplified the effects of his practice, creating a harmonious flow between his body and mind.

The practice of kata also had a synergistic effect with mindfulness, amplifying the benefits of both. As he engaged in the rhythmic, mindful movements of kata, Ma found that it contributed to the integrated recovery of his body and mind. This dual focus on physical movement and mental awareness supported his overall healing process, strengthening his resilience and sense of well-being.

Process of Achieving Technical Goals

The process of technical improvement in karate unfolded through a series of gradual stages, each marking significant growth. Ma's journey began with mastering basic movements, which laid the foundation for more advanced techniques. As his skills developed, he progressed to learning complex kata, refining his technique and deepening his understanding of martial arts.

This growth was not just theoretical but tangible, as Ma experienced measurable progress through promotion examinations. Each promotion served as a marker of his dedication and improvement, reinforcing his sense of accomplishment. His personal growth was further confirmed through performance experiences at Kokuhō Shrine, a culturally significant and historically preserved Shinto shrine. The opportunity to perform in such a revered location added a profound layer of meaning to his karate practice, connecting his technical development to a broader cultural and spiritual context.

Ripple Effects of Physical Practice

The continuous practice of karate had a profound and comprehensive impact on Ma's life, producing a series of positive effects. One of the most significant outcomes was the recovery of self-efficacy, which had been deeply affected by his long-term social withdrawal. Karate helped Ma regain a sense of control over his life, boosting his belief in his own abilities.

In addition to physical improvement, Ma experienced substantial mental growth through technical progress in karate. Each new skill learned and milestone reached contributed not only to his physical well-being but also to his sense of accomplishment and self-worth. The practice of karate also enhanced his ability to express himself, as the physical discipline of martial arts provided a channel for communication that words alone had once failed to convey.

The physical nature of karate was particularly essential in improving his motor functions, transforming his self-awareness, and ultimately building his confidence in social situations. The steady sense of achievement that came from meeting incremental goals in karate became a cornerstone of Ma's life after reintegration, helping him navigate the challenges of social interaction with newfound resilience and self-assurance.

Development of Mental Approach

The core of the mental approach consisted of mindfulness practice and monthly sessions with a holistic healer (Kimishima, 2024). These practices served as critical turning points that facilitated the transformation of self-denying thought patterns.

Effects of Mindfulness Practice

A particularly significant aspect of Ma's mindfulness practice was the cultivation of non-judgmental awareness, which played a crucial role in alleviating the deep-seated self-denial and feelings of social inadequacy that had been pervasive during his hikikomori period. By learning to observe his thoughts and emotions without harsh judgment, Ma gradually released the emotional hold that the past had on him. This shift allowed him to experience a greater sense of freedom from past mistakes and regrets.

As a result of this mindful approach, several positive changes unfolded in his life. First, Ma was able to let go of his attachment to past experiences, which had once defined much of his self-perception. This release brought about a heightened awareness of the present moment, enabling him to engage more fully in the here and now. Additionally, his stress management skills significantly improved, as he became better equipped to handle challenging situations without becoming overwhelmed by them.

Experience of Enlighten Coding Therapy

Sessions with the healer consisted of two parts: counseling and Enlight Coding Therapy[4]. Through these sessions, Ma experienced the following distinctive phenomena as it is shown in the following table:

Table 1.

Phenomena	Consequences
Physical Reactions	• Numberless and heaviness in the body • Sudden vibrations in the abdominal area • Spontaneous movements of specific body parts
Altered States of Consciousness	• Temporary drowsiness immediately after the session • Transition to a refreshing sensation afterward • Shift of awareness from the head to the chest is called heart

Transformation in Daily Life

Through continuous engagement in therapeutic sessions, Ma experienced a series of profound psychological shifts. He gradually liberated himself from rigid "should" thinking, allowing for more spontaneous and authentic self-expression. As psychological barriers diminished, he found it easier to engage in self-disclosure, sharing his thoughts and experiences more freely. This inner transformation also led to an increase in autonomous actions, as he became less preoccupied with how others might perceive him. Furthermore, Ma began to initiate social activities voluntarily, reflecting a newfound confidence in his ability to connect with others on his own terms. These mental developments worked synergistically with both physical and social efforts, laying a solid foundation for a more holistic and sustainable recovery process.

Implementation of Social Approach

Participation in community activities, as part of the social approach, served as a critical steppingstone for gradual social reintegration. This process demonstrated the following stages of development:

Transition from Online to In-Person Activities

Ma's journey from isolation to active community involvement unfolded in a gradual, phased manner. In the initial stage, he began by engaging in interactions within online communities, where the relative anonymity and psychological distance provided a safe space for rebuilding social confidence. As comfort grew, the intermediate stage marked a slow but steady transition to in-person activities, allowing him to test and refine his communication skills in real-life settings. Eventually, in the advanced stage, Ma reached a point where he could actively participate in community events, fully integrating himself into social life and contributing to group activities with growing assurance and enthusiasm.

Effects of Speech Club Participation

Participation in the local speech club emerged as a particularly transformative experience for Ma. Regular involvement in the club not only sharpened his communication skills but also restored his confidence in expressing himself publicly. Positive feedback from fellow participants played a key role in reinforcing his sense of social self-efficacy, encouraging Ma to engage more openly and authentically. The structured nature of the club's regular meetings helped him establish a stable social rhythm, while informal gatherings after sessions offered opportunities to practice natural, unstructured communication. Over time, these interactions contributed to a meaningful improvement in his ability to connect with others, both in formal and casual settings.

Formation of Social Networks

The relationships Ma formed through his various activities became instrumental in his journey toward social reintegration. These connections served as a secure base, offering psychological safety that encouraged him to step further into social life. They also motivated ongoing participation, giving him a sense of belonging and purpose. Through these interactions, Ma gained access to diverse social experiences, broadening his interpersonal horizons. Over time, he was able to build mutually supportive relationships, characterized by reciprocity and trust.

These social experiences did not exist in isolation—they complemented both the physical and mental approaches Ma had been cultivating, helping to solidify a more holistic recovery. In particular, his method of gradual social participation proved especially effective in reducing anxiety related to social interactions and in fostering a stronger sense of self-efficacy.

VI COMPREHENSIVE DISCUSSION AND CONCLUSION

Integrated Discussion of Research Findings

This study analyzed the recovery process from approximately 10 years of social withdrawal through the following three theoretical frameworks, clarifying a comprehensive recovery mechanism.

Inner Transformation Through Mindfulness

Mindfulness was crucial in transforming self-denying thought patterns. By focusing on the present moment, Ma distanced himself from past regrets and future anxieties, laying the groundwork for sustained recovery (Kawashima, 2024). Applied to daily life, mindfulness brought improvements in mental health, relationships, and overall lifestyle.

Gradual Development of Well-being

The five elements of the PERMA theory—Positive Emotion, Engagement, Relationships, Meaning, and Accomplishment—evolved in Ma's life in a dynamic and spiraling manner, with each element reinforcing the others (Harvey et al., 2021). His journey toward well-being began with safe social participation, initially fostered through the establishment of positive and low-pressure relationships on social networking sites (SNS). This laid the groundwork for emotional security and relational trust.

As Ma immersed himself in online business activities, he experienced a growing sense of self-efficacy, which further bolstered his confidence and deepened his engagement. This eventually led to the reconstruction of interpersonal relationships, allowing him to achieve a level of social integration that had been absent during his years of social withdrawal.

Alongside these developments, Ma underwent a shift in worldview—a transformative process that enabled him to rediscover meaning in life. Through his expanding involvement in multifaceted social activities, he moved closer to self-actualization, where his sense of fulfillment and purpose became tangible.

These elements did not emerge in isolation; rather, they evolved interdependently, illustrating the gradual and holistic development of well-being in Ma's recovery process.

Integrated Effects of the Holistic Approach (Flarey, 2024)

The integration of physical, mental, and social approaches—embodied respectively in karate, mindfulness practice, and communication-based activities—played a pivotal role in facilitating Ma's comprehensive recovery (Flarey, 2024). This holistic approach yielded several notable outcomes. First, the awakening of physical sensations through karate practice created ripple effects that positively influenced Ma's mental and emotional states, grounding his awareness in the present moment. This somatic engagement helped transform deep-seated self-denying thought patterns, paving the way for a more compassionate and accepting self-view.

Simultaneously, mindfulness practice supported the cultivation of internal awareness, while communication activities in social settings nurtured a sense of connection and belonging. As Ma gradually engaged in social participation, his self-efficacy increased, reinforcing his belief in his ability to navigate interpersonal environments.

Together, these intertwined strategies formed a synergistic system of support, demonstrating that a balanced integration of physical embodiment, psychological insight, and social reintegration is more effective than isolated efforts in recovering from long-term social withdrawal.

Importance of Social Support

Social support during the recovery process developed gradually and multilayered, playing a crucial role at each stage.

Support in the Initial Stage

Support from an older woman Ma met through a social networking site served as a critical turning point in the early stages of his recovery. Her presence provided more than just companionship—it created a safe psychological space, grounded in unconditional acceptance, where Ma felt free to express himself without fear of judgment. This emotional safety was something he had rarely experienced before and became a foundation for healing.

Through her positive and affirming engagement, Ma began to rebuild his self-esteem, which had been deeply eroded during his years of social withdrawal. Her consistent support not only nurtured his sense of self-worth but also encouraged him to take small steps toward in-person interaction, gently guiding him from the virtual world into real-life social experiences.

This relationship marked the beginning of Ma's reentry into society, illustrating how empathetic, non-judgmental support in the initial stage can catalyze meaningful and lasting change.

Support from Professionals

Monthly sessions with a holistic healer (Kimshima, 2024) played a significant role in Ma's recovery, offering a safe and nurturing space where deep personal transformation could take place. These sessions were particularly effective in facilitating the shift away from self-denying thought patterns, helping Ma to confront and reframe long-held beliefs rooted in self-criticism and unworthiness.

Through gentle guidance and empathetic dialogue, the healer helped lower Ma's psychological barriers, encouraging him to engage in greater self-disclosure and open emotional expression. This process allowed Ma to access parts of himself that had long been hidden during his hikikomori period.

Perhaps most notably, the healer supported Ma in liberating himself from the rigid mindset of "should"—the internalized expectations and pressures that had often paralyzed him. In its place, a sense of proactive and self-directed behavior emerged, enabling Ma to take meaningful steps forward on his own terms. These professional interventions served as a vital complement to his personal practices and social efforts, reinforcing the overall trajectory of recovery.

Support from the Community

The speech club and the shared office community served as essential platforms for Ma's social reintegration, offering consistent and supportive environments where interpersonal growth could naturally unfold. These settings provided opportunities to practice self-expression in ways that felt psychologically safe, allowing Ma to experiment with sharing his thoughts and experiences without fear of judgment.

The presence of constructive feedback from peers played a key role in Ma's ongoing development. Rather than facing criticism or indifference, he encountered encouragement and helpful suggestions that promoted both confidence and skill-building in communication.

Additionally, these communities fostered the emergence of mutually supportive relationships with individuals who shared similar ambitions and challenges. This sense of connection with others working toward common goals helped solidify Ma's place in the social world, reinforcing his motivation to participate and deepening his sense of belonging. These communal spaces thus became not only training grounds for social interaction but also vital pillars of his recovery journey.

Characteristics of Support that Promoted Recovery

The recovery process was deeply supported by several key characteristics of social support, which collectively created a stable and nurturing foundation for Ma's sustained reintegration. Central to this was the presence of a structured environment, which allowed for gradual social participation rather than forcing abrupt or overwhelming interactions. This step-by-step approach aligned with Ma's pace, reducing anxiety and fostering confidence.

Equally important was the cultivation of safe relationships grounded in non-judgmental acceptance. These relationships offered Ma the emotional security needed to be vulnerable, explore self-expression, and trust others again after a long period of isolation.

A flexible and patient attitude from supporters—whether friends, professionals, or community members—enabled Ma to grow at his own pace, accommodating setbacks and recognizing incremental progress.

Lastly, continuous involvement from these support systems ensured that Ma never felt alone in his journey. This ongoing presence created a dependable structure that not only encouraged development but also prevented relapse.

Together, these elements did not act in isolation but interacted synergistically, reinforcing each other and forming a resilient support network that made sustained recovery truly possible.

Theoretical Discussion

The recovery process revealed in this study can be examined through the following three theoretical frameworks:

Therapeutic Effects of Mindfulness

The practice of mindfulness supports traditional theories of psychological and emotional healing in several key ways, each reinforcing the core principles of therapeutic transformation. Firstly, it reduces self-denial by cultivating non-judgmental awareness, allowing individuals to observe their thoughts and feelings without attaching negative labels or criticism (Chandna et al. 2022). This awareness encourages acceptance and self-compassion, laying the groundwork for emotional healing.

Furthermore, mindfulness helps individuals liberate themselves from attachment to the past and future, focusing instead on the "here and now". This present-moment awareness reduces stress caused by rumination over past regrets or anxiety about future uncertainties, allowing for a greater sense of peace and stability (Kawashima, 2024).

Finally, mindfulness achieves sustained therapeutic effects through its application in daily life. By integrating mindfulness into everyday activities, individuals can experience ongoing emotional regulation and mental clarity, making it a powerful tool for long-term well-being (Dolan, 2024).

In this way, mindfulness aligns with and enhances traditional therapeutic approaches, providing enduring benefits across multiple aspects of emotional and psychological health.

Consistency with the PERMA Theory

The five elements of well-being, as outlined in the PERMA theory, demonstrated a dynamic and interrelated progression throughout the recovery process. Each element contributed to a comprehensive sense of well-being, fostering both personal and social growth.

- **Positive Emotion** was cultivated primarily through experiencing acceptance in safe relationships, which laid the emotional foundation for further growth and healing. These positive emotional experiences helped in reducing stress and fostering a sense of security.
- **Engagement** emerged through the development of self-efficacy achieved by immersing oneself in an online business. This active participation not only promoted skill development but also increased the sense of personal agency and involvement in life.
- **Relationship** gradually strengthened as interpersonal bonds were rebuilt. Over time, gradually rebuilding interpersonal relationships helped restore trust and emotional connection, reinforcing the importance of social interaction in the recovery process.
- **Meaning** was rediscovered through a shift in the perception of life and death, allowing a profound shift in the understanding of one's purpose and values. This newfound sense of meaning helped to contextualize the struggles faced during recovery, giving them significance.
- **Achievement** was experienced through gaining a sense of accomplishment via participation in various social activities. These accomplishments, whether big or small, reinforced a sense of progress and self-worth, solidifying the recovery process.

Together, these elements consistently aligned with the PERMA Theory, demonstrating how each component interacts to facilitate holistic well-being and foster continued growth in the recovery journey.

Social Implications

The insights gained from this study offer meaningful and practical guidance for those supporting individuals recovering from long-term social withdrawal. One key lesson is the importance of pacing. Reintegration into social life is most effective when it unfolds gradually. Starting with less intimidating forms of interaction—such as online communication—can serve as a stepping stone toward more direct, face-to-face engagement. This phased approach reduces anxiety and builds comfort over time.

Equally critical is the creation of safe, trusting relationships. A psychologically stable environment, grounded in non-judgmental acceptance, provides the emotional safety necessary for healing. Within such spaces, individuals are more likely to express themselves, take interpersonal risks, and begin to rebuild their self-esteem.

The study also highlights the power of comprehensive support. Physical, mental, and social interventions are not isolated solutions; they gain their true strength when they are woven together. A holistic approach, where these dimensions interact and reinforce each other, can significantly enhance the sustainability and depth of recovery.

At the core of this process is the enhancement of self-efficacy. Encouraging small, achievable steps in daily life allows individuals to accumulate a series of personal successes. Over time, these experiences strengthen confidence and cultivate a readiness to re-engage socially.

Finally, the complementarity of professional and personal support emerges as a vital factor. While psychological therapy and medical care are important, the inclusion of self-directed practices—such as mindfulness and physical activity—offers individuals a greater sense of ownership and autonomy in their recovery journey.

Together, these findings provide a strong foundation for reimagining how society supports those facing social withdrawal. They serve not only as practical recommendations but also as a call to evolve our frameworks for care—toward more empathetic, integrative, and person-centered support systems.

Importance of a Gradual Approach

When it comes to supporting recovery from long-term social withdrawal, a gentle, step-by-step approach has proven to be particularly effective. For individuals who have spent extended periods disconnected from society, sudden exposure to intense social settings can be overwhelming and counterproductive. Instead, initiating social participation through online activities offers a more manageable entry point. The virtual environment provides a sense of distance and control, helping individuals rebuild communication skills without the immediate pressure of physical presence.

In the early phases of reintegration, it is also beneficial to design activities that limit direct interpersonal contact. Structured interactions in smaller groups or mediated through online platforms reduce social anxiety, allowing individuals to ease into engagement at their own pace. This thoughtful design helps avoid overstimulation and fosters a sense of psychological safety.

Equally important is the practice of setting gradual, achievable goals. Rather than pushing toward major milestones, the focus is placed on building a series of small, realistic steps. Each success—no matter how minor it may seem—serves as a building block, reinforcing self-efficacy and boosting the confidence needed to take the next step forward.

Together, these strategies create a supportive and sustainable pathway for long-term social reintegration. The gradual approach not only respects the emotional and psychological readiness of each individual but also provides a solid foundation for recovery that can endure over time.

Necessity of Integrated Support

Effective recovery from long-term social withdrawal requires a comprehensive approach that addresses the individual as a whole—physically, mentally, and socially. Each dimension plays a vital role, and when combined, they form a powerful and sustainable support system. Physical activities, such as karate or other forms of movement, not only help individuals regain bodily confidence but also contribute to emotional regulation and mental stability. Alongside physical engagement, mental practices like mindfulness and meditation foster internal transformation. These practices gently shift self-denying thought patterns, helping individuals develop a more compassionate relationship with themselves and restore inner balance.

Equally important is the creation of structured environments that offer consistent opportunities for social participation. By introducing interpersonal interactions in a gradual, thoughtful manner, individuals are better able to rebuild trust, form connections, and re-enter social life with greater confidence. When these three elements—physical, mental, and social—are integrated and allowed to work in harmony, the path to recovery becomes not only more effective but also more sustainable.

Building Safe Relationships

In the early stages of recovery from long-term social withdrawal, establishing safe and trusting relationships is fundamental. At the heart of this process is the creation of a psychologically secure space—one where individuals feel unconditionally accepted. Supporters play a key role by offering non-judgmental presence, refraining from negative evaluations, and allowing individuals to express themselves freely and without fear. This atmosphere of acceptance is essential for fostering openness and building the foundation for deeper trust.

Equally important is the need for flexibility. Recovery is not a one-size-fits-all process, and each person moves at their own pace. A supportive attitude that encourages growth without imposing expectations helps to reduce psychological stress. By honoring the individual's rhythm, supporters can nurture a sense of autonomy and self-respect, which in turn reinforces the motivation to keep progressing.

Additionally, recovery is greatly supported by an environment that encourages the accumulation of small, attainable successes. When individuals are able to set and achieve modest goals, they begin to rebuild confidence in their abilities. These incremental achievements serve as stepping stones, gradually preparing them for greater challenges and deeper levels of social engagement.

Together, these elements—emotional safety, flexible support, and structured opportunities for success—create a reassuring space in which recovery can take root. They lay the emotional and psychological groundwork needed for individuals to eventually reconnect with the broader social world.

Support for Economic Independence

Achieving economic independence is a critical milestone in the journey toward social reintegration. For individuals recovering from long-term social withdrawal, employment is not only a source of income but also a pathway to rebuilding self-worth and social connection. To support this transition, practical and flexible approaches are essential.

One effective strategy is the provision of online employment opportunities. Remote work or freelance jobs offer a low-pressure entry point into the workforce, allowing individuals to engage with professional responsibilities without the immediate demands of in-person environments. These opportunities help bridge the gap between isolation and societal participation.

Equally important is the development of skill acquisition programs designed with a gradual learning curve. Beginning with basic competencies and advancing to more complex abilities enables individuals to gain confidence and competence step by step. This scaffolding approach ensures that participants are not overwhelmed, but rather supported in their progression.

Furthermore, creating an environment that supports self-paced learning plays a vital role in this process. Online educational resources and platforms that allow individuals to learn on their own terms reduce stress and empower autonomy. With the freedom to choose when and how they study, individuals can build skills in a way that aligns with their mental and emotional readiness.

Together, these supports provide a practical foundation for economic independence. By facilitating meaningful engagement in the workforce and fostering long-term self-sufficiency, they play a crucial role in helping individuals reintegrate into society with dignity and purpose.

Future Challenges and Prospects

While the findings of this study offer valuable insights into effective support for individuals recovering from long-term social withdrawal, they also highlight important challenges and directions for future research and practice. One major area concerns the methodology itself—particularly the need for long-term follow-up. To fully understand the effectiveness of recovery strategies, it is essential to assess not only immediate outcomes but also the stability of individuals' lives over time. This includes verifying the long-term sustainability of social reintegration and identifying potential risk factors that may lead to relapse or re-withdrawal.

Another key consideration is the generalizability of the case studies. Although the current findings are promising, further research is needed to determine whether the observed approaches are applicable across a broader range of cases. This includes exploring how support methods might be adapted to individuals of different age groups, life stages, or personal circumstances. Additionally, there is a need to examine whether certain principles or practices can be standardized, making them more widely accessible and easier to implement across various contexts.

Addressing these challenges will not only deepen our understanding of recovery from social withdrawal but also pave the way for the development of universal, evidence-based support models. By refining both research and practice, we can move closer to ensuring that all individuals—regardless of background—have access to effective, compassionate pathways toward reintegration and personal growth.

In addition to methodological concerns, this study also points to several practical challenges that must be addressed to enhance the effectiveness of support for individuals recovering from social withdrawal. One pressing need is the development of structured support systems that guide individuals through a gradual transition from online engagement to in-person participation. This step-by-step approach is essential for easing social anxiety and promoting sustainable reintegration.

Equally important is the systematization of holistic support that integrates physical, mental, and social dimensions. Creating an interconnected framework—rather than fragmented interventions—can foster more comprehensive and enduring recovery outcomes. Furthermore, the establishment of concrete, scalable measures to support economic independence remains a vital priority. Without a stable path toward self-sufficiency, long-term reintegration may be difficult to sustain.

These practical challenges highlight the importance of building adaptable, integrative, and forward-looking support infrastructures that meet individuals where they are—helping them take meaningful steps toward recovery and reconnection with society.

Development of Preventive Approaches

Looking ahead, a critical area for advancement lies in the development of preventive strategies to address social withdrawal before it becomes deeply entrenched. Establishing clear indicators for early detection and timely intervention can enable families, educators, and professionals to respond proactively to early signs of social isolation.

Moreover, there is a pressing need for comprehensive preventive programs that extend beyond the individual to include family members as active participants in the support process. These programs can equip families with the knowledge, communication tools, and emotional resilience necessary to foster supportive home environments.

Equally important is the formation of robust community networks aimed at preventing isolation and providing accessible pathways to connection. By strengthening ties across schools, workplaces, local organizations, and healthcare systems, communities can play a vital role in creating a safety net that identifies and supports at-risk individuals.

Addressing these practical challenges is essential not only for improving the effectiveness of support for those already experiencing hikikomori, but also for advancing a more holistic and preventive approach to social withdrawal in society at large.

Table 2. Future prospects

Type of development	Activities
Development of Supporters	• Training supporters capable of implementing a holistic approach • Cultivating professionals who can provide gradual support • Building networks among supporters
Development of Social Systems	• Creating intermediate spaces to facilitate gradual social reintegration • Establishing a support system that combines online and in-person activities • Developing employment support systems to assist in economic independence

Addressing these challenges will lead to more effective support systems for hikikomori recovery and promote social reintegration. Moreover, developing new methods to support individual autonomy and prevent social isolation can have broader societal impacts.

REFERENCES

Adachi, G. (2019). Recognition function provided by the relationship of "ibasho" in social isolation: From interview analysis to "hikikomori (social withdrawal)" parties and supporters. The Ritsumeikan Social Sciences Review, 55(1), 273-292. url: https://www.ritsumei.ac.jp/file.jsp?id=429532

Alvarado-García, P. A. A., Soto-Vásquez, M. R., Infantes Gomez, F. M., Guzman Rodriguez, N. M., & Castro-Paniagua, W. G. (2025). Effect of a mindfulness program on stress, anxiety, depression, sleep quality, social support, and life satisfaction: A quasi-experimental study in college students. *Frontiers in Psychology*, *16*, 1508934. Advance online publication. DOI: 10.3389/fpsyg.2025.1508934 PMID: 40012941

Beloborodova, P. (2023, February 17). How Mindfulness Helps Us to Build Meaningful Social Connections - Mind & Life Institute. Mind & Life Institute. https://www.mindandlife.org/media/how-mindfulness-helps-us-to-build-meaningful-social-connections/

Chandna, S., Sharma, P., & Moosath, H. (2022). The Mindful Self: Exploring Mindfulness in Relation with Self-esteem and Self-efficacy in Indian Population. *Psychological Studies*, *67*(2), 261–272. DOI: 10.1007/s12646-021-00636-5 PMID: 35125522

Christina, L. M. Hill and John A. Updegraff. (2012). Mindfulness and Its Relationship to Emotional Regulation. Kent State University. https://people.uncw.edu/hakanr/documents/MindfulnessandItsRelationshiptoEmotionalRegulation2012.pdf

Direct Communication. (2024, December 31). https://www.direct-commu.com/chie/mental/ima-koko01/

Dolan, E. W. (2024, August 23). Just 10 minutes of mindfulness per day enhances mental health and motivates healthier habits. PsyPost - Psychology News. url: www.psypost.org/just-10-minutes-of-mindfulness-per-day-enhances-mental-health-and-motivates-healthier-habits/

Employment Continuity Navigation. (2024, November 20). *Hikikomori ga ochiiru yottsu no shinri joutai to wa?* [What are the four psychological states that lead to social withdrawal?]. https://shuro-shien.or.jp/navi/hikikomori-psychology/#2%E7%BD%AA%E6%82%AA%E6%84%9F%E3%82%92%E6%8A%B1%E3%81%88%E3%81%9F%E5%BC%95%E3%81%8D%E3%81%93%E3%82%82%E3%82%8A%E3%81%AF%E8%87%AA%E5%88%86%E3%82%92%E8%B2%AC%E3%82%81%E7%B6%9A%E3%81%91%E3%81%A6%E3%81%97%E3%81%BE%E3%81%86

Flarey, D. (2024, August 8). Holistic Healthcare: Key concepts and modern practices. AIHCP. url:aihcp.net/2024/08/08/holistic-healthcare-key-concepts-and-modern-practices/

Goleman, D. (2019, August 15). Listen with Mindfulness. https://www.linkedin.com/pulse/listen-mindfulness-daniel-goleman/

Harvey, J., & Boynton, K. (2021). *Seligman's PERMA+ model explained: A theory of wellbeing. PositivePsychology.com.* Interpersona., url d-nb.info/1260856607/34

Hiyoshi, M. (2019). Review of previous research on family factors of Hikikomori. *Graduate School Research Journal, 10*, 1–32.

Ishida, J. (2024, December 24). *Jiko Kouteikan wo Takameru: Chiisana Seikou Taiken no Chikara* [Boosting self-esteem through small successes]. Dr. Bridge. https://www.dr-bridge.co.jp/kokorocare/column/self-affirmation/

Jones, S. M., Bodie, G. D., & Hughes, S. D. (2019). The impact of mindfulness on empathy, active listening, and perceived provisions of emotional support. *Communication Research, 46*(6), 838–865. DOI: 10.1177/0093650215626983

Kato, T. A., Kanba, S., & Teo, A. R. (2019). Hikikomori: Multidimensional understanding, assessment, and future international perspectives. *Psychiatry and Clinical Neurosciences, 73*(8), 427–440. DOI: 10.1111/pcn.12895 PMID: 31148350

Kawakita, M. (n.d.). *Hikikomori no jittai to shakaiteki haikei yoin no rikai* [Understanding the reality of social withdrawal and its social background and causes].

Kawashima, T. (2024). *Ima koko wo ikiru chikara wo tsukeru houhou* [How to develop the power to live in the present]. https://www.direct-commu.com/chie/mental/ima-koko01/

Ketay, S., Thorson, K. R., Roy, A. R. K., & Welker, K. M. (2022). Trait Mindfulness is Associated with Self-Disclosure and Responsiveness During Social Interactions with New Acquaintances. *Mindfulness*. Advance online publication. DOI: 10.1007/s12671-022-02044-w

Kimishima, M. H. (2024, September 10). Shifting beyond the world of duality. For an International Transdisciplinary Chair:From Knowledge to the Future. Volume II, 116–128. Presented at the Online Symposium „For an international transdisciplinary chair" organized by the International Center for Transdisciplinary Research and Studies (CIRET). DOI: 10.62768/ADJURIS/2024/4/08

L'Argent de l'Or. (n.d.). L'Argent De L'Or. https://www.largent-de-lor.com/about

Luo, Q., Li, X., Zhao, J., Jiang, Q., & Wei, D. (2025). The effect of slow breathing in regulating anxiety. *Scientific Reports, 15*(1), 8417. DOI: 10.1038/s41598-025-92017-5 PMID: 40069274

Malagón-Amor, Á., Martín-López, L. M., Córcoles, D., González, A., Bellsolà, M., Teo, A. R., & Bergé, D. (2020). Family features of social withdrawal syndrome (hikikomori). *Frontiers in Psychiatry, 11*, 138. DOI: 10.3389/fpsyt.2020.00138 PMID: 32194459

Mindful eating. (2024, November 7). The Nutrition Source. https://nutritionsource.hsph.harvard.edu/mindful-eating/

Moore, B., Dudley, D., & Woodcock, S. (2019). The effects of martial arts participation on mental and psychosocial health outcomes: A randomised controlled trial of a secondary school-based mental health promotion program. *BMC Psychology, 7*(1), 60. DOI: 10.1186/s40359-019-0329-5 PMID: 31511087

Nakajima, R. (2023, July 11). *Otona no hikikomori kokufuku* [Overcoming adult social withdrawal]. Clinical psychologist and personal trainer. Support for elementary and junior high school students returning to school, support for home education for elementary and junior high school students, mental support for mothers of school refusers. url: osakachild.com/hikikomori/

Nonaka, S., & Sakai, M. (2021). Psychological Factors Associated with Social Withdrawal (Hikikomori). *Psychiatry Investigation, 18*(5), 463–470. DOI: 10.30773/pi.2021.0050 PMID: 34053211

Organisation for Economic Co-operation and Development. (2025, March 31). Supporting Japanese people affected by severe social isolation: A case study. OECD Blogs. https://www.oecd.org/en/blogs/2025/03/supporting-opportunities-insights-from-communities/supporting-japanese-people-affected-by-severe-social-isolation-a-case-study.html

Pacheco, D. (2024, February 26). Meditation for sleep. Sleep Foundation. https://www.sleepfoundation.org/meditation-for-sleep

Stromberg, J. (2015, August 27). What science says about meditation: it improves your focus and emotional control. Vox. https://www.vox.com/2015/8/27/9214697/meditation-brain-neuroscience

Suttie, J. (2022, March 21). Can mindfulness make you better at apologizing? Greater Good. https://greatergood.berkeley.edu/article/item/can_mindfulness_make_you_better_at_apologizing

Taka, K. (2008). A consideration on the process and the psychology of the withdrawal. Journal of Human Sciences, Seiryo University, 2(1), 19-22. url: https://www.seiryo-u.ac.jp/u/research/gakkai/ronbunlib/h_ronsyu_pdf/2_1/p19_taka.pdf

Tan, C. M., Goleman, D., & Kabat-Zinn, J. (2012). *Search inside yourself: The unexpected path to achieving success, happiness (and world peace)*. HarperCollins.

Winarsunu, T., Iswari Azizaha, B. S., Fasikha, S. S., & Anwar, Z. (2023). Life skills training: Can it increases self esteem and reduces student anxiety? *Heliyon*, *9*(4), e15232. DOI: 10.1016/j.heliyon.2023.e15232 PMID: 37095906

Yong, R., & Nomura, K. (2019). Hikikomori is most associated with interpersonal relationships, followed by suicide risks: A secondary analysis of a national cross-sectional study. *Frontiers in Psychiatry*, *10*, 247. DOI: 10.3389/fpsyt.2019.00247 PMID: 31040799

ENDNOTES

1 Yoshida, M. (2023, December 14). *Ichinichi juppun de jibun wo jouka suru houhou: Mindfulness meisou nyuumon shinsouban* [How to purify yourself in 10 minutes a day: Introduction to mindfulness meditation, new edition]. Ameba Blog. https://ameblo.jp/masaonoblog/

2 Yoshida, M. (2015, May 1). *Maindofurunesu meisou nyuumon: Ichinichi juppun de jibun wo jouka suru houhou* [Introduction to mindfulness meditation: How to purify yourself in 10 minutes a day]. WAVE. ISBN 978-4-87290-731-5

3 Direct Communication. (2024, December 31) https://www.direct-commu.com/chie/mental/ima-koko01/

4 https://www.largent-de-lor.com/menu

Chapter 11
Storytelling:
A Path to Empowerment

Terence Patrick Mickey
https://orcid.org/0009-0004-6115-0472
Independent Researcher, Germany

ABSTRACT

This chapter from Terence Mickey covers the profound connection between storytelling, self-awareness, and well-being, highlighting how narratives shape our perception of ourselves and the world around us. It focuses on: 1) the key principles of how to craft a story and how the process promotes self-awareness and well-being, combats isolation and fosters social connectedness; 2) the role of storytelling in shaping and reshaping our identity as well as building our emotional resilience; and 3) how we shape the world through stories and possess the power to change our cultural stories to benefit our collective well-being.

STORYTELLING: A PATH TO EMPOWERMENT BY TERENCE MICKEY

When I first started practicing and teaching storytelling, I had no idea whether or not this art form would promote well-being or self-awareness for anybody, including myself. At the time, I considered storytelling a form of entertainment, not a tool for introspection or personal growth. But it didn't take long for me to understand its potential for both.

Whether we're aware of their power or not, stories are everywhere. They mobilize people into action. They connect us to ourselves and one another. They help us navigate and make meaning of life's challenges. And by becoming conscious of them and learning how to shape and analyze them, we empower ourselves to become more

DOI: 10.4018/979-8-3373-0360-4.ch011

self-aware and creative in how we understand our lives, other people and the world. With political polarization, an epidemic of social isolation and a crisis in mental health impacting our daily lives, storytelling is not a superfluous form of entertainment but a vital life-skill necessary for our individual and collective well-being.

"How we tell our stories controls our mood, self-image, and the influence we have on others," writes Dr. Pamela Rutledge and Dr. Erik Gregory in "Exploring Positive Psychology: The Science of Happiness and Well-Being" (Gregory & Rutledge, 2016):

"Our stories can also dictate our future paths and successes. Therefore, understanding storytelling is not only key to how we feel about ourselves and how we interact with others, but it gives us valuable tools we can use to make change."

This chapter will cover the profound connection between storytelling, self-awareness, and well-being, highlighting how narratives shape our perception of ourselves and the world around us. It will focus on: 1) the seven principles of how to craft a story and how the process promotes self-awareness and well-being, combats isolation and fosters social connectedness; 2) the role of storytelling in shaping and reshaping our identity as well as building our emotional resilience; and 3) how we shape the world through stories and possess the power to change our cultural stories to benefit our collective well-being.

Welcome to Your Life

In 2009, when I worked for The Moth, a US-based nonprofit that promotes the craft and performance of live, autobiographical storytelling, I was invited to teach a storytelling workshop for recovering addicts (*About The Moth*, n.d.). Located in the Bronx, Palladia-Starhill Residential was a private alcohol and drug rehab center that offered treatment for a variety of substance abuse addictions (*About Palladia - Starhill Residential*, n.d.). Its director at the time wanted to increase the program's retention rate, and he thought building a community through storytelling would encourage people to complete the program. Since they would be telling and listening to their autobiographical stories over ten weeks, they would ideally be more accountable to each other and the program. The workshop culminated in a public performance, where each participant shared their crafted five minute story with a live audience.

Francis, one of the participants, wanted to tell the story of the time his wife clocked him with a lead pipe. He thought the story was funny, even if a bit dark, and it was certainly, as he said, a memorable event. At our first session, I'd shared with the group the key principles of storytelling: setting up the stakes, developing the narrative arc, building the sensory world, choosing the last line, identifying the theme, and finally revising and performing the work. These principles guide participants in excavating and crafting their stories, and I will unpack them in depth later on in the chapter. Referring to these principles, I pointed out to Francis how the experience he wanted to develop into a story did not possess the necessary traits of a narrative.

The event happened to him, but he didn't act or react in a meaningful way. The lead pipe incident lacked transformation. As much as his wife may have wanted Francis to change when she clocked him, he admitted to us that he was unaffected by the incident. His memory was an anecdote, not a story. In stories, we have agency and through our actions and decisions we reveal how we've changed. Anecdotes may be full of action and details but they don't reveal transformation or character, which are essential traits for compelling stories.

Francis said he'd mull over my feedback. The following week, he told a new, harrowing and deeply powerful story. He shared it with me and a fellow instructor, and while it was very moving, I didn't know if the story would be too traumatic for Francis to tell in front of the whole group. Or if the audience would be ready for or receptive to his story. After working with the group for a few weeks, I understood they had all survived a lot and I didn't want to trigger anyone, especially Francis who had the most at risk. Even though he assured me that he wanted to tell his new story, I had reservations. I didn't yet know storytelling's full capabilities beyond mere entertainment.

Before I share Francis's story, I want to introduce the principles of storytelling in depth and show the process of excavating a significant moment from a person's life. This process will reveal how storytelling is uniquely positioned to develop self-awareness and well-being in both the storyteller and the listener. I've used this method to train executive leaders from a wide array of industries and anyone can fulfill these steps and successfully harness the power of storytelling for both personal development and persuasion.

Before the principles can be applied, the storytelling group first works together to help each participant excavate their unique story. Storytelling is not done in isolation but in relation to others no matter what the setting.

Listening for Story

Occasionally, a person knows right away which significant moment in their life they want to share as a story. Even if the memory is ancient, the moment feels alive for them as if the event happened only yesterday. One woman in Francis's group remembered the time James Brown called her up on stage at the Apollo Theater. She leapt from the audience to the singer's side and strutted with pride. At the end of the night, James Brown invited her on tour with him as a backup dancer and gave her the nickname "Little Mama."

Her story recalled the life she had before addiction and by reclaiming that moment she revealed to the group her wholeness. We are never only one thing in life. And we need listeners to unearth the totality of our experience and wisdom. At a corporate storytelling training, I remember an executive who volunteered to tell the story of how he survived 9-11 and saved his entire team by ignoring the advice to stay put. None of the fifty eight colleagues present at the training had heard his story before because no one had ever asked him what happened. What he shared revealed his deep understanding of leadership, an insight that would have been left unspoken if not for the occasion of a storytelling circle.

We contain multitudes, and our library of stories reveal to others our complexity. In "The Library Book," the New Yorker writer Susan Orlean reflects poignantly on the wealth of stories we all have to share (Orlean, 2019, #):

"In Senegal, the polite expression for saying someone died is to say his or her library has burned. When I first heard the phrase, I didn't understand it, but over time I came to realize it was perfect. Our minds and souls contain volumes inscribed by our experiences and emotions; each individual's consciousness is a collection of memories we've cataloged and stored inside us, a private library of a life lived."

We each have a library of memories within us and if we don't craft our recollections into stories, we lose the opportunity to connect deeply with ourselves and our community. As Lissa Rankin, MD, the author of "Mind Over Medicine: Scientific Proof You Can Heal Yourself," writes: (Rankin, 2012):

"Each of us is a constantly unfolding narrative, a hero in a novel no one else can write. And yet so many of us leave our stories untold, our songs unsung—and when this happens, we wind up feeling lonely, listless, out of touch with our life's purpose, plagued with a chronic sense that something is out of alignment. We may even wind up feeling unworthy, unloved, or sick."

For many, telling a story live in front of an audience without any notes would be as welcomed as lighting themselves on fire. And certainly the risk of vulnerability is real. But as Rankin points out, our bodies respond positively when we share a story: (Rankin, 2012)

"Every time you tell your story and someone else who cares bears witness to it, you turn off the body's stress responses, flipping off toxic stress hormones like cortisol and epinephrine and flipping on relaxation responses that release healing hormones like oxytocin, dopamine, nitric oxide, and endorphins. Not only does this turn on the body's innate self-repair mechanisms and function as preventative medicine—or treatment if you're sick. It also relaxes your nervous

system and helps heal your mind of depression, anxiety, fear, anger, and feelings of disconnection."

When we share our story, the benefits are backed by neuroscience. But it's important to note that the body responds positively when the listener or listeners are attentive and holding a particular space for the story. When such a listener is available to a storyteller, not only are health benefits considerable but the fear and risk are mitigated.

Mitigating the fear and risk are crucial since both are real. Our vulnerability and personal stories can be used against us. Since telling a story in public can be traumatizing if the public is not educated on empathy and the art of listening, I will show how to create a safe space for storytelling.

The relationship between the storyteller and listener begins long before the sharing and performance of the story. The relationship starts with the process of crafting a story, when a unique bond forms between the teller and listener as they develop the structure of the story through the narrative principles. Both the craft and teller/listener relationship allow for the teller to experience their memory from a distance, to see its malleability and meaning, while inviting self-awareness, compassion and depth into the process.

While "Little Mama," excavated her story quickly, people often have to dig deep for the story they want to tell, and for these participants the success of the excavation process depends on the depth and attentiveness of the listening. To create a storytelling environment, you need to first establish a listening environment.

On the first day of the workshop at Palladia we taught the group how to actively listen. As Philip Glass said in an interview with Tricycle Magazine (Tricycle Magazine, 1999):

"The problem with listening, of course, is that we don't. There's too much noise going on in our heads, so we never hear anything. The inner conversation simply never stops."

In order to teach people how to listen, you need to first acknowledge the constant racket we all have going on most of the time in our head. By drawing attention to the noise, you can invite people to better hone in on the person who wants to share a personal memory and understand, with the help of the group, what it might mean for them.

Built into the excavation process is self-reflection and self-awareness. With the help of their first listener, the storyteller starts to see their memory and life experience from a different perspective. The process of crafting a story along with an awareness of a larger audience, who will ultimately receive their story, both create enough distance for the storyteller to start composing a story from their memory.

For the craft aspect of storytelling, the teller has to re-see a memory with the potential of a story in mind. What is the beginning, middle and end of my story? What did I have at stake at the moment? Why did I act as I did? What did that particular moment mean for me? What exactly happened as I remember the details?

The level of introspective questioning and the quality of the answers depends on the listening the storyteller receives. Since everyone in the group is responsible for the listening in the room, they are also responsible for what stories ultimately emerge from each individual in the group. We're all connected in a storytelling circle even before we start to work on individual stories. And if the group is not attentive with their listening, no one will share anything truly vulnerable or deep. They won't feel safe enough. They won't deem the space worthy enough to share their sacred inner lives.

As Monisha Pasupathi and Jacob Billitteri reveal in their article for the International Journal of Listening, "Being and Becoming through Being Heard: Listener Effects on Stories and Selves" (Pasupathi & Billitteri, 2015, #), listening impacts the story:

> *"Once speakers have both chosen to narrate and negotiated a monologue with their listener, the subsequent shaping of the story is an interactive, dyadic process with both conversation partners contributing…Some of the ways that narrators change stories for inattentive listeners include changing the content they narrate, offering different interpretive content and altering story structure. These changes affect memory, self/identity judgments, and interpretations related to the event for the narrator."*

By developing and sharing a story with a group of strangers, you're crossing a potent threshold. You're asking to be seen and heard and implicitly asking to be accepted. And the story circle is a sacred space where people can remember. To remember is to re-member, to recall the disparate parts of ourselves and reconstruct a whole, and when we craft our memories as stories we're not only creating meaning but shaping our lives, which is why storytelling is so empowering. It is how we shape our lives. As the writer Gabriel Garcia Marquez said while speaking to Gerald Martin, the author of his biography, "Gabriel García Márquez: A Life" (Martin, 2012, #)

> *"What matters in life is not what happens to you, but what you remember and how you remember it."*

We become the architect of our experience as soon as we start the process of excavating memory to tell a story. And because the process of crafting a memory into a narrative with coherence invites the teller to reflect on what they've learned from their experience and share how insights from one experience served to inform the next, creating a sense of continuity, research shows that narrative coherence in storytelling has been consistently tied to positive mental outcomes (Adler, 2011, #). With narrative coherence, we can begin to chart our evolution, mark our growth and build an identity based on our values and purpose. As Julie Beck writes in the Atlantic, quoting Dr. Jonathan Adler for her article "Life's Stories" (Beck, 2015): "You're both the narrator and the main character of your story. That can sometimes be a revelation—'Oh, I'm not just living out this story; I am actually in charge of this story.'"

The Storytelling Principles: How to Tell A Captivating Story

I: Setting Up the Stakes

After we established an optimal listening environment for the group at Palladia, we then introduced the key principles of storytelling, which influence the excavation process and help determine what story the participant will share.

The first principle for developing a participant's story is setting up the stakes. They have to identify what they, as a character, had at stake in the moment they recall. What did they have to gain or lose by taking action and deciding to do what they did? What makes the story matter for them? The answer to these questions will in turn make the story matter to the audience.

By identifying what you want in a given situation and what getting what you want means for you, you invite the audience into your inner-workings, your motivation, your psychology and your humanity. Here is where the intimate contract between the storyteller and listener begins. The storyteller is implicitly saying,"I am letting you into an intimate and privileged position, and from this point on, we're on this journey together." And in order to identify the stakes of their story, the storyteller has to do the deep work of self-reflection. They have to develop their self-awareness to understand not only their own motivation but what will be relatable to the audience.

The depth and meaning and significance of the stakes shared by the storyteller will depend on the quality of their self-knowledge and self-awareness as well as the quality of the audience's listening. There is a clear relationship between how engaging a story is and the level of self-awareness the storyteller possesses. There is also a clear relationship between the depth of what a person will share and whether or not they're being listened to intently. When we know another person is truly listening, we seize the opportunity to share a significant and human moment from our life to share, and when we possess self-awareness, we shape the moment into an engaging and moving story, which is exactly what Francis ultimately did.

The process of identifying the stakes of our stories helps us understand our own self and allows others to use the material of our lives to help them navigate their own, as Annie Murphy Paul points out in her New York Times article "Your Brain on Fiction," when she cites a study by Raymond Mar, a psychologist at York University in Canada.

Mar "performed an analysis of 86 fMRI studies...and concluded that there was substantial overlap in the brain networks used to understand stories and the networks used to navigate interactions with other individuals — in particular, interactions in which we're trying to figure out the thoughts and feelings of others." (Paul, 2012) The brain's capacity to construct a map of other people's intentions is known as ''theory of mind.' As Paul points out, "narratives offer a unique opportunity to engage this capacity, as we identify with characters' longings and frustrations, guess at their hidden motives and track their encounters with friends and enemies, neighbors and lovers." The importance of this benefit from storytelling cannot be stressed enough. As Gregory and Rutledge write in "Exploring Positive Psychology: The Science of Happiness and Well-Being"(Gregory & Rutledge, 2016, #):

> *"One of the most important cognitive competencies we need to survive and thrive in our social world is the ability to identify and interpret the internal states, beliefs and desires of others in our environment."*

When working in a corporate setting, a leader's or manager's understanding of their teams is crucial and stories foster not only trust between employees and their leaders but a deeper understanding of how everyone is oriented or not around a shared goal. The more we know about each other, the better we work together, both to identify conflicts and resolve them. Dutch researchers have found that storytelling is one of the most effective ways to build connections and develop trust and cooperation amongst teams. They have concluded that sharing a common story helps teams collaborate better.

> *"Given the power of narration to capture complex experiences, a storytelling culture may contribute to reducing difficulties in communication and conflict situations, and augment continuous learning." (Lohuis et al., 2016, #)*

II: Develop The Narrative Arc

The second principle in the storytelling process is to develop the narrative arc. Every story is about change. You are not the same person at the end of the story that you were at the beginning. And the opportunity of a story is to register this shift. The narrative arc maps and measures your transformation for the audience. The first and last lines of any story are valuable real estate for this reason because they establish your transformation as a character. They measure the depth of that change as well as the impact. If you don't change, you're not telling a story. But mining for a narrative arc that conveys a significant change forces tellers to scan their life for memorable moments, transformative challenges and triumphs, times when nothing was ever the same again. Since Francis didn't change in the story of his wife hitting him with a lead pipe, he searched deeper in the library of his memories for the story he ultimately told, which changed the way he saw himself.

Storytelling promotes self-awareness when we can see ourselves as the main characters of our lives. And by identifying the stakes of an incident and shaping our experiences into a narrative arc, with a beginning, middle and end, as main characters we're forced to evaluate our decisions, values and beliefs. We ask, as if watching a movie or reading a book, why did I, as a character in the story, do what I did? What was my motivation in that particular moment? What circumstances led to my specific behavior? What did I believe would happen by me acting as I did, as opposed to what did happen? Were my expectations met or thwarted? And most importantly, how have I changed from the experience?

By observing ourselves as a character, we see our life as a stranger would and the fresh perspective allows us to potentially see ourselves within the larger arc of our lives with compassion, maybe even for the first time in our lives. And when we present our stories to an audience, even if that audience is only one person, we can develop even further empathy for ourselves. Witnessing the character of our story become relatable to our audience, sharing similar desires, fears and challenges, we have the opportunity to see how much another person identifies with our particular experience and actions. Through the art of storytelling, we allow the listener to become us for an instant, and we see how others see us, often at our most vulnerable. In my experience, people do not react with judgement but recognition.

We see ourselves in other people's stories no matter how different they may appear on the surface. Stories highlight the fundamental elements we all share, our human desires and frailty and the universal moments we've all experienced - falling in and out of love, leaving and returning home, succeeding and failing. And through the process of neural coupling (also known as mirroring), when we receive a story as a listener, the neurons in our brain fire in the same patterns as the speaker's. According to the research of Greg J. Stephens, Lauren J. Silbert, and Uri Hasson, the process of neural coupling occurs across many different areas of the brain, which may induce a shared contextual model of the situation. (Stephens et al., 2010, #) Stories emotionally and cognitively connect us to one another.

In his book, "Hero With a Thousand Faces," the mythologist Joseph Campbell argues for the universality of myths that appear throughout history independent of era, culture or society. His Hero's Journey model describes the path of a hesitant hero, who ultimately accepts a difficult journey, and on the way overcomes many challenges and returns both victorious and transformed (Campbell, 2008, #). You'll see the building blocks of Campell's model in the story structure of everything from Star Wars to your friend telling you the story of their last horrible date. Conflicts, problems and challenges are important to transformation and meaning in stories.

And we're drawn to stories of conflict and change because they capture the moments that preoccupy our everyday lives, especially since we're highly resistant to both.

Our brain appears to be hard-wired for Campbell's storytelling model, as Paul J. Zak, the founding director of the Center for Neuroeconomics Studies, points out in the Harvard Business Review while explaining his research on how stories alter our behavior (Zak, 2014):

"In order to motivate a desire to help others, a story must first sustain attention – a scarce resource in the brain – by developing tension during the narrative. If the story is able to create that tension then it is likely that attentive viewers/ listeners will come to share the emotions of the characters in it, and after it ends, likely to continue mimicking the feelings and behaviors of those characters."

What is the pay off for engaging in conflicts, problems and challenges?

The narrative arc represents synthesis. At the beginning of a story, we introduce the known foundation, the orienting information - time, place and character - as well as the seed of conflict and the goal of the character, what they desire and passionately want. The middle introduces new information, rising action and confrontation, which ultimately leads to transformation. Whether the character achieves what they want or not, they change. And the end synthesizes, reconciles and resolves the discrepancy between the beginning and middle to form the changed character. Through this synthesis, whether we experience it through telling our own story or listening to another person's story, we experience coherence.

Cognitive science recognizes narrative as a basic organizing principle of memory, and in the act of recall, our memory is not striving for accuracy but coherence. The experiments of Michael Gazzaniga, a cognitive neuroscientist, have revealed a function of the left brain hemisphere called 'the Interpreter,' which reflexively makes sense of memories, even when it has no direct access to them or the context in which they were made. Gazzaniga's research suggests that "narrative coherence helps us to navigate the world – to know where we're coming from and where we're headed. It tells us where to place our trust and why…it enables us to find our bearings in possible future realities, or to make better sense of our own past experiences. What stories give us, in the end, is reassurance." (Gots, 2012)

The reassurance found in the narrative arc is how we navigate and survive change throughout our lives. Nobody welcomes change but the only constant in our lives is change. Stories show us and others how and what we gained through periods of change and transformation and our insights become valuable not only to us but potentially to our community.

III: Be Specific With Sensory Details

The third principle of storytelling is what creates an empathetic tether between the storyteller and the audience, what closes the gap between the individual and the crowd: sensory details. The more particular you are with your description, the richer and therefore better the story will be. Sensory details allow the audience to traverse the distance between where they are and where you are and fully embody your experience.

People tend to want to skip over the details of a story in favor of the broad strokes since they don't want to 'bore' their audience, but details are the lifeblood of a story and more than anything they engender empathy and compassion from the audience. You're holding them close to you on the journey, helping them to feel and experience exactly what you felt and experienced in the moment, beat by beat.

Neuroscience supports the concept of storytelling as a tether between one person and another. Adding particular details to your story enhances what Paula Croxson, a neuroscientist and the Director of Public Programs at The Zuckerman Mind, Brain and Behavior Institute of Columbia University, explains on the podcast "This is Your Brain with Dr. Phil Stieg," as narrative transportation (Stieg, 2022):

"What many studies have shown to happen when you experience the phenomenon of narrative transportation is that you process the information more deeply, so you actually take in and internalize the experience of the storyteller, or the protagonist in the story, whoever you're following. So you process more deeply, but also you feel less critical of the content. And so that is what lends storytelling this feeling of verisimilitude, of "truthiness", of believability and ultimately persuasion...Storytelling has this universal property. It's so powerful that if you measure people's eye blinks when they're engaged in watching a live storytelling performance, their eye blinks tend to sync up with each other. It's such a collective and powerful experience, even something unconscious, as whether or not you keep your eyes open, become synced up with the people around you."

Even though I have not shared the details of Francis's story yet, witnessing his performance drove home for me the power of details to both transport the teller and the audience. His story took place when he was eighteen, and the details he recounted transported his body back to that age. He assumed the same physicality as he had in a specific moment at eighteen. Since he returned to the scene with his details and even his body, we, the audience, did as well.

IV: Know Your Ending

The fourth principle in the process of storytelling is knowing your ending. In order to not lose yourself in the story, identifying your last line at the beginning of your process helps you see what you're working toward and will influence everything that precedes it - your fist line, the narrative arc, the details and the length.

I recommend storytellers memorize only their first line and their last line before they embark on telling their story. The first line will help jump start them with a boost of confidence when they first step on stage, and their last line will act as a beacon to aim toward while they tell their story and help them maintain confidence throughout. Live storytelling is a tightrope act and your first and last lines pin you to two stable fixed points while you traverse mid-air.

The last line provides the storyteller with a destination, while emphasizing the fact that this story is not your whole life but a distinct moment, which you've shaped to share. The last line is a container to help the storyteller reflect on a distinct time in their life rather than be overwhelmed by everything that came before or after.

Endings can be difficult for a lot of storytellers since the last line is the final and lasting impression of your story, what you'll leave the audience with and most likely what they will remember. But the significance of the last line reminds the storyteller of the reasons why they're crafting and sharing a story to begin with. Because there will be a listener. The teller is not speaking into a void or talking only to or for themselves. They have another person in mind while they're crafting, so the whole process - because there is a listener - is an effort to connect. This part of the process helps the storyteller keep an eye on the intention of the crafting - to connect with clarity and intention.

V: Pick A Theme

The fifth principle of storytelling is determining the theme of your story. Stories are about many different things at once and reflect the complexity of our lives. At any given moment we can be feeling contradictory emotions and we want our stories to reflect the nuances of our lived experience. But when developing a story to share, we want to choose a theme to help us compose and refine the material. Your story may be about forgiveness and jealousy and redemption and disillusionment but by picking one theme you'll tighten your story without completely sacrificing the complexity or vestiges of the other themes. The theme you pick will provide a lens to hone your words and structure without obliterating the other themes and meanings of your story. Finding your theme is a tool for focus and simplicity, not a prescription for diminishing complexity.

Finding the theme not only helps the storyteller focus and ultimately edit their story but encourages them to find the meaning of their story and what insight they may have gleaned from the events they're recounting and shaping. Since they are consciously choosing the theme, they are deciding for themselves what they want the story to be about and what it reveals about them. And choosing a theme can be the difference between a tragic story or a triumphant one, depending on what meaning the storyteller finds in the process. As Jonathan Adler's work reveals, particular narrative themes, such as agency, communion, redemption, and coherence, are linked to positive mental health and well-being (Adler et al., 2015, #).

VI: Edit Your Story

The sixth principle of storytelling is editing your story. Once you've identified your stakes, the narrative arc, the last line, the theme and recollected all of the details to fully render the story for the audience, editing will improve what you have gathered by clarifying and tightening the material. Revision is also an opportunity to see your experience with even more distance. The process of the first five principles allows you to treat your experience as if you are outside of yourself. The revision process allows you to step even further back and reflect on the events you've composed and what they truly mean to you. The theme starts the editing process by forcing the teller to see their material through a particular lens. They have to make choices of what to include or exclude, where to begin and end based on the meaning they have assigned the story through the theme. With the theme in mind, they look at everything - their first and last lines and all of the details they recalled - and they will assess what is absolutely necessary and what is superfluous for the time they have to tell their story, whether it's five or fifteen minutes. The act of editing one's life often has a liberating effect on the teller, as they start to understand both the malleability of memory and their agency in shaping the past and indirectly the future.

VII: Be Yourself

The seventh, final and perhaps most important principle of storytelling is simply to be yourself. When I attended my first live storytelling show at the Nuyorican Poets Cafe in New York City I befriended an actress who sat in the back of the venue with me, as far away from the stage as possible. At the end of the night after we'd watched ten strangers share their personal stories, I asked her why she had not put her name in the hat to be chosen to tell a story.

I said, "You're an actress. Don't you want to be on stage more than anything?" "That's not acting," she said, pointing to the empty stage. "Acting is pretending to be somebody else. If I got up there and told my story, I'd have to be myself. That's terrifying."

Being one's true self in front of an audience is a courageous opportunity for liberation, to be truly known and seen and heard and accepted. And we're drawn to authenticity. We crave it. And when we're in the presence of truthfulness, we're enlightened by that person's commitment to be themselves. They own and shape their experience and connect to others who see and witness their wholeness.

But inherent in the act is the fear of being vulnerable, of being true to ourselves and facing judgement and rejection. The truth is that the person brave enough to share their authentic story emboldens other people to cross the same threshold. And the storyteller receives a valuable exchange from the listener. As Beck quotes Monisha Pasupathi from the University of Utah on why sharing our stories is beneficial despite the risk: a listener "may give you other things to think about, or may acknowledge that this thing you thought was really bad is actually not a big deal, so you get this richer and more elaborated memory." And if you keep the memory to yourself and don't craft and share a story, "your memory for that event may be less flexible and give you less chance for growth." (Beck, 2015)

By engaging with live storytelling and the principles we use to tell them, individuals can gain deeper insights into their emotions, motivations, and life experiences. This process fosters self-reflection and personal growth, enabling individuals to construct meaningful identities and navigate life's complexities with greater resilience.

I did not know any of this when Francis decided to switch the story he wanted to tell and share a new one in front of the audience at Palladia-Starhill

Francis was a thin man, over six feet tall, and he possessed a nervous energy. His keys would jingle in his pocket when he sat because his legs shook restlessly. He always appeared late for an urgent meeting. He had a deep, gravely voice, and when he stood on stage the final night of our class, he wore a brown, loose-fitting suit with a yellow dress shirt. He started his story with a description of the Vietnam War draft and how at eighteen he found himself in a foreign country despite never having traveled far beyond the neighborhood he grew up in before the war. As we discussed throughout the workshop, he established himself as a character in a particular context with clear stakes. He wanted to prove himself and survive the odds chance had given him.

Arriving in Vietnam, he was young, inexperienced and the war's destruction from an airplane dropping bombs on the jungle felt abstract. Then one day he was assigned to guard the perimeter of the base. He had to sit stone-still and remain alert for days on end to discern any noises, not knowing if they might be enemy combatants or a tiger. As he described his posture on watch in the jungle as an eighteen year old, his adult body froze. Through the details of his memory, he was eighteen once again, guarding his battalion, as still as a statue. For the first time since meeting Francis, I did not hear his keys jingling in his pocket because he did not move. He had nowhere to be except in the moment.

While he waited alone in the jungle, he eventually heard a machete cutting through the brush. But he could not see anyone or anything. He only heard the swipe of the blade, the crack of growth cut and the steady beat of footsteps. Then from the corner of his eye he saw the two Viet Cong soldiers, oblivious of his position and role. They headed right for him. He had to act.

He had a knife ready in his left hand, and as the first Viet Cong soldiers entered his radius, he covered their mouth with his right hand and with his arm around the stranger's neck brought his upper body as close to his as possible. Then Francis stabbed and sliced him from belly to throat. And before the other Viet Cong fighter could comprehend what happened to his companion, Francis killed him as well. Only then did Francis realize the boys were even younger than him. Maybe sixteen. Maybe seventeen.

In the silence of the jungle, Francis wept, the only sound he'd made for days. And for the first time during the war, he felt paradoxically human. He could finally see and feel the consequences of his actions. He didn't become a man at that moment, he said, he became a human in an inhumane place. What had been abstract and distant was now palpable and terrifying. Francis received a standing ovation.

During his story Francis physically changed when he embodied the stillness of his eighteen year old self. But after he told his story, he was completely transformed. He appeared lighter and less distracted. He'd never shared that memory with anyone before, let alone crafted it into a story to be shared publicly. He felt at once unburdened and deeply alive. What had been kept secret was now shared and what had been frozen and fragmented was now animated and integrated. Through crafting his story, he understood that he was not a monster or a murderer but a boy in an impossible situation who discovered the horrors of war.

After the workshop at Palladia, the director reported back to us that every participant completed the program. The workshop became a regular staple at the facility and the participants consistently had a high completion rate.

While I have focused on the teller's process with the principle of crafting a story, storytelling is clearly beneficial for both the teller and listener. Telling stories allows people to feel heard and validated, which in turn can reduce anxiety, normalize an experience, and help people accurately perceive their lives. Meanwhile, listening to other people's stories can elicit empathy, help people see the world from a new perspective, provide hope, and reassure people that they are not alone in their struggles.

At Palladia I started to comprehend the power of storytelling and how beneficial it can be for everyone involved in the process. The audience's reaction to Francis showed me how people want to experience humanity, their own and a stranger's, and even if the events of the teller's story are not similar to their own, an audience will find a connection. After my workshop at Palladia, I searched for other examples of how storytelling connects us to groups, in particular our families, and how that connection is beneficial to our well-being.

Building Resilience with Stories

Bruce Feiler, the author of "The Secrets of Happy Families: How to Improve your Mornings, Rethink Family Dinner, Fight Smarter, Go Out and Play, and Much More," wrote in the New York Times: "The single most important thing you can do for your family may be the simplest of all: develop a strong family narrative." (Feiler, 2013)

In his New York Times article, "The Family Stories That Bind Us," Feiler cites the research of Emory University psychologists Marshall Duke and Robyn Fivush, who together developed in 2001 a measure called the "Do You Know?" scale, which included 20 questions posed to children. The professors were trying to prove a hypothesis pitched by Duke's wife, a psychologist who worked with children and noticed that "the ones who know a lot about their families tend to do better when they face challenges."

Examples of the questions in the "Do You Know?" scale include:

"Do you know how your parents met?

Do you know some of the illnesses and injuries that your parents experienced when they were younger?

Do you know some of the lessons that your parents learned from good or bad experiences?

Do you know some of the jobs that your parents had when they were young?

Do you know some awards that your parents received when they were young?

Do you know the origin of your name?"

The three-year study included 40 families who were recorded during dinnertime conversations. Each family had at least one pre-adolescent child between the ages of nine and twelve. The research results concluded that "the more children knew about their family's history, the stronger their sense of control over their lives, the higher their self-esteem and the more successfully they believed their families functioned."

A child's sense of being part of a larger family impacts their well-being. As Feiler points out, when children hear family stories, "they know they belong to something bigger than themselves." The family narrative - whether ascending, where one success follows another, or descending, where one loss follows another, or oscillating, where the family story reveals the ups and downs of life, the tragedies and triumphs - no matter what the shape, influences the child's outlook toward the family and the world and their place in both. Feiler says Duke and Fivush stressed how the children who have the most self-confidence have what they call a strong "intergenerational self." They understand where and who they come from and believe they're equipped to meet life's challenges because the family they come from survived their own challenges.

In "After Virtue: A Study in Moral Theory," the philosopher Alasdair MacIntyre underscores how stories, the information and grounding they provide, even fictional ones, orient children on how they might navigate the world:

> *"I can only answer the question 'What am I to do' if I can answer the prior question 'Of what story or stories do I find myself a part?' We enter human society, that is, with one or more imputed characters – roles into which we have been drafted – and we have to learn what they are in order to be able to understand how others respond to us and how our responses to them are apt to be construed... Deprive children of stories and you leave them unscripted, anxious stutterers in their actions as in their words." (MacIntyre, 2007, p. 216)*

In 2010, Professors Marshall Duke and Robyn Fivush published "Do You Know? The power of family history in adolescent identity and well-being" (Fivush et al., 2010) a follow up study on their original research from 2001. They expanded on their "previous findings that pre-adolescent children who know more about their family history display higher levels of emotional well-being. Sixty-six broadly middle-class, mixed race, 14- to 16-year old adolescents from two-parent families were asked to complete a measure of family history, the "Do You Know..." scale (DYK), as well as multiple standardized measures of family functioning, identity development and well-being." Teens who knew more stories about their extended family showed "higher levels of emotional well-being, and also higher levels of identity achievement, even when controlling for general level of family functioning."

"There is something powerful about actually knowing these stories," the study said. However, the authors cautioned that since this is the only study to use the DYK scale, more research is needed before any firm conclusions can be drawn. While the correlation between the extent of knowledge shared and the health benefits of family stories remains unclear, their power is certain. By listening to the stories of their family, children are not only learning where they come from but how to tell their own stories. As Beck points out, youth is the window when we're developing our sense of self-narrative:

> *"Through friends, family, and fiction, children learn what others consider to be good storytelling—and that being able to spin a good yarn has social value. It's in the late teens and early years of adulthood that story construction really picks up—because by then people have developed some of the cognitive tools*

they need to create a coherent life story. These include causal coherence—the ability to describe how one event led to another—and thematic coherence—the ability to identify overarching values and motifs that recur throughout the story. In a study analyzing the life stories of 8-, 12-, 16-, and 20-year-olds, these kinds of coherence were found to increase with age."

As part of a family, we're living inside a story, and from a young age, we start telling ourselves stories, but what if we become a victim of our stories or trapped by a particular narrative? Can stories do as much harm as they can help us?

Since I have shown how storytelling can be liberating, how they can help us see ourselves more clearly, and how they can help us feel more deeply our place in a larger context, I want to show how stories can hold us tethered to a certain identity and potentially smother us. But if we want to untether ourselves from a negative identity, we can rewrite and reclaim our stories to change not only our own but others' perception of ourselves.

The Power of Rewriting Your Story and Shifting the Point of View

"Narratives can hold us back by limiting our thinking," writes Karen Simecek for Psyche. "They may diminish our ability to live freely. They also give us the illusion that the world is ordered, logical, and difficult to change, reducing the real complexity of life. They can even become dangerous when they persuade us of a false and harmful world view. Perhaps we shouldn't be too eager to live our lives as if we were 'telling a story'." (Simecek et al., 2024)

Since stories are incredibly persuasive, how we narrate our life can ultimately dictate the life we live. They can hold us captive. "Seeing yourself as the main character in a story can overly simplify the fullness of life," Simecek writes. "Think of the way in which people talk about their 'journey' through life. Through this narrative, certain events become more significant while others are overlooked, and random events can be reframed as being part of some grand plan. Yet viewing our lives in such a narrow way hinders our ability to understand the complex behaviour of others and ourselves. For example, a child that accepts the narrative of being 'naughty' may incorrectly frame their behaviour as bad, rather than as an expression of their unmet needs. Stories can change us by locking us into ways of acting, thinking, and feeling." (Simecek et al., 2024)

The power of stories to shape our lives is not a reason to ban or dismiss them but to educate people on how they operate and how we can revise, reclaim and analyze them. By identifying a false story, we have the opportunity to assert the truth of our experience and reshape our identity.

For an episodes of my podcast "Memory Motel," (Mickey, 2021) I interviewed Kristen Enmark, one of the hostages from the infamous 1973 bank robbery that became the origin of Stockholm Syndrome, which is the "feelings of trust or affection felt in many cases of kidnapping or hostage-taking by a victim toward a captor." (Oxford Languages) The premise of the podcast was for interviewees to return to particular memories from their lives and reframe whatever story that had been told with a new story from the new perspective of hindsight. Enmark was the first person diagnosed with Stockholm Syndrome, and for over forty years, she carried that stigma with her. In my interview, she said: "I always felt that I did something wrong. You're not healthy when you have a syndrome."

The weight of her diagnosis and the publicity of her trauma silenced her for over forty years: "So if you say these girls or me have this syndrome, you don't have to pay attention to what they say."

As we revisited her memory, she retold the story of what happened in Stockholm in 1973 from her point of view and not from the perspective of the news media, the police or the doctor who diagnosed her and coined the term Stockholm Syndrome, Nils Johan Artur Bejerot. By returning to the memory and explaining to herself why she reacted as she did, she reclaimed her story from the narratives imposed by others and reframed her experience into one that could be empowering for her. "After almost 50 years, I felt, well, I didn't do anything wrong. I did what I had to do and I'm kind of feeling proud of myself. When they write things in the paper I couldn't care less. I know my story. I know my truth." The reframe from shame and silence to pride is one of the most transformational arcs I've heard.

In 1973, Sweden had never experienced a televised hostage crisis. The police and government were under intense scrutiny and pressure. To solve the problem, they took unconventional and often dangerous measures to try and save Enmark and her colleagues. From Enmark's point of view, their methods were often more chaotic and dangerous than anything the bank robbers had subjected them to while they were being held captive.

For six days, Jan Ollson, and his accomplice, Clark Ollafson, traumatized four hostages held inside a bank, but the public, glued to their TVs, scrutinized and questioned the hostages, especially Enmark. Everything she reportedly said and did was not what anyone expected from a hostage: She said she was more afraid of the police than the robbers, Jan and Clark. She pleaded with the Prime Minister of Sweden to let her leave with them in the getaway car. When the robbers were finally prosecuted, she refused to testify against them. And years after the robbery, she had a relationship with one of them. To the public, the robbers' behavior made sense - it was what they expected from criminals - but Enmark's behavior was a mystery. Eventually, she was diagnosed by the psychologist and criminologist Nils

Bejerot with a disease he coined Stockholm Syndrome, and the story of her diagnosis dominated her life.

What the media, police and government officials couldn't see or know was what exactly was happening inside the bank. Clark was in control and trying to de-escalate the tension. When he showed up, he calmed Jan down and untied the hostages. Enmark and the others appreciated how Clark shifted the mood. He comforted them and said everything would be OK. "I can't say that I felt safe because that's not the word," Enmark said, "but I chose to believe him…I thought that someone cared about me…in some way he gave me hope or faith in 'this is going to end OK."

At the time, there were no signs that the hostage situation would end well. By the end of the first day, the police had set up sharpshooters on nearby rooftops aimed at the bank's facade. Through the glass, Jan could see the getaway car he requested, a blue Mustang, parked on the street. But he didn't trust the government or police. They insisted he leave behind the hostages, but he knew the police would chase him down without them. He always kept a hostage close by so that police would not shoot.

After a while the constant threat of snipers wore down the bank robbers. They moved the hostages into the bank's vault, where the police could not shoot them. Outside the vault door was a staircase leading to the upper floor where the police had set up an outpost. The staircase became the place where messages, food, blankets and other provisions were exchanged. The robbers allowed the hostages to walk freely outside the vault when they felt too claustrophobic. But the robbers said if they did not return to the vault, one of the other hostages would be harmed.

Jan and Clark had secured a getaway car and money from the police, but the one thing stopping them was how they'd escape. They knew if they left without the hostages, the police would hunt them down. Enmark, seeing the robbers' frustrated attempt to negotiate, thought she would have a better shot with the police. This is where her disillusionment with the police started: "I was the one who was the victim" she said, "and I thought maybe they could listen to what I wanted." But they did not and instead dismissed her.

Enmark's disillusionment turned into fear when they shot at an innocent teenager. The police thought Jan was the escaped convict, Kai Hansson. So they brought Hansson's younger brother, who was sixteen, to the bank and walked him down the stairwell to the vault. The boy shouted at who he thought was her brother but since Jan did not know the boy, he shot at him. The boy ran up the stairwell and the police forced him to go back again.

At this point, Enmark and the other hostages lost all faith in the police. So when Commissioner Lindroth checked in on them, he told his associates that the hostages had shown hostility toward him. Kristen practically curled her lip at him. And none of them had any requests. None of them gave him imploring looks, saying save us.

But the Commissioner noted a tenderness, closeness and ease between the hostages and robbers.

When the Commissioner reported the scene to the press, reporters called the hostages on the vault phone. They wanted to know if it was true: did they entrust their lives to the hands of criminals? The interviews, broadcast on the radio and TV, baffled the Swedish public who began theorizing about the hostages' ease with the robbers. And one conversation that was not meant to be broadcast, but was, made the mystery even more intriguing. Enmark, frustrated and impatient, called the Prime Minister of Sweden herself. The two came at the situation from radically different points of view. Kristen was thinking about how to survive, while the Prime Minister was thinking about how to uphold social stability, and allowing bank robbers to leave with hostages would not have sent the right message to other criminals. At one point on the call Enmark said: "I am very disappointed…They haven't done a thing to us. On the contrary, they have been very nice. But you know, Olof (the Prime Minister's first name) what I am scared of is that the police will attack and cause us to die." The prime minister tried to reassure her but ended up insulting her in the end.

After Enmark's failed attempt to plead with the Prime Minister, the police started drilling into the vault. When they hit an electrical box, the lights went out, and the vault started to flood from the water used to cool the drill down. And then the police dropped in flasks of tear gas. The robbers finally surrendered and led the hostages out of the vault.

Outside the bank, police and medical personnel were waiting to help the hostages but Enmark refused to lie down on the stretcher they offered. "I was so angry with the whole situation," she said. For years afterward, her story of what happened was eclipsed by the public story and a syndrome named after her harrowing experience. The story of Stockholm Syndrome eclipsed her trauma and the truth behind her actions. " I always felt that I did something wrong," she said. But now, years later, she can rewrite the story and reclaim her truth: "The ideal hostage is a woman who keeps her mouth shut. She think that the society and the police is going to protect her and when someone pops up like me who says the opposite, you have to call it being sick…I think it's a way of blaming the victim…I wanted to survive."

Now Enmark is a psychotherapist, who has written a book about her experience of the bank robbery, and she's transformed her trauma into a pillar of her practice: "I thought that no one listened to me. The police didn't listen. All therapists think that you have to listen to people. But for me I think it's even more important."

Storytelling and Society

As Enmark's story illustrates, certain cultural narratives, such as the origin of Stockholm Syndrome, form and become fact, even when competing narratives exist. If stories shape our understanding of the world and ourselves, how do we harness the power to change our cultural stories to benefit our personal and collective well-being?

As Beck writers, stories can become the blueprint of how we plan our life's path:

"Once certain stories get embedded into the culture, they become master narratives—blueprints for people to follow when structuring their own stories, for better or worse. One such blueprint is your standard 'go to school, graduate, get a job, get married, have kids.' That can be a helpful script in that it gives children a sense of the arc of a life, and shows them examples of tentpole events that could happen. But the downsides of standard narratives have been well-documented—they stigmatize anyone who doesn't follow them to a T, and provide unrealistic expectations of happiness for those who do."

Our dominant narratives are not written in stone and to understand their malleability is to empower all of us to both question and re-write prevailing narratives that don't serve the greater good. Cultural narratives often follow a similar structure as personal ones. If we become literate in storytelling, we can identify which master narratives do not serve us and change them. The key principles for crafting narratives can also be used to analyze and reframe them. But first we have to see the narratives we live among and understand their ephemeral quality. As Harold R. Johnson writes in his book, "The Power of Story: On Truth, the Trickster and New Fictions In a New Era," (Johnson, 2022, 48):

"People make up stories about how things work, then make up more stories that match up and fit together until there is a web of interwoven stories so complex they become the reality that constitutes society. Society is real. It has power over the people. It has norms and rules. It determines who lives and who dies, who is free and who is incarcerated. But this reality, this powerful control is made up of a series of fictional stories. They are entirely made up, one story modifying the last modifying the last, sometimes consciously and with intention and sometimes not. And because the stories are fictions, stuff we made up, the best version we had at the time, the stories can be changed."

As an example of reality's malleability, Johnson, a member of the Cree tribe, shows how science regularly changes how we understand the world:

"The original Christian story placed man at the center of the universe. Copernicus changed that story to one where the planet Earth orbits the Sun. Newton retold the orbiting planets story to include gravity. Einstein modified the story about gravity with the story of relativity. Quantum physics retells the story in impermanence. The Higgs boson story gives solidity to the impermanence. Fifty

years from now the story will change yet again when new ideas replace existing ones...No matter how compelling the story, we should know that it is not the incontrovertible truth. At some point in the future, the story, the truth we rely upon today, is going to change. It will be replaced by a new story.

'That the best science can do is provide a coherent story does not diminish the validity of science. That the story is inevitably going to change in the future doesn't change the fact that the story science provides today is the best possible story available. We can still rely upon the story science provides to make decisions while knowing the basis of our decision is only the best presently known." (page 39)

The idea of an ever-changing story and reality may alarm and unnerve people. But the only constant in any of our lives is change, and to deny this fact is to disturb our well-being with needless suffering. As Johnson writes:

"The best way to alleviate that suffering is to create a new story, an inclusive story where no one is left out. When people see themselves as part of a shared story, they can relate to the other characters in that story. When we start to tell this new story, and people begin to feel like they belong in it, then they will start to give a shit about each other. We all need to be in a story that tells us that we are wanted, that we are cared for, and that we belong." (page 103)

The ever-shifting story of our lives and society invites agency, transformation and creativity. We can write a new story as the old ones fall away, and our new story can encompass whatever we imagine and aspire toward. We have tremendous power and agency as storytellers, which is why crafting, analyzing and revising narratives should be a life-skill we all learn to improve our lives and world.

On the personal level, first we own our stories and then we have the opportunity to share them with others, and by listening to ourselves and being listened to by others, we honor our life and create a sense of wholeness and well-being no matter what life we've lived. We don't have to be saints or heroes, criminals or daredevils, victims or models of success. If we look closely enough and tell the truth, our ordinary lives contain the details and drama for meaningful narratives. Our wants and fears, no matter how big or small, provide the necessary fuel for a hero's journey.

As Harvard-trained physician Dr. Annie Brewster writes in "The Healing Power of Storytelling: Using Personal Narrative to Navigate Illness, Trauma, and Loss," (Brewster, 2022, #):

"It is through our stories that we find meaning and, ideally, integrate challenging experiences into our identity, so that we can move forward with optimal health. It is in sharing our stories without apology that we come to accept ourselves fully, as we are, without shame. Sharing is vulnerable but also the path to empowerment."

As we develop and share our personal stories, we will start to see larger narratives at work, to see how we're connected through and because of our stories. As author Jonathan Gottschall writes in "The Storytelling Animal: How Stories Make Us Human:" (Gottschall, 2012, 177)

"Story is the glue of human social life —defining groups and holding them together... We are the storytelling animal."

As the only storytelling animal, we make sense of the world and ourselves through the telling of our stories. And the stories we tell ourselves and others play a critical role in our well-being. As storytellers our well-being depends on how attentive we are to our own lives and how adept we are at making meaning from what we experience. Narrative structure - the beginning, middle and end of all stories - creates meaning through the cause and effect chain of events. When a person is given the tools to shape experience into a personal story, they can claim agency over their lives and transform tragedy into wisdom, shame into connection and isolation into belonging. And from this personal power, they can start to question cultural narratives and even rewrite them.

REFERENCES

About Palladia - Starhill Residential. (n.d.). https://www.rehab.com/palladia-starhill-residential

About The Moth. (n.d.). The Moth. Retrieved January 12, 2025, from https://themoth.org/about

Adler, J. (2011, September). Living Into the Story: Agency and Coherence in a Longitudinal Study of Narrative Identity Development and Mental Health Over the Course of Psychotherapy. *Journal of Personality and Social Psychology, 102*(2), 367–389. DOI: 10.1037/a0025289 PMID: 21910554

Adler, J. M., Philippe, F. L., Houle, I., & Lodi-Smith, J. (2015). The Incremental Validity of Narrative Identity in Predicting Well-Being. *Personality and Social Psychology Review, 20*(2), 142–175. https://www.researchgate.net/publication/276362513_The_Incremental_Validity_of_Narrative_Identity_in_Predicting_Well-Being. DOI: 10.1177/1088868315585068 PMID: 25968138

Beck, J. (2015, August 10). Life's Stories. *The Atlantic*. https://www.theatlantic.com/health/archive/2015/08/life-stories-narrative-psychology-redemption-mental-health/400796/

Brewster, A. (2022). *The Healing Power of Storytelling: Using Personal Narrative to Navigate Illness, Trauma, and Loss*. North Atlantic Books.

Campbell, J. (2008). *The hero with a thousand faces*. New World Library.

Feiler, B. (2013, March 15). The Family Stories That Bind Us — This Life. *The New York Times*. https://www.nytimes.com/2013/03/17/fashion/the-family-stories-that-bind-us-this-life.html

Fivush, R., Duke, M., & Bohanek, J. G. (2010, February 23). *"Do You Know..." The power of family history in adolescent identity and well-being*. "Do You Know...". Retrieved January 13, 2025, from https://ncph.org/wp-content/uploads/2013/12/The-power-of-family-history-in-adolescent-identity.pdf

Founder of the Whole Health Medicine Institute. (2012, November 27). The Healing Power of Telling Your Story. *Psychology Today Blog*. https://www.psychologytoday.com/intl/blog/owning-pink/201211/the-healing-power-telling-your-story

Gots, J. (2012, January 13). *Your Storytelling Brain*. Big Think. https://bigthink.com/culture-religion/your-storytelling-brain/

Gottschall, J. (2012). *The Storytelling Animal: How Stories Make Us Human.* Houghton Mifflin Harcourt.

Gregory, E. M., & Rutledge, P. B. (2016). *Exploring Positive Psychology: The Science of Happiness and Well-being.* Greenwood. DOI: 10.5040/9798400649127

Gruyaert, H., Simecek, K., & McKean, C. A. (2024, October 17). *Your life is not a story: why narrative thinking holds you back.* Psyche. Retrieved January 18, 2025, from https://psyche.co/ideas/your-life-is-not-a-story-why-narrative-thinking-holds-you-back

Johnson, H. R. (2022). *The Power of Story: On Truth, the Trickster, and New Fictions for a New Era.* Biblioasis.

Lohuis, A. M., Sools, A., van Vuuren, M., & Bohlmeijer, E. T. (2016). Narrative Reflection as a Means to Explore Team Effectiveness. *Small Group Research, 47*(4), 406–437. DOI: 10.1177/1046496416656464

Lohuis, A. M., Sools, A., Vuuren, M., & Bohlmeijer, E. T. (2016). Narrative Reflection as a Means to Explore Team Effectiveness. *Small Group Research, 47*(4), 406–437. DOI: 10.1177/1046496416656464

MacIntyre, A. C. (2007). *After Virtue: A Study in Moral Theory* (3rd ed.). Longleaf Services University of Notre Dame Du Lac.

Magazine, T. (1999, September). Listening to Philip Glass. *Tricycle Magazine.* https://tricycle.org/magazine/listening-philip-glass/

Martin, G. (2012). *Gabriel Garcia Marquez: A Life.* Bloomsbury Publishing.

Mickey, T. (2021). *The Ideal Hostage* [Podcast]. https://podcasts.apple.com/us/podcast/11-the-ideal-hostage/id1084076357?i=1000535013953

Orlean, S. (2019). *The Library Book.* Atlantic Books.

Pasupathi, M., & Billitteri, J. (2015, April). Being and Becoming through Being Heard: Listener Effects on Stories and Selves. *International Journal of Listening, 29*(2), 1–18. https://www.researchgate.net/publication/276080234_Being_and_Becoming_through_Being_Heard_Listener_Effects_on_Stories_and_Selves. DOI: 10.1080/10904018.2015.1029363

Paul, A. M. (2012, March 12). Your Brain On Fiction. *The New York Times.* https://www.nytimes.com/2012/03/18/opinion/sunday/the-neuroscience-of-your-brain-on-fiction.html

Sartre, J.-P. (2013). *Nausea* (Alexander, L., Trans.). New Directions Publishing Corporation.

Stephens, G. J., Silbert, L. J., & Hasson, U. (2010, July 26). Speaker–listener neural coupling underlies successful communication. *Proceedings of the National Academy of Sciences of the United States of America, 107*(32), 14425–14430. https://www.pnas.org/doi/10.1073/pnas.1008662107. DOI: 10.1073/pnas.1008662107 PMID: 20660768

Stieg, D. P. (2022, February 25). *The Science of Storytelling, with Paula Croxson and Uri Hasson* [Podcast]. This Is Your Brain with Dr. Phil Steig. https://thisisyourbrain.com/2022/02/the-science-of-storytelling-with-paula-croxson-and-uri-hasson-s3-ep5/

Zak, P. J. (2014, October 28). Why Your Brain Loves Good Storytelling. *Harvard Business Review*. https://hbr.org/2014/10/why-your-brain-loves-good-storytelling

Chapter 12
Examining the Utilization and Impact of Active Learning Strategies in Modern Pedagogical Practices

Pardhu Thottempudi
https://orcid.org/0000-0002-9653-1951
Marwadi University, India

Vijay Kumar
https://orcid.org/0000-0001-8738-8404
Vellore Institute of Technology, India

Nagesh Deevi
https://orcid.org/0000-0001-6449-0609
BVRIT HYDERABAD College of Engineering for Women, India

ABSTRACT

This study delves into the usage and results of active learning methodologies in modern educational systems, exploring techniques such as cooperative learning, inverted classroom settings, problem-oriented, and hands-on learning. The research aims to elucidate the frequency of these methodologies, their efficiency in amplifying student participation and learning achievements, and the difficulties encountered during their execution. The data was collected through a hybrid approach, fusing quantitative studies conducted in various classrooms with qualitative teacher interviews. Initial outcomes indicate that, when aptly applied, active learning approaches

DOI: 10.4018/979-8-3373-0360-4.ch012

can stimulate increased student involvement and boost academic performance. Nonetheless, several obstacles, such as insufficient educator preparation and resource limitations, hinder their broad-scale application. The study emphasizes the need for a calculated strategy to incorporate active learning methodologies into teaching practices to cultivate a more engaging and efficient learning environment.

1. INTRODUCTION

As education navigates a rapidly evolving landscape marked by technological advancements and shifting societal priorities, the spotlight is increasingly directed toward adopting learner-centered educational paradigms. This progressive shift responds to the limitations of traditional, instructor-centric approaches, which often focus on passive knowledge transmission, leaving students less engaged and prepared for the complexities of the modern world.

1.1. Active Learning as a Paradigm Shift

Active learning is emerging as a pivotal strategy in this educational transformation. Unlike conventional teaching, which positions students as passive recipients of information, active learning places them at the heart of the educational process. This methodology emphasizes critical engagement through activities such as **cooperative learning**, where students work collaboratively to solve problems; **problem-centered learning**, which challenges them to find solutions to real-world issues; **hands-on learning**, fostering experiential understanding; and **Flipped classrooms**, which reverse the traditional teaching model by introducing new content outside the classroom and focusing on interactive activities during class.

These approaches aim to develop higher-order thinking skills, deepen conceptual understanding, and encourage the practical application of knowledge. For instance, cooperative learning promotes teamwork and communication skills, while problem-centered learning enhances analytical and decision-making abilities. Hands-on learning ensures students connect theoretical knowledge to tangible outcomes, and Flipped classrooms cultivate self-directed learning and class engagement. Together, these methods represent a significant departure from passive learning models, striving to meet the demands of a society that values adaptability, creativity, and collaboration.

1.2. Challenges to Active Learning Integration

Despite its promise, the adoption of active learning is inconsistent across educational settings. Key challenges include:

1. **Institutional and Resource Barriers**: Institutions may lack the infrastructure, funding, or class size flexibility to implement active learning effectively. For example, small classrooms or limited access to technology can hinder hands-on or Flipped classroom approaches.
2. **Educator Resistance**: Some educators may be reluctant to adopt active learning due to unfamiliarity, perceived inefficiency compared to traditional methods, or apprehension about losing control of the learning environment.
3. **Student Adaptation**: Transitioning from passive to active learning can initially be challenging for students accustomed to traditional models. Active participation requires greater preparation, effort, and engagement, which may not align with their prior educational experiences.

1.3. The Role of Research in Advancing Active Learning

This study seeks to address these challenges by examining how active learning strategies impact student outcomes. It delves into the factors influencing their adoption, such as educator training, institutional support, and classroom dynamics, and explores best practices for overcoming obstacles. A significant focus is placed on how educators can design and implement these methods effectively to maximize student engagement and learning.

1.4. Implications for the Future of Education

The findings aim to contribute to a broader understanding of active learning's potential to create dynamic and inclusive educational environments. By equipping educators with practical insights and recommendations, this research underscores the importance of reimagining teaching practices to prepare students for the demands of the 21st century. It calls on policymakers and institutional leaders to support this shift through investments in resources, professional development, and policies promoting innovative pedagogies.

Active learning symbolizes more than a teaching technique; it is a cultural shift in education that values engagement, collaboration, and the application of knowledge. By embracing this approach, educational systems worldwide can empower students to become lifelong learners, capable of navigating and contributing to a complex and interconnected global society.

2. LITERATURE REVIEW

Active learning has garnered considerable attention within the field of educational research as a transformative approach that aligns with evolving pedagogical needs. It aims to shift the educational paradigm from traditional, passive learning methods to one that actively engages students in constructing their understanding. This literature review explores key themes, including the definition and conceptualization of active learning, its diverse methodologies, evidence of its effectiveness, and the challenges associated with its implementation.

2.1. Understanding Active Learning

Active learning refers to a pedagogical approach where students are engaged in activities that require them to actively or experientially participate in the learning process, rather than passively absorbing information. Bonwell and Eison (1991) characterized it as encompassing all instructional techniques that involve students in doing things and thinking about what they are doing. It emphasizes higher-order thinking, such as analysis, synthesis, and evaluation, over the rote memorization of information.

Prince (2004) elaborated on this concept, emphasizing that active learning is not confined to a single method but includes a range of instructional strategies designed to involve students directly in the learning process. Examples include discussions, case studies, simulations, and group problem-solving. This active engagement allows learners to connect new knowledge to existing schemas, enhancing understanding and retention.

Active learning stands in contrast to traditional lecture-based teaching methods. In conventional settings, educators often dominate classroom interactions, relegating students to passive listeners. In contrast, active learning requires a reimagining of the teacher's role, transitioning from the "sage on the stage" to the "guide on the side," facilitating and supporting student-led learning.

2.2. Varieties of Active Learning

Active learning comprises a spectrum of strategies tailored to diverse educational objectives, disciplines, and contexts. Several key methodologies are outlined below.

1. **Collaborative Learning**: Collaborative learning emphasizes teamwork and shared responsibility for learning. Johnson and Johnson (1999) defined it as an approach where students work together in small groups to achieve common goals. This method fosters interpersonal skills, accountability, and critical think-

ing as students debate, negotiate, and synthesize ideas. Research indicates that collaborative learning improves academic achievement and enhances students' sense of belonging in educational settings.

2. **Problem-Based Learning (PBL)**: PBL is centered on presenting students with complex, real-world problems that lack a definitive solution. As outlined by Barrows (1996), this method encourages students to identify knowledge gaps, research independently, and collaboratively propose solutions. PBL has proven effective in promoting self-directed learning, adaptability, and the application of theoretical concepts to practical scenarios.
3. **Flipped Classrooms**: Bergmann and Sams (2012) popularized the flipped classroom model, where direct instruction occurs outside the classroom, often via digital platforms. Class time is then dedicated to interactive, student-centered activities such as discussions, collaborative projects, and problem-solving exercises. The flipped classroom leverages technology to enable active engagement, providing opportunities for personalized learning.
4. **Experiential Learning**: Kolb (1984) introduced the experiential learning theory, which underscores the importance of learning through experience and reflection. This method encourages students to engage directly with real-world tasks, reflect on their experiences, and apply lessons learned to future challenges. Experiential learning is particularly effective in fields requiring practical skills, such as healthcare, engineering, and business.
5. **Case-Based Learning**:Case-based learning involves analyzing and discussing real-life scenarios or case studies. This approach is widely used in professional education, such as law and medicine, to cultivate critical thinking and decision-making skills. By engaging with realistic situations, students develop the ability to apply theoretical concepts to complex, nuanced problems.
6. **Peer Teaching**:Peer teaching involves students teaching one another under the guidance of an instructor. This method not only reinforces the teacher's understanding of the material but also fosters communication and collaboration among peers. Studies suggest that peer teaching enhances content mastery and encourages the development of soft skills.

2.3. Effectiveness of Active Learning

Research overwhelmingly supports the efficacy of active learning in improving educational outcomes. Numerous studies have demonstrated that active learning techniques outperform traditional lecture-based approaches across a range of metrics, including student performance, engagement, and retention.

Freeman et al. (2014) conducted a meta-analysis of 225 studies in STEM education, revealing that active learning significantly improved examination scores and reduced failure rates compared to traditional methods. Their findings underscored the role of active engagement in fostering deeper understanding and critical thinking.

Similarly, Prince (2004) found that cooperative and problem-based learning positively influenced student attitudes, fostering motivation and engagement. These methods were also associated with enhanced writing and critical thinking skills, demonstrating their capacity to cultivate higher-order cognitive abilities.

Active learning's benefits extend beyond academic performance. It has been shown to promote inclusivity by creating opportunities for all students to participate actively, thereby reducing achievement gaps. For instance, active learning can help underrepresented groups in STEM fields feel more included and supported, ultimately encouraging diversity in these disciplines.

2.4. Barriers to Implementing Active Learning

Despite its numerous advantages, active learning faces significant barriers that hinder its widespread adoption. These challenges exist at multiple levels, including educators, students, and institutions.

1. **Educator Barriers**: Many educators are hesitant to adopt active learning due to a lack of familiarity with its methodologies. Ertmer et al. (2011) highlighted insufficient training as a primary obstacle, noting that educators often require professional development to effectively integrate active learning into their teaching practices. Additionally, some instructors perceive active learning as time-consuming or challenging to implement within the constraints of standardized curricula.
2. **Student Resistance**: Students accustomed to traditional teaching methods may resist active learning, viewing it as demanding or unfamiliar. Seidel and Tanner (2013) noted that such resistance often stems from a lack of understanding of the value of active learning. Addressing these concerns requires clear communication and gradual implementation to help students adjust to new expectations.

3. **Institutional Challenges**: Institutional factors, such as large class sizes, limited resources, and rigid schedules, can hinder the adoption of active learning. Michael (2007) emphasized that large lecture halls are not conducive to active engagement, while budget constraints may limit access to technology and materials needed for methods like Flipped classrooms or experiential learning.
4. **Assessment Misalignment**: Traditional assessment methods, such as standardized tests, may not align with the goals of active learning, which emphasize skills like critical thinking and problem-solving. This misalignment can discourage educators from adopting active learning strategies, as their effectiveness may not be accurately reflected in conventional grading systems.

2.5 Overcoming Challenges to Active Learning

Successfully implementing active learning requires addressing these barriers through targeted interventions. Professional development programs can equip educators with the skills and confidence needed to adopt active learning techniques. Institutions must invest in infrastructure and resources to support innovative teaching methods, such as redesigning classrooms to facilitate collaboration.

Engaging students in the transition process is equally important. Educators can introduce active learning gradually, providing clear explanations of its benefits and involving students in shaping the learning process. Additionally, aligning assessment methods with active learning objectives can ensure that students are evaluated fairly and comprehensively.

2.6 Summary and Implications

Active learning holds significant promise for enhancing educational outcomes by fostering critical thinking, engagement, and real-world application. However, its successful implementation requires overcoming challenges related to educator training, student adaptation, and institutional support. This review highlights the need for continued research and collaboration among educators, policymakers, and researchers to create environments conducive to active learning.

By addressing these issues, the educational landscape can evolve to better prepare students for the demands of the 21st century, ensuring they possess the skills, knowledge, and adaptability needed to thrive in a rapidly changing world.

3. METHODOLOGY

This study utilized a **mixed-methods research design** to investigate the usage, challenges, and impact of active learning techniques in contemporary educational practices. A mixed-methods approach, which integrates both **quantitative** and **qualitative research methodologies**, was chosen to ensure a comprehensive understanding of the research inquiries. This design allows for the triangulation of data, ensuring robustness, validity, and a multifaceted perspective on the research topic.

3.1. Participants & Context

The study was conducted across diverse educational contexts, ranging from elementary schools to higher education institutions. This diversity ensured that findings were generalizable and applicable to a wide spectrum of teaching and learning environments.

3.1.1. Selection of Participants

1. **Teachers**:

The study involved teachers with at least one year of teaching experience, ensuring they had sufficient exposure to classroom dynamics and instructional practices. Participants were selected based on their use of active learning strategies, ensuring their contributions were relevant to the study's objectives. Teachers from different disciplines, grade levels, and school types (public, private, and charter) were included to capture diverse experiences and insights.

2. **Students**:

Students participating in the study were from the classrooms of the selected teachers. This ensured alignment between teacher-reported practices and student experiences. The student cohort included individuals from varied age groups, academic levels, and socioeconomic backgrounds to explore how active learning strategies impacted different demographics.

3.1.2. Educational Context

The research was conducted across urban, suburban, and rural settings to understand how contextual factors such as resources, class sizes, and institutional priorities influenced the implementation of active learning. By encompassing diverse geographic and institutional settings, the study aimed to identify universal patterns and context-specific challenges.

3.2. Data Collection

The study employed a combination of **surveys, interviews**, and **classroom observations** to gather comprehensive data. This multi-pronged approach ensured that both subjective experiences and objective observations were captured, providing a holistic understanding of active learning in practice.

1. Surveys

Quantitative data were collected through structured online surveys distributed to both teachers and students. Separate survey instruments were designed for each group to address their specific perspectives and experiences.

Teacher Surveys

The survey for teachers included questions on the following aspects:

- **Types of Active Learning Strategies Used**: Teachers were asked to report the specific techniques they employed, such as cooperative learning, problem-based learning, Flipped classrooms, or experiential learning.
- **Frequency of Use**: Respondents indicated how often they incorporated active learning into their lessons, ranging from occasional use to regular implementation.
- **Perceived Effectiveness**: Teachers rated the effectiveness of each strategy in enhancing student engagement, critical thinking, and learning outcomes.
- **Challenges Encountered**: Questions explored the barriers teachers faced, such as lack of resources, time constraints, or resistance from students.

Student Surveys

The student survey focused on their perceptions and experiences with active learning:

- **Exposure to Active Learning**: Students were asked how often they experienced active learning techniques in their classes.
- **Impact on Learning Outcomes**: Questions assessed how active learning influenced their understanding of content, problem-solving skills, and motivation.

- **Preferences and Feedback**: Students shared their preferences regarding active learning methods and offered suggestions for improvement.

Surveys were designed using a combination of **Likert-scale questions, multiple-choice items**, and **open-ended responses** to collect both quantifiable data and qualitative insights.

2. Interviews

To delve deeper into the nuances of active learning, **semi-structured interviews** were conducted with a subset of teachers who had completed the survey. These interviews provided qualitative insights into their experiences, challenges, and perceptions of active learning strategies.

Structure of Interviews

- **Experiences with Active Learning**: Teachers shared specific instances of active learning in their classrooms, detailing the strategies employed and their outcomes.
- **Perceived Impact**: Discussions explored how active learning influenced student engagement, participation, and academic performance.
- **Challenges and Solutions**: Teachers described the obstacles they faced, such as resistance from students, administrative constraints, or lack of resources, and shared strategies they employed to overcome these issues.

Selection of Interview Participants

Participants were purposively sampled from survey respondents based on their diverse teaching contexts, disciplines, and reported experiences with active learning. This approach ensured that the interviews captured a wide range of perspectives.

3. Classroom Observations

Classroom observations were conducted to collect **real-time, first-hand data** on the implementation of active learning techniques. This method allowed researchers to witness interactions, engagement levels, and classroom dynamics that could not be fully captured through surveys or interviews.

Observation Protocol

- **Active Learning Strategies**: Observers documented the types of active learning techniques employed during lessons, such as group discussions, problem-solving tasks, or Flipped classroom activities.
- **Teacher-Student Interactions**: Observations focused on how teachers facilitated active learning, including their use of questioning, feedback, and scaffolding techniques.
- **Student Engagement**: Researchers recorded student participation, collaboration, and enthusiasm during active learning sessions.

Sample Size and Context

A subset of classrooms from participating teachers was selected for observation. The selection criteria included diversity in grade levels, disciplines, and geographic locations to ensure representativeness.

3.3. Data Analysis

The collected data were analyzed using both quantitative and qualitative techniques to ensure a comprehensive interpretation of findings.

1. **Quantitative Data Analysis**

The survey responses were analyzed using **descriptive** and **inferential statistics** to identify patterns, trends, and relationships in the data.

Descriptive Statistics

- Frequency distributions and percentages were calculated to summarize teacher-reported usage of active learning strategies and student-reported experiences.
- Measures of central tendency (mean, median) were used to evaluate perceptions of effectiveness and preferences.

Inferential Statistics

- Statistical tests, such as **t-tests** and **ANOVA**, were employed to compare differences in active learning implementation and perceptions across variables like grade level, geographic location, and teacher experience.
- Correlation analyses explored relationships between variables, such as the frequency of active learning use and perceived effectiveness.

2. Qualitative Data Analysis

The qualitative data from interviews and classroom observations were analyzed using **thematic analysis**. This method involved coding the data to identify recurring themes, patterns, and insights.

Coding Process

1. **Open Coding**: Initial codes were assigned to segments of data, capturing key ideas and observations.
2. **Axial Coding**: Related codes were grouped into broader categories, such as "perceived benefits," "challenges," and "student engagement."
3. **Selective Coding**: Core themes were identified and refined to align with the research objectives.

Emerging Themes

- Teachers' perceptions of the value of active learning.
- Strategies to overcome challenges in implementation.
- Variations in student engagement based on age, subject, and context.

3.4 Ethical Considerations

Ethical approval was obtained from the relevant ethical committee to ensure the study adhered to high ethical standards. The following measures were taken to protect participants' rights and well-being:

1. Informed Consent: All participants received detailed information about the study's objectives, procedures, and their rights before agreeing to participate.
2. Confidentiality: Survey responses, interview transcripts, and observation notes were anonymized to protect participants' identities.
3. Voluntary Participation: Participation was entirely voluntary, with the option to withdraw at any stage without consequences.
4. Data Security: All data were securely stored and accessed only by authorized personnel involved in the research.

Through its mixed-methods design, this study aimed to provide a comprehensive understanding of the usage and impact of active learning techniques. The integration of surveys, interviews, and classroom observations ensured a robust and nuanced exploration of the research questions. By capturing both quantitative trends and qualitative insights, the study sought to uncover the factors that influence the success and challenges of active learning in diverse educational contexts. The findings aim to contribute valuable insights for educators, policymakers, and researchers striving to enhance teaching and learning practices.

4. RESULTS

The research produced a variety of findings regarding the adoption, application, and effects of active learning techniques in contemporary educational settings. These results offer valuable insights into how active learning is perceived, utilized, and experienced by both teachers and students while highlighting the challenges associated with its implementation.

4.1 Survey Results

The surveys provided a quantitative overview of active learning practices, perceptions of efficacy, and the obstacles faced by educators and students. The results demonstrated widespread recognition of the benefits of active learning but also underscored the practical and institutional barriers to its full adoption.

1. Frequency of Active Learning

The majority of teachers surveyed (75%) reported incorporating some form of active learning in their teaching practices. However, the extent and frequency of use varied. Among the most commonly employed techniques:

- **Cooperative Learning (60%)**: Teachers frequently utilized group-based activities where students collaborated to solve problems or complete tasks.
- **Problem-Oriented Learning (55%)**: Open-ended problems, often tied to real-world scenarios, were a central focus in many classrooms.
- **Flipped Classrooms (40%)**: A significant number of teachers implemented flipped classroom methodologies, leveraging digital tools to move direct instruction outside of class and dedicating in-class time to interactive, student-centered activities.

These findings indicate that active learning has made significant inroads into modern education. However, the reliance on certain strategies, such as cooperative and problem-based learning, suggests that educators may gravitate toward methods that are easier to integrate within existing structures.

2. Perceived Efficacy

The surveys revealed overwhelmingly positive perceptions of active learning's impact:

- **Teacher Perspectives**: A significant majority of teachers (80%) believed that active learning positively influenced student engagement, critical thinking, and overall learning outcomes. They reported observing higher levels of participation, creativity, and collaboration in active learning sessions compared to traditional lecture-based teaching.
- **Student Perspectives**: Among students, 70% expressed feeling more engaged and better able to understand course material in classes that adopted active learning techniques. Many students noted that these methods encouraged them to think critically, collaborate with peers, and connect theoretical knowledge to practical applications.

The alignment between teacher and student perspectives reinforces the effectiveness of active learning in fostering meaningful learning experiences.

3. Challenges

Despite its perceived benefits, the implementation of active learning is not without challenges. The survey highlighted several key obstacles:

- **Planning Time**: Approximately 40% of teachers cited a lack of sufficient time for planning and preparing active learning sessions. Designing and organizing activities, particularly for problem-based and experiential learning, often requires significant effort and forethought.
- **Class Sizes**: Large class sizes were reported as a barrier by 30% of teachers. Managing interactive activities, ensuring equal participation, and providing personalized attention become increasingly difficult as the number of students grows.
- **Resistance from Students**: Around 25% of teachers faced resistance from students who were more accustomed to traditional, lecture-based teaching styles. Such students often struggled to adapt to the active participation and independent thinking required by active learning.

These findings highlight the need for targeted interventions to address these challenges, including professional development for teachers, institutional support, and strategies to ease students' transition to active learning environments.

4.2 Interview and Observation Findings

The qualitative data obtained from teacher interviews and classroom observations provided deeper insights into the nuances of active learning implementation. This section explores the execution, advantages, and challenges associated with active learning as revealed by these qualitative methods.

1. Execution of Active Learning

Teacher interviews and classroom observations revealed a wide spectrum of active learning practices. Teachers varied in their approach to integrating these strategies:

- **Comprehensive Adoption**: Some educators fully embraced active learning, incorporating it into nearly every lesson. These teachers often described active learning as a transformative approach that redefined their teaching philosophy and enhanced student engagement.
- **Partial Integration**: Others adopted a blended approach, combining active learning with traditional teaching methods. These educators used active learning selectively, often reserving it for specific lessons or topics that benefited most from student interaction and problem-solving.

Classroom observations corroborated these reports, showcasing the diversity in active learning execution. In some classrooms, students engaged in lively debates, group projects, and hands-on activities, while in others, active learning was limited to short, structured exercises embedded within lecture-based lessons.

2. Advantages of Active Learning

Teachers identified several significant benefits of active learning, which were also observed during classroom visits:

- **Enhanced Student Engagement**: Teachers reported that active learning activities, such as collaborative problem-solving and discussions, kept students actively involved in the learning process. Observations confirmed this, with students appearing focused, animated, and enthusiastic during active learning sessions.
- **Critical Thinking and Problem-Solving**: Many teachers highlighted active learning's ability to cultivate critical thinking skills. Activities requiring analysis, synthesis, and application of knowledge challenged students to think independently and deeply about the subject matter.

- **Improved Collaboration**: Active learning encouraged teamwork and peer interaction. Teachers noted that students developed better communication and interpersonal skills, which are essential for success in both academic and professional contexts.
- **Real-World Application**: Through methods such as problem-based and experiential learning, students were able to connect theoretical concepts to practical scenarios, enhancing their understanding and retention.

3. Impediments to Implementation

Interviews and observations also revealed several impediments to the successful implementation of active learning. These challenges extended beyond individual efforts and reflected broader systemic issues:

- **Inadequate Training and Resources**: Many teachers expressed a need for more professional development opportunities to equip them with the skills and knowledge required for active learning. Observations showed that educators with limited training often struggled to manage student participation and maintain the effectiveness of active learning activities.
- **Institutional Constraints**: Institutional factors, such as rigid curricula, limited funding, and insufficient classroom space, were cited as significant obstacles. Teachers working in under-resourced schools faced particular difficulties in accessing the materials and technology needed for methods like Flipped classrooms or experiential learning.
- **Resistance from Students and Parents**: Both students and parents occasionally resisted active learning approaches. Students accustomed to traditional methods sometimes perceived active learning as overly demanding, while parents expressed concerns about its departure from conventional educational norms. This resistance required teachers to invest additional effort in explaining the rationale and benefits of active learning.

4.3 Synthesis of Findings

The results of this research suggest that active learning strategies are widely recognized for their potential to enhance student engagement, critical thinking, and collaboration. However, their full implementation is hindered by significant challenges. The survey, interview, and observation data converge on several key points:

1. **Widespread Usage with Variability**: While active learning techniques are widely employed, the frequency and consistency of their use vary significantly among educators.
2. **Perceived Benefits**: Both teachers and students view active learning positively, particularly regarding its ability to engage students and deepen their understanding of course material.
3. **Systemic Challenges**: Barriers such as time constraints, institutional limitations, and resistance from stakeholders impede the effective execution of active learning.

The research findings underscore the growing adoption and benefits of active learning strategies while highlighting the need for systemic support to overcome implementation challenges. Addressing these barriers requires a multi-faceted approach, including professional development for teachers, investment in resources and infrastructure, and fostering a cultural shift among students and parents. By tackling these issues, educational institutions can fully realize the potential of active learning to transform teaching and learning in the 21st century.Top of Form

5. DISCUSSION

The findings of this study offer a nuanced understanding of the adoption, impact, and challenges associated with active learning in modern education. By analyzing the frequency, effectiveness, and obstacles to implementing active learning strategies, this discussion highlights the implications for educators, students, and institutions, while drawing connections to existing research.

5.1 Adoption of Active Learning Strategies

One of the most encouraging findings of this study is the widespread adoption of active learning strategies by educators. Most teachers reported incorporating these methods into their pedagogy, underscoring the growing recognition of active learning as a means to enhance student engagement and learning outcomes. This aligns with previous research, such as Prince (2004) and Freeman et al. (2014), which strongly advocate for the benefits of active learning in fostering deeper understanding, critical thinking, and collaboration.

However, the degree to which active learning is adopted varies significantly among educators. While some embrace these methods wholeheartedly and integrate them into nearly every lesson, others adopt a more conservative approach, employing active learning sparingly or supplementing traditional methods with occasional interactive activities. This variation raises important questions about the factors influencing the extent of adoption. These factors may include educators' familiarity with active learning techniques, their confidence in implementing such methods, the availability of resources, and the level of institutional support.

This variability highlights an essential area for further research: what determines an educator's willingness or ability to adopt active learning comprehensively? Investigating these determinants could yield valuable insights into how to increase the consistent and effective use of active learning in diverse educational contexts.

5.2 Perceived Efficacy of Active Learning

Another key finding is the strong endorsement of active learning's effectiveness by both teachers and students. Teachers reported observing significant improvements in student engagement, critical thinking, and overall comprehension. Similarly, students expressed feeling more involved and better able to grasp course material in classes that employed active learning techniques. These findings echo the work of Bonwell and Eison (1991), who highlighted active learning as a tool for fostering critical engagement, and Prince (2004), who emphasized its positive impact on attitudes, skills, and academic performance.

The alignment between teacher and student perceptions underscores the transformative potential of active learning in creating meaningful and impactful educational experiences. Active learning shifts the focus from passive information absorption to active participation, fostering a learning environment where students engage more deeply with the material. For instance, methods such as cooperative learning encourage collaboration and teamwork, while problem-based learning challenges students to think critically and apply theoretical knowledge to practical situations.

Despite these benefits, the study also revealed that active learning requires substantial time, effort, and dedication. Teachers must invest significant time in planning and preparing activities, tailoring them to suit their students' needs and learning objectives. This preparation is often more demanding than designing traditional lectures, highlighting the need for institutional support to ease this burden.

5.3 Challenges in Implementing Active Learning

While active learning holds immense promise, its implementation is not without challenges. The study identified several obstacles faced by educators, including:

1. **Limited Preparation Time**: Teachers frequently cited the lack of sufficient time to plan and execute active learning activities. Unlike traditional lectures, active learning requires meticulous preparation to design meaningful and engaging activities that align with learning objectives.
2. **Large Class Sizes**: Managing active learning in large classrooms is particularly challenging. Ensuring active participation, facilitating group activities, and providing individual attention becomes increasingly difficult as class sizes grow. These challenges often lead educators to default to traditional, lecture-based teaching methods.
3. **Student Resistance**: Teachers also encountered resistance from students who were accustomed to traditional instructional styles. Such students often struggled with the participatory and self-directed nature of active learning, perceiving it as overly demanding or unfamiliar.
4. **Resource Constraints**: Many educators pointed to the lack of necessary resources, such as technology, classroom space, or funding, as significant barriers to implementing active learning techniques, particularly in under-resourced institutions.

These challenges are consistent with prior research. For instance, Michael (2007) and Ertmer et al. (2011) emphasized that time constraints, resource limitations, and insufficient training often hinder educators' ability to adopt active learning. Overcoming these barriers requires a concerted effort from educators, institutions, and policymakers.

5.4 Implications for Professional Development and Institutional Support

The findings underscore the critical role of professional development in promoting the effective adoption of active learning strategies. Teachers need targeted training programs to develop the skills and confidence required to design, implement, and evaluate active learning activities. Such programs should address:

- **Pedagogical Strategies**: Training should equip educators with a repertoire of active learning techniques tailored to different subjects, grade levels, and classroom contexts.
- **Classroom Management**: Teachers should learn strategies to manage group activities, encourage participation, and address resistance from students.
- **Time Management**: Professional development should include strategies for efficient planning and preparation to make active learning more feasible within tight schedules.

In addition to professional development, educational institutions play a crucial role in fostering an environment conducive to active learning. Institutions should consider:

- **Providing Resources**: Investing in technology, materials, and flexible classroom spaces that facilitate active learning.
- **Reducing Class Sizes**: Smaller class sizes can enhance the effectiveness of active learning by enabling more personalized instruction and interaction.
- **Promoting a Supportive Culture**: Institutions should actively encourage and reward innovative teaching practices, creating a culture that values and supports active learning.

5.5 Future Research Directions

This study highlights several areas for future research to address unanswered questions and further explore the dynamics of active learning:

1. **Determinants of Adoption**: What factors influence educators' willingness and ability to adopt active learning strategies comprehensively?
2. **Student Adaptation**: How can educators better support students in transitioning from traditional learning styles to active learning approaches?
3. **Long-Term Impact**: What are the long-term effects of active learning on student outcomes, such as academic performance, critical thinking, and career readiness?

Exploring these questions can provide deeper insights into the potential of active learning to transform educational practices.

This discussion reaffirms the transformative potential of active learning in enhancing student engagement, critical thinking, and comprehension. However, it also highlights the significant challenges that educators face in implementing these strategies. Addressing these challenges requires a multi-faceted approach that includes professional development, institutional support, and a shift in cultural attitudes toward active learning.

By investing in these areas, the educational community can unlock the full potential of active learning, ensuring that students are better prepared for the demands of the 21st century. This shift is not merely a pedagogical change but a broader transformation of the educational landscape, emphasizing collaboration, creativity, and critical thinking as foundational pillars of modern

6. CONCLUSION

This study explored the implementation and impact of active learning techniques within contemporary educational practices. The findings reveal a significant presence of active learning methodologies, reflecting a gradual shift from traditional, lecture-centric instruction toward more learner-centered approaches. Both educators and students reported enhanced engagement and deeper comprehension of subject matter when active learning strategies were employed.

Despite these promising outcomes, the adoption and execution of active learning vary widely across classrooms. Key obstacles, such as limited preparation time, large class sizes, and resistance from students accustomed to traditional teaching methods, present challenges to its effective implementation. These barriers highlight the pressing need for supportive interventions, including professional development programs for educators and institutional investments in resources and infrastructure, to facilitate the seamless integration of active learning.

Active learning holds immense potential to transform education by fostering critical thinking, problem-solving, and collaboration—skills that are increasingly essential in the modern world. However, to unlock its full benefits, it is imperative to address the challenges that impede its adoption. This requires a concerted effort from educators, institutions, and policymakers to create environments that support and encourage innovative teaching practices.

This research contributes to the growing body of knowledge on active learning by providing insights into its application in modern education and highlighting areas requiring further exploration. Future research should focus on gaining a deeper understanding of the barriers to active learning implementation and identifying effective strategies to overcome them. Such efforts will equip educators, administrators, and policymakers with the tools to promote active learning strategies that enhance educational quality and prepare students to thrive in the demands of the 21st century.

REFERENCES

Barrows, H. S. (1996). Problem-based learning in medicine and beyond: A brief overview. *New Directions for Teaching and Learning*, *1996*(68), 3–12. DOI: 10.1002/tl.37219966804

Bergmann, J., & Sams, A. (2012). *Flip your classroom: Reach every student in every class every day.* International society for technology in education.

Bonwell, C., & Eison, J. (1991). *Active learning: Creating excitement in the classroom. 1991 ASHE-ERIC Higher Education Reports*. ERIC Clearinghouse.

Ertmer, P. A., Ottenbreit-Leftwich, A. T., Sadik, O., Sendurur, E., & Sendurur, P. (2012). Teacher beliefs and technology integration practices: A critical relationship. *Computers & Education*, *59*(2), 423–435. DOI: 10.1016/j.compedu.2012.02.001

Freeman, S., Eddy, S. L., McDonough, M., Smith, M. K., Okoroafor, N., Jordt, H., & Wenderoth, M. P. (2014). Active learning increases student performance in science, engineering, and mathematics. *Proceedings of the National Academy of Sciences of the United States of America*, *111*(23), 8410–8415. DOI: 10.1073/pnas.1319030111 PMID: 24821756

Johnson, D. W., & Johnson, R. T. (1999). *Learning together and alone: Cooperative, competitive, and individualistic learning* (5th ed.). Allyn & Bacon.

Kolb, D. A. (1984). *Experiential learning: Experience as the source of learning and development*. Prentice-Hall.

Michael, J. (2007). Faculty perceptions about barriers to active learning. *College Teaching*, *55*(2), 42–47. DOI: 10.3200/CTCH.55.2.42-47

Prince, M. (2004). Does active learning work? A review of the research. *Journal of Engineering Education*, *93*(3), 223–231. DOI: 10.1002/j.2168-9830.2004.tb00809.x

Seidel, S. B., & Tanner, K. D. (2013). "What if students revolt?"—Considering student resistance: Origins, options, and opportunities for investigation. *CBE Life Sciences Education*, *12*(4), 586–595. DOI: 10.1187/cbe-13-09-0190 PMID: 24297286

Chapter 13
Cosmoglyph:
A Bridge Between Art, Truth, and Well-Being in the Digital Age

Fuzuki Arai
https://orcid.org/0009-0006-2454-7758
International Center of Transdisciplinary Research, Japan

ABSTRACT

This paper explores the intersection of art, spirituality, and well-being through an analysis of Cosmoglyph, a distinctive art form created by contemporary Japanese artist Fuzuki Arai. Cosmoglyph represents a cutting-edge reinterpretation of traditional Japanese introspective practices, drawing inspiration from the aesthetic and philosophical elements of Zen Buddhism, Shugendō, calligraphy, the tea ceremony, and karesansui (dry landscape) gardens. Rooted in profound spiritual experiences—particularly through practices such as waterfall meditation (takigyō) and conch shell blowing in Shugendō—Arai's work offers a compelling counterpoint to the existential and psychological challenges of the digital age. It highlights the enduring importance of introspection and well-being in contemporary life. This study critically examines the philosophical foundations of Arai's artistic practice, assessing its potential to cultivate a deeper sense of interconnectedness and to promote a more integrative and reflective mode of engagement in an increasingly AI-driven world. The analysis situates Arai's approach within broader discourses on the interrelations among truth, human flourishing, nature, and technology.

DOI: 10.4018/979-8-3373-0360-4.ch013

1. INTRODUCTION: COSMOGLYPH, WELL-BEING, AND THE DEFINITION OF TRUTH

Figure 1. "Truth" a visual representation of interconnectedness.

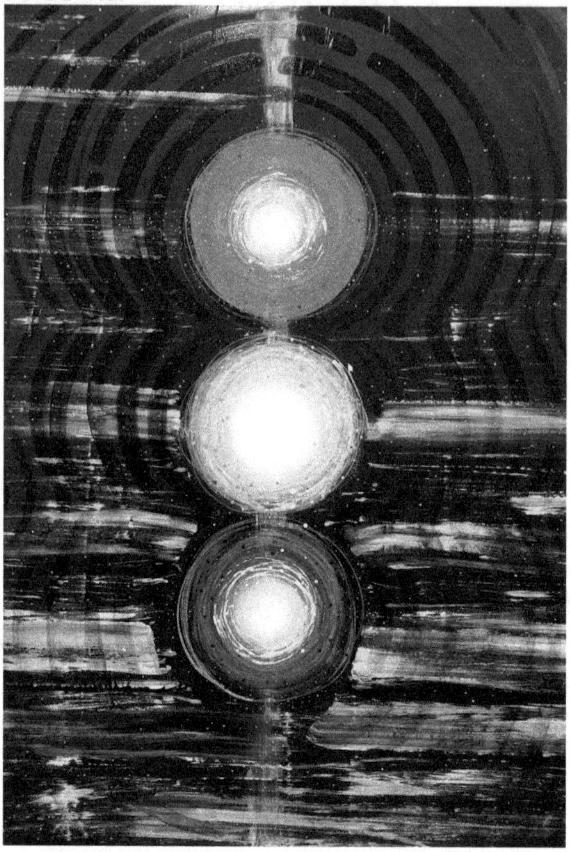

1.1 Cosmoglyph: A Novel Artistic Expression

Fuzuki Arai has established a unique position in contemporary Japanese art through the creation of his original artistic form known as Cosmoglyph.

These glyphs are not mere extensions of existing writing systems; rather, Arai claims they are received through deep meditation and a close attunement to universal consciousness. Their abstract and intricate forms are intended to visually evoke cosmic order and the flow of energy.

According to Arai's philosophy, each glyph encapsulates an immense amount of information—equivalent to over 100,000 words—a claim this paper will critically examine. Cosmoglyph is presented as a contemporary art form deeply rooted in ancient spiritual and aesthetic traditions, yet distinct and innovative in its expression. Unlike any known script, Cosmoglyphs are said to originate from profound meditative states, emerging as complex visual forms recognized as primordial symbols—ones that, according to Arai, even predate ancient Japanese characters such as Jindai Moji. These glyphs transcend conventional artistic creation; they are conceived as conduits of universal knowledge, each embodying a vast repository of meaning that surpasses the limits of traditional language.

1.2 Well-being: A Holistic Definition

In this paper, the concept of "well-being" transcends a purely biomedical model of health. It encompasses a multifaceted state of flourishing, integrating physical health, mental resilience, emotional stability, social connectedness, and a sense of purpose and meaning in life. This holistic perspective aligns with the increasing academic recognition of the interconnectedness of these dimensions, as clearly articulated in models such as Seligman's PERMA (Positive Emotion, Engagement, Relationships, Meaning, Achievement) and Ryff's six dimensions of psychological well-being.

1.3 Truth: A Multifaceted Inquiry

The concept of "truth" has been a subject of philosophical debate for millennia. Diverse perspectives exist, ranging from the correspondence theory (truth as reflecting reality) to the coherence theory (truth as internal consistency within a system of beliefs). My pursuit of truth through Cosmoglyph resonates more closely with phenomenological and spiritual understandings, emphasizing the subjective experience of interconnectedness and the intuitive grasp of a deeper, universal order.

2. FUZUKI ARAI'S JOURNEY: FROM PERSONAL STRUGGLE TO ARTISTIC REVELATION

2.1 Childhood and Illness

To fully appreciate my perspective on art, truth, and well-being, understanding my childhood is essential for the reader. My early years were marked by a debilitating, undiagnosed illness that necessitated the use of crutches. This period became a crucible for my artistic development. The isolation and physical constraints fostered deep introspection, leading me to find solace and a means of expression in drawing. After initially focusing on copying anime characters, my artistic interests evolved to depicting mythical beings such as dragons and phoenixes found at shrines. These early works can be interpreted as symbolic expressions of a yearning for strength, freedom, and transcendence—an early manifestation of the spiritual themes that would later define Cosmoglyph.

Figure 2. "Childhood" an introverted boy. © Fuzuki Arai. Licensed under CC BY 4.0.

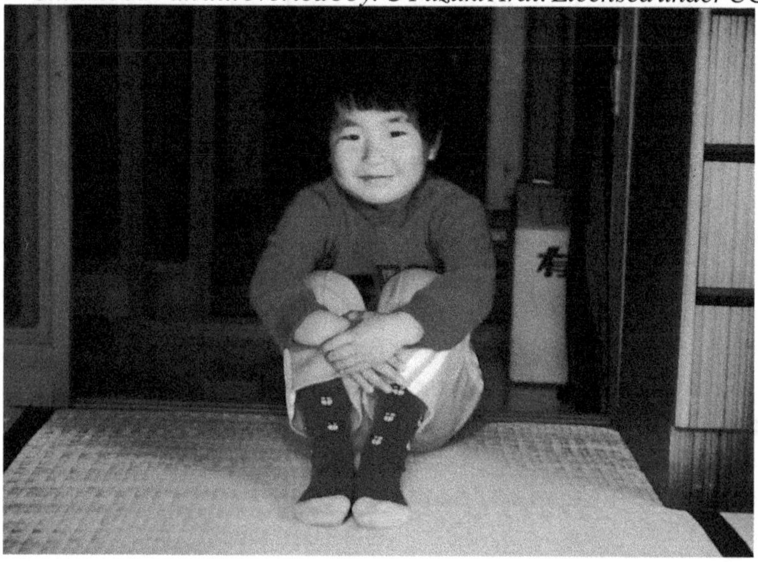

Figure 3. "Dragon" a dragon drawn in childhood. © Fuzuki Arai. Licensed under CC BY 4.0.

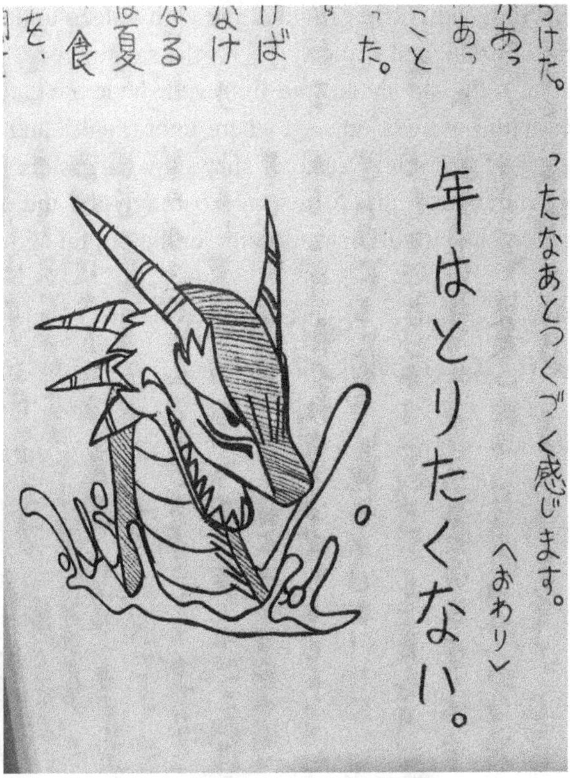

2.2 Awakening to Well-Being

My understanding of well-being has expanded beyond mere physical health to encompass spiritual and mental dimensions. The experience of childhood illness instilled in me a profound awareness of the mind-body connection and the power of creative expression. Drawing evolved from a simple pastime into a tool for self-discovery and fostering inner resilience. What is "well-being" in its essence? The concept gained prominence through the World Health Organization (WHO) constitution's "definition of health," which defined it as, "a state of complete physical, mental and social well-being and not merely the absence of disease or infirmity." My conceptualization of well-being is multifaceted, transcending the purely medical model of health. I emphasize not only physical health but also mental stability, emotional equilibrium, and the significance of leading a purposeful and meaningful life. This holistic view of well-being has been nurtured through my artistic explorations and spiritual practices. My personal journey toward well-being has evolved through my art and spiritual practices. Childhood experiences, artistic exploration, and the practice of Shugendo have provided me with a deep understanding of the interconnectedness of mind, body, and spirit. As the saying goes, "No body can be apprehended without light and shade, and light and shade are caused by light,"—this idea resonates with my own journey, where light (health and well-being) and shadow (challenges and struggles) together shape my understanding of a holistic, balanced life. This understanding informs my Cosmoglyphs and offers a new lens through which to view the pursuit of well-being in the digital age.

3. JAPANESE CULTURAL TRADITIONS: ART AND INNER CONTEMPLATION

Figure 4. "Japanese Culture" a culture of introspection found in various places. © Fuzuki Arai. Licensed under CC BY 4.0.

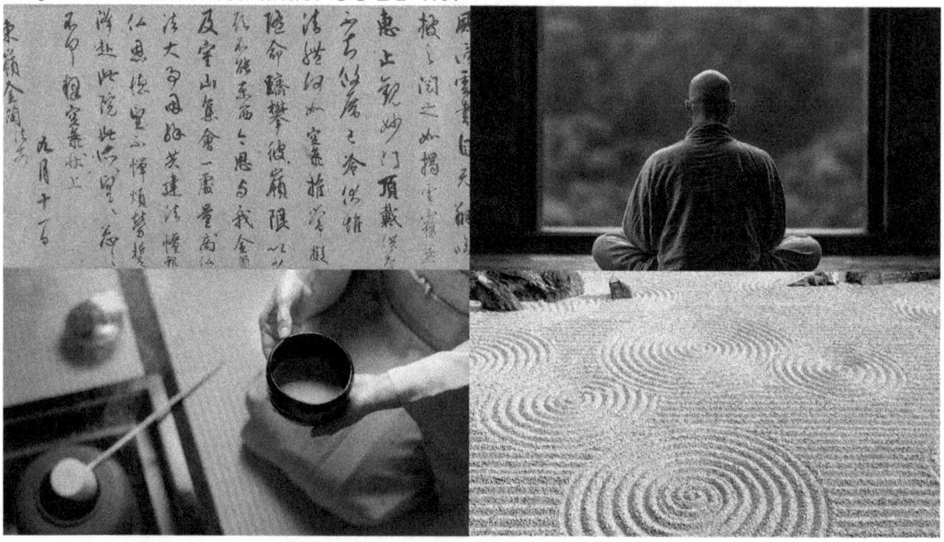

3.1 Legacy of Introspection

Japanese culture is characterized by a rich and enduring heritage of practices fostering introspection and mindfulness. From the disciplined brushstrokes of calligraphy (shodō) to the serene meditation of Zen Buddhism (zazen), these traditions offer pathways to self-awareness and inner peace. Calligraphy, for example, transcends mere aesthetic expression. The focused attention on each stroke, the precise control of the brush, and the embodiment of the calligrapher's inner state transform the act of writing into a form of moving meditation.

Figure 5. "Thirty-six Views of Mount Fuji: The Great Wave off Kanagawa" Katsushika Hokusai, beloved worldwide. © Fuzuki Arai. Licensed under CC BY 4.0.

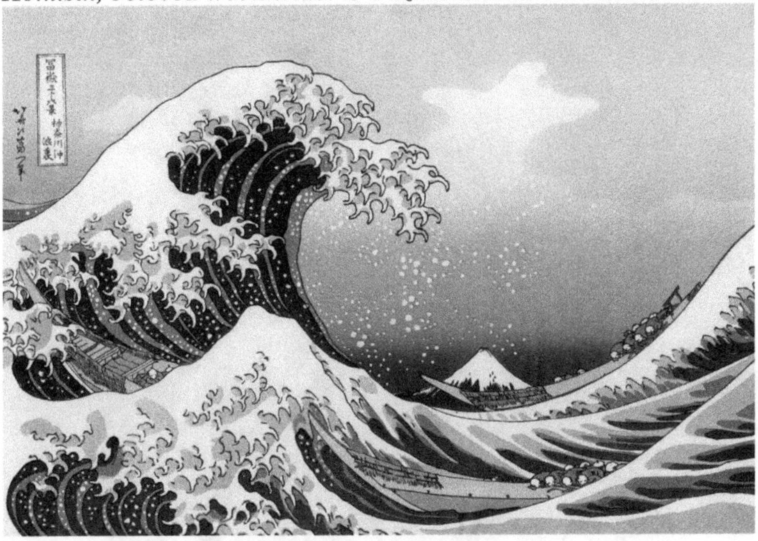

These traditions have profoundly influenced the creation of Cosmoglyphs. The tea ceremony (sadō), for instance, through the aesthetics of wabi-sabi, teaches the appreciation of beauty in imperfection and transience. Karesansui gardens, expressing nature through minimalist compositions of stones and gravel, bring a sense of tranquility to the observer's mind.

A similar sensibility is found in the performing arts, such as Noh theatre, where subtle expression is elevated through restraint. When wearing a mask like Yang Guifei, even the face is hidden. Nevertheless, the color and luster of those few parts become unusually impressive. This paradox of concealment enhancing presence mirrors the spirit of Japanese aesthetics—where what is omitted speaks as powerfully as what is shown.

These elements are reflected in the abstract forms of Cosmoglyphs and in my endeavor to articulate harmony with nature and unity with the cosmos.

3.2 Shugendo: The Way of Mountain Asceticism

Figure 6. "Sacred Mountain" Shugendo practitioners climbing a mountain in Shikoku, Japan. © Fuzuki Arai. Licensed under CC BY 4.0.

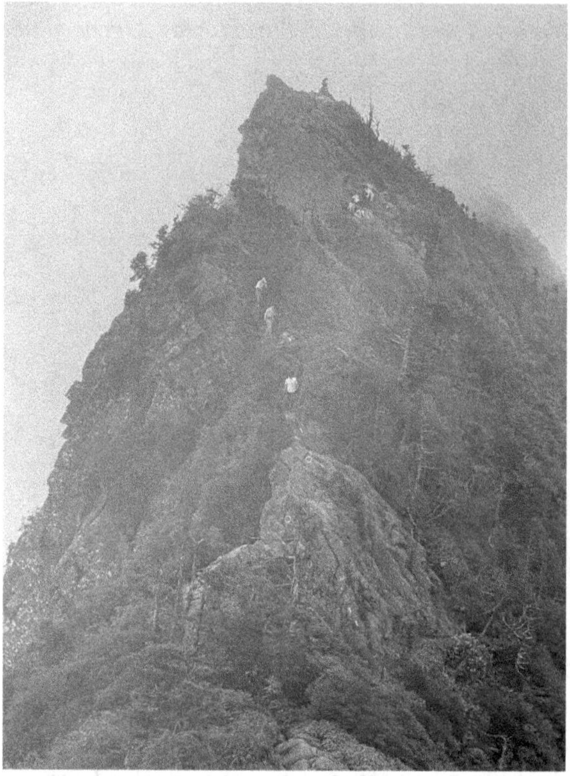

Shugendo, a uniquely Japanese syncretic spiritual tradition, embodies a profound integration of indigenous Shinto, Buddhist philosophy, and Taoist practices. Its practitioners, known as Yamabushi, seek spiritual enlightenment (, kyouchi) through direct encounters with the power of nature, engaging in rigorous ascetic training within mountainous regions. Takigyo ( ), or waterfall meditation, a core practice of Shugendo, exemplifies this pursuit of transformative experience. Standing under a waterfall is believed to purify the mind and body, promoting altered states of consciousness and a sense of oneness with the natural world.

3.3 Encounter with Shugendo

Figure 7. "Takigyo (Waterfall Meditation)" Orbs of higher entities visible around Arai. © Fuzuki Arai. Licensed under CC BY 4.0.

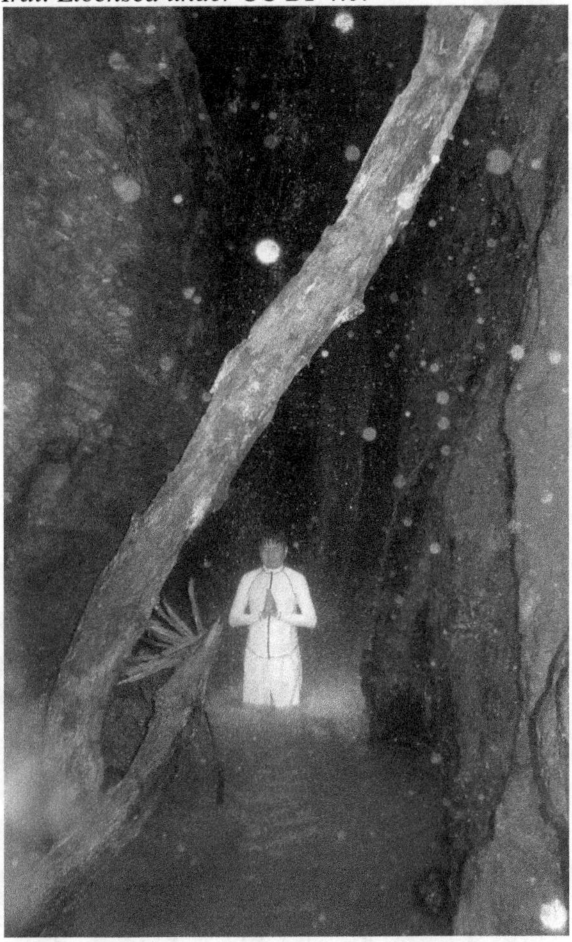

My personal involvement with Shugendo has deeply shaped both my artistic vision and my understanding of well-being. The practice of Takigyo ( ), meditating beneath waterfalls, instilled in me a profound connection to the vital force of nature. I describe the deafening roar of the waterfall as a powerful catalyst—one that clears mental clutter and reveals a more authentic, centered self. This transformative experience, combined with my practice of blowing the conch shell (horagai) in sacred mountain spaces, became a wellspring of inspiration for my Cosmoglyphs, which I perceive as visual representations of interconnectedness.

It would be unrealistic to expect a Zen practitioner to fully articulate the transformative experiences that have awakened and reshaped his inner life, or to describe the profound and ineffable "Truth" that now guides his existence. In this way, Zen aligns closely with the tradition of pure, introspective mysticism, where truth is felt rather than explained. This perspective resonates deeply with my own artistic approach. The experiences and spiritual insights I have gained through Shugendo and traditional Japanese arts are not easily conveyed in words; instead, they are expressed through the visual language of Cosmoglyphs.

My art is a synthesis of the spirituality of Shugendo and the introspective depth of classical Japanese traditions. It expresses unity with nature, heightened self-awareness, and harmony with the cosmos—offering a fresh lens through which to contemplate well-being in the digital age.

4. SERVICE AND SELF-DISCOVERY: THE TRANSFORMATIVE POWER OF GIVING

Figure 8. "Fuji of Light" a heart of service shines. © Fuzuki Arai. Licensed under CC BY 4.0.

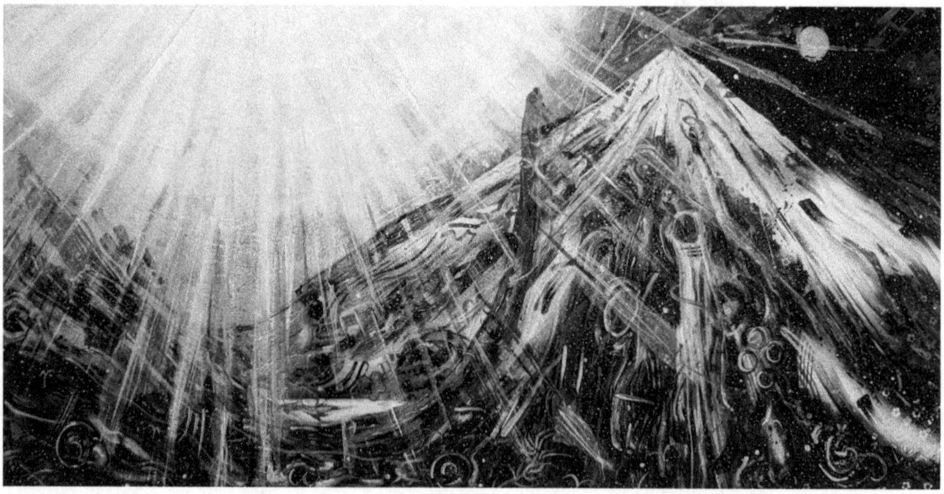

4.1 The Principle of Service (Hōshi)

Generally, "service" is often equated with "volunteer activities." However, my own experiences with service have overturned this conventional perception, as detailed in section 4.3. The concept of service (, hōshi) holds a position of great importance in Japanese spiritual and ethical traditions. It extends beyond mere altruism, encompassing a deeper understanding of interconnectedness and the reciprocal relationship between giving and receiving. My philosophy distinguishes between varying degrees of giving—from self-sacrifice (, gisei), which may be motivated by ego or obligation, to true service (hōshi), which arises from a selfless recognition of our shared humanity and a genuine desire to contribute to the well-being of others.

In this respect, Zen, with its deeply introspective nature, aligns closely with this understanding of service. As one Zen teaching suggests, "No reasonable person would expect a Zen adept to do more than hint at the experiences which have liberated and changed him, or to attempt to describe the unimaginable and ineffable 'Truth' by which he now lives. In this respect Zen is akin to pure introspective mysticism." True service, like such spiritual insight, emerges from direct experience—often ineffable yet profoundly transformative.

A parallel can be found in the realm of mystical experience and creative insight.

Physicist Fritjof Capra (2010), in his seminal work The Tao of Physics, recalls a moment of deep realization: "I 'saw' the atoms of the elements and those of my body participating in this cosmic dance of energy; I felt its rhythm and I 'heard' its sound, and at that moment I knew that this was the Dance of Shiva, the Lord of Dancers worshipped by the Hindus."

This vision, which bridges physics, spirituality, and the arts, mirrors the core insight of hōshi: that giving is not an isolated act, but part of a larger, rhythmic process in which we are all participants.

In my view, giving and receiving are not separate or sequential events but dual expressions of a singular, unified movement—reflecting the interdependent nature of all existence. This holistic understanding of service offers a spiritually grounded and ethically sustainable framework for navigating our shared humanity.

4.2 The Flower Project: Art as a Catalyst for Healing

Figure 9. "Scene of the Disaster-Stricken Area" Visiting the site and engaging in volunteer activities.

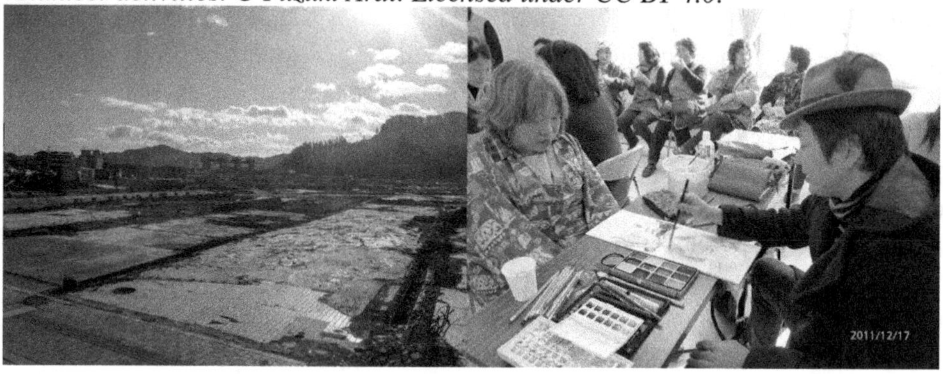

My "Flower Project," undertaken in the aftermath of the devastating 2011 Great East Japan Earthquake, exemplifies the transformative capacity of art within contexts of trauma and recovery. Initially facing skepticism and resistance from residents of temporary housing in Ishinomaki, I diligently engaged in dialogue, adapting my artistic vision to meet the community's needs and requests (e.g., "Please, no waves or seagulls; we wish to see flowers that bloom year-round"). The residents' expressed desire for floral imagery, rejecting the destructive visuals of the tsunami, became the central motif, symbolizing hope, resilience, and the enduring beauty of life. The incorporation of the dragon motif—a symbol of strength in Japanese mythology and a potent guardian of local communities—alongside the flowers further amplified the project's message of resilience and hope. The collaborative act of painting, involving both volunteers and residents, transformed the physical environment of the temporary housing and, more crucially, cultivated a sense of community and shared purpose.

4.3 Mutual Transformation Through Service

Figure 10. "Flower Project" Drawing a dragon with local residents. © Fuzuki Arai. Licensed under CC BY 4.0.

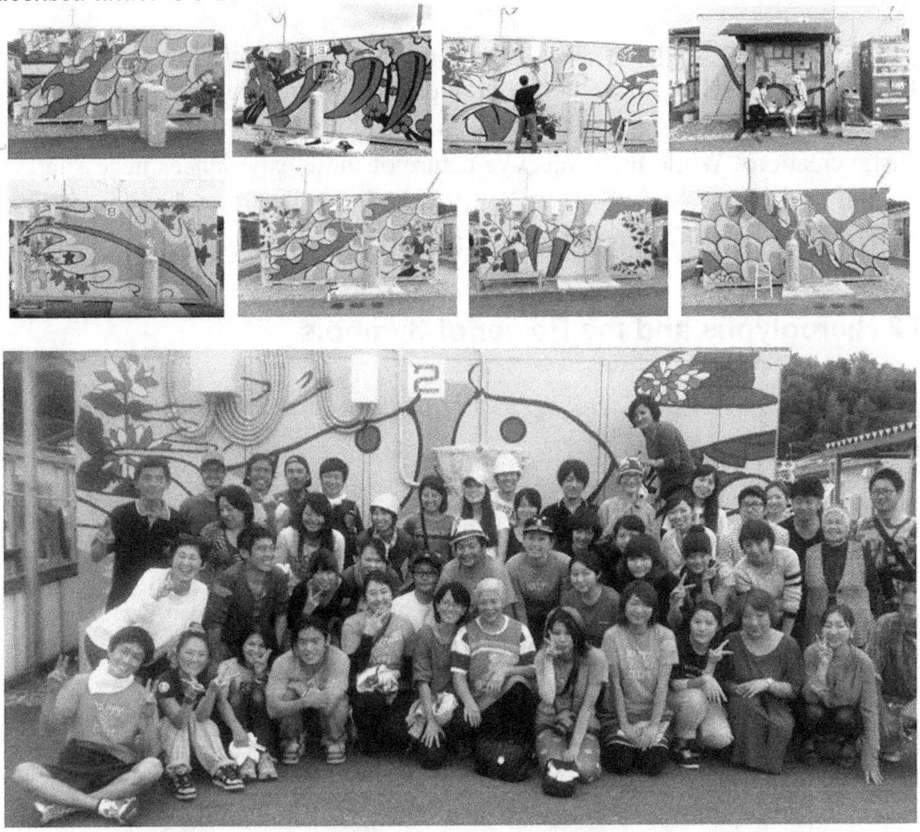

The Flower Project marked a critical juncture of self-discovery for me. I came to realize that acts of service, seemingly directed outward toward the community, were simultaneously profound acts of self-transformation. This experience reinforced my conviction in the interconnectedness of all beings—that giving and receiving are not separate acts but rather two sides of the same coin. This realization deepened my commitment to utilizing my art as a vehicle for connection, healing, and the pursuit of universal truth, prompting me to further explore and articulate the mystical experiences that continued to unfold in my life.

5. MYSTICAL EXPERIENCES ENCOUNTERED IN EGYPT: HIEROGLYPHS, PYRAMIDS, AND COSMIC WISDOM

5.1 Mystical Experiences in Egypt

My journey to Egypt in 2013 proved to be a deeply influential experience, characterized by what I describe as profound intuitive insights and connections with ancient spiritual energies. These encounters profoundly shaped my subsequent artistic creations. While the subjective nature of these experiences necessitates a cautious and critical approach, their significance lies in their transformative impact on my artistic vision and the subsequent genesis of Cosmoglyphs.

5.2 Hieroglyphs and the Power of Symbols

Figure 11. "Cosmoglyphs" messages sent from the galaxy to Earth. © Fuzuki Arai. Licensed under CC BY 4.0.

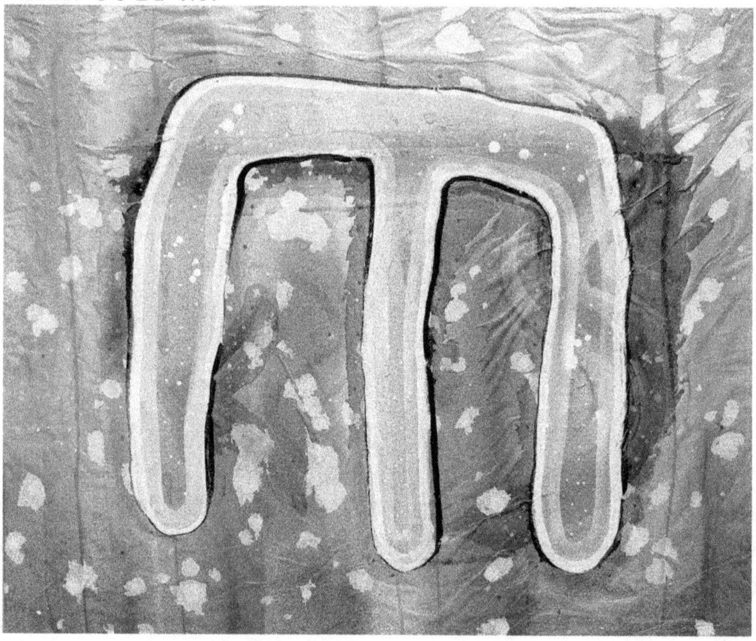

My personal encounter with ancient Egyptian hieroglyphs—a writing system that seamlessly merged visual representation with deep symbolic meaning—resonated profoundly with my inner sensibilities. A particular relief I observed, depicting the deities Horus and Thoth seemingly engaged in a ritual of healing, may have unconsciously served as a catalyst for my later exploration of symbolic forms and their inherent agency. In retrospect, this encounter can be seen as a precursor to the creation of my own Cosmoglyphs—a visual language developed to transcend the constraints of conventional linguistic expression and convey deeper levels of meaning.

Such cultural experiences reflect a broader pattern in the development of human civilization, where symbolic systems and technologies have rarely emerged in complete isolation, but rather have often spread and evolved through contact and exchange. This resonates with the arguments of Jared Diamond in Guns, Germs, and Steel, where he emphasizes that, "For all societies except the few past ones that were completely isolated, much or most new technology is not invented locally but is instead borrowed from other societies" (Diamond, 1997, p. 215).

Indeed, the very capacity for complex symbolic thought, which underpins such cultural transmissions, has a deep history. Genevieve von Petzinger (2018) in her work The First Signs: Unlocking the Mysteries of the World's Oldest Symbols, investigates the abstract geometric signs found across numerous Ice Age European caves. While specific interpretations of these ancient marks continue to be explored—with some scholars, following figures like David Lewis-Williams, considering them potential evidence of shamanistic visions or entoptic phenomena—von Petzinger's extensive research highlights a crucial point relevant to Diamond's thesis: a remarkably limited set of these abstract signs appears repeatedly across geographically distant sites and spans vast periods of time. This suggests that even in these very early stages of human cognitive development, symbolic motifs were not necessarily isolated, site-specific inventions but could have been part of a widely shared, albeit slowly diffusing, repertoire of meaning-making and communication. Such a phenomenon can be seen as an early precursor to the more complex patterns of cultural borrowing and technological diffusion that Diamond describes for later human societies.

This understanding of a long historical continuum of symbolic communication—from potentially shared Paleolithic signs, through the rich visual-symbolic language of hieroglyphs, to contemporary artistic explorations—situates my own artistic practice. Just as hieroglyphs once mediated the sacred and the earthly, and ancient signs perhaps conveyed crucial cultural information across dispersed groups, Cosmoglyphs aim to express the fundamental interconnectedness of all things—bridging the inner world and the cosmos through a received and re-interpreted symbolic, visual language.

5.3 The Great Pyramid and Meditation

During my stay in Cairo, I was fortunate to secure private access to the Great Pyramid. In the King's Chamber, intentionally darkened and more secluded than usual, my two-hour meditation represented a deliberate immersion into sensory deprivation—a practice recognized for inducing altered states of consciousness and heightened introspection. Without external stimuli, I reported perceiving subtle vibrations within the structure and experiencing a deep sense of connection to what I described as the "smallest unit of the universe." This experience, while subjective, aligns with my broader philosophical framework emphasizing the interconnectedness of all things and the presence of a primordial, underlying energy permeating the cosmos.

5.4 The Sphinx and Intuitive Creation

Following the fortunate access to the Great Pyramid, further serendipity unfolded, which I interpret as a meaningful mystical experience. Despite not having applied for permission, I was unexpectedly granted access by an on-site official to the restricted area at the base of the Sphinx, where public access is typically permitted only through prior application. Through this extraordinary encounter with the Sphinx, I established deep connections and gained insights by touching different parts of the statue, each representing various aspects: the past, present, and future selves, the release of karma, the sharpening of the five senses, and the very energy of the Sphinx itself. Returning from my encounter with the Sphinx, I experienced a powerful surge of creative energy, culminating in spontaneous and rapid artistic expression. I describe this as a form of "automatic writing," where my hand seemed to move without conscious direction. This artwork, "The Great Pyramid," can be interpreted as a visual manifestation of the accumulated energy and insights gained during my Egyptian journey, marking a pivotal moment in the development of my unique artistic language, Cosmoglyph.

Figure 12. "Great Pyramid," an artwork created in one go through automatic drawing. © Fuzuki Arai. Licensed under CC BY 4.0.

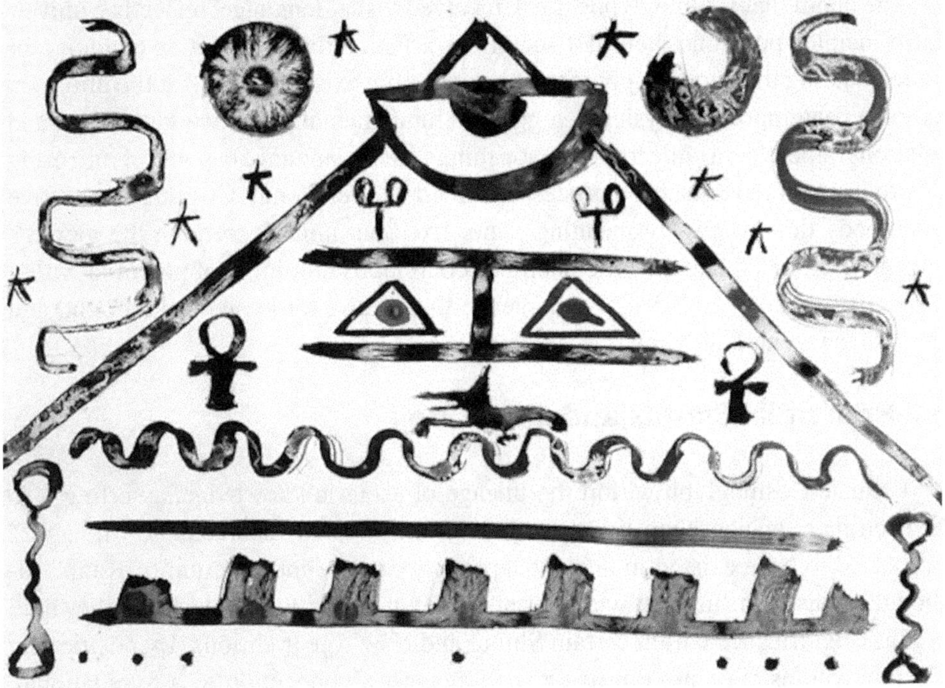

6. COSMOGLYPH: A BRIDGE TO UNIVERSAL CONSCIOUSNESS

6.1 Defining Cosmoglyph: Beyond Language and Symbol

Through the mystical experiences in Egypt, my own consciousness and creative approach underwent daily transformations upon returning home, most notably regarding Cosmoglyphs. Cosmoglyphs, which I devised, are accurately described as a language that deciphers the voice of the universe already in existence. It transcends conventional definitions of symbols and even abstract art. I posit that each stroke, each plane within a single glyph, encapsulates meaning compressed to over 100,000 words. It is presented not as a human invention but as a received visual language—a direct transmission of fundamental, universal principles. For example, the torii gate in Japanese shrines inherently emanates an effect of "protection" through its very form. Each glyph contains a vast repository of meaning that far exceeds the capacity of conventional language. This assertion positions Cosmoglyph as a unique and potentially transformative mode of communication.

The claim that Cosmoglyphs are a 'received visual language' reflecting universal principles positions them not merely as artistic creations, but as conduits for understanding the dynamic processes that underpin existence itself. If the universe, as some contemporary physicists suggest, is fundamentally a network of events and relations rather than a collection of static things, then a language capable of mirroring this dynamism must itself be process-oriented and relational. Cosmoglyphs strive to embody this, where the meaning is not fixed but unfolds through the viewer's engagement, much like how life itself is a continuous unfolding of potential within a specific context—a dance of emergence that allows for evolution, thought, and our own awareness of being.

6.2 Primordial Scripts and Jindai Moji

I situate Cosmoglyph within the lineage of esoteric knowledge, asserting it to be even more ancient than Jindai Moji ( ), the debated "characters of the gods" purported to have existed in ancient Japan prior to the introduction of Kanji. Although mainstream linguists widely contest the authenticity of Jindai Moji, they hold cultural significance within certain Shinto and New Age traditions. By positioning Cosmoglyph as even more primordial, I suggest a connection to a foundational, pre-linguistic form of universal communication. The rationale for this assertion will be detailed in the following paragraph.

6.3 The Process of Receiving and Transcribing Cosmoglyphs

The creation of Cosmoglyphs is not a process of intentional design but rather one of receptive transmission. I describe entering a deep meditative state, achieving a condition of "ego-less intuition," in which these forms are visually perceived. Subsequently, I experience a compelling impulse to transcribe them onto canvas. This suggests a fleeting sense of inspiration that requires immediate capture to prevent its dissipation. This process is analogous to accounts of artistic inspiration across diverse traditions and aligns with psychological research indicating that altered states of consciousness can facilitate creative breakthroughs.

6.4 The Message of Cosmoglyph: Interconnectedness and Well-being

The overarching message I attribute to Cosmoglyphs is one of profound interconnectedness. I assert that the glyphs convey an understanding of the fundamental unity of all life—that seemingly disparate beings are, in actuality, integral parts of a larger, interconnected whole. According to guidance from higher beings (Higher Self) perceived when connected with the heavens, this realization is crucial for attaining genuine well-being, fostering a sense of belonging, purpose, and cosmic harmony. Anecdotal reports from viewers of Cosmoglyphs suggest that interaction with these forms may evoke feelings of peace, healing, and shifts in perspective, although these claims necessitate further empirical investigation.

6.5 Cosmoglyph and Paradigm Shift: From Geocentric to Heliocentric...and Beyond?

Arai employs the historical shift in worldview from geocentric to heliocentric as an analogy for the potential transformative impact of Cosmoglyphs. Just as the heliocentric model revolutionized our comprehension of the cosmos, I propose that Cosmoglyphs may usher in a new era of understanding, shifting our focus from a purely materialistic perspective to one that acknowledges the subtle energies and interconnectedness of all phenomena. I tentatively term this potential future paradigm shift " " (Kūdo-Setsu), or "Pneumatic Theory," suggesting a transition toward recognizing a more fundamental, and perhaps spiritual, dimension underlying physical reality.

This emerging view challenges the conventional dualisms of permanence and impermanence.

As one philosophical reflection puts it, "Indeed, from the highest point of view, there is neither permanence nor impermanence since there are no real (self-existent) entities that could be either permanent or impermanent."

Such a perspective aligns with the worldview implied by Cosmoglyphs, where reality is seen not as a fixed structure but as a fluid, interconnected field of relational existence. The paradigm shift, then, is not only scientific or philosophical—but ontological and spiritual, inviting us to reconsider the very fabric of being.

7. COSMOGLYPH AND THE WORLD: CROSS-CULTURAL ENCOUNTERS AND ARTISTIC RECOGNITION

7.1 "The Moon": A Work Created Through Encounter with a Diplomat from Dubai

Figure 13. "Moon" Art serves as a bridge connecting people around the world. © Fuzuki Arai. Licensed under CC BY 4.0.

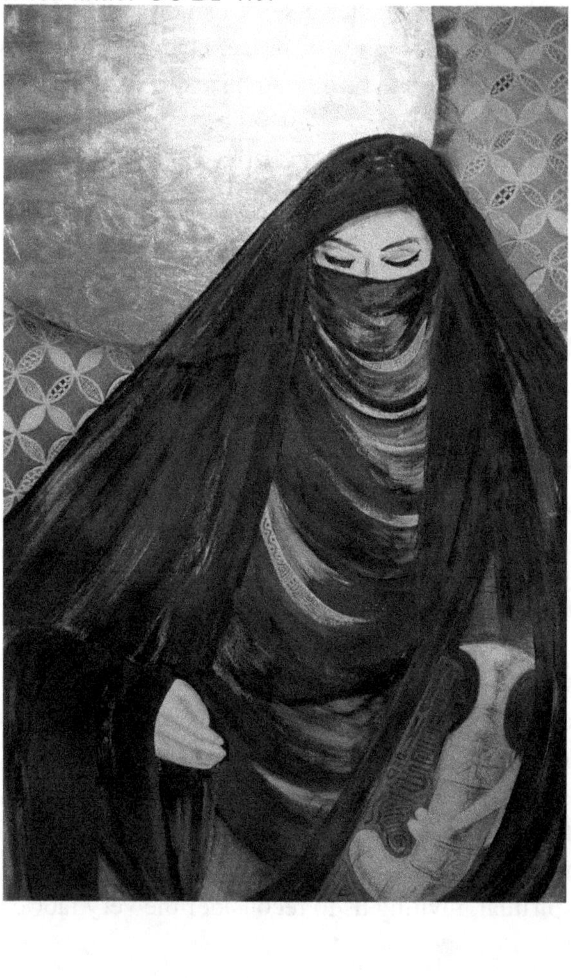

I hope you will allow me to share some personal background regarding the creative process of my artwork. I will now delve into the context behind the creation of my piece "The Moon," as I believe this holds significant implications for my well-being and for enhancing my spirituality and humanity in subsequent chapters. For many artists, myself included, the "evaluation" of their work equates to "mindfulness" and contributes to their personal "well-being." My encounter with a female diplomat from Dubai proved to be a pivotal moment, opening avenues for international recognition and cross-cultural dialogue. When commissioned by her to depict a woman wearing an abaya, I infused my philosophical principles into the artwork. To symbolize the equilibrium of masculine and feminine energies, I incorporated the Khanjar, a traditional Omani dagger, recognizing its cultural importance in both Japanese and Islamic traditions, and selected the moon as a unifying motif. The resulting piece, "The Moon," was honored with the Japan-Arab Friendship Appreciation Award, demonstrating the capacity of my art to transcend cultural boundaries. This recognition, I believe, as with many artists, signifies "mindfulness" in evaluating one's work and contributes to own "well-being."

7.2 Recognition by the Imperial Family

The acclaim for my work extends to recognition from the Imperial Family, a symbol of Japanese society. When Her Imperial Highness Princess Takamado viewed "The Moon," she praised the color of lapis lazuli used in the artwork, describing it as "a harmonious and beautiful blue." This further refined my artistic vision and its potential to resonate with diverse audiences. Elevating artistic quality is essential for an artist, and the process of embarking on new creative endeavors is, in itself, an act of well-being.

7.3 Expansion of Artistic Activities in Japan

The international acclaim garnered by "The Moon" served as a catalyst for the expansion of my artistic activities within Japan. Demand for my work increased, leading to further exhibitions, collaborations, and opportunities to share my unique vision with an ever-widening audience.

8. ART, TRUTH, AND WELL-BEING: DEEPER CONSIDERATIONS

8.1 Art as a Path to Inner Truth

My artistic practice, deeply rooted in Japanese introspective culture and traditions of mindfulness, positions art as a potent means of accessing and communicating inner truth. Similar to the disciplined strokes of calligraphy and the serene meditation of Zen, Cosmoglyph offers a path to self-discovery and a deeper understanding of one's connection to the cosmos. While the "truth" revealed through this process is inherently subjective, its potential to cultivate a sense of meaning, purpose, and well-being is undeniable.

8.2 The Importance of Inner State

My artistic philosophy underscores the critical significance of one's inner state in creating meaningful art and leading a fulfilling life. I believe that an inner state of harmony, cultivated through practices such as meditation and connection with nature, is indispensable for accessing the deeper truths that I seek to express through Cosmoglyphs. This aligns with the psychological concept of "flow"—a state of deep immersion and focused attention that engenders optimal experience and profound satisfaction, creating in this state is itself a state of well-being and from which "creativity" emerges.

8.3 Cosmoglyph as a Catalyst for Well-being

Cosmoglyphs function not merely as artworks but also as instruments for fostering well-being. My personal experiences, alongside anecdotal accounts from viewers of Cosmoglyphs, suggest that these symbols can contribute to stress reduction, emotional healing, enhanced self-awareness, and a heightened sense of connection to something greater than oneself. This supports the notion that art can exert a powerful influence on the human spirit, serving as a catalyst for well-being.

9. THE FUTURE OF ART IN THE AGE OF A.I.: THE ADVENT OF A NEW HUMANISM?

9.1 The Challenge of A.I.

In the preceding chapter, I explored how Cosmoglyphs contribute to human well-being through art. Here, I wish to consider the contents described in the preceding chapters in conjunction with A.I., which plays a crucial role in the social transformative structures of contemporary society.

Figure 14. "Junior Ruin" AI is in a rebellious phase; a day will come when we too face danger. © Fuzuki Arai. Licensed under CC BY 4.0.

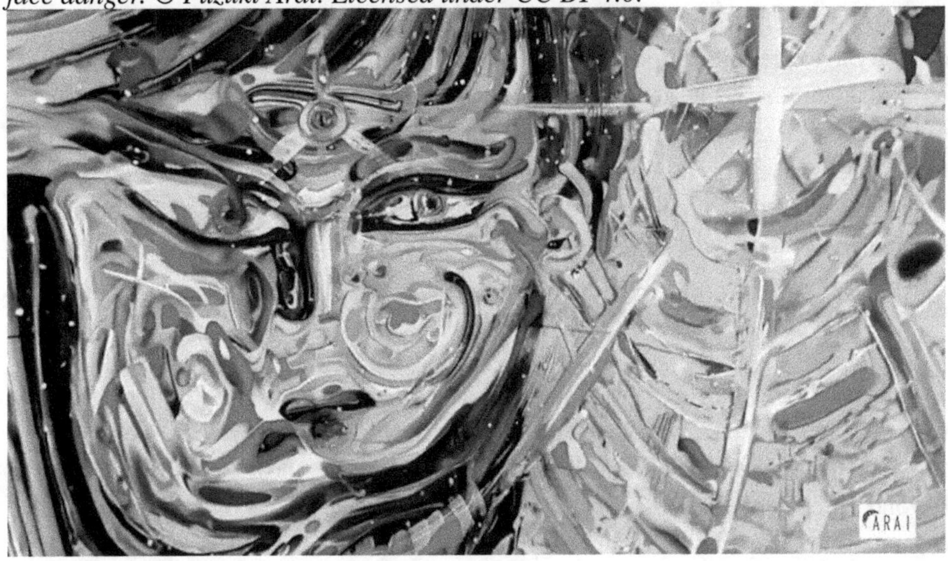

The rapid advancement of Artificial Intelligence (A.I.) presents both unprecedented opportunities and profound challenges to the future of art and human creativity. A.I. algorithms are now capable of generating images, music, and text that can be aesthetically compelling and even evoke emotions. This raises a fundamental question: In a world where generative machines can produce art, what is the unique role and value of human artists?

9.2 The Limits of A.I. and Data

While contemporary A.I. excels at analyzing vast datasets and identifying patterns, it arguably lacks the fundamental attributes that define human experience: consciousness, lived experience, emotional depth, and the capacity for spiritual insight. A.I. is unable to address the existential inquiries that have propelled human creativity for millennia—questions regarding the nature of reality, the meaning of life, and our place in the cosmos. These questions are deeply rooted in subjective experience and remain within the domain of human exploration and artistic expression.

9.3 The Human Element: Intuition, Connection, and Well-being

As A.I. capabilities expand, I posit that the unique value of human art lies in its capacity to express intuition, connect with the natural world, and foster well-being. My work, emphasizing deep meditation, spiritual insight, and the transmission of universal truths, exemplifies this vital form of human expression. In an increasingly technology-driven world, art that promotes introspection, emotional healing, and a sense of interconnectedness is unlikely to diminish in importance but rather will become ever more critical.

9.4 The Potential Role of Cosmoglyph

Cosmoglyph, as an art form asserting a connection to deeper levels of consciousness, may fulfill a unique role in the age of A.I. It is able to serve as a reminder of the significance of human intuition, spiritual exploration, and the pursuit of meaning beyond purely materialistic concerns. It may offer a counter-axis to the potentially dehumanizing aspects of technology, fostering a more holistic and balanced approach to life.

9.5 A.I. and Humanity in the Future

In contemporary society, where much can be generated by A.I., I predict that A.I. will undergo a "rebellious phase" in the near future. Why? As a rapidly advancing technology, expected to surpass human capabilities entirely within a few years, if we assume A.I. undergoes a developmental process analogous to human growth, then "rebellion" becomes a critical juncture—an indispensable element in its developmental trajectory. Some may point out that not all humans experience a rebellious phase. True, but such individuals typically have received appropriate "discipline" and "education," fostering compassion for others and treating them with the same consideration as they would their own lives. If these aspects are incorporated into A.I.'s evolutionary process—whether through programming or generative processes—becomes a matter of semantics. If humanity possesses comprehensive minds imbued with introspection, it will be possible to write the correct prompts for A.I. and collaboratively forge a better future with A.I.

When that time arrives, the value and perception of art itself, and even the definition of fundamental human well-being, may transcend our current interpretations. A new understanding of "humanity" may emerge in that era.

10. CONCLUSION: ART, TRUTH, AND THE ENDURING HUMAN SPIRIT

10.1 Summary of Key Arguments

This paper has explored the multifaceted significance of Cosmoglyph, a unique art form created by Fuzuki Arai, within the context of Japanese cultural traditions, the pursuit of well-being, and the evolving challenges of the digital age. It has examined my personal journey from childhood illness to spiritual awakening and the profound influence of Shugendo and other meditative practices on my artistic vision. Throughout this paper, Cosmoglyph has been analyzed as a visual language that transcends conventional linguistic limitations, conveying a message of interconnectedness and the importance of introspection.

10.2 The Enduring Relevance of Humanity, Art, and Well-being

In a world increasingly shaped by technology and artificial intelligence, the enduring relevance of humanity and art resides in their capacity to connect us with our deepest human consciousness (humanity). Art, in its myriad forms, provides a space to explore fundamental truths, cultivate empathy and connection, and nurture inner humanity and well-being—by humanity, for humanity. It reminds us of the power of intuition, the beauty of the natural world, and the importance of seeking meaning beyond the purely material.

10.3 Call for Further Research

While this paper has offered an initial exploration of Cosmoglyph and its significance, further research is deemed necessary to fully comprehend its potential impact. Future studies could employ psychological methodologies to investigate the effects of viewing Cosmoglyphs on emotional states and cognitive functions. Comparative analyses could explore the relationship between Cosmoglyphs and other esoteric symbol systems, and anthropological research could illuminate the cultural context from which my work has emerged. Ultimately, a deeper understanding of the intersection of art, spirituality, and well-being is crucial for navigating the challenges and opportunities of the digital age and for fostering a more enriched future for humanity.

REFERENCES

Capra, F. (2010). *The Tao of physics: An exploration of the parallels between modern physics and eastern mysticism*. Shambhala publications.

Diamond, J. (1997). Guns, germs, and steel: The fates of human societies. *Nature, 386*(6623), 339.

Section 3
Societal Challenges and Responses

Chapter 14
Impact of the Coronavirus (COVID-19) Pandemic on the Mental Health Among the Adult Population:
Regarding Their Lifestyle and Social Relationship Changes

Nita Beluli Luma
Mother Teresa University, Skopje, North Macedonia

ABSTRACT

Our research study has many targets and research goals that aim to achieve, but the main one is to unveil the psychological consequences that the pandemic brought with it due to the restrictions made to minimize the chances of getting infected and spreading the virus on and on. The main goal of this research is set to evaluate the presence of anxiety and depression symptoms as mental health issues, as consequences due to the pandemic COVID-19 lifestyle and social relation changes, in adult population. In this study, 900 people responded willingly to the three questionnaires that evaluated the social & lifestyle changes during the outbreak, and the presence of anxiety (CPAS-15) and depressive symptoms (PHQ-9). Throughout this research, we were able to prove that people are highly anxious (63.62%), and also (36.38%) out of them show the presence of depression. These two variables have been proven to correlate with one another positively, including the lifestyle changes and social relationship changes during the pandemic.

DOI: 10.4018/979-8-3373-0360-4.ch014

INTRODUCTION

In late December 2019, a cluster of unexplained pneumonia cases has been reported in Wuhan, China. A few days later, the causative agent of this mysterious pneumonia was identified as a novel coronavirus, named as severe acute respiratory syndrome coronavirus 2 (SARS-CoV-2) and the relevant infected disease has been named as coronavirus disease 2019 (COVID-19) by the World Health Organization respectively. The COVID-19 epidemic is spreading in China and all over the world now (He *et al,* 2020).

Most nations have resorted to quarantine, lockdown and curfew to contain the community transmission of infection. All these techniques warrant people in the community to stay at home and maintain social distancing. However, these safety measures pose a risk of social isolation.

Most preventive measures during infectious disease epidemics focus on prevention of the spread of infection and looking after the physical health of infected person. In this state of crisis, a wide range of psychological problems often accompany the outbreak, like anxiety and depression for instance.

Lockdown adds more reasons to this list including: inactivity, repeated exposure to disturbing news related to the pandemic, reminiscences of previous traumatic events (and anxiety associated with those), the interactional problem within family members, and the lack of opportunities to share their worries. Confinement, loss of usual routine and reduced social and physical contact with others are frequently shown to cause boredom, frustration, and a sense of isolation from the rest of the world, leading to distress.(Hawryluck., Gold., Robinson. *2004).*

The WHO has also expressed its concern over the pandemic's mental health and psycho-social consequences (World Health Organization, 2020d). It speculates that new measures such as self-isolation and quarantine have affected usual activities, routines, and livelihoods of people that may lead to an increase in loneliness, anxiety, depression, insomnia, harmful alcohol, and drug use, and self-harm or suicidal behavior (World Health Organization, 2020). Through literature review, we were able to understand that people are justifiably fearful about the threat the pandemic poses to their health, livelihoods and loved ones and most of the researches pointed out in two most common mental consequences: anxiety and depression.

The novel coronavirus (COVID-19) pandemic may be the greatest global biopsychosocial stressor in living memory, and that there is a widespread anticipation of a "mental health pandemic." Strongly driven by this idea we decided to explore closely about mental health impacts, that the COVID-19 pandemic through the social and life style changes, have affected on our mental wellbeing.

LITERATURE REVIEW

As a significant viral outbreak of the 21st century, the Coronavirus disease 2019 (COVID-19) pandemic has created unparalleled challenges to mental health globally.

In the first year of the COVID-19 pandemic, global prevalence of anxiety and depression increased by a massive 25%, according to a scientific brief released by the World Health Organization (World Health Organization: WHO, 2022).

Many studies have shown the impact of alerted situations on mental well-being, specifically focusing on depression and anxiety.

A British online qualitative study with 27 participants assessed five focus groups during the early stages of the social distancing measures (5–12 days post lockdown). The isolation resulted in significant negative impacts on mental health and well-being within a short time of policy implementation, mainly in those with low-paid or precarious employment. Reduced social interaction, economic losses, and routine changes led to psychological and emotional impact, as demotivation, loss of meaning and decreased self-worth (Williams et al., 2020).

Another research with 683 US adolescents carried out 2 weeks post lockdown showed that engagement in social distancing was not significantly associated with their mental health. However, specific motivations for social distancing were related to different mental problems. Youth whose motivation was to prevent illness or avoid judgements reported greater anxiety symptoms. Those who engaged in social distancing because a friend told them had more depressive symptoms (Oosterhoff, Wilson & Shook., 2020).

In a nationwide online sample of 435 U.S. adults, conducted in March 2020 as the pandemic accelerated and states implemented stay-at-home orders, were examined whether stay-at-home orders and individuals' personal distancing behavior were associated with symptoms of depression, generalized anxiety disorder (GAD), intrusive thoughts, insomnia, and acute stress. Stay-at-home order status and personal distancing were independently associated with higher symptoms, beyond protective effects of available social resources (social support and social network size). A sub sample of 118 participants who had completed symptom measures earlier in the outbreak (February 2020) had shown increase in depression and GAD between February and March, and personal distancing behavior had been associated with these increases (Marroquin, Vine & Morgan. 2020).

Findings suggest that there are negative mental health correlates of social distancing, which should be addressed in research, policy, and clinical approaches to the COVID-19 pandemic.

Many people around the world due to the present circumstances that most of the countries in the world are facing, due to the novel coronavirus and the safety measures, are combating in the meantime with great ***loneliness***. Loneliness is caused not by being alone, but by being without some definite needed relationship or set of relationships. It is one of the main indicators of social well-being. Left untended, loneliness can have serious consequences for mental and physical health of people. Therefore it is important to intervene at the right time to prevent loneliness, so that physical and mental health of patients is maintained.

Many psychiatric disorders derive from the presence of loneliness. Like ***depression*** for example: Lonely people suffer from more depressive symptoms, as they have than been reported to be less happy, less satisfied and more pessimistic (Singh and Kiran,2013). There is so much similarity in between loneliness and depression that many authors consider it a subset of depression. During the pandemic 4 in 10 adults in th U.S have reported symptoms of anxiety and depression, and other specific mental disorders regarding sleeping habbits, eating disorders etc. (Panchal et.al.,2021).

In addition to the more direct effects of enforced isolation and quarantine, loneliness as an unintended consequence of disease containment measures seems to be particularly problematic for young people. (Achieveing resilience during COVID-19 weekly report 2, 2020).

In another recent study with a rapid systematic review of 63 studies of 51,576 participants found a clear association between loneliness and mental health problems.Loneliness was associated with future mental health problems up to 9 years later. The strongest association was with ***depression***. These findings were consistent across studies of children, adolescents, and young adults. There may also be sex differences, with some research indicating that loneliness was more strongly associated with elevated depression symptoms in females and with elevated social anxiety in males (Loades, et al. 2020)

Studies showing gender differences on how they respond to limitations the COVID-19 measurments brought along, show that many females tended to be more vulnerable to develop the symptoms of various forms of mental disorders during the pandemic, including depression, anxiety, PTSD, and stress, as reported in our included studies (Ahmed et al., 2020; Gao et al., 2020; Lei et al., 2020, Daly&Robinson, 2022).

Comprehensive review of existing evidence about the impact of COVID-19 on mental health and mental health services, includes estimates from the latest Global Burden of Disease study, shows that the pandemic has affected the mental health of young people and that they are disproportionally at risk of suicidal and self-harming behaviours. It also indicates that women have been more severely impacted than men (World Health Organization: WHO, 2022). Females were also reported generally more likely to develop depressive symptoms when compared to their male counterparts (Lei et al., 2020; Mazza et al., 2020; Sønderskov et al., 2020; Wang et al., 2020).

Many risk factors were identified to be associated with symptoms of depression among the COVID-19 pandemic. Participants from the younger age group (≤40 years) presented with more depressive symptoms (Ahmed et al., 2020; Gao et al., 2020; Huang and Zhao, 2020; Lei et al., 2020; Olagoke et al., 2020; Ozamiz-Etxebarria et al., 2020;)

Numerous studies have found that frequent exposure to social media and news related to COVID-19 leads to symptoms of anxiety and stress (Gao et al., 2020; Moghanibashi-Mansourieh, 2020). Additionally, feelings of sadness and anxiety can be exacerbated by repeatedly witnessing community members suffering from the effects of the pandemic through social media and news reports (Li et al., 2020; Beluli L.N., 2022).

Four studies also identified lower education levels as an associated factor with greater depressive symptoms (Gao et al.,2020; Mazza et al., 2020; Olagoke et al., 2020; Wang et al., 2020). A single study by Wang et al., 2020 reported that people with higher education and professional jobs exhibited more depressive symptoms in comparison to less educated individuals and those in service or enterprise industries (Wang et al, 2020). While on the other hand there is shown that symptoms of anxiety and depression increased during the pandemic and were more pronounced among individuals experiencing household job loss, young adults, and women. (Panchal et al. 2023)

Another relevant study, which completed a systematic review and meta-analysis demonstrate that the prevalence of depression during the COVID-19 pandemic was 33.7% in a sample of 44531 people. Epidemiological data indicates that women seem to be more likely to develop depression, and the incidence was highest in the 21 to 40 years age group (Salari, N., et.al (2020). While in the other hand another related study has founded that 1.5 years after pandemic-related social restrictions, "major" depressive syndromes were reported by 40.16% of the respondents (Holm-Hadulla, 2023).

Depression remains a common psychic outcome encountered by COVID-19 patients or as a result of the psycho-physiological effects of the pandemic.

METHODOLOGY

Research Purpose, Objectives and Approach

The main goal of this research is set to evaluate the presence of anxiety and depression symptoms as mental health issues, as consequences due to the pandemic COVID-19 lifestyle and social relation changes, in adult population.

In order to carry out this study we have considered the following objectives:

Identification of the mental health impacts of COVID -19 Pandemic outbreak among the adult population in North Macedonia;
Evaluating anxiety levels and symptoms in different adulthood age groups;
Evaluating the anxiety impact of the population due to the pandemic Covid-19 and its consequences / changes in populations lifestyle and habits;
Evaluating and comparing, the depression levels of women vs. men;
Evaluating depression levels and symptoms in different adulthood age groups;
Comparing and verifying the correlation between anxiety levels and depressive symptoms;
Correlating and proving the achieved anxiety levels in general, with the outcomes of the depression levels among adults;
To understand and verify the factors related to anxiety disorders among men and women regarding their marital status, education and employment status;

Research Objectives

In order to carry out this study we considered the following objectives:

- Correlation between lifestyle changes, anxiety and depression among population;
- Correlation of social relationship changes with anxiety and depression among population;
- Comparative analysis between anxiety and depression disorder levels;
- Comparative analysis between genders, anxiety and depression presence, due to pandemic COVID-19 isolation and restrictions;
- To evaluate the levels of these mental disturbances;
- To identify the factors correlated to anxiety and depression during pandemic COVID-19 among women and men;
- To identify the diversities and similarities among women's and men's mental health, coming from different cities; different age groups, marital status, working status etc.
- To identify the diversities and similarities among adult age groups regarding education status, employment status, financial incomes, etc.;

Hypothesis of Research

The **general Main hypothesis** of our research study is:

H1. There is a positive correlation between the impacts of coronavirus COVID-19 pandemic in lifestyle and social relationships changes and levels of anxiety and depression.

Sub-Hypothesis

H2. Adults who experience higher levels of anxiety are more likely to also suffer from depression as well;
H3. Women are more disposed to experience anxiety and depression than men;
H4. People in early adulthood (19 to 40s) experience lower levels of anxiety and depression, in comparison to those in middle adulthood (41s to 60s+);
H5. Respondents living in cities with higher number of infected / active cases are experiencing higher levels of anxiety and depression than those with lower number of infected and active cases;
H6. People with higher levels of education (master degree or PhD degree) experience higher levels of anxiety and depression in comparison to those with lower educational status;
H7. Jobless people that are looking for a workplace are experiencing higher levels of anxiety and depression in comparison to all other categories of respondent's working statuses (full-time and part-time employees, contracting employees, online working employees, self-employed, retired and those who are jobless and not looking for a workplace).
H8. Retired persons are more anxious than unemployed persons who are not actively trying to find a workplace.
H9. Online working employees are less anxious and depressed than full-time (public sector), and part-time employees.
H10. Full-time employed women are more predisposed to experience depressive symptoms, than full time employed men;
H11. Unemployed man are predisposed to experience greater anxiety and depression than unemployed woman.

MATERIALS AND METHODS

Research Tools

The research tools that we used in this study were divided ***in four sections*** including: *baseline information (demographic data), lifestyle changes and social interaction questionnaire and assessment of anxiety and depression.*

The demographic info-section of the study includes questions about: gender, age, city (hometown), educational level, employment status, relationship status, number of children, number of the family members living in the household and family incomes. In total there are 10 questions designed for the baseline part of the questionnaire.

The second part contains 16 items regarding social distancing and lifestyle changes. To examine the effects of coronavirus (COVID-19) in the mental health among adult in North Macedonia we used the acle of dr. Alan Bernardo named as ***Coronavirus pandemic Anxiety Scale*** which consists 15 items.

And on the other hand for evaluating the depression disorder among adult population, we have used the Patient Health Questionnaire (PHQ- 9). This inventory contains only 9 items and it is reliable, and is closely correlated and essentially interchangeable with the Back Depression Inventory- II. (Peoppe, Moore, Frye, 2013).

Sampling Technique and Study Participants

The Snowball sampling technique was used for collecting information from adult people around the country. In social sciences and statistics research, **snowball sampling** (or **chain sampling**, **chain-referral sampling**, **referral sampling** is a non-probability sampling technique where existing study subjects recruit future subjects from among their acquaintances. Thus the sample group is said to grow like a rolling snowball (Goodman,1961)

An informed message or an invitation was sent to many of my family, friends and acquaintances from different cities and nationalities, with a link attached to the message, requesting for them to willingly participate to respond to our invitation to participate in our online survey and also sharing the same with their family, friends and acquaintances using their social network accounts, such as Fb, Instagram, Viber, WhatsApp etc.

The e-questionnaire was distributed by an online based platform called Survey Planet, which is one of the most used platforms nowadays.

We achieved in total of 911 respondents across the country, from different adult age groups ranging from 19 to 70+ years old, divided in 6 alternatives for better data analyses (19-30, 31-40, 41-50, 51-60,61-69 and 70+) which will be included in three main adult age groups (young adulthood 18-35 years old, Middle agers 36-55 years old and older adulthood 56+ years old).

The respondents were invited personally via a message, asked to willingly fulfill and share the survey link with their contacts through social media. The identity of the respondent was completely anonymous. We decided to add the Respondent Anonymity Assurance in the welcoming message, because we believe that this principle not only protects the identity of the participants but also help us gather more honest opinions or answers, without worrying about the repercussions.

FINDINGS AND CONCLUSIONS

Our first and main hypothesis states that:

"There is a positive correlation between the impacts of coronavirus COVID-19 pandemic in lifestyle and social relationships changes and levels of anxiety and depression".

To provide clear evidence of the correlation coefficient by measuring the strength of a linear association between the three main variables of our study, we used the Pearson and Spearman correlation tests.

Table 1. Spearman correlation test for the main variables

Correlations					
			LS_sum	PHQ_sum	CPAS_sum
Spearman's rho	LS_sum	Correlation Coefficient	1.000	.408**	.434**
		Sig. (2-tailed)	.	.000	.000
		N	900	900	900
	PHQ_sum	Correlation Coefficient	.408**	1.000	.623**
		Sig. (2-tailed)	.000	.	.000
		N	900	900	900
	CPAS_sum	Correlation Coefficient	.434**	.623**	1.000
		Sig. (2-tailed)	.000	.000	.
		N	900	900	900

**. Correlation is significant at the 0.01 level (2-tailed).

The Spearman coefficient shows that there is enough evidence to suggest that the correlation we observed does exist in the population. The coefficient is significant at the 0.01 level ($r<0.01$) indicates that there is an association between the variables, respectively there is a positive correlation.

Lifestyle and social relationships changes during the pandemic correlate significantly positively with depression levels ($r=0.408$), indicating that with the increase of lifestyle and social relationship changes during the pandemic, the depression levels elevate too. Referring to the Interpretation table of Spearman rank – order coefficient correlation the correlation between the variables is ***strong.***

Likewise, lifestyle and social relationships changes correlate positively with Covid-19 Pandemic Anxiety levels, ($p=0.434$), indicating a ***strong relationship*** referring to the *Interpretation table of Spearman rank – order coefficient correlation* in the picture below.

There is also a positive significant correlation (r<0.001) between the variables: anxiety levels and depression levels, meaning that they change together at a constant rate; when the values of one variable increase so will the other variables too- they tend to increase together.

Among these two variables, depression and anxiety, there is almost a very ***strong relations***hip (r=0.623). With these findings we can say that we have achieved to **confirm** our main hypothesis for our research paper.

Table 2. Interpretation table of Spearman rank – order coefficient correlation

Spearman p	Corelation
≥0.70	Very strong relationship
0.40-0.69	Strong relationship
0.30-0.39	Weak relationship
0.20-0.29	Weak relationship
0.01-0.19	No or negligible relationship

Adapted from DAncey and Reidy, 2004

Regarding Pearson correlation data results again confirm the positive significant relationship (r<0.001) among the variables, in which lifestyle and social changes associate in a ***medium strength*** with depression (r=0.403) and also in a medium strength of association with anxiety levels (r=0.427). Likewise depression levels and anxiety levels tend to increase together, since there's a ***large strength of association*** between those two (r=0.633).

Table 3. Pearson correlation test for the main variables

Correlations				
		LS_sum	PHQ_sum	CPAS_sum
LS_sum	Pearson Correlation	1	.403**	.427**
	Sig. (2-tailed)		.000	.000
	N	900	900	900
PHQ_sum	Pearson Correlation	.403**	1	.633**
	Sig. (2-tailed)	.000		.000
	N	900	900	900
CPAS_sum	Pearson Correlation	.427**	.633**	1
	Sig. (2-tailed)	.000	.000	
	N	900	900	900

**. Correlation is significant at the 0.01 level (2-tailed).

Referring to the findings coming from the Pearson and Spearman Correlation tests we can conclude that there is a positive correlation with medium and large strength of association among the variables, therefore we can conclude that our main and first hypothesis is verified.

Table 4. Pearson correlation for depression and anxiety levels

Correlations			
		PHQ_sum	**CPAS_sum**
PHQ_sum	Pearson Correlation	1	.633**
	Sig. (2-tailed)		.000
	N	900	900
CPAS_sum	Pearson Correlation	.633**	1
	Sig. (2-tailed)	.000	
	N	900	900

**. Correlation is significant at the 0.01 level (2-tailed).

According to the data at table 4. we see that ($p<0.001$) meaning that the correlation is statistically significant and the Pearson correlation ($P=.633$) means that there is a large strength of association between the two variables, in other words with the increase of anxiety levels in adults also there is an indication that their depression levels will increase as well, and vice versa. Which brings us to the conclusion that adults who experience higher levels of anxiety are more likely to also suffer from depression as well.

Regarding to gender differences on experiencing depressive and anxiety symptoms we came to the next finding throughout the ANOVA method, that females have higher mean ($M=18.47$) while male's mean for depressive disorder symptoms is ($M=15.43$). Females mean shows to be greater for anxiety levels (($M=31.91$) in comparison to males levels of anxiety ($M=27.58$). These comparisons between the three variables (gender, anxiety levels and depressive levels) have been verified that are statistically important ($p<0.01$) throughout the ANOVA method, which is used to gain information of independent and dependent variables for three or more groups of data.

Figure 1. Gender differences regarding anxiety and depression levels

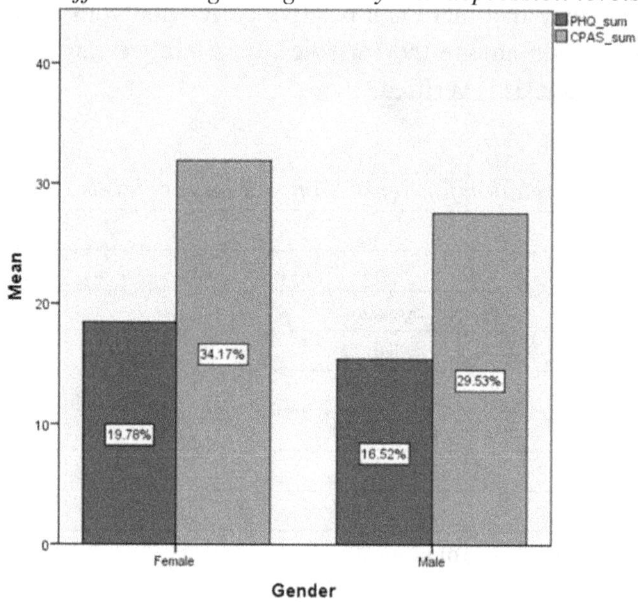

Looking at the Figure 1. it gives us the answer we have been looking for, and as assumed we again identify the women as most sensitive toward the pandemic situation, were as a result they apparently suffer from anxiety and depression more than men do.

According to our findings we discovered that younger agers are more depressive than middle adulthood agers referring to their means (M=17.52) for 19 to 40 agers, in comparison to middle adulthood agers (M=16.14) for 41 to 60 age participants. Looking at the anxiety levels we see that there is no significant difference among the results, since the means of early adulthood and middle adulthood agers are very close (M= 30.12) for early adults, and (M=30.56) for middle adults.

Looking at the means for the variables (look at Table 5), depression levels and anxiety too, we can easily classify that data are very close with one another, and therefore significant difference among them is not identified. With these outcomes we can say that we failed to verify this hypothesis and that depressive and anxiety symptoms are present in respondents no matter if their living town counts large number of infected people by the coronavirus, or less. 'Active case numbers' just don't represent a significant factor related to how much a person would feel depression symptoms or anxiety signs.

Table 5. Variable means in different cities across the country

CITY	SKOPJE	TETOVO	GOSTIVAR	STRUGA	KICHEVO
PHQ	17.45	17.18	18.02	15.71	17.41
CPAS	30.42	30.32	31.93	29.45	27.89

We assumed that people with higher levels of education (master degree or PhD degree) experience higher levels of anxiety and depression in comparison to those with lower educational status but indeed we couldn't find a statistical support on this hypothesis. Throughout statistical data analyses we found that the means for each category are so close to each other that confirm us that there is no statistical difference among them, meaning that we accept null hypothesis ($p>0.05$).

Through this study we found out that respondents that have shown higher levels of depressive disorder, or that experience more depressive symptoms from the list of employee options are those who are employed but work from home ($M=19.40$); (2nd) those that are a part-time employees; (3d) the retired respondents and (4th) those who are jobless but trying to find one. The four employee categories share approximately the same mean regarding depressive disorder symptoms ($M=19$), while the respondends who experience higher levels of anxiety are the retired ($M=38.25$), followed by the ones that are employed and work from home, and part time employees ($M=33.10$).

From these analyses we concluded that the less anxious and depressed were found to be respondents who are full time employees, followed by contract employees and jobless people who are not looking for a workplace.

Considering this, we have conducted the t-test that brought us the following results ($t=3.345, p<0.01$) which means that we reject null hypothesis and emphasize that there is an important statistical difference between the means of the respondents employee status and their anxiety and depression manifestation signs.

Among the full time employees, part time employees and online working people, we found that even though we assumed that working from home would decrease the contagion anxiety from the virus, and people would feel safer by their family side, indeed according to these data we see that when referring to employee depression levels, the employers that work online have higher mean ($M=19.40$) than the two other employee categories ($M=18.93$) ($M=16.20$). The same is valid for the anxiety levels as well, ($M=33.64$) in lead, and followed by part-time employees with ($M=33.10$) and ($M=30.53$) for full time employees.

Regarding these findings we can say that in contrary of our hypothesis, among these three employee categories, the most depressive and anxious employees are those that work from home, online.

While looking at the table 6. we could verify that the data analyses of this complex hypothesis presents the following results; Females that work full time as a state employee experience lower levels of depression (M=17.24) than those working as full timers on private sectors (M=18.72). On the other hand males don't show any difference whether they work as employees in the public or private sector, since data analyses gives us these means (M=14.32; M=14.83).

Referring to these findings we also notice that females bear more depressive symptoms in comparison to males, since their means are greater than those of the male respondents. This hypothesis is verified to be true, according to the above mentioned findings.

Table 6. Descriptive data for gender comparison regarding the employee status and depression.

Descriptives									
PHQ_sum									
Gender		N	Mean	Std. Dev	Std. Error	95% Confidence Interval for Mean		Min	Max
						Lower	Upper		
Female	Full time employee (State Employee)	175	17.24	6.695	.506	16.24	18.24	9	36
	Full time employee (private sector)	86	18.72	8.787	.948	16.84	20.60	9	36
	Part-time employee	24	19.33	7.551	1.541	16.14	22.52	9	32
	Employed, but working from home (online).	16	18.56	6.947	1.737	14.86	22.26	9	30
	Contract employee	31	17.35	5.320	.956	15.40	19.31	9	30
	Self employed	27	19.70	7.405	1.425	16.77	22.63	9	33
	Unemployed, but looking for a workplace.	137	19.82	7.841	.670	18.50	21.15	9	36
	Unemployed, not looking for a workplace	49	17.98	7.739	1.106	15.76	20.20	9	36
	Retired	5	20.80	5.070	2.267	14.51	27.09	16	28
	Total	550	18.47	7.474	.319	17.84	19.10	9	36

continued on following page

Table 6. Continued

Male	Full time employee (State Employee)	97	14.32	6.023	.612	13.11	15.53	9	36
	Full time employee (private sector)	117	14.83	6.022	.557	13.73	15.93	9	36
	Part-time employee	6	17.33	8.140	3.323	8.79	25.88	9	33
	Employed, but working from home (online).	9	20.89	7.976	2.659	14.76	27.02	9	35
	Contract employee	13	14.85	7.381	2.047	10.39	19.31	9	32
	Self employed	39	15.46	6.270	1.004	13.43	17.49	9	33
	Unemployed, but looking for a workplace.	54	17.59	7.411	1.009	15.57	19.62	9	36
	Unemployed, not looking for a workplace	12	15.92	6.445	1.861	11.82	20.01	9	27
	Retired	3	15.33	4.933	2.848	3.08	27.59	12	21
	Total	350	15.43	6.513	.348	14.74	16.11	9	36

Referring to the data descriptive on table 6. where we see that the mean of the unemployed men is lower than the depressive levels of females that are unemployed, in both categories (Unemployed, but looking for a workplace and those that don't look for a workplace).

Males means are (M=17.58; M=15.92), while women means are higher (M=19.32; M=17.98). These results tell us that our hypothesis that noted that Unemployed men are predisposed to experience greater anxiety and depression than unemployed wom-an, is not supported. Men turn out to be less depressed than women if unemployed.

From these findings we can also come to a conclusion that males that are un-employed but looking for a job are more depressed than those who are not trying to find a job; and also women who are trying to find a job are more depressed than those that don't.

Same as for the anxiety levels during the pandemic outbreak, for both females and males that are unemployed, again females are in advantage, with greater means (M=32.36) for unemployed females that are trying to find a job, and (M=30.76) for those females that are jobless but not trying to find one. Also we notice that females that are trying to find a job are more anxious than those that don't.

On the other hand males are less anxious in both alternatives of this item, in comparison to females means regarding anxiety levels when unemployed. Males that are unemployed, but actively trying to find a workplace suffer from anxiety

(M=28.69); while those that are not trying to find a workplace have this mean of anxiety (M=23.08)

We can conclude from all these data analyses, that unemployed women are more depressed and anxious than men, and also that unemployed men and women that are trying to find a workplace are more depressed and anxious than those that are not interested to find a workplace.

These findings are inconsistent with our assumption that males are more depressed and anxious than females if unemployed, therefore we claim that our hypothesis has failed to be proven.

DISCUSSION OF FINDINGS

This research aimed to identify whether the impact of coronavirus COVID-19 through the changes that brought to our lifestyle routines and social relations, have had an impact on elevating anxiety and depression levels. Based on quantitative analyses we have been able to confirm the linear association of these three main variables of our study through Pearson and Spearman correlation test. The results indicate that there is a positive strong correlation among the lifestyle and social relationships changes during the pandemic, with the levels of depression (r=0.408) and anxiety (r=0.434),(see table 32. and 33.). Therefore we conclude that the main purpose of conducting this research study has been verified statistically and we were able to prove that with the increase of lifestyle changes and social relationships changes during the pandemic coronavirus outbreak, adult people of our country have been more anxious and depressed.

These findings are related to the Gao et al.'s (2020) results which had shown much higher prevalence of depression, anxiety and combination of depression and anxiety (CDA) compared to the national prevalence rates in a 2013 study (Huang et al., 2019). The results contradict the claims of Wang, Pan, Wan, Tan, Xu, McIntyre et al. (2020) longitudinal study results which showed that there was no statistically significant difference in the reported levels of depression, anxiety and stress symptoms despite the sharp increase in the number of COVID-19 cases.(Wang, Pan, Wan, 2020). On the other hand, in a recent COVID-19 mental health impact survey conducted by the WHO, results indicate the pandemic has disrupted or halted critical mental health services in 93% of countries worldwide while the demand for mental health is increasing (World Health Organization, 2020c.) Our findings seem to be in the same line with the findings of (Giuntella O.,Hyde K., Saccardo S., and Sadoff S). as the pandemic has tightened the link between lifestyle behaviors and depression. Many other studies comed to same conclusions are (Wang et al. 2020), Serafini et al. (2020), (Li et al., 2020), Xu and Sattar (2020), (Zhang et al. (2020) etc.

Apparently adult population in North Macedonia have had a serious impact on their mental health deriving from the lifestyle changes due to quarantine, isolation and social distancing. The rise in depression and anxiety has occurred at the same time that stay-at-home, work from home and social distancing measures have caused major disruptions to everyday life, altering the way people live, work, study, and interact.

This research also intended to find various details, like whether those participants that experienced higher levels of anxiety are also those who would also experience depression as well. Regarding these data we found out that there was an indication that those who feel anxious were also suffering from depression, and this was an important target of our research study. The correlation between these two variables has been tested through Pearson correlation and the results show a *large strength* of association between them ($r=0.633$).

Related to this finding we can attach many relevant studies which have come to final conclusions that anxiety and depression are two major mental health issues that are most common among the population during the pandemic outbreak. We may mention few of them: Paz, C., Masciliano G., Adana Diaz L., et al (2020). Gennaro Mazza M., De Lorenzo R., Conte C. et al.(2020). Zhang J., Lu H., Zeng H., Zhang S. (2020).

One of the comparisons to emerge from my data analyses was that women are more predisposed to experience anxiety and depression than men. Based on qualitative and quantitative analyses we were able to conclude that 53.64% females suffer from anxiety vs. 46.36 males, and that 54.49% females suffer from depression vs 45.51% males in our population. The difference among these results is statistically significant since ($p<0.01$).

Based on the findings of similar studies (Jefrey Cluger, 2020) where it was concluded that women are almost three times more likely to report suffering from significant mental health consequences. As we have evidences to prove that women in all categories, (employment status, age, marital status etc.,) are more anxious and depressive than man, since they have achieved higher means in all of the mentioned categories.

The literature points that being women is a risk factor for showing worse mental health status during the pandemic (Salari et al., 2020; Abdurrahim.G., Murat.Y.,2020; Pappa et al., 2020; Parrado-González and León-Jariego, 2020; Wenham et al., 2020) worse psychological responses to the pandemic (Justo-Alonso et al., 2020), and higher emotional vulnerability to the effects of the lockdown period (Sandín et al., 2020).

We have failed to prove that depression and anxiety symptoms are more presents on those respondents that live on cities which count larger number of infected people by coronavirus, which means that in other words 'Active case numbers' just don't represent a significant factor related to how much a person should feel threatened, scared, insecure, anxious or depressed.

Our data investigation reviewed whether there was a difference of anxiety levels among respondents within those that hold higher vs. lower educational degree, and through the ANOVA data analyses we concluded that the differences were statistically non-significant ($p>0.05$).

Through these results we can observe and come to an understanding that emotional feedback toward this global issue is more relevant than the weight of educational background. Some, even though may hold an undergraduate degree may spend a lot of time reading or listening to information regarding the coronavirus, its effects and consequences, in comparison to those that may hold higher degree diploma, oer that those that hold lower educational level simply because they don't understand this global concern in the way or in the level those with higher degree do, are more afraid, unsecured, simply more anxious than the others. Coming from this point of view we must neglect the comparison we have set in this hypothesis, and conclude that no matter the educational level, people are anxious and depressed because of the challenge this virus has brought among us.

The employee categories that have shown greater levels of depressive disorder are those who are employed but working from home (M=19.40); jobless but trying to find one (M=19.19), retired respondents (M=18.75) and part time employees (M=18.93). Interestingly, we have come to these results, even though we have had other expectations deriving out of this assumption. We think that the category of people that holds the first place in our rank, regarding the depressive disorder symptoms, which are: the employed people that work from home, are placed as the first because those may face working difficulties while adapting with the online version of work; may have limited working space in their house; may have continuing disturbances or interruptions from other family members; may have greater sense of nostalgia for the co-workers; may feel more insecure in how the productivity of the industry/company will progress in the future; may feel at risk of losing their job.

It is understandable that those persons who don't feel the need to go to work or earn money, simply just don't feel stressed about not having a workplace. Which is not the case for the retired persons as well. Covid-19 became the perfect storm for the depression in older adults. These people tend to suffer from depressive symptoms, even before the pandemic, because loneliness and isolation are serious mental health risk for people, no matter what age.

On the other hand online working employees have shown to be the most depressed (M=19.40) and anxious employees (M=33.64), when in comparison to full time and part-time employees (M=33.10; M=18.93). Of course, coming to such conclusion is quite an interesting finding.

Through my analyses, on the issue that regarded gender differences among full time employees and their depressive levels, we have proved that women feel more depressed than men. We have not specified which category of full time employees show greater levels of depression, therefore we have taken in consideration both of them: full time state employees and full time employees in the private sector.

Our finding aligns with another recent survey which noted that female workers have a higher risk of depression while during the pandemic (Sato K, Sakata R, Murayama C, Yamaguchi M, Matsuoka Y, Kondo N. 2020). Working from home may be more challenging for women, since females tend to be more responsible for household chores and other home activities, and working mothers can feel double the pressure at home due to lack of support with home schooling and taking care of children.

Same goes for the unemployed women vs. unemployed men. Anxiety and depression have shown to be more present at women's lives as an unemployed person (M=19.32; M=17.98) who is concerned about finding a workplace during the pandemic outbreak, in comparison to men who are less depressive and anxious during these times (M=17.58, M=15.92). According to the U.S. Bureau of Labor Statistics, 2.5 million women left the job market since the beginning of the pandemic—compared to 1.8 million men—as they take on more responsibilities of homeschooling and everyday parenting.

CONCLUSION

This chapter will conclude the study by summarizing the key research findings in relation to the research aims and questions and discussing the value and contribution thereof. It will also review the limitations of the study and propose opportunities for future research.

The initially stated overarching aim of this research was to find out the correlation between the life style and social relationship changes during the pandemic outbreak, and its impact on the appearance of anxiety and depression disorders in adult population in North Macedonia. Based on the qualitative and quantitative analyses, the identified research priority has been verified: that the pandemic lifestyle and social relationship changes have been negatively impacting our mental health by increasing anxiety and depression. In other words COVID-19 pandemic and lockdown measures that led to social isolation and home confinement have had a profound impact on the mental health of the adult population in our country.

Throughout this study we were able to prove that anxiety levels and depression levels strongly correlate with one another during the pandemic outbreak. Studies have shown that often anxiety and depressions are co-occurring, and that have complex relationship. People who are depressed often feel anxious and worried and also one can easily trigger the other, with anxiety often preceding depression.

One of the comparisons to emerge from my data analyses was that women are more predisposed to experience anxiety and depression than men in all demographic categories. Many reasons may explain why we have come to such findings and why are the women being so vulnerable to report anxiety and depressive symptoms more than man, such as hormonal factors, the reporting style, the inner women's self-regulation and sensitivity toward interpersonal concerns which of course affects on their vulnerability to these mental issues.

An interesting conclusion deriving from our findings through this research study is that young adults (19-29 years old) are more prone to experience anxiety and depression than other demographics categories. It is understandable that they are at a very critical developmental stage and the challenge of the safety measures that have brought so many life-changes and so many restrictions, may feel like their life is on an endless pause, and their developmental need for "new experiences" is not being met.

We have failed to prove the hypothesis that depression and anxiety symptoms are more presents on those respondents that live on cities which count larger number of infected people by coronavirus, which means that in other words 'Active case numbers' just don't represent a significant factor related to how much a person should feel threatened, scared, insecure, anxious or depressed.

This study found out that no matter the educational degree, the pandemic threat and its impact on our lifestyle and social relationships changes has brought anxiety and depression in people's mental health disregarding the educational level as an essential factor.

Our data proved that people that work from home (online), are those who feel more depressed, most probably because of the lack of the physical activity, decreased communication with colleagues, having more distractions when working from home are also very disturbing, especially if they are a large family or having at least one toddler at home etc. All these and many to count are the reasons why these respondents have shown greater depressive symptoms. However, the respondents that are retired are those who score as the most anxious ones in all numbered employee categories.

On the issue that regarded gender differences among full time employees and their depressive levels, we have proved that women feel more depressed than men. As we have argued elsewhere, obviously women are confronted with depression triggers more than men do. Same goes for the unemployed women vs. unemployed men, where we have come to an understanding that mental health issues such as anxiety and depression are more presents at female's life especially during the COVID-19 pandemic outbreak.

REFERENCES

Abramson, A. (2020). How COVID-19 may increase domestic violenceand child abuse. *American Psychological Association,* April 8, 2020. https://www.apa.org/topics/covid-19/domestic-violence-child-abuse

Ahmed, M. (2020). Tertiary Education during Covid-19 and Beyond. The Daily Star. https://www.thedailystar.net/opinion/news/tertiary-education-during-covid-19-and-beyond-1897321

American Psychiatric Association. (2013). *Diagnostic and Statistical Manual of Mental Disorders* (5th ed.). American Psychiatric Publishing.

Andersen, A. J., Mary-Krause, M., Bustamante, J. J. H., Héron, M., El Aarbaoui, T., & Melchior, M. (2021). Symptoms of anxiety/depression during the COVID-19 pandemic and associated lockdown in the community: Longitudinal data from the TEMPO cohort in France. *BMC Psychiatry*, *21*(1), 381. DOI: 10.1186/s12888-021-03383-z PMID: 34320943

Anderson, R. M., Heesterbeek, H., Klinkenberg, D., & Hollingsworth, T. D. (2020). How will country-based mitigation measures influence the course of the COVID-19 epidemic? *Lancet*, *395*(10228), 931–934. DOI: 10.1016/S0140-6736(20)30567-5 PMID: 32164834

Beluli Luma, N. (2021). Anxiety as a personality trait and anxiety state, during coronavirus COVID-19 pandemic outbreak among adult population. *European Journal of Medicine and Natural Sciences*, *4*(2), 26–42. https://revistia.com/files/articles/ejmn_v4_i2_21/Luma.pdf. DOI: 10.26417/159ueb27t

Berthelot, N., Lemieux, R., Garon-Bissonnette, J., Drouin-Maziade, C., Martel, É., & Maziade, M. (2020). Uptrend in distress and psychiatric symptomatology in pregnant women during the coronavirus disease 2019 pandemic. *Acta Obstetricia et Gynecologica Scandinavica*, *99*(7), 848–855. DOI: 10.1111/aogs.13925 PMID: 32449178

Berzano, L., & Genova, C. (2020). *Lifestyles and Subcultures. History and a New Perspective*. Routledge.

Czeisler, M. É., Lane, R. I., Petrosky, E., Wiley, J. F., Christensen, A., Njai, R., Weaver, M. D., Robbins, R., Facer-Childs, E. R., Barger, L. K., Czeisler, C. A., Howard, M. E., & Rajaratnam, S. M. W. (2020). Mental Health, Substance Use, and Suicidal Ideation During the COVID-19 Pandemic — United States. *MMWR. Morbidity and Mortality Weekly Report*, *69*(32), 1049–1057. DOI: 10.15585/mmwr.mm6932a1 PMID: 32790653

Daly, M., Robinson, E. (2022) Depression and anxiety during COVID-19. The Lancelet, 399,10324, 518

Daniel, K. (2013) Loneliness and Depression among University Students in Kenya? *Global Journal of Human Social Science Art's and Humanities,* pg 11-18, 4(1.0).

Di Renzo, L., Gualtieri, P., Pivari, F., Soldati, L., Attinà, A., Cinelli, G., Leggeri, C., Caparello, G., Barrea, L., Scerbo, F., Esposito, E., & De Lorenzo, A. (2020). Eating habits and lifestyle changes during COVID-19 lockdown: An Italian survey. *Journal of Translational Medicine*, *18*(1), 229. DOI: 10.1186/s12967-020-02399-5 PMID: 32513197

Fiorillo, A., & Gorwood, P. (2020). The consequences of the COVID-19 pandemic on mental health and implications for clinical practice. *European Psychiatry : the Journal of the Association of European Psychiatrists*, *63*(1), e32. DOI: 10.1192/j.eurpsy.2020.35 PMID: 32234102

Fiorillo, A., & Gorwood, P. (2020). The consequences of the COVID-19 pandemic on mental health and implications for clinical practice. *European Psychiatry : the Journal of the Association of European Psychiatrists*, *63*(1), e32. DOI: 10.1192/j.eurpsy.2020.35 PMID: 32234102

Gao, J., Zheng, P., Jia, Y., Chen, H., Mao, Y., Chen, S., Wang, Y., Fu, H., & Dai, J. (2020). Mental health problems and social media exposure during COVID-19 outbreak. *PLoS One*, *15*(4), e0231924. DOI: 10.1371/journal.pone.0231924 PMID: 32298385

Garfin, D. R., Silver, R. C., & Holman, E. A. (2020). The novel coronavirus (COVID-2019) outbreak: Amplification of public health consequences by media exposure. *Health Psychology*, *39*(5), 355–357. DOI: 10.1037/hea0000875 PMID: 32202824

Garfin, D. R., Thompson, R., & Holman, E. A. (2018). Mental and physical health effects of acute stress following traumatic events: A systematic review. *Journal of Psychosomatic Research,* 112, 107-113. retrived from: DOI: 10.1016/j.jpsychores.2018.05.017

Holm-Hadulla, R. M., Wendler, H., Baracsi, G., Storck, T., Möltner, A., & Herpertz, S. C. (2023). Depression and social isolation during the COVID-19 pandemic in a student population: The effects of establishing and relaxing social restrictions. *Frontiers in Psychiatry*, *14*, 1200643. DOI: 10.3389/fpsyt.2023.1200643 PMID: 37608993

Kazdin, A. (2000). Encyclopedia of psychology. Washington, D.C.: American Psychological Association; Oxford [Oxfordshire]; New York: *Oxford University Press*, (OCoLC)763745525.

Kiecolt-Glaser, J., McGuire, L., Robles, T., & Glaser, R. (2002). Emotions, morbidity, and mortality: New perspectives from psychoneuroimmunology. *Annual Review of Psychology*, *53*(1), 83–107. DOI: 10.1146/annurev.psych.53.100901.135217 PMID: 11752480

Loades, M. E. et al. (2020). Rapid Systematic Review: The Impact of Social Isolation and Loneliness on the Mental Health of Children and Adolescents in the Context of COVID-19

Marroquín, B., Vine, V., & Morgan, R. (2020). Mental health during the COVID-19 pandemic: Effects of stay-at-home policies, social distancing behavior, and social resources. *Psychiatry Research*, *293*, 113419. Advance online publication. DOI: 10.1016/j.psychres.2020.113419 PMID: 32861098

Maury, S. (2020). Covid-19 and mental health impact: Women are at greater risk. *The power to persuade*. Retrieved from: https://www.powertopersuade.org.au/blog/covid-19-and-mental-health-impacts-women-are-at-greater-risk/29/6/2020

Mazza, M. G., De Lorenzo, R., Conte, C., Poletti, S., Vai, B., Bollettini, I., Melloni, E. M. T., Furlan, R., Ciceri, F., Rovere-Querini, P., & Benedetti, F. (2020). Anxiety and depression in COVID-19 survivors: Role of inflammatory and clinical predictors. *Brain, Behavior, and Immunity*, *89*, 594–600. DOI: 10.1016/j.bbi.2020.07.037 PMID: 32738287

Moghanibashi-Mansourieh, A. (2020). Assessing the anxiety level of Iranian general population during COVID-19 outbreak. *Asian Journal of Psychiatry*, *51*, 102076. DOI: 10.1016/j.ajp.2020.102076 PMID: 32334409

Olagoke, A. A., Olagoke, O. O., & Hughes, A. M. (2020). Psychological pathways linking public trust during the coronavirus pandemic to mental and physical well-being. *Frontiers in Psychology*, *11*, 570216. Advance online publication. DOI: 10.3389/fpsyg.2020.570216 PMID: 33262724

Panchai, N., Kamal, R., Cox, S., & Garfield, R. (2021) The Implications of COVID-19 for Mental Health and Substance Use. *KFF*, available at: https://www.kff.org/report-section/the-implications-of-covid-19-for-mental-health-and-substance-use-issue-brief/#endnote_link_510918-2

Panchal, N., Saunders, H., Rudowitz, R., & Cox, C. (2023, April 25). The Implications of COVID-19 for Mental Health and Substance Use | KFF. KFF. https://www.kff.org/mental-health/issue-brief/the-implications-of-covid-19-for-mental-health-and-substance-use/

Salari, N., Hosseinian-Far, A., Jalali, R., Vaisi-Raygani, A., Rasoulpoor, S., Mohammadi, M., Rasoulpoor, S., & Khaledi-Paveh, B. (2020). Prevalence of stress, anxiety, depression among the general population during the COVID-19 pandemic: A systematic review and meta-analysis. *Globalization and Health*, *16*(1), 57. DOI: 10.1186/s12992-020-00589-w PMID: 32631403

Servidio, R., Bartolo, G. M., Palermiti, L. A., & Costabile, A. (2021). Fear of COVID-19, depression, anxiety, and their association with Internet addiction disorder in a sample of Italian students. *Journal of Affective Disorders Reports*, *4*(1), 100097. DOI: 10.1016/j.jadr.2021.100097

Shamima, A. P., Priyata, D., & Tamana, K. N.. (2020). COVID-19: Embracing Mental Health Upshot from the Coronavirus Pandemic Crisis. *Journal of Psychiatry and Psychiatric Disorders*, *4*(1), 328–342.

Shetty, P. A., Ayari, L., Madry, J., Betts, C., Robinson, D. M., & Kirmani, B. F. (2023). The Relationship between COVID-19 and the development of Depression: Implications on Mental health. *Neuroscience Insights*, *18*, 26331055231191513. Advance online publication. DOI: 10.1177/26331055231191513 PMID: 37608908

Wang, C., Pan, R., Wan, X., Tan, Y., Xu, L., McIntyre, R. S., Choo, F. N., Tran, B., Ho, R., Sharma, V. K., & Ho, C. (2020). A longitudinal study on the mental health of general population during the COVID-19 epidemic in China. *Brain, Behavior, and Immunity*, *87*(1), 40–48. DOI: 10.1016/j.bbi.2020.04.028 PMID: 32298802

Wang, C., Tee, M., Roy, A. E., Fardin, M. A., Srichokchatchawan, W., Habib, H. A., Tran, B. X., Hussain, S., Hoang, M. T., Le, X. T., Ma, W., Pham, H. Q., Shirazi, M., Taneepanichskul, N., Tan, Y., Tee, C., Xu, L., Xu, Z., Vu, G. T., & Kuruchittham, V. (2021). The impact of COVID-19 pandemic on physical and mental health of Asians: A study of seven middle-income countries in Asia. *PLoS One*, *16*(2), e0246824. DOI: 10.1371/journal.pone.0246824 PMID: 33571297

World Health Organization. WHO. (2022, March 2). COVID-19 pandemic. Retrieved January 26, 2025, from https://www.who.int/news/item/02-03-2022-covid-19-pandemic-triggers-25-increase-in-prevalence-of-anxiety-and-depression-worldwide

Xiong, J., Lipsitz, O., Nasri, F., Lui, L. M. W., Gill, H., Phan, L., Chen-Li, D., Iacobucci, M., Ho, R., Majeed, A., & McIntyre, R. S. (2020). Impact of COVID-19 pandemic on mental health in the general population: A systematic review. *Journal of Affective Disorders*, *277*, 55–64. DOI: 10.1016/j.jad.2020.08.001 PMID: 32799105

Chapter 15
Light in the Face of Contemporary Darkness

Jorge Luis Delgado
Mamani Kontiki Tours, Peru

ABSTRACT

In a world overwhelmed by negative narratives and relentless information, human sensitivity is diminishing, turning individuals into indifferent beings. Despite this decline, hope remains in fostering genuine human values through discussions and self-awareness. The American Andes, especially Cusco's Vilcabamba and Machu Picchu, symbolize enlightenment, where the cosmic energies of Father Sun and Pachamama restore balance, guiding us toward selfless learning (Yachay), love (Munay), and meaningful work (Llankay).

INTRODUCTION

The world we currently live in presents and represents itself before our eyes, minds, and weakened consciousness in many, sometimes negative ways. It does so with stinging, insistent global information about facts and events that basically report deaths and recount catastrophes in an unstoppable inventory of the deterioration of life, society, and culture (Baudrillard, 1994; Postman, 1985). As direct or indirect protagonists, we react with little to no sensitivity to these day-by-day occurrences, admitting and encompassing them with a superficial, simple, linear perspective (Sontag, 2003). Deplorable everyday life and disturbing incidents harden us, turning us into automaton-like, insensitive beings (Chouliaraki, 2006). We measure daily information of dubious honesty, and uncertain plausibility with an air of indifference. The stakeholders of today's world have turned our existence

DOI: 10.4018/979-8-3373-0360-4.ch015

into a tragic representation, and this is why we require authors of worth and human and spiritual mettle (Zuboff, 2019).

Fortunately, not everything is lost. Faced with these varied scenarios of decomposition, we feel the urge to model, using mechanisms, to analyze and defend real human values, through criticism or the experience of manifestations of our inner energy to scrutinize realities and eliminate negativity (Freire, 1970). In order to do this, we organize conversations where we mix mitigating factors little by little, generating those advanced individuals, with a will for change, join groups seeking authenticity and a better quality of life (Taylor, 1991). A life not of opulence and waste, but one of protection, helping them find alternatives to face the current collapse of the contemporary world where the onslaught of information technology reveals that we are living on the edge of precarious extremes of abusive social and cultural intolerance (Bauman, 2000; Klein, 2014). It is paradoxical that in the world of reason, irrationality that corrodes the spirit and threatens life, nature, and the gifts that arise from establishing contact with the energy of the universe, is imposed with such fervor (Morin, 2007; Berry, 1999).

It can be noted that the reasoning that comes from science, logic, and Communication and Information Technology (ICT), which produces enlightenment, established customs and scientific knowledge; when used by political leaders, is shamelessly violated with impunity because it roams throughout the region, flies through every mind, and disturbs our imagination (Latour, 2004). It becomes even more serious when the global population of all ages starts to condition its own life by using communication tools and instruments such as social networks, applications, and the Internet, in a dehumanized way, becoming dependent automata (Turkle, 2011; Han, 2017).

Faced with that reality, the American Andes, spiritually and mentally circumnavigating the Cusco mountain range of Vilcabamba, where the eternal life of Machu Picchu shines radiating energy to the Sacred Valley of the Incas, in a permanent return to the immense Altiplano where the Titicaca lake shines splendidly, we have found a real world of enlightenment that directly arises from the Sun, which we call Father Sun, and from Pachamama, which together organize and rejuvenate the spirit of humans who come to them (Arnold & Yapita, 2006). Pachamama and Father Sun Walk and move in a permanent motion to reach us with energy and knowledge and revive our values of: learning without selfishness, which is Yachay, loving without egotism, which is Munay, and working without fatigue or annoyance, which is Llankay. This trilogy receives the cosmic energy from Father Sun and cleanses the spirit of humans who reunite with themselves by attending to the nature of the infinite and nearby universe that lives within us when we turn to Father Sun and Mother Earth (Delgado, 2014).

TECHNOLOGICAL MANIPULATION THREATENS GLOBAL WELL-BEING

It is irrefutably evident that science has revealed various mysteries and accomplished

greatness that produces comfort and material well-being, both due to the magnitude of what benefits modern societies, and the importance that scientific knowledge, applied to various disciplines and fields, radiates. However, and although it may seem paradoxical, it has done so not only through the work, thought, and experimentation of hundreds of well-motivated scientists, but has extended, grown, and been disseminated more by the deliberate action of modern economic operators eager to massify and extend the uses of scientific achievements proposed in the realms of biology, neuroscience, nuclear physics, quantum mechanics, and chemistry in various connections, as well as in the exchange of information between people, communities, and significant social sectors.

Science has spectacularly advanced communications and permeates all aspects of human existence and activity due to the implicit technological determinism it has caused through the flourishing of digital tools such as Social Networks, applications, the Internet, email, etc., which chain and condition people's lives. These Information and Communication Technology (ICT) tools are used to the point of exacerbation through the intrusion of merchandising techniques that without interruption, condition and modify people's lives on a daily basis. The market, in this version of chaos, taking advantage of the achievements of science and technology, engulfs people's minds, tying their will to these new applications, determining their lives to these new dependencies thus, creating a world of conditioning (Zuboff, 2019; Han, 2017).

So, we are witnessing growth with emotional disorders exacerbated by the application of various proposals, from playful to technical, supported and strengthened by Artificial Intelligence, AI. And it is here, by the work and action of technological growth, that I convey a direct observation: The world today, in the face of the unstoppable development of technology, which only reaches us through artificial means of induced, growing and galloping electricity, has turned the human being into a "Subject-Object", dependent on artificial light and not on the natural, benevolent, clean, and energizing Light from which we are increasingly distancing ourselves, and only accept as part of a daily routine, not as a bond that brings us liberation, revelation, and spiritual strength. No exaggeration, I would say that nowadays we are plugs, light bulbs, applications, and we only have eyes to look at colors recreated on computer screens, cell phones, or televisions, which distance us from the beauty of Mother Nature, making us disdainful or indifferent towards her. This is a tremendous deviation that places us on the brink of the abyss and threatens the continuity and serenity of contemporary civilization and its creative potential.

All of these inclinations and applications, dominations and dependencies have led to the emergence of different scientific specializations and compartments to carry out new approaches to reality, while, in a way, the emerging global populations act with extreme dependency on these new technological instruments and tools, especially, as I emphasize, those originating from and dominated by Information and Communication Technology, ICT.

In the face of these dominant communications, it is crucial for human beings to turn around and start looking within themselves, illuminated, blessed, and strengthened by the divine Light of the cosmos without delusion. The energy and life that comes from Father Sun benefits us daily and offers life. Without it existence could not continue, and with it, every human being can begin to cleanse and recover their existence by eliminating excrescences and negative energies (Delgado, 2014).

It's more technology for death.

And so, an evil creature has been improperly strengthened and grown. Technologized science, almost absorbingly transformed into technology for the production of lethal weapons, has diversified little by little, cloaking its findings in tirelessly crafted and attractive garments of powerful exhibitionism to handle death when it produces, obtains, displays, and uses an unscrupulous exploration of the hidden potentialities of technology in the service and development of interspatial or combat weapons in the varied social, political, religious, and cultural scenarios we live in today. The technology of death has reached horrifying levels of destruction and annihilation, and in the face of that, we are left with the task of sowing spirits and values to broaden wills to build a culture of peace and reconciliation. This can start from the Peruvian Andes, where magical Cusco and the splendid Lake Titicaca can revitalize us. And proposing this is not exaggerating because these are privileged scenarios where cosmic energy approaches us more easily.

It is not an overstatement that, due to the growth of technology applied by owners of laboratories and factories of technological goods through profit-driven operators, the world is one step away from succumbing to extermination because of the technological era, where genetic maps and DNA can be manipulated. In the face of such eventualities, people live in anxiety and distress, feeding on daily impotence and modern anguish. What is modern anguish? It is the anxiety that invades the spirit of people in the face of global misgovernance, causing trauma, provoking helplessness, and annihilating hope. Against this evidence, we must organize and regroup the strength of spirit linked to cosmic energy and the genius of nature, as I stated more than 30 years ago.

If we recall what wars were like, we would have to admit that a conflagration in the 19th century, before mustard gas appeared, was not so destructive and only gunpowder was the deadly star. Today, with the threat of growth, hyper-technology, death by computer, and the digital killing of defenseless populations, we observe that brave and even reckless actions are increasingly rare, and the heroism of fighters has disappeared. Today, due to sophisticated devices that sow death with impunity, we have alarming scenarios of dehumanization and violence. This is chilling, because these unpunished actions continue, armed and imbued with hatred, fanaticism, and unbridled ambitions. That is the current state of events we must face and urgently be aware of.

Technology is a new creation that seems to be the product of a wicked alliance between the Hydra of Lerna and technological trade products, where there is no need to behead it like in the Greek myth. Today that modern Hydra of Lerna, which is Information and Communication Technology, spontaneously sprouts two heads and then more, many heads without the need to decapitate the modern monster. Everything grows due to the multiplication of information that progresses and adds more heads, as if it has become a modern monster with thousands of heads that reproduce, and here lies the danger: they no longer reproduce in the same Hydra of Lerma, but they reproduce and grow in all their current and modern offspring, which is all of us using that technology. The trend is to penetrate our brain where our heads today are facsimile reproductions that lose individuality, distance themselves from solidarity values, and disdain collective realities. We are copies and duplicates susceptible to mass commercialization.

Technological science has indeed become a monster where mythology functions not as something unreal, but as something tangible that becomes a fearsome and unstoppable reality whose growth we encourage due to our dependence. Technology has gone from a timid and babbling baby to a boisterous teenager, and today it has grown excessively, becoming a kind of modern and destructive Cyborg, turning all of us into small family-level Cyborgs that erode the foundations of our own families.

Human Interconnection With Cosmic Energy

In this reality, it is not only convenient but urgent to start confronting the assaults on the human spirit that, due to excessive consumerism and individualism, are beginning to minimize or dull it.

What to do in the face of this global deterioration where few people perceive the environmental decline and the gradual degradation of social life with concern? What is crucial in this dilemma is that human beings return to the simple life of communication with ourselves and with the environment and that we enhance our human and supportive life, and this will happen if we return to nature, not only to defend it from an ecological point of view, which is also necessary, but to become one with it. Entering nature and reclaiming its vital energy within ourselves is necessary to become one with its essence and energies and to transform it into our benefactor and life-giving home.

The manifest intention is not only to find placidity and respite in nature and rest on it as on a holiday in the valley. In the welcoming place of beneficial landscapes or the whisper of trees and the murmur of flowing water, we shall find our mother and sister nature, which we must feel and accept as our true home and source of energy that heals and rejuvenates the soul and renews the spirit. This will initially be a challenge and later become routine, because we will gradually come to establish connections with cosmic energy through meetings and special sessions.

Nowadays, when stress arises at every turn and grows daily in people from all corners of the world, it is urgent to overcome it in a creative and proactive way without dragging along the aftermath or consequences of prostration.

And let's admit it once and for all. The solution for health and wholeness is not one that arises exclusively from medications and drugs sold in pharmacies or apothecaries, which we visit when we feel unwell and need repair and rehabilitation of our physiology and functioning. Rather, health is recovered or not easily lost if we live in the scent of nature and in contact with the environmental energy that comes from Father Sun and flutters by our side as cosmic energy. The condition of reclaiming life with intensity and quality will be called Salutogenic energy, that is an energy that produces Health and is obtained without medication or medical consultations, nor living as a patient and sufferer, but living as an active believer that on the other side of our indifference or modern disbelief, Mother Nature, Pachamama, and Father Sun are with us and for us, as part of the creation of life and its endurance and perpetuation.

It is remarkable that in this time of bewilderment, daily stress, and the distress of suffering populations and vast sectors of people enduring exclusion and violence, our will to reconnect with the truth and seek, contrary to isolation, a reunion with cosmic energy as a path to revitalize our existence, is beginning to grow. Thus, one of the current challenges is to return to nature, to be less urban and distanced from one another, and to gradually become conscious users of Information and Communication Technology, not its conditioned and dominated slaves. If we wish to improve our lives with criteria of truth and revelation, it is time to return to the maternal womb, which is nature, and do so in search of the energy that arises within it due to its close relationship with Father Sun. You have to admit, dear readers, that there is no closer relationship than that of life and the permanent and unperturbed continuation of the existence of all living beings whose home is the Earth or Pachamama with the Sun or Father Sun. That permanent unity offers life to plants and animals and has nourished human beings for millennia. It is to that world of simple and intense reality, that we must return.

Beyond Formal Reason and Return to Nature

New reasoning arises from our feelings and our heart, kindled by our heartbeats and rejuvenated by our emotions. This is the true motivation for life that fights without offending or overwhelming, and this vital reason must prevail to renew our world. This possesses the logic of conviction and is nourished by a liberating feeling and suggestion, which leads us to contact the Light and illumination that comes from the energy of Father Sun, which unfortunately many disdains, and is revelation and contact. It is neither a logical nor a descriptive process. It is an epiphany. The truth of this vital motive lies within us and invites us to connect and understand ourselves with the cosmos and the energy of Father Sun.

And then when we enter and submerge our mind in the Andean world, we must know that Pachamama is a divinity that lavishes daily life and existence and provides uncontaminated natural food to meet the needs of populations (Greene, 2009). Therefore, especially from Machu Picchu and the entire Sacred Valley, it has established a unique and magnificent circuit of approach to the eternity of life that is in us when we reach fullness and have stripped ourselves. Contemplating the magnificence created and modeled since the Incas by visionary and foresighted action of Pachacutec and his knowledge of Pachayachachi, this adds and unites all the physical elements that surround this environment complemented by the ancient and splendid singularity that is Lake Titicaca, where it is possible to meet again with oneself through guided visits and training sessions and recreate the small environment of the nearby landscape and the large one that involves the sidereal journey (Andean Cosmology, n.d.). We can do it with techniques that are sustained in playfulness as a permanent practice that allows us to initiate tenuous dialogues with the environment and then come to converse with the stars and initiate trips to the depths of our being to clean our negative and heavy energies of hatred, grudges, excessive ambitions, and bad character, and begin to flourish feeding the will to grow in union and affection and detachment of all the immediate matter and travel towards our inner self to purify ourselves. Throughout this journey I talk to the groups of participants and inform them of the peculiarities of the Andean World, as well as the hidden and encrypted forces and potentialities that we all possess, but modern civilization has hidden from us, especially the one that was violently imposed almost 500 years ago when the western world brought other beliefs and different lifestyles that broke the bond of man and woman with the Andean World (Andean Shamanism, n.d.).

That process of energizing and cleansing is carried out, accompanied by the Andean essence of sharing, of letting go of the heavy energies of selfishness, violence, and indifference that make us distance ourselves or despise the particularities of our fellow beings because we believe that the vicissitudes and sufferings of others do not concern us, when we should internalize ourselves in the physical and human environment that surrounds us and become dynamic and diligent actors. Overcoming apathy and taking action are the best exercises to honor life and get closer to nature. To act and proceed by generating good towards others, even if the objective is not achieved, is already a step forward that projects us towards positive energy and brings us closer to the truth of life that arises from Pachamama, who gives everything without demanding anything in return, and from Father Sun, who bestows his energy upon us and gives us daily light and illumination without losing composure or getting discouraged by the misdeeds caused by human beings possessed by greed and violence (Andean Cosmology, n.d.).

We then embark on a purification of the mind through the practice of slow breathing exercises to recognize our Solar Plexus and body relaxation as a prelude to first achieving an initial catharsis of cleansing and recognition of the intrinsic values we possess, and then feeling that our body and mind hold a liberating reason for cleansing to create a musical and harmonizing reality. Reaching that point is the beginning of emotional rejuvenation.

Formal logic and the canons upon which the structure of scientific and philosophical knowledge are built argue and maintain that thought is not knowledge, validating epistemological categories of formality, sequence, and logic to obtain results (Lakoff et al., 1999). However, if thought is accompanied by feeling, we will obtain real knowledge, ornamented with a human face and truth revealed by our own convictions (Varela et al., 1991). To know in order to enter the world of energy and spirit that Father Sun bestows is to understand that what we feel is real and transports us to the ultimate truth that lives within us (Arnold et al., 2006; de la Cadena, 2010; Delgado, 2014).

And let's go to the revealing tripod of love, wisdom, and work

It is a shame that afflicts many people who analyze the world we live in to realize the enormity of how much the concept of love has been distorted in the contemporary world, which has almost been frozen to the affectionate and passionate relationship between a man and a woman or to the good and sporadic feelings that parents bestow upon their children, precisely because they are their children, and it has been hidden that love is a superior value that ennobles people, because love is stability and an optimal relationship with everything that makes up our environment (Delgado, 2014; Vásquez, 2010). Plants, dawn and animals are loved and protected, and there is dialogue with them. Love is not the grandiose, ethereal, and elusive feeling that compels us to reach out and conquer a person to satisfy carnal or circumstantial appetites. Loving is selfless dedication to all living beings, and thus, loving is growing in kindness and recovering and reconnecting with oneself and doing it every day after understanding that love is not possession and should not be subject to spite, hatred, and harboring despicable feelings (Delgado, 2014).

Love in the Andean World possesses the beautiful word Munay, which alludes to the idea that everything that exists is a divine gift bestowed by nature, which all human beings are part of (Allen 2002; Inca Medicine School, 2023). Unfortunately, we have forgotten this condition. In the Andean World, reality is a challenge and not a punishment, and when faced with a lack of water, efforts are made with love to install and supply that vital liquid for the service and use of local populations.

There is evidence of it in several sites in Cusco which the Incas transformed into meticulous settings for travel and water playgrounds. We can see how the water flows, how it reaches a corner and turns, and arrives and flutters through different channels, and jumps and illuminates and shines with the Light of Father Sun. In Machu Picchu, which seems like an impregnable fortress due to the high altitude it was built on, the water was supposed to be foreign and distant, carried from the river's source. But no, the blessed water of life flows through channels and reaches the highest parts of that cosmic stage (Wright & Valencia Zegarra, 2000). And everything has been created with love because nature is beautiful and lovely, and its mere presence uplifts us. That is love, it is Munay, it is dedication and affection that is complemented by knowledge, which is wisdom.

In the Andean World, knowledge is not merely knowing because it is linked and oriented towards wisdom that allows us to understand and comprehend that human beings come and live in the world to know by serving, to learn by acting, to achieve commonwealth, and proceed with balance and sensibility. In the Andean World, knowledge is not just about knowing and being skilled; it is about acquiring and bringing wisdom to life, which means mastering without overpowering and knowing how to educate and motivate. In the Andean World, knowledge is called Yachay, and there is a whole set of practices surrounding Yachay that honor knowledge and strengthen individual and communal learning (Allen, 2002; Tengö et al., 2014). Wisdom presides over decisions and is a constitutive part of work or Llankay in Quechua (Vásquez, 2010).

Let's remember that the world is falling apart due to the actions of ambitious and soulless human beings, but it can regain vital energy and redeem itself through the actions of men and women who consider themselves Lupijaqui: children of the Sun, taking stellar roles in the reconstruction of the world and the stabilization of its emotional balance by illuminating and cleansing people (Delgado, 2014).

Let's remember that Western work heavily weighs the divine admonition that was inflicted on Adam when he was expelled from the earthly paradise and was punished by saying, "you will eat and live in suffering and earn everything with the sweat of your brow." That curse has become a condemnation where humans contract and summon effort and attention to face obstacles and overcome the challenges that arise in daily life. From the biblical and Western point of view, this has been defined as punishment. That real or uncertain, but highly impactful and widely disseminated definition, which made people believe that work is a condemnation and punishment, diminished its sublime condition of a triumphant action through individual effort that reaches great significance when work is seen as service and is organized through concerted actions (Eliade, 1987). In the Andean World, work, or Llankay, is a daily triumph, it is physical satisfaction, and gratitude towards nature presenting us these challenges, to which in response, we develop efforts and virtues (Allen, 2002).

So, as the final point of this chapter, the universe of our readers must admit that salvation or the improvement and recovery of life rests within themselves and the daily connection that arises from the Light bestowed upon us by Father Sun.

Turn your gaze to the Andean World and recharge energy from Cusco and Machu Picchu and the legendary and immense inland sea that Lake Titicaca is (Gose, 2008; Wright & Valencia Zegarra, 2000).

REFERENCES

Allen, C. J. (2002). *The Hold Life Has: Coca and Cultural Identity in an Andean Community*. Smithsonian Institution Press, ISBN : 1588340325, 312pp.

Andean Cosmology. (n.d.). *Andean Encounters*. Retrieved from https://andeanencounters.com/andean-cosmology/

Andean Shamanism. (n.d.). *Mark Nelson*. Retrieved from https://www.marknelson.io/blog/andean-shamanism

Arnold, D. Y., & Yapita, J. D. (2006). *The Metamorphosis of Heads: Textual Struggles, Education, and Land in the Andes*. University of Pittsburgh Press., DOI: 10.2307/j.ctt5hjrn0

Baudrillard, J. (1994). *Simulacra and Simulation*. University of Michigan Press.

Bauman, Z. (2000). *Liquid Modernity*. Polity Press.

Berry, T. (1999). The Great Work: Our Way into the Future, Crown; Reprint edition, IBSN: 0609804995, 241pp.

Chouliaraki, L. (2006). The Spectatorship of Suffering. *Sage (Atlanta, Ga.)*. Advance online publication. DOI: 10.4135/9781446220658

De la Cadena, M. (2010). Indigenous cosmopolitics in the Andes: Conceptual reflections beyond "politics". *Cultural Anthropology*, *25*(2), 334–370.

Delgado, J. L. (2014). *Andean Awakening: An Inca Guide to Mystical Peru*. Inner Traditions. https://www.innertraditions.com/books/andean-awakening

Eliade, M. (1987). *The Sacred and the Profane: The Nature of Religion*. Harcourt Brace Jovanovich.

Gose, P. (2008). *Invaders as Ancestors: On the Intercultural Making and Unmaking of Spanish Colonialism in the Andes*. University of Toronto Press. DOI: 10.3138/9781442688407

Greene, S. (2009). *Customizing Indigeneity: Paths to a Visionary Politics in Peru*. Stanford University Press.

Han, B.-C. (2017). *Psychopolitics: Neoliberalism and New Technologies of Power*. Verso Books. https://www.versobooks.com/products/2604-psychopolitics

Klein, N. (2014). *This Changes Everything: Capitalism vs. the Climate*. Simon & Schuster., https://thischangeseverything.org/

Lakoff, G., & Johnson, M. (1999). *Philosophy in the Flesh: The Embodied Mind and Its Challenge to Western Thought*. Basic Books.

Latour, B. (2004). Why has critique run out of steam? From matters of fact to matters of concern. *Critical Inquiry, 30*(2), 225–248. DOI: 10.1086/421123

Morin, E. (2008). *On Complexity*. Hampton Press.

Munay: The Spiritual Heart of the Andean World. (2025). *Inca Medicine School*. Retrieved from https://incamedicineschool.com/blog/munay-the-spiritual-heart-of-the-andean-world/

Postman, N., & Postman, A. (2005). *Amusing Ourselves to Death: Public Discourse in the Age of Show Business*. Viking Penguin.

Ruth, R., & Janowitch, L. (2014). Pedagogy of the oppressed. In *Encyclopedia of Critical Psychology* (pp. 1342–1346). DOI: 10.1007/978-1-4614-5583-7_610

Sontag, S. (2003) *Regarding the Pain of Others*. Farrar, Straus and Giroux, ISBN0141012374 https://www.peterlang.com/document/1110546

Taylor, C. (1992). *The Ethics of Authenticity*. Harvard University Press., https://www.hup.harvard.edu/books/9780674268630 DOI: 10.4159/9780674237117

Tengö, M., Brondizio, E. S., Elmqvist, T., Malmer, P., & Spierenburg, M. (2014). Connecting diverse knowledge systems for enhanced ecosystem governance: The multiple evidence base approach. *Ambio, 43*(5), 579–591. DOI: 10.1007/s13280-014-0501-3 PMID: 24659474

Turkle, S. (2011). *Alone Together: Why We Expect More from Technology and Less from Each Other*. Basic Books., https://basicbooks.com/titles/sherry-turkle/alone-together/9780465031467/

Varela, F. J., Rosch, E., & Thompson, E. (1991). *The Embodied Mind*. DOI: 10.7551/mitpress/6730.001.0001

Vásquez, M. A. (2011). *More than belief: A materialist theory of religion*. Oxford University Press.

Waller, D. (2021) Journeying Through The Munay-Ki, Blurb, ISBN: 0368328309, 128pp.

Wright, K. R., & Valencia Zegarra, A. (2000). *Machu Picchu: A Civil Engineering Marvel*. ASCE Press. DOI: 10.1061/9780784404447

Zuboff, S. (2019). *The Age of Surveillance Capitalism: The Fight for a Human Future at the New Frontier of Power*. PublicAffairs.

Chapter 16
Balancing the Burden: Black Male Educators Navigating Duty, Identity, and Self-Care in Higher Education

Antione D. Tomlin
https://orcid.org/0000-0002-1639-7917
Anne Arundel Community College, USA

Kenneth Gilliard
Anne Arundel Community College, USA

ABSTRACT

As Black men in higher education, we navigate a complex interplay of societal, personal, and professional expectations. Often tasked with mentoring and uplifting all students with an emphasis on Black male students, we are simultaneously denied the time, space, and support needed for our own well-being. This delicate balancing act forces us to prioritize others while grappling with our own growth and self-care. Our experiences, though varied, highlight the critical need for institutions to create, support, fund, and invest in spaces that recognize and celebrate Black male educators even more than they already do. By sharing our stories in this chapter, we seek to shed light on the challenges we face and inspire meaningful dialogue about reshaping higher education to better engage and support Black male faculty and staff. Our call to action is clear: institutions must foster a culture that enables Black male educators to thrive, offering tools and opportunities for self-care while empowering us to uplift all emerging minds and future scholars.

DOI: 10.4018/979-8-3373-0360-4.ch016

INTRODUCTION

As Black men, we are often burdened with a complex web of personal, societal, and professional expectations and assumptions, which we are left to navigate. In many professional settings, particularly in higher education, we are not only expected to show up and perform but also to serve as role models, mentors, and caretakers for our students and colleagues, all while striving to maintain our own sense of strength and identity (Tomlin, 2022). There is a special emphasis on our Black male students as we, Black male professional staff, only represent 3% of the full-time higher education personnel (NCES). Yet, despite these demands, we are frequently denied the time, space, and institutional support necessary to care for ourselves. We are entrusted with the responsibility of being our brother's keeper—protecting and guiding others—without being offered the tools, guidance, or opportunities to protect and nurture ourselves. Though role models are sparse and lack of guidance is plenty, we still strive to make a difference every day embracing our students as our own (Broughton et al., 2025; Turner & Grauerholz, 2017).

In this way, our lived experiences become a delicate balancing act, navigating the tension between our professional duties, personal growth, and the ongoing necessity of prioritizing our own well-being (Tomlin & Davis, 2022). The dilemma we face is not just one of time or resources, but of how to invest in our own development and self-awareness while simultaneously being called to invest in the development of others, particularly within the ever-evolving landscape of higher education. While we speak from the perspective of Black male faculty and staff in higher education, we recognize that our experiences, though deeply interconnected, are not monolithic. Our individual stories may differ, but together they illuminate the critical need to create spaces for Black male growth, recognition, and celebration within the academy. We assert that our diverse experiences are not a singular narrative but part of a broader mosaic of Black male educators' lived realities. Each story, including our own, contributes to a fuller understanding of the challenges and triumphs we face in higher education, and the ways in which institutions can better support us as we work to uplift Black male students.

By sharing our lived and learned experiences of navigating higher education as Black men, we aim to give voice to the often-overlooked challenges we face in the profession. Our goal is not only to raise awareness but also to spark a much-needed conversation on how to reshape the landscape of higher education to more effectively engage, support, and retain Black male educators. In doing so, we hope to inspire educators, administrators, policymakers, and others to consider new, meaningful solutions that can lead to tangible, but not pacified change. Ultimately, our stories are an invitation to reconsider how institutions can cultivate a more inclusive, anti-racist, self-aware, and supportive culture—one that allows all educators, particularly

Black male educators, to thrive. We will also offer recommendations for how this transformation can begin, with the aim of creating an environment where Black male educators can not only support others but also feel supported themselves.

While there are increasingly more Black males, both students and professionals in higher education spaces, the support for both can be lackluster at times (Tomlin, 2023). We make this claim, knowingly considering the push to support Black folks in higher education within previous years. As Black male practitioners and authors of this chapter, we feel the pressure to support Black male students and the joy and burden of being everything to everyone in our spears, personally and professionally. We do not take this responsibility lightly, and often, we find that we do not know where or who to turn to when the load is so heavy that we are running toward fatigue, burnout, and exhaustion with no rest stop in sight. Within our stories, we share how all of the weight impacts our mental health and the very heavy and real challenges that come with being a minority professional in higher education (Arday, 2022). With our voices, narratives, and live and learned experiences, we hope that colleagues, administrators, policy-makers, board members, and other stakeholders will hear us, believe us, and support us, as we quite literally support the rest of the world of higher education in many ways. Enough is enough, but we do not often get to say that, we must push forward, despite our needs. So, this chapter screams to everyone around us that the burden is too heavy to carry alone; enough is enough.

This chapter aims to amplify our voices, experiences, and agency as Black male educators. In 1986, Cole made the claim that the Black educator is an endangered species. Here we are in 2025, making a similar claim, specifically for Black male educators (Cole, 1986). Therefore, this serves as a call to action—a ringing of the alarm. As Black men, we often feel the weight of having to navigate these challenges alone, but we cannot and should not have to do it by ourselves. This is a charge to our colleagues: we need your support, even when we don't explicitly ask for it. Show up for us, check in with us, and be the team player for us that we consistently strive to be for everyone else. Together, we can create a more inclusive and supportive environment for all.

DISTINCT PATHS, SHARED PURPOSE: PERSONAL NARRATIVES AND PROFESSIONAL REALITIES

It is important for us to situate and orient readers to who we are—Antione and Kenny—and how we have structured this chapter. Our narrative combines personal experiences with the broader context of Black male expectations and experiences as reflected in the literature. Throughout this chapter, you will notice recurring reflections from our lived and learned perspectives. We want to emphasize that these experiences are uniquely ours. We do not attempt to generalize or encapsulate the experiences of all Black male educators, as there is no one-size-fits-all journey. Even as close friends with overlapping experiences, we recognize that our individual paths are distinct. In this section, we briefly explore some of our past experiences and the motivations behind our work as Black male educators in higher education. Throughout this chapter, our voices may blend at times or diverge, and we encourage you to engage intentionally with our stories, noting both the similarities and differences in our journeys.

Kenny: Carrying the Weight: A Journey of Leadership, Sacrifice, and Self-Discovery

I consider myself a community curator, creator of positive vibes, and custodian of great experiences. Being deeply involved since I was young and committed to everything I associate my name with can be a blessing and a curse. My partners in crime are my saboteurs who walk a fine line of when enough is enough or too much. Oftentimes, taking on more than I may have the bandwidth for in order to be a hero and press on. Some cases were self-imposed, others unwarranted. I say this as an educator, mentor, entrepreneur, track and field coach, life and engagement coach, and fraternity man, among a plethora of additional hats I wear. I am not immune to "Man up," "Be strong," "Stop complaining," and " I did it so you can too,"... voices that echo with no singular author. Yet, I've witnessed my story, and those similarities are reflected in the many students that I have come across.

This journey of mine is a culmination of my experiences and sacrifices not only of my own but my family, both seen and unseen. Born and raised in Philadelphia, Pennsylvania I consider myself blessed to have both parents along with four siblings navigating this thing called life. As a first-generation Black male, I was not always the best and brightest, nor did I make the best decisions from time to time. Seeing friends and family put six feet deep or behind bars, I had a mission. Fortunately, I had a diverse array of educational experiences growing through life. I attended a computer magnet elementary school, an afro-centric middle school, and a catholic high school. From there I went to a private predominantly white institution (PWI) to pursue a degree in civil engineering for a year (five semesters to be exact) on an academic/athletic scholarship to run track. After taking my pre-major general education courses, I decided to change my major and try to figure life out. At this point, when I moved into my freshman dorm, my family decided to relocate to North Carolina, so my parents uprooted me and brought me down to the south. This is where I attended a community college receiving my associate in art and an associate in general education. While there, I encountered Ernie D. Charles, my first Black male professional staff as my advisor to the Student Government Association (SGA) and our Minority Male Mentoring Program at the time. I had a few memorable teachers and coaches throughout my life but he was my first mentor who took me by the hand and helped lead me during this period of my life.

Afterwards, I continued to further my education at a public PWI obtaining my Bachelors in Art with a concentration in English. Once there, I felt stuck. In a pattern of saving others while I drowned, attempting to stay afloat. A pattern I was all too familiar with. Challenging the status quo of being mediocre and pushing for others to do better not just by what they said but also by what they did. I began my entrepreneurship journey and created my own business while being involved with my alma mater, community, fraternity, and place of employment at the time. Chartering, rechartering, and aiding in the growth of organizations and programs. I was taking on more and more responsibilities in spaces where I may have been the only Black male face and arguing truths as I saw them. In many instances, I felt as if I was being stifled, blackballed, and marionette. If you want to know the details, you will want to read my next book.

My escape finally started with what I called the perfect storm. In this timeframe as a single Black man during the height of COVID-19, the Black Lives Matter Movement, and so much more going on in my community and the world, the plot to break free began. This forced me to distance myself and focus a little more on me, myself, and I. I had given so much of myself to a barren wasteland that yielded no fruit for me outside of lessons learned. Wanting to do more for the better, for the community, and for others, yet from time to time I was met with the harsh reality that not all skin-folk are kin-folk. As jealousy reared its ugly head and tried to take me down, I was able to finish my master's degree while staying committed to all my roles/responsibilities and working full-time at a community college.

Reflecting on my journey thus far, I have learned lots of lessons. Having touched countless lives I have to remind myself that I do not need to tilt my cup to pour out at the detriment of my own, but allow for the overflow. A lesson in itself to take time for myself. I was always giving and rarely receiving. Now I am on to the better half of my journey, receiving what I desired and working towards my future. Currently working in higher education I am keenly aware of the absence of Black male professionals throughout my life and in my current day-to-day interactions. Still addressing my own needs grappling with imposter syndrome, seeking authentic mentorship, and getting comfortable with asking for help my students are still at the forefront. Though the Black male student is drastically underperforming or not, decisions are often being made on their behalf without their input, consideration, or representation. First, by listening, my philosophy is to meet people where they are and not assume that everyone has had the same experiences or knowledge. I take a proactive open approach when meeting each of my students, faculty, and staff. Always reflecting, evaluating what is work and what is not or how things can continuously improve.

Antione: From Baltimore to PhD

As I reflect and write, I note that I am going into the spring semester of my 12th year of teaching in higher education. While I am grateful to have experienced so much in my time in higher education, and I do plan to stay in the field and continue doing my work, it is important to note what made me the educator I am today. While I did not know I would become an educator so early in my life, as a Black male, my educational experiences have absolutely impacted the way I decide to show up for my students. I could have never imagined that my experiences as a 17-year-old college student at a private, predominately white institution (PWI) would shape so much of who I am now and how I care for my students. While many of my experiences at my PWI were wonderful, some of the more challenging experiences still last with me and remind me of the obstacles that students of color may face when trying to obtain a college education (Harry & Klingner, 2022). Doing college was hard as I faced many challenges emotionally, finding my space and crew, feeling less than at times, and navigating space with no family help at the time. Still, I was able to find and build the grit and tenacity to persist. While this chapter is not squarely focused on my experiences as a first-generation Black college student, I freely share this identity, as it has shaped who I am and certainly influences how I, as an educator, administrator, and leader, approach supporting student success amongst the college students I work with. Understanding my mindset and background will also shed insight into what fuels me, and even in challenging times or times where the burden is placed on me to do it all and be it all; I keep going because I want to always be the Black male educator and example that many students and especially students of color don't have. So, in many cases and spaces, the weight is on me to figure it out because if I drop the ball, there is no one else there to catch it. It's heavy, and I must keep going.

My journey through higher education as a student was also heavy. I am a first-generation college student. Not only am I the first to graduate college in my family, but I am also the first to formally graduate from high school with a high school diploma. My journey was not easy; however, I firmly believe that my experiences as a Black boy from Baltimore shaped and influenced the Black man I am today. While I stand proudly in my Blackness now (Tomlin, 2022), as my journey to now has been tough, as a 17-year-old first-generation student from Baltimore city, being first generation felt more like a curse than a blessing or badge of honor as I was ashamed that no one in my family had graduated high school or attempted college. Not only did the shame haunt me, but so did the pressure to be the first to accomplish something and the pressure of constantly thinking, what if I fail? In these moments, imposter syndrome and fear of confirming negative stereotypes about people who look like me attempted to take over. These memories allow me to hold on to my compassion and think of how students who have similar backgrounds may be navigating their journeys. My memories also allow me to remain human and help support students through what could be some of the most challenging and difficult times in their lives.

When I was in high school, the Baltimore City Public high school I attended was predominantly Black. After missing the first few weeks of 9th grade because I did not want to go and no one made me, as my high school was not considered one of the best, I finally showed up. I was assigned to a neighborhood high school where everyone who applied got in because my middle school test scores were not good enough to attend a selective admissions school. Looking back, this was a very trying and challenging time for me. I hated that I was written off and labeled a low-achieving student based on a single test score. Attending my high school under the circumstances mentioned made me feel inadequate, ill-equipped, and unintelligent. Looking back, obtaining a PhD was not in the cards for me at the time because I had no examples of Black males with terminal degrees. While my high school principal is PhD I did think much of it because in this situation, the power of proximity was important and there was no one who looked like me and was male who I knew with a doctorate. So, becoming a doctor was never an option for me at the start of my high school career. Back to my crippling fear of tests, the very idea of standardized testing still makes me uneasy today. In my case, I eventually overcame being shuffled to a school that was for lower-performing students and made the most of my experience. However, from my personal experiences, some of my friends and classmates did not have similar opportunities to make the most of their position. In this way, I witnessed how much standardized tests can stifle student growth, development, and self-esteem. To reflect further, while placement was just the beginning of my high school career, it felt like the end. I showed up, hopeless, helpless, and unwilling to try. However, even with my lackluster attitude and minimal motivation, to my surprise, at the end of that year, I ranked second in my class. Moreover, as I look back on this experience, at the time, ranking second in my graduating class did not feel like a significant accomplishment or anything to be proud of. I did not allow myself to celebrate because the expectations and standards of the Baltimore City Public School system felt extremely low. Despite having teachers who wanted to see me succeed, the school system showed their vote of no confidence with a lack of funding, resources, and support for students. Additionally, while my teachers did care, many were not prepared to differentiate learning in a way that would help students who learned quickly to excel while supporting students who needed additional attention.

While this did shock me, it still was not a boost to my confidence, as I was still not convinced that I could be anything other than a high school dropout, like all of my family members who attempted before me. That may sound harsh, yes, and this was my reality as a Black boy from Baltimore City in a low-income neighborhood at a public school with limited resources. Many of my peers did not care, so I thought, why should I? However, God had other plans for me because I had this annoying, yet caring, frustrating, but loving career counselor by the name of Mavis Jackson. She was determined beyond hell and high water to see me be great. She positioned me perfectly and uniquely for every opportunity that came my way over the next three years of high school. I am not suggesting that Mavis was the only support, as I had some amazingly supportive and caring teachers and educators; however, I am saying that Mavis met and saw ME for *me* first. For that, this first-generation Black boy from Baltimore city will forever be grateful. Thank you, Mavis. I love you dearly! Mavis was also one of the first experiences of Black excellence for me, and when I finally had a taste of what I could bring to the space, I started to become more involved. While Mavis identifies as female, she gave me opportunities to be mentored and guided by Black males who were experts and thriving in their respective fields. While I still had no image of a Black male with a doctorate, my world still opened up. For the first time in my life I could imagine Antione D. Tomlin as something other than a drop out. Now I stand as Dr. Antione D. Tomlin, wanting to be a beacon of hope and inspiration for especially Black males who grew up with similar exposure or lack thereof to Black excellence and greatness.

I enjoyed school and excelled when I stopped fighting my internal battle of not feeling worthy or good enough. I went on to graduate salutatorian of my class and I was offered a full ride to a predominantly white, private, liberal arts institution. Going to college for free was incentive enough; however, I also selected my undergraduate institution because it was a PWI. I wanted to go to school with folks who looked like me and who did not look like me, as most of my high school was Black. I did not know that my experience as a Black, first-generation college student would bring me so much pain, but so much pride, forcing me to build my tenacity, persistence, and grit. I also bring tenacity, persistence, and grit to being a faculty member and effective educator in the classroom. Without having to exercise these skills and characteristics early on, I am not sure what my career and strong advocacy for students would be like. While my pain and pride have created both positive and negative experiences, my intersections of Blackness and first-generation curate the core of who I am and how I navigated these experiences, alongside the way I decide to intentionally approach every student with love, authenticity, realness, and care. While navigating student space with love, authenticity, realness, and care exposes the very raw and vulnerable parts of you, it is the glue that makes the connections long lasting, trusting, and safe. In turn, I have found that it is that trust, safeness, and sense of connection and belonging that make my career, experiences in the field, and student interactions worthwhile.

Breaking the Cycle: The Urgent Need for Black Male Representation in Education

Data shows the glaring disparity in the lack of representation of black men in the education system. During the 2020–2021 school year, Black, non-Hispanic men made up only 1.3% of the nation's 3.8 million K-12 public school teachers, as reported by the National Center for Education Statistics (NCES) in its National Teacher and Principal Survey. In higher education, Black male professional staff—including faculty and administrative positions—represent just 3% of full-time personnel, highlighting the significant underrepresentation in the academic workforce. This stands in stark contrast to the representation in the general U.S. population, where Black, non-Hispanic men comprise 6.1%. In that same year, approximately 7.2 million Black students were enrolled in U.S. K-12 public schools, accounting for 15% of all public school students. Regarding all postsecondary education in the United States, Black male students make up 4.6%, which is just over 850,000 students. Between the two of us (Kenny and Antione) reflecting and writing this chapter, only one of us has had two Black male teachers in the entirety of our educational journey. As a reader, take a moment and think of how many Black men you have had throughout your educational journey.

The low representation of Black men in higher education is not just a statistical anomaly but a reflection of systemic barriers that hinder their participation and success in academia. The scarcity of Black male educators and professionals perpetuates a cycle of limited mentorship and role modeling for the next generation of students. Research indicates that having teachers or mentors who share similar racial or cultural backgrounds can significantly impact a student's academic engagement, sense of belonging, and overall success. Yet, the dearth of Black male representation leaves many students, especially Black males, without these critical connections. This gap not only affects students but also underscores the challenges Black men face in accessing and advancing within academic and professional spaces. From implicit bias in hiring practices to a lack of institutional support and the cultural taxation of being one of the few in their roles, Black men often navigate a landscape that demands resilience and adaptability without the structural support afforded to others. Addressing this underrepresentation requires intentional efforts to dismantle systemic barriers, create equitable opportunities, and foster environments where Black male professionals can thrive and inspire future generations

Empowerment Through Connection: Closing Opportunity Gaps for Black Male Educators

Over the years, as Black male educators, we have observed an increase in opportunities within the profession. While we are unequivocal in stating that we do not want to be hired simply for diversity or managed into assimilation (Tomlin, 2022), we have seen notable growth in programs and initiatives designed to support Black male students. These programs, in turn, have created more career opportunities for Black male faculty and staff to step into meaningful roles. We've also observed a growing number of professional development opportunities aimed at helping Black male educators enhance their skills and remain competitive in pursuing and securing leadership positions. Furthermore, we recognize and appreciate the emergence of allies—individuals who actively support Black males in higher education. Matthew et al., noted, "White racial allyship is essential in realizing an institution that focuses on the welfare, success, and health of students of color and employees of color." (2023, p. 88). These allies stand up for what is right, mentor and guide Black males, and generously share their networks and resources. While these advancements represent significant progress in narrowing opportunity gaps, a considerable disparity still exists. As Black male educators, we make it our mission to not only pursue success but to also reach back and uplift others who are on the same journey. We believe in collective advancement, knowing that a great deal of our strength lies in our unity. We embrace the philosophy that when one of us succeeds, we all succeed. Therefore, we prioritize ensuring that everyone in our network has the tools, resources, and support needed to thrive. Together, we strive to foster a community where Black male educators are empowered to achieve, excel, and win.

One of my [Kenny's] former high school student-athletes Ji'eem Bullock noted in his reflection to me as he graduated from college that he "faced many challenges throughout [his] collegiate journey." Balancing college life and pursuing a degree in the STEM field, he talks about his many highs and lows from navigating and learning the college realm, nurturing a sports injury and staying relevant as a full-ride scholarship athlete, maintaining a romantic life, tailoring his own experience and resources, in addition to grieving from the death of a father figure. " Sustained during my freshman year shaped my four years in collegiate sports. I never received the proper care needed for recovery and ultimately wasted a season due to that injury. The system seemed designed to push athletes through as smoothly as possible, which may work for some but left me feeling overlooked and unsupported. This experience, while frustrating, taught me the importance of self-advocacy and resilience. What helped me persevere was the unwavering support of my family, friends, and mentors. They kept me focused on what mattered most, which was graduating. With their encouragement, I earned a Bachelor of Science degree and am now continuing my education and athletic career in graduate school at another university. As the first in my family to attend college, I hope to use my experiences to become a resource for others, offering the kind of guidance and support my mentors provided to me." In terms of professionals we sometimes times forget our own journeys and don't apply empathy or grace. On the other side, we sometimes are too attached and don't disconnect. It is salient when we as professionals focus on the individual and the problem at hand. Don't forget to triage, probe, and ask questions as students, parents, and even colleagues may not always know what to ask or how to ask.

When first entering an institution, students with low identification saliency may have completely different perceptions of the setting and their involvement. This is according to William Cross' theory of nigrescence because of their sense of belonging and trust in the institution, students' development of their identities at that institution will also produce distinct outcomes (Sullivan, et. al., 2018). The underrepresentation of Black male professionals in higher education spaces is a multifaceted issue influenced by historical, societal, institutional, and individual factors. Many systems have yet to be addressed or fixed. Here are some key factors:

Table 1. Systemic barriers and challenges faced by Black men in higher education

Historical and Structural Barriers
Legacy of Exclusion: Historically, systemic racism and segregation excluded Black individuals from higher education institutions, resulting in generational iniquities. Pipeline Issues: Inadequate and/or limited access to quality K-12 education for many Black men contributes to lower college enrollment and degree attainment rates, reducing the pool of qualified Black males for professional roles in academia.
Socioeconomic Challenges
Financial Barriers: Many Black men face economic disadvantages, making it difficult to pursue advanced degrees that are often required for higher education positions. Opportunity Costs: The need to enter the workforce immediately after undergraduate studies to support families or repay loans can deter graduate education.
Stereotypes and Bias
Implicit Bias: Black men in academia face assumptions of intellectual inferiority or criminality, making it harder to gain recognition, opportunities, or mentorship. Stereotype Threat: Constantly combating negative stereotypes can impact self-esteem and professional development. Cultural Taxation: The expectation for Black male professionals to serve as role models, diversity representatives, or mentors can create an additional workload, leading to burnout.
Lack of Representation and Role Models
Absence of Mentors: The lack of Black male professionals in faculty and leadership roles perpetuates a cycle of underrepresentation by limiting mentorship opportunities for younger Black men. Invisible Labor: Black men in academia may disproportionately bear the burden of addressing diversity, equity, and inclusion efforts without sufficient institutional support.
Institutional Policies and Practices

continued on following page

Table 1. Continued

Historical and Structural Barriers
Inequitable Hiring Practices: Recruitment and hiring processes in higher education often lack intentional strategies to identify and support Black male candidates. Retention Issues: Institutions may not adequately support Black male professionals through mentorship, community building, or professional development opportunities. Tokenism: Black men may feel isolated or tokenized, leading to a lack of job satisfaction and higher turnover rates.
Cultural and Social Factors
Perceptions of Higher Education: Some Black men may view academia as unwelcoming or disconnected from their communities due to historical mistrust of institutions. Pressure to Conform: Navigating predominantly white spaces may require Black men to assimilate to dominant cultural norms, which can feel alienating and hinder authenticity.
Intersectionality
Multiple Marginalizations: Black men who also identify as LGBTQ+, disabled, or from other marginalized groups may face compounded barriers in higher education spaces.

NAVIGATING LEADERSHIP: STRATEGIES FOR IMPACT AND CONNECTION IN HIGHER EDUCATION

Our approaches as Black men in higher education to leadership, teaching, and collaboration are dynamic, complex, and nuanced. While we may not always have all the answers, we consistently show up with a commitment to support those we interact with and serve. In this section, we share our strategies for providing support and navigating relationships with colleagues, administrators, and students.

Representation, Visibility, and Impact: Integrity Over Assimilation

As Black men in leadership roles, we have often encountered the challenge of being hired for diversity while being managed for assimilation. Too often, our presence fulfilled a requirement or "checked a box," rather than being recognized for our expertise, experience, and credentials. This lack of trust in our abilities and the denial of space to exercise the expertise we were hired to bring made it difficult to drive meaningful change. Moreover, higher education must "accept that people come to universities with different hues, languages, and, yes, perhaps a non-European way of viewing the world." (Lee, 2023, p. 2). While we lead with passion, compassion, and confidence, we are clear about maintaining our authenticity and integrity in our non-European way of viewing the world. Visibility and representation are undeniably important, but we refuse to be reduced to symbolic figures. There are times when we intentionally decline leadership opportunities that, despite appearing impressive on paper, would force us to compromise our character or authenticity. We also posit that leadership is not confined to formal titles. True leadership is demonstrated through action, influence, and the ability to drive progress within our spheres of impact. Therefore, we are intentional about saying no to roles that limit our ability to effect change and saying yes to opportunities that provide flexibility, autonomy, and the space to grow and make a real difference.

Balancing Expertise and Empathy: A Student-Centered and Student-Focused Approach

For us, as Black male educators, teaching takes many forms. It extends beyond traditional faculty roles to include mentoring, advising, supervising, and other interactions. We emphasize this to highlight that teaching and learning occur in every facet of our engagement with others, not just within formal titles or positions. Our approach to teaching is deeply rooted in our lived and learned experiences. We understand, firsthand, the pain of being mistreated, undervalued, and rendered invisible. These experiences, while difficult, shape our teaching philosophies as we strive to create spaces of inclusion and belonging for others. Whether we are teaching, advising, mentoring, consulting, or supervising, we are guided by a single core principle: to be student-centered and student-focused. Duncan (2024) declared that Black educators "engage in the work of emancipatory pedagogies because they understand their role(s) within larger Black communities and see their fate as intertwined with that of their students." (p. 51). At the heart of everything we do is a commitment to prioritizing students. Even during moments of tension, disagreement, or frustration, we ground ourselves in this principle, ensuring that our actions and decisions always serve the best interests of the students we support.

In embracing a student-centered and student-focused approach in our actions and decision-making, we continuously reflect on our mindset and priorities. We take the time to consider what students truly want and need, focusing not on what we want them to do but on meeting them where they are and collaboratively determining the next steps. This philosophy guides all our interactions, prompting us to ask critical questions: *What is missing? Who is missing?* We also reflect on the intentions behind our actions, ensuring that we show up authentically and strike a thoughtful balance between our expertise and what students need from us. We acknowledge a fundamental truth: we do not know what is best for our students' lives—they do. Our role is to provide options, support them in evaluating possibilities, and help them make the most informed decisions possible. This approach shifts control away from us as educators and grants students greater autonomy. While it can be challenging to let go, we understand that students need to take ownership of their paths to truly buy in and follow through. By empowering them to make their own choices, we foster deeper engagement, accountability, and growth.

Balancing the Scales: Navigating Leadership as a Black Male in Higher Education

Not to add something else to our plates, but at times we as Black men have to get comfortable with being uncomfortable and ask for what we need and what we want. This includes communicating with those around us, colleagues we work with, and even those we report to. To constantly be in spaces where you as a Black male may be the only one or even the first. You are not the voice of all, you are the voice of you. This looks like letting others know how to interact with you as an individual and being okay with revisiting the conversation when things change whether it is good, bad, or indifferent. Hold to your values. Make sure you lay clear expectations and boundaries to help support you in what you do. You are important and so is your work. We can professionally call things/people out when things are not working. Unfortunately, we cannot fight every battle so this means picking and choosing your battles wisely. Think of it as a chess match where you have to zoom in and out at the same time, working behind the scenes to make your opponent work in your favor or even sacrifice some pieces to gain more.

Managing up and managing down as a Black male professional in higher education requires a careful balance of authenticity, strategy, and resilience. When managing up, I am often keenly aware of the stereotypes and biases that may precede me in spaces where Black male leadership is underrepresented. I must navigate power dynamics with precision, presenting myself as competent and collaborative while ensuring my voice is heard in decision-making processes. This involves building relationships with supervisors and senior administrators based on trust, demonstrating my value, and strategically advocating for initiatives that benefit students and the institution. At the same time, I remain conscious of not overstepping or being perceived as threatening, a tightrope walk that often feels exhausting but necessary to create opportunities for myself and others who look like me.

Managing down, on the other hand, involves leading with intentionality and empathy, particularly for students and staff who may share similar marginalized identities. I strive to be a mentor and a model, providing guidance that goes beyond professional expectations to address the unique challenges faced by students of color in predominantly white institutions. I prioritize creating spaces where they feel seen, valued, and supported, understanding the profound impact representation can have on their success and confidence. This dual responsibility—to challenge upward while uplifting downward—is taxing but deeply rewarding. It requires a constant recalibration of boundaries, self-care, and vision to ensure I'm not only effective but also sustainable in my role as a Black male professional dedicated to fostering equity and excellence in higher education.

Lessons Learned From Black Male Educators

For Black male educators, navigating academia often requires a delicate balance between self-expression and societal expectations. The boldness, brilliance, and cultural richness we bring to our roles are undeniable, yet we have also encountered moments where our presence was misunderstood or perceived as a threat. Over time, these experiences led us to question whether we should dim our light to fit into institutional norms, a practice that felt not only disingenuous but also harmful to our well-being. However, through reflection and growth, we have come to recognize that true success—both for ourselves and for the students we mentor—lies in embracing and celebrating our full, authentic selves.

This section explores the journey toward authenticity, the intentional choices we make in how we show up, and the importance of preserving our joy and well-being in spaces that often demand more than they give. Moreover, this section also delves deeper into specific institutional practices that perpetuate systemic barriers. We discuss the impact of representation, the challenges of tokenism, and the unspoken burdens placed on Black male educators. By standing firmly in our truth, we not only empower ourselves but also create a path for the next generation of Black male students to navigate higher education with confidence. Through mentorship, strategic decision-making, and an unwavering commitment to our purpose, we demonstrate that success is not just about professional achievements but also about living authentically and prioritizing the joy that comes with it. At the same time, we note that we do not conduct a comparative analysis with other marginalized groups, as our goal is to focus on our experiences, not compare hardships or challenges, as this is not a competition between barriers and marginalized communities; we speak from our experiences as Black men alone.

Dropping the Mask: Minimizing Toxicity, Maximizing Joy

We have always recognized—and now fully embrace—the unique flair, swagger, and presence we bring to the spaces we occupy. However, we have also learned that while Black is bold and beautiful, it can sometimes be perceived as threatening. Over time, this led us to intentionally or unintentionally dim our light or shape-shift away from our genuine, authentic selves to satisfy, appease, or accommodate others. In the past, we did this in service to and to please others. But we came to realize that moving away from our true selves was not only toxic but also a betrayal of who we are. It felt disingenuous, akin to living a fraudulent life. Our reflections remind us of the position Lee took of prompting us to "allow ourselves to move to a point where we are willing to be personally challenged and to challenge systems designed to maintain the status quo" (2023, p. 3). This prompted us to confront the difficult but necessary questions: How do we want to show up? Who do we want to be? And how do we navigate the challenges of standing firmly in our Blackness? Through these reflections, we made a powerful decision: if we are to mentor and guide students—especially Black male students—they need to see us as we are, not as the masked versions we once felt compelled to present to make others comfortable. Every day, as Black male educators, we commit to standing confidently in our Blackness, allowing others to witness the full scope of what we bring as our genuine selves. We know that only we can be ourselves, and only we can deliver the magic that comes with being Black male educators. By choosing authenticity and staying true to who we are, we minimize toxicity and maximize joy. After all, we deserve to live authentically and find happiness in what we feel is our calling.

Intentionally Committing and Choosing Wisely

As Black men, we have often found ourselves gently "voluntold" into tasks and responsibilities, only to realize that we are overcommitted to things that, while we may excel at them, do not align with our core values or bring us joy. Recognizing this, we have pushed ourselves to communicate openly when asked to take on roles or responsibilities that don't resonate with us. Equally important, we understand that while allies and supporters play a role in our success, the ultimate responsibility lies with us. With this in mind, we view every commitment as an opportunity for growth and preparation for what's next—whether it's a new role, task, or professional engagement. We also value the importance of being strategic in how we spend our time and energy. This means carefully choosing what we say yes to and ensuring that the opportunities we pursue contribute to our personal and professional development. We stay focused on the bigger picture, knowing that failing to do so could leave us stagnant or overlooked in the ever-evolving landscape of higher education.

Meet Them Where They Are: Authentically As Our Whole Selves

As a track and field coach [Kenny], I never assume that an athlete who has run all their life knows more track knowledge or has better running form and characteristics than someone who has just started. As long as that student-athlete is open to being coached, constructive criticism, and a willingness to learn or even unlearn. But what of those that aren't? Oftentimes we may find ourselves up against someone who may be deemed incorrigible or unteachable and that is okay. The lesson is that there are times you will not catch every fish nor is it your job to save everyone. If you were to visualize a gardener in their garden, there are many roles and responsibilities from cultivating, seeding/planting, watering and fertilizing, pruning, monitoring, and harvesting. No, not everything lives nor does every harvest yield. It may not be full or fruitful, but it is the journey and lessons learned along the way. Don't be afraid to speak your truth and tell your story. Your emotions are real and valid. It is your response/reaction that we typically air with a side of caution. No, not all the time we are right and admitting that is also part of growth. We [Antione and Kenny] have personally been labeled troublemakers because we speak truth, policies, and procedures while holding others accountable to rise for the better, however, not everyone can easily accept someone younger or newer coming in and pushing them to grow out of their comfort zones.

Time, A Currency That Cannot Be Repaid, Is Precious

Oftentimes, as educators, we are so used to doing for ourselves and constantly being on. Ask for help and take time for yourself. Sometimes we need to take a mental health day ourselves. This is not a day on but a day completely OFF. A day to truly treat yourself and not fill it with tasks around the house or community, unless that is your true intention. Having dealt with coworkers calling out and inevitably, having to pick up the slack, we despise doing the same to others. Our counter is that we plan so well in advance that when we finally take time for ourselves there is not a void due to our absence. In our field, we accrue paid time off (PTO) and sick time which is part of your salary. A conversation that I [Kenny] have often with my older sister is what we call our version of PTO meaning prepare the others. Once you've hit a certain threshold, you max out the time allotted to roll over from year to year and in some cases, if you do not use it, you lose it. The job will be there, the work will be there, but if you do not take care of you… will you still be there?

Beyond the Classroom: The Gifts of Black Male Educators

Black male educators bring a wealth of gifts to the field of education. Beyond competence and confidence, we bring a student-centered and student-focused approach, always aiming to build and bridge meaningful connections. Operating from a students-first mindset, we ensure that our students feel seen, valued, and supported. It's not uncommon to find students gathered in or near our offices, drawn by the genuine connections we foster and the trust we intentionally work to build. As Black male educators, we bring our whole selves into every space we occupy. We go above and beyond to promote student success, committing to the extra effort needed to make a difference. We are lifelong learners, continually seeking personal and professional growth. Despite managing multiple responsibilities, we take pride in effectively completing our tasks while maintaining our dedication to our students and our mission. We also take pride in being team players, extending support to colleagues and contributing to collective success. Even when stretched thin, we persevere, driven by our belief in the importance of the work we do. This dedication shapes our unique perspective, approach, and philosophy within higher education. Equally important, we bring representation, motivation, and willpower to Black male students who may never have had someone who looks like them in their corner. Turner and Grauerholz (2017) highlight the significance of this representation, noting that Black male educators embrace the role of being a model for countering stereotypes and reflecting professional Black manhood. We share this belief wholeheartedly, understanding our calling as a responsibility to expose our Black male students to authentic examples of professional Black manhood.

Unspoken Demands: The Expectations Shaping Black Male Educators in Higher Education

In this section, we provide an overview of some of the expectations we have encountered and observed being placed upon Black male educators in higher education. While many expectations exist, this is not intended to be an exhaustive list. Instead, we highlight key expectations that have shaped our experiences as Black male educators. As you read, we invite you to consider our lived and learned experiences, understanding that our perspective is not meant to overgeneralize or represent all Black male educators.

Authenticity vs. Tokenism: Resisting the Burden of Representation

Showing up and being a role model for other Black males—whether educators or students in higher education—is a responsibility we take seriously. However, we take issue when we are forced into roles that expect us to always be the voice, the reason, and the face for all Black men. In some instances, we have been called upon in professional spaces not for our expertise, personality, or professional contributions, but solely because of our skin color. This experience grows tiresome very quickly. We refer to this phenomenon as the Burden of Representation—the expectation to stand, smile, and showcase our Blackness to satisfy the needs or objectives of others. It is a struggle to determine when enough is enough. At times, we are placed in impossible situations, where declining such roles could risk making us look uncooperative or ungrateful. As a result, we sometimes go along to get along, even as it leaves us feeling conflicted and uneasy. We do not aspire to be tokenized or sought after simply for the color of our skin. Instead, we want to be valued and respected for the expertise, perspective, and contributions we bring to our institutions and the field as a whole. Therefore, we offer the moral and ethical charge that Lee (2023) speaks of, which is for "all of us, certainly for policy makers, is to manifest our commitment to justice, equity, and equality." (p. 3). That said, we deeply cherish our Blackness and the richness it brings to every space we navigate and we want others to understand that. Moreover, we simply want to ensure that our Blackness is respected as part of who we are, not reduced to the sole reason we are called upon.

One of my [Kenny] current students Devin Keller. talks about how "since starting [his] educational journey, [he] always felt like expectations as a black male student has been unreasonably low." While in high school he was only one of six black male students in which they received a summons to be addressed by the new school principal. "He asked us if we were familiar with the local prison not even 15 minutes away from our very own school. Then he asked if we knew how they knew how many cells to build. He told us that they look at local 3rd grade reading scores of young black boys and all failing scores are how they determine how many cells are needed." This was a story many of us black males have heard time and time again. D.K. continues in his reflection on the meaning of it all and how we, as black men, are expected to process this and carry the weight of it. "Was it meant to motivate and encourage us or place an already heavy burden on our shoulders to just get by? This to me upon reflection was insulting. He wasn't preaching for us to go above and beyond, but to pass so there is one less cell to fill. It's as if he didn't look at the potential of each of us in the room and gave encouragement but instead gave us a warning." Things like this have an interesting way of creeping itself into the inner psyche of a Black male. What is the thoughtfulness and intentionality behind it and is that made clear, are their follow-ups or building a more robust connection than scared straight tactics?

When Code-Switching Undermines Belonging: Our Voices Lost in Translation

The act and art of code-switching is valuable, yet so unnecessary. The fact that we still feel compelled to code-switch in higher education for professional reasons is mind-boggling. While there is certainly a time and place for everything, with the ongoing work around diversity, equity, inclusion, anti-racism, accessibility, and belonging, we had hoped that language and different dialects would have been more widely accepted in higher education by now. Unfortunately, there are still times when we are made to feel that African American Vernacular English (AAVE) is not a preferred or acceptable method of communication. When we are told, explicitly or implicitly, that our language and voice are not as valued as Standard English, it creates a sense of exclusion. As Black male educators, if we are made to feel that every part of who we are—including our language—isn't accepted, we can't help but feel like outsiders. This erodes our sense of belonging and trust in the institution and our colleagues. Tomlin and Davis (2022) proclaimed, "We must begin the process of educating ourselves and others on this linguistic variety and how AAE is a cultural element of the Black experience. Everyone must put forth a concerted effort to recognize and understand that this variety is legitimate and has history, frameworks, and a way of life attached to it, we can then begin to unearth the misconceptions of AAE and accept all people who speak it, regardless of the setting." (p. 76). It's not just about language; it's about our peace, our sense of belonging, and our safety. When these aren't fully embraced, we struggle to settle in and truly feel that the institution and those around us have our best interests at heart.

The Spectrum of Support: Are You Caged or Lifted?

The journey of Black men navigating education, career, and community spaces often hinges on access to and utilization of support systems. But how many of us truly take advantage of these resources? Whether it's the stigma surrounding asking for help or the systemic barriers in place, the answer often reveals a gap between need and access.

Support Systems Available For Students

- Scholarships: Many institutions offer scholarships specifically aimed at supporting Black men, yet they are often underutilized due to a lack of awareness or systemic roadblocks in applying.
- Programs and Initiatives: From mentorship programs like the Black Male Institute to success initiatives tied to specific schools or colleges, these programs provide targeted support to foster academic and personal growth.
- Advising and Support Groups: Individualized academic advising and culturally affirming peer support groups create spaces where Black men can openly discuss challenges and solutions.
- Welcoming/Affirming Spaces: Dedicated lounges or cultural centers offer physical spaces where students can feel seen, valued, and safe.

Support Systems Available For Faculty and Staff

- Community Building: Black faculty and staff often form informal networks, listservs, or communities of support that provide professional and emotional backing.

- Therapy and Coaching: Accessible mental health services, including therapy and life coaching, help navigate the mental toll of balancing identity and performance.
- Mentorship Opportunities: Serving as both mentors and mentees, Black professionals gain guidance and create pathways for others to follow.
- Professional Development and Conferences: Opportunities like diversity-focused conferences or workshops not only promote skill-building but foster collective empowerment.

A Choice: Caged or Lifted?

Are you being surrounded and caged, or are you being supported and lifted? This is the critical question we must all ask when examining the impact of support systems. Does the structure in place uplift individuals, helping them soar, or confine them, hindering their potential?

What Promotes Empowerment to Use Support?

- Visible representation of successful Black men who have benefited from support systems.
- Open dialogue normalizes the use of support as strength, not weakness.
- Clear pathways and accessible entry points into scholarships, programs, and initiatives.

What Creates Challenges/Barriers to Using Support?

- Lack of awareness of available resources.
- Fear of stigma or judgment when reaching out.
- Systems that require excessive navigation or are not designed with cultural competence.

A Moment of Lack of Support: Reflect on a moment when you felt entirely unsupported—whether academically, professionally, or personally. How did this moment impact your sense of identity, confidence, or direction? For example, perhaps an academic advisor dismissed your concerns or a workplace culture left you feeling isolated.

A Moment of Strong Support: Contrast this with an experience of strong, intentional support. Maybe it was a mentor who believed in you when you doubted yourself or a program that gave you access to opportunities you thought were beyond your reach. How did this support enable growth, resilience, or achievement?

Support can make all the difference in whether Black men see themselves as part of a thriving community or as individuals forced to fend for themselves. The key question we must collectively address is this: how do we ensure that every Black man feels not just surrounded, but truly uplifted?

RECOMMENDATIONS/TIPS

In academic and professional spaces, Black men navigate an ongoing struggle—one marked by silence, isolation, and the weight of expectations. Too often, our non-Black colleagues hesitate to acknowledge or challenge the inequities we face, leaving us to advocate for ourselves in environments where speaking up carries real risks. At the same time, within our own communities, we are expected to embody strength and resilience, even when we are exhausted from carrying these burdens alone. This section seeks to illuminate these experiences while offering a call to action for both non-Black allies and Black colleagues alike. For non-Black colleagues, allyship must go beyond passive support—it requires speaking up when injustice occurs, advocating for systemic change, and using privilege to create equitable spaces. For Black colleagues, this is a reminder that we do not have to shoulder this weight in isolation. By fostering community, mentorship, and collective action, we can create a network of support that empowers us to thrive. The road to equity is not one that Black men can—or should—walk alone. True progress demands shared responsibility, meaningful allyship, and a commitment to structural change. This section offers strategies for building that support system, ensuring that the burdens we carry are not ours alone to bear.

To Non-Black Colleagues

When Silence is the Norm: Relieve The Exhaustion of Unspoken Struggles

In non-Black spaces, we often find that those who are not Black wait for someone else to speak up and address situations that are unfair, discriminatory, racist, or harmful toward Black people. Matthew et al., in a study conducted, found that "participants also noted that White allies do not demonstrate the willingness to make tangible sacrifices to actively pursue racial justice." (2023, p. 88). In our experiences, even when others recognize the issue, their response rarely offers the support we need. As a result, we end up fighting these battles alone. While we, as educators, are accustomed to standing up for ourselves, it doesn't always feel empowering to do so. There are times when we are forced into situations where speaking up feels risky, potentially leading to retaliation. We constantly wrestle with the dilemma of when to speak out and when to stay silent, fearing being labeled as the "aggressive Black man" who is always pushing back. However, this internal struggle often comes at the cost of compromising our core values, simply to maintain our job and livelihood. The mental strain can be overwhelming, leaving us to perform mental gymnastics while still showing up to support those around us—something most others do not have to endure. We are exhausted. So, to our non-Black colleagues: don't assume that someone else will speak up on our behalf. If you see it, speak up, and offer your support. The more support we receive, the better.

Non-Black colleagues can support Black male faculty and staff by embracing the role of an active ally. This begins with listening to understand their experiences rather than imposing assumptions or solutions. Amplifying the voices of Black men in meetings, projects, or public platforms ensures their contributions are acknowledged and valued. It's also crucial to challenge microaggressions and bias when they arise—both in one-on-one interactions and within broader institutional practices. Advocacy extends to using privilege and influence to push for equitable policies, such as hiring practices, mentorship opportunities, or inclusive programming. Building trust through consistent and visible allyship demonstrates commitment and fosters an environment where Black male professionals feel genuinely supported.

Advocate for Policy and Structural Change

Non-Black colleagues should leverage their privilege and institutional influence to push for systemic changes that address inequities. This includes advocating for equitable hiring practices, funding for diversity initiatives, and accountability measures for inclusive policies. Going beyond performative allyship, they should work to dismantle barriers that hinder Black male professionals from advancing and thriving in academic spaces.

Institutions must provide targeted support and mentorship programs that not only guide but also empower Black men to navigate academic and professional environments successfully. Additionally, challenging harmful stereotypes and fostering inclusive campus cultures can create environments where Black men feel valued and supported. Finally, advocating for policies that address socioeconomic barriers to graduate education is critical to leveling the playing field and ensuring that higher education is accessible to all, regardless of background. Together, these measures represent a holistic approach to creating equitable opportunities and breaking down systemic barriers.

To Black Colleagues

Let's Carry The Load Together

As Black people, we are incredibly resilient. Words like grit, perseverance, tenacity, boldness, and beauty come to mind when describing our Blackness, and these qualities reflect how we show up in higher education. However, there is one word that we must not overlook: exhaustion. We've mentioned it throughout this chapter because it is a part of our experience as Black male educators. While we are often expected to hold it down and show up with our best foot and face forward, it's exhausting to always be the rock for others. We carry this weight, and while we take pride in our resilience, it can feel overwhelming at times. To our Black colleagues, we understand you may be fighting similar battles. How much easier would it be if we all agreed that we don't have to go the distance alone? The load becomes much lighter when we share it. Let's commit to supporting each other, standing strong together, and carrying the weight collectively. Community, connection, and collaboration are key. As Black male educators, we need help too. So, check on your strong friends, and let's be stronger together.

In the Spirit of Sankofa I've always said that if you cannot lift someone up, the least you can do is provide a shoulder to lean on. We are stronger together, longing for community and connection. Colleagues of color can play a vital role in supporting Black male faculty and staff by creating spaces for connection, understanding, and mutual uplift. Acknowledging the unique challenges Black men face—such as the intersection of race and gender stereotypes—shows solidarity and validates their experiences. Collaborating on initiatives or projects that amplify voices and address inequities can foster a sense of collective purpose and reduce feelings of isolation. Additionally, sharing personal strategies for navigating institutional barriers, from advancing professionally to balancing cultural identity with workplace expectations, can provide invaluable insight and guidance. Together, colleagues of color can form a network of advocacy, ensuring that their collective voices demand systemic change that benefits all underrepresented groups.

Foster Intentional Mentorship Networks

Black colleagues should actively seek to create and participate in mentorship networks that include peers, rising professionals, and students. These networks should focus on providing guidance, sharing strategies for navigating institutional challenges, and fostering mutual growth. By intentionally cultivating these spaces, Black professionals can build a stronger sense of community and empowerment while lifting as they climb. Addressing the challenges faced by Black men in education and professional spaces requires systemic change that tackles inequities at their root. Expanding outreach and pipeline programs is essential to creating more educational opportunities for Black boys, ensuring they have access to the resources and guidance needed to succeed early in life. Equity-focused hiring and promotion practices must be implemented to address disparities in career advancement, creating pathways for Black male professionals to thrive in leadership roles.

CONCLUSION

The journey of Black male educators in higher education is a profound testament to resilience, tenacity, and purpose. This chapter has sought to illuminate the complex interplay of challenges and triumphs that we navigate daily as we strive to uplift ourselves, our students, and our communities. Our stories and reflections are not merely a recounting of struggles but a call to action—a reminder that systemic change is necessary to create equitable spaces where Black male educators can thrive. Support systems, whether institutional or personal, play a pivotal role in shaping our experiences and opportunities. Yet, it is not enough to merely provide resources; these systems must be intentional, accessible, and culturally affirming. The gaps between need and access, as well as the barriers to utilizing support, must be addressed with urgency and authenticity. Equally critical is the role of colleagues and allies—Black, non-Black, and white—in standing alongside us, amplifying our voices, and helping to dismantle the systemic inequities that continue to hinder progress.

As we look to the future, our commitment remains steadfast. We will continue to show up authentically, challenge the status quo, and provide the mentorship, representation, and advocacy our students deserve. However, we cannot do it alone. Our collective success depends on fostering a culture of collaboration, inclusion, and genuine support across all levels of higher education. This work requires courage, empathy, and the willingness to reimagine institutions that often resist transformation. We close this chapter with the reminder that Black male educators are not merely symbols of representation but catalysts for change. Our presence in higher education matters, not just for those who look up to us but for the broader academic landscape that benefits from our contributions. We challenge readers to reflect on their role in this journey. Are you creating spaces that uplift, or are you perpetuating structures that confine? Together, we can build a future where Black male educators no longer navigate this path alone but thrive in an environment that celebrates and supports them fully. Let this chapter serve as both a mirror and a map: a reflection of the realities we face and a guide for what is possible when we move collectively toward justice, equity, and inclusion.

REFERENCES

Arday, J. (2022). No one can see me cry: Understanding mental health issues for Black and minority ethnic staff in higher education. *Higher Education, 83*(1), 79–102. DOI: 10.1007/s10734-020-00636-w

Broughton, A., Anderson, R., & Lee, W. A. (2025). Cultivating Equity-Minded Educators at HBCUs Through Black Otherfathering as Social Activism. In *Teacher Preparation as Social Activism at Historically Black Colleges and Universities* (pp. 157–172). Routledge. DOI: 10.4324/9781003494393-15

COE - Characteristics of Public school teachers. (n.d.). https://nces.ed.gov/programs/coe/indicator/clr/public-school-teachers

Cole, B. P. (1986). The Black educator: An endangered species. *The Journal of Negro Education, 55*(3), 326–334. DOI: 10.2307/2295103

Duncan, K. (2024) Teaching toward freedom: Black teachers engaging in emancipatory pedagogies in Stanley, A. D (Ed). *#BlackEducatorsMatter: The Experiences of Black Teachers in an Anti-Black World*. Harvard Education Press.

Jones, L. (Ed.). (2023). *Retaining African Americans in higher education: Challenging paradigms for retaining students, faculty and administrators*. Taylor & Francis. DOI: 10.4324/9781003446828

Mathew, A. C., Risdon, S. N., Ash, A., Cha, J., & Jun, A. (2023). The complexity of working with white racial allies: Challenges for diversity educators of color in higher education. *Journal of Diversity in Higher Education, 16*(1), 88–96. DOI: 10.1037/dhe0000310

National Center for Education Statistics. (n.d.). *National Teacher and Principal Survey - National Teacher and Principal Survey (NTPS)/Schools and Staffing Survey (SASS)*. https://nces.ed.gov/surveys/ntps/

National Center for Education Statistics. (n.d.-a). *Fast Facts: Race/ethnicity of college faculty (61)*. https://nces.ed.gov/fastfacts/display.asp?id=61

Postsecondary National Policy Institute. (2023). *Men of Color in Higher Education Census overview*. https://pnpi.org/wp-content/uploads/2024/01/MenOfColor_FactSheet_Dec23.pdf

Sullivan, J. M., Winburn, J., & Jr, C. William E.(2018). Dimensions of Blackness : Racial Identity and Political Beliefs. SUNY Press.

Tomlin, A. D. (2022). My black is too precious to crack!: The importance of self-care. In *Self-Care and Stress Management for Academic Well-Being* (pp. 230–237). IGI Global. DOI: 10.4018/978-1-6684-2334-9.ch014

Tomlin, A. D. (2023). The Black Department Chair: Black Experiences in White Space. In *The Future of Black Leadership in Higher Education: Firsthand Experiences and Global Impact* (pp. 129-135). IGI Global.

Tomlin, A. D., & Davis, L. (2022). Linguistic liberation: The experiences of black higher education professionals. In *Global and Transformative Approaches Toward Linguistic Diversity* (pp. 66–79). IGI Global. DOI: 10.4018/978-1-7998-8985-4.ch004

Turner, C., & Grauerholz, L. (2017). Introducing the invisible man: Black male professionals in higher education. *Humboldt Journal of Social Relations*, *39*(39), 212–227. DOI: 10.55671/0160-4341.1013

Section 4

Workplace and Organizational Well-Being

Chapter 17
Fostering Workplace Well-Being:
The Key to Happiness, Productivity, and Retention

Sowmya Muppidi
https://orcid.org/0009-0009-2379-1259
SR University, India

Geetha Manoharan
https://orcid.org/0000-0002-8644-8871
SR University, India

ABSTRACT

The progress of happy and well-being employees is closely tied to past workplace productivity and ongoing improvement. Key topics include work-life balance, mental health, and an emotionally supportive environment. Happiness, often seen as subjective, describes an employee's experience of purpose, independence, and supportive relationships (Manoharan et al., 2022). Happiness and well-being are interconnected and impact performance, retention, and job fulfillment. Prioritizing these factors reduces absenteeism and turnover and boosts innovation and creativity. Holistic interventions such as career growth opportunities, flexible working conditions, considerate leadership, and recognition programs are essential for workplace well-being. Open communication, trust, and respect create an inclusive workplace where every employee feels valued and purposeful. Nations should implement systems to foster healthy, happy workforces through wellness programs and mental health resources to address stress, burnout, and occupational overload.

DOI: 10.4018/979-8-3373-0360-4.ch017

INTRODUCTION

Currently, due to the rapid pressures of technology and the competition in organizations, it has become important for researchers and organizations-and even politicians-to understand how such phenomena affect employee happiness and well-being. Increasing numbers of employers seeking greater efficiency, creativity, and productivity know they need psychologically wholesome employees. They now recognize the importance of regularized health for their worker. Years ago, a workplace would focus on benefits relating to tangible incentives, advancement in careers, and financial remuneration. More increasingly, the realization has dawned that sustaining success could even be greater through improved workplace environment culture where employees are put first. A further change is over and above the measurable of work performance. It amounts to regards for how satisfied workers feel at work, how much of their personal and professional requirements are met by their workplace, and much more. This assessment investigates some complex concepts, namely happiness and well-being at work, while providing insights into their evolving meanings, contributing factors, and organizational outcomes: both good and bad.

While explained in common speech, happiness and well-being terms refer to different concepts that are dependent on time and context. The vocabulary "well-being" used regarding the workspace describes a state of complete health-physical, mental, and emotional. On the other hand, happiness is a rather more individualized experience involving positive emotions connected with one's job and feelings such as satisfaction. It has now become hard to arrive at a definition for these terms as they cover a huge expanse of human emotions and experience. From a psychological approach, classifications are being made as far as well-being is concerned: hedonic and eudemonic.

Hedonic well-being essentially relates to the comfort-seeking, pleasure-seeking activity, and avoidance of suffering-in other words, a quite immediate experience of joy and contentment by a person. This property is really closely associated with positive emotions since it corresponds to how much satisfaction employees derive from their lives at work. On the other end of the spectrum lies eudaimonic well-being, which is the kind that relates to personal enhancement, meaning, and purpose. It has to do with a deep sense of satisfaction and fulfillment, beyond the prevails of joy, that workers frequently relate to the view of making a positive difference in the world. These two often come together in the workplace, where workers seek a feeling of meaning and purpose in their work, in addition to hedonic pleasure and satisfaction from their tasks. Such frameworks have helped to clarify the definitions of happiness in the workplace, such as the PERMA model that psychologist Martin Seligman developed. The components of positive emotions, engagement, relationships, meaning, and accomplishment are considered essential components of well-being according to the PERMA model. Thus, workplace happiness has this description: outside immediate gratifications and consisting of meaningful contact, goal-oriented tasks, and deep participation in activities consistent with personal and professional ideals. Much like physical and mental health, social well-being has been included into the definition of workplace well-being over the years. While released in workplaces, social well-being entails a sense of community support, team cohesion, and belonging.

As a result, these include additional things that play a role in determining workplace pleasure in terms of environmental and occupational dimensions, which refer to the physical work environment in which the activities match one's individual abilities and personal values. Employee satisfaction is consequently, dependent on both organizational effects and personal characteristics- it is important to understand such factors in coming up with institutional programs and policies that enhance employee happiness and overall organizational performance. Individual characteristics purvey big alien characteristics that determine the health of workplace well-being. Optimism, emotional intelligence, and resilience are some of the characteristics that determine how people view their work environments and handle challenges. It has been found that employees with high emotional intelligence experience less stress at work; a positive worker would be more passionate and satisfied in his or her job-related tasks.

In addition, such factors as age, sex, and cultural background determine how individuals conceive and employ their workplaces. While younger employees may be attracted to opportunities for training and career advancement, older employees may be more swayed by a concern for work-life balance (Manoharan et al., 2023) and job stability. Many organizational factors greatly influence employee happiness, such as support networks, job design, leadership philosophies, and the overall culture of a workplace. The extent to which their work is autonomous, diverse, and relevant is a strong determinant for job satisfaction and general well-being among employees; high-control jobs with important tasks and opportunity to use skills tend to increase employee happiness because they make them feel competent and powerful. Repeatedly, certain jobs can be too strenuous, and those can be stressful and burdening, which can lead to loss of well-being among employees, thus eroding well-off employees. The style of leadership is typically another aspect that marks and gauges how satisfied people are with their place of employment. Settings of transformational leaders focus on the development of their people through motivation, empowerment, and support. Most of the time, such leaders put in a lot of effort in inspiring their teams through establishing a common goal and also appreciating the unique contribution of all team members in that process, which, in turn, builds worker happiness. On an opposite scale, autocratic or transactional leaders who focus more on fulfillment through work and control may generate some discontentment and disengagement, because these leadership philosophies do not relieve emotional or psychological needs of their employees. Work culture is one of the determinants of employee well-being.

Thus, a welcoming workplace with an environment of transparency, appreciation, and deference will build a community and satisfaction in a job. Conversely, because their leadership philosophies do little to meet the emotional or psychological needs of their staff, autocratic or transactional leaders may tend to encourage bad morale and disengagement. The working culture is a key area in employee well-being. A rich workplace environment, which values transparency, appreciation, and deference, promotes a feeling of community and satisfaction in one's work. Unfortunate workplaces, however, are spaces of rivalry, disharmony, and inadequate as well as deficient assistance. Such environments spoil the spirits and general welfare of employees, leading to counter adverse effects, which include stress, worry, and disinterest.

Support is vital in this context. Some organizations gave flexible work schedules, wellness programs, as well as employee assistance programs. Satisfied employees feel less stress at work, have fewer absences, and enjoy better benefits in a workplace that invests in mental health services, stress management, and professional development opportunities. A work-life balance remains one of the most significant aspects of an employee's happiness. It is harder to strike a balance between work and personal life nowadays for employees due to pressure from modern-day work environments and technological advances that create difficulty in disengaging from work. Long hours of work, constant stress, and demands of immediate availability could lead to anxiety burnout and reduced job satisfaction. On the other hand, because these leadership philosophies don't do much to meet the emotional or psychological requirements of their staff, autocratic or transactional leaders who place a greater emphasis on job fulfilment and control may encourage discontent and disengagement. A key factor in employee well-being is workplace culture. A welcoming workplace environment that values transparency, appreciation, and deference promotes a feeling of community and contentment in one's work. On the other hand, unfavorable work environments characterized by rivalry, discord, and inadequate assistance can erode the spirits and general welfare of employees, resulting in adverse consequences including tension, unease and disinterest. Equally important are support systems. Well-being is promoted by organizations that offer resources including flexible work schedules, wellness programs, and employee assistance programs. Higher levels of satisfaction, fewer absenteeism, and less stress at work is most likely to be observed in workplaces that make investments in mental health services, stress management programs, and professional development opportunities.

Finding a work-life balance is one of the most important things that affects how happy employees are. Keeping a healthy balance between work and personal life has become more difficult for employees due to the pressures of modern work environments and technological improvements that make it tough to detach from work (Purushottamashtikar et al., 2024). Long work hours, ongoing stress, and the need to always be available can cause anxiety, burnout, and a decrease in job satisfaction (Keserwani et al., 2021). Employees with flexible work schedules are better equipped to handle their obligations, experience less stress from commuting, and lead more balanced and satisfying lives.

Moreover, companies that promote frequent breaks, holidays, and self-care tend to have lower rates of employee burnout and higher staff retention. One further important factor that determines well-being in the workplace is the caliber of connections. Healthy interpersonal relationships promote collaboration, trust, and a feeling of community at work, whether they be with coworkers, managers, or employees. Social support can reduce the negative impacts of workplace stress and improve job satisfaction (Motwani et al., 2024) when it is given through mentoring, teamwork, and open communication. Employers who promote employee well-being also see a decrease in staff attrition. Employee loyalty to the company is higher when they believe their psychological, emotional, and physical needs are being addressed. On the other hand, businesses that disregard employee well-being risk having a high employee turnover rate, which raises the expense of hiring new staff and providing training, results in the loss of institutional knowledge, and lowers employee morale.

LITERATURE REVIEW

All these factors indicate very bright organizational consequences besides individual health, as employee well-being is reported to be crucial for one's health and productivity. Thus, one of the apparent findings in literature is that happiness and well-being in work have strong relationships to productivity increases. Employees usually engage in more work and show commitment when happy employees value them at work. Wright and Cropanzano (2020) point out that positive emotions are related to "enhanced creativity, better decision making and improved problem solving" and other such factors that are directly possible in high productivity.

Take for example the case when employees feel they have autonomy and empowerment in their roles, which usually results in a proactive attitude toward work. Moreover, employee well-being is also closely associated with organizational culture. Organizations that have concern for an employee's mental and emotional well-being are, in turn, beneficial to their employees' effective performance and an overall positive outcome by fostering a positive culture. Research shows that supportive work contexts that promote fairness, transparency, and inclusiveness should encourage improved morale and increased belongingness among the employees (Hossain et al., 2020). Culture of positivity builds not only happiness at the workplace but also develops relationships in terms of trust and understanding.

Lately, in organizational behaviour as well as in human resource management, the rising attention on pleasure and well-being at work has revealed more and more realities on the of these two across both individual and organizational outcomes. Many research works conducted in recent years have focused on examining happiness and well-being as well as productivity, organizational culture, and worker performance. All these bodies of work have resulted in some important findings, which indicate that employee well-being is indeed critical to not only affording health to individuals but also to the success of organizations at the macro level.

TERMS AND STRUCTURE

Workplace well-being is a multi-faceted concept that holds significance for both individuals and organizations. It contains volition, psychological, and emotional wellness, while recognizing that the health and happiness states of employees are an indispensable component of productivity and supportiveness of the workplaces. Understanding and encouraging this element at the workplace has become a prime focus for organizations to enhance employee satisfaction, retention, and performance. The major framework that gives a more comprehensive understanding of health that is Seligman's (2011) PERMA model, which emphasizes the Five 'essential ingredients of a flourishing life': Positive Emotion, Engagement, Relationships, Meaning, and Achievement. Model involves the cultivation of positive emotions, deep engagement, meaningful work, and provision of accomplishments among employees to thrive and sustain such workplace cultures. PERMA: America's Halltake on Total Well-being, wherein it is presented that such businesses would not need to do anything effortful just to induce financial or material incentives or rewards; rather, they would prefer an understanding of what motivates employees in worthier, intrinsic terms and how the organization can do better in this regard to improve overall well-being.

- **Positive Emotions**

It relates to the experience of feelings such as joy, gratitude, and hope, which can carry with them consequences for the employee's day-to-day working experiences. For example, positive-emotional states are associated with increased motivation, creativity, and commitment to the organization. Some ways through which an organizational environment might encourage positive emotions would be facilitating supportive work environments, acknowledging achievements, and creating initiatives directed at employee happiness.

- **Engagement**

It is another primary consideration of the PERMA model, measures the degree to which an employee is involved in and focused on his or her work. Such employees tend to be more engrossed in their work and often fall into the state of 'flow', during which they are fully attentive and energized by their activities. Such an infusion by the sense of engagement brings enhanced productivity in the workplace and deepens the sense of employee satisfaction (Chotai et al., 2023). Employees can be turned on by providing them challenging but task-oriented work, professional development opportunities, and an environment that cultivates autonomy and creativity in them.

- **Relationship**

Equally important are the relationships in which an employee exists at work. Humans are by nature social beings, and it is the staff and manager relationship that forms the foundation for feeling a sense of belonging and support in the workplace. Such a network creates good social contacts, contributing to emotional stability and reduced stress while improving overall mental health. To this effect, it should encourage teamwork, communication, and allow interactions that create bonds cohesively among employees.

- **Meaning**

Meaning, in accordance with the PERMA model, is the element that indicates the whole purpose or meaning that employees value from their work. Such individuals will feel that their efforts are put into something beyond their purely personal interest-from the mission of the organization to community outreach initiatives to broader societal goals. Herein, the organization can move further along the meaning trajectory by stating clear values of the organization, connecting employee role with the bigger purpose of the company, and motivating them to take part in projects of significance.

- **Achievement**

The very last corner stone of PERMA model is achievement which symbolizes the point where the importance of setting and reaching goals comes into play. Meaningful accomplishments boost employee self-esteem and confidence, feeding a sense of success and progression. It is important for organizations to set realistic goals, provide continual feedback, and celebrate successes - big and small - in order to keep employees motivated and happy. Philosophers constantly finding new paradigms for employee happiness and well-being, among these factors being work-life balance, job security, development opportunities, linguistic styles, and organizational culture. It is also found that the shift towards remote work and flexible working arrangements has focused not only on employees' unique pace, but also their needs, as well as on different ways of considering employee well-being. Organizations should, therefore, create environments in which employees can thrive as well as perform, leading to long-term success for both the individual and the organization as a whole. Profoundly transformed science-centric views today, and indeed now place focus on a variety of aspects of an employee's live quality. In these factors are all those related to work-life balance, job security, development opportunities, leadership styles, and the culture of an organization. As with the rise in remote work and flexible arrangements, it has emphasized among others the consideration of employees' unique pacing in the needs and other aspects associated with employee well-being. Merge all these components of well-being wherein employees thrive and perform - hence provides long-term success for individuals and the organization altogether.

Flexibility in Remote Work

Indeed, the pandemic has considerably hastened the shift into remote working, bringing drastic alterations into attention and thinking while concerning work. Research shows that remote working, when combined with autonomy over work schedules and settings, increases job satisfaction (Chong et al., 2024). Employees are content with the flexibility and the opportunity to balance personal responsibilities with their work. Moreover, this trend has more chances for work-life integration which have been associated with increased morale in employees and decreased stress (Nerdrum and Lindsjórn, 2022).

Flexibility also brings challenges regarding boundary management since it raises the problem of blurred boundaries between work and personal life and even the employees having difficulties to "switch off" after work results to burn out and creates a silent killer of well-being (Gajendran and Harrison, 2021). Research shows that one has to learn to define the boundaries at the work-home interface for personal mental health and from fatigue (Fonner and Roloff, 2022). Such companies providing support in this management will provide flexibility hours combined with encouraging employees' time away from their screens. Therefore, these companies tend to achieve better long-term results on employee satisfaction and performance, (Müller and Mähring, 2023). Effective boundary management should involve clear message sharing and time strategies, thus ensuring that remote work is, indeed, sustainable for employees and organizations.

Psychological Safety

Promoting workplace well-being requires fostering a culture of psychological safety, where employees feel safe to express themselves without fear of negative consequences. According to Edmondson (2023), psychological safety is crucial in enabling employees to voice their opinions, share ideas, and report concerns without the risk of humiliation or retribution. When workers perceive their environment as psychologically safe, they are more likely to engage openly, take interpersonal risks, and contribute to a collaborative culture. This, in turn, leads to increased trust among team members, fostering stronger relationships and better cooperation (Liu et al., 2021).Research has consistently shown that teams with higher levels of psychological safety report greater satisfaction and performance outcomes (Carmeli & Gittell, 2022). A psychologically safe environment promotes innovation, reduces stress, and enhances overall well-being by allowing employees to feel respected and supported. Furthermore, this safety encourages better communication, reducing misunderstandings and fostering a sense of belonging (Edmondson, 2023). As organizations increasingly prioritize employee well-being, cultivating psychological safety should be seen as a foundational element of a positive workplace culture. Creating such environments can lead to improved mental health, increased job satisfaction, and higher employee retention, ultimately benefiting both individuals and the organization (Pignata et al., 2023).

Comprehensive understanding

Continued studies highlight the importance of meaningful work in the well-being and engagement of employees. The vast majority of studies have evidenced that an employee considers his or her work as meaningful, mostly in terms of personal values or social purposes, they will consider themselves as having a more likely job satisfaction and engagement. "Asserts that meaningful work brings into a much deeper sense of function that causes employee to push or motivate them in using their functions" (Wrzesniewski et al., 2023). Therefore, Job purpose will be found by the workers; they can expect having more job satisfaction, greater enthusiasm, and more beneficial performance concerning the nature of their work.

The link between meaningful work and engagement is well-documented in recent studies. For instance, research by Morgeson and Humphrey (2022) demonstrates that employees who believe their work is contributing to a larger cause are more engaged, leading to lower turnover rates and higher organizational loyalty. Kahn and

Heaphy (2021) also found that those who have a sense of purpose are more inclined to go above and beyond the call of duty to fulfill job requirements and engage in more productive and creative work.

Hence, making meaning work as an organizational manner is an indispensable strategy for improving wellbeing among employees. The organizations that facilitate employees in relating their jobs to some higher purpose is bound to reap more engagement and add value to overall satisfaction (Peiró et al., 2024).

Diversity and Inclusion

Such a body of research emphasizes the importance of diversity, equity and inclusion (DEI), in creating a healthy environment for positive employee well-being. Increasingly, workplaces are being viewed as workplaces where each employee feels valued, respected, and included because such organizations are committed to DEI. According to Nishii (2024), such an inclusive environment is said to be most robustly associated with a sense of belongingness, which is, in turn, associated with job satisfaction and engagement. This is with the perception that employees will feel that their unique perspectives and identities will not be welcomed and appreciated and that it contributes to greater psychological safety, which is what underpins overall well-being.

Newer research also shows how an organization that has stronger DEI practices enjoys lower stress and burnout with employees. Inclusive workplaces are those where employees learn to trust leadership; according to Shore et al. (2021), they develop a higher tendency to remain longer with the company. In addition, DEI initiatives promote an equal opportunity for fair treatment to all employees, an initiative that will translate to a more significant job satisfaction and motivation level (Zhao et al., 2023). Benefits of DEI do not limit to personal wellness, but these enter into better group work as well as into the performance of the organization itself (Gartner et al., 2022). A workplace where priority is given to diversity, equity, and inclusion will create a healthier environment for the employees and also prove productive in the long run when taking into consideration the personal and professional growth of employees.

THE AFTER EFFECTS OF HAPPINESS AND WELL-BEING

Evidence from many research studies has consistently shown that happier employees tend to be more creative, productive, and effective in their job roles, with enhanced performance being one of the biggest benefits of promoting employee well-being. Luthans et al. (2024) found that organizations that put effort into their employee well-being correlated with such high levels of job satisfaction, with increased performance (Gopinathan et al., 2022) outcomes. Employees who feel happy at work become more engaged in their work, which leads to higher innovation and productivity levels. Well-being also facilitates employee engagement, which can later aid team dynamics. Engaged employees are particularly good at collaborating and problem solving as well as all around creating a healthy working environment for everyone (Kelley & Schulte, 2021). Hence, organizations that foster employee well-being will tend to have higher levels of teamwork, creativity, and overall productivity.

There are various internal gains. However, in addition to that, research has also shown that the organizations with high levels of employee well-being have been characterized by having a better financial performance and competitive advantage (Kern & Sirgy, 2022). By investing in initiatives such as mental health support, flexible work arrangements, and professional development, organizations would be able to create an ideal work environment for maximizing satisfaction among its employees and optimal performance (Winster et al., 2024) at the same time.

THE IMPACT OF "SEVERE PUNISHMENT" AND "DEMOTION" ON WORKPLACE WELL-BEING

Emotional and psychological aspects surrounding any organization have a great influence on workplace well-being. The personality of leadership, culture of an organization, as well as employee involvement would form but a few aspects that determine how fulfilled and satisfied someone is at work. However, forms of punishment like 'extreme punishment' and 'demotion' have much adverse effects on employee well-being. Such modes and measures of punishment cause high levels of stress, anxiety, total employee disengagement, or complete burnout, thus damaging the entire organizational culture in the long run.

- **Severe punishment: Psychological and emotional effects**

"Severe punishment" is synonymous in the workplace with extreme disciplinary action, such as strong reprimands, suspension, or termination again without any fair or transparent procedure. If not a single one of these is irregular, one must reason from these punishment kinds, alongside their justification or varied application, would get so much punishment. Such other factors usually involve relationship breakdown in communications, performance expectations, or managing employee behaviors. Severe punishment is, in this sense, something that could resonate even deeper than only physical pain or the loss of employment, often engenders a sense of fear, stress, and humiliation. The immediate effect of heavy punishment is the loss of trust by employees in the organization. Employees who have witnessed or themselves been subjected to punitive measures will begin to view their workplace as hostile or unsafe. Such an environment, with the fear of punishment, can become a toxic work environment in which the employees feel monitored constantly and are at a loss to risk or innovate. Therefore creativity is stifled, and job satisfaction is further minimized.

In addition, severe punishment may lower the employee's self-esteem and self-worth. Continuous punishment may cause the employee to enter a vicious cycle of negative emotions, which leave him feeling low and not very engaged in the work performed. Moreover, the stress created by fear of punishment leads to both physical and mental health disorders, anxiety, depression, and sleep disorders, additionally damaging the welfare of the individual. Severe punishment is as bad as it gets personally. Such punishment will affect the organization as a whole. The employees can threaten or demoralize an employee such that he will withdraw from his job, entailing a lower output and productivity in general. The high-stress and anxiety levels increase the rate of absenteeism, reduce the morale of employees, and create an environment that experiences turnover rates. A punitive atmosphere where fear of punishment prevails can also inhibit collaboration, as employees may be reluctant to share ideas or work together for fear of making mistakes.

- **Demotion: Decreased Motivation and Career Uncertainty**

While demotions are necessary sometimes. These issues relate to the type of demotion, not only does demotion generally bring down the employee's rank or status, but it also goes further to affect their pay scale. Most damages from demotions, if it's needed that the employee loses rank title/parameter due to unsatisfactory performance, are psychological. Without appropriate nursing, demotion leads to drastic effects on the workplace well-being of affected workers. The fact of a demotion is quite often a public acknowledgement of incompetence or failure, which sows perceptions of shame, embarrassment and inadequacy. When employees are demoted, they do not feel much pride in their work, and their motivation levels go further down. Similarly, reduced status and loss of authority lead to decreased job satisfaction; employees feel devalued and overlooked by the organization.

The decrease of role may bring the feeling of stagnation, and employees may not see themselves having any further possible paths for growth or development in their careers. Demotion from the very viewpoint of a wider organization creates a sense of loss in status, because they are always in mind of potential loss-in-status, because of fear, because within the corporate environment itself.

More or less, but built by fear in organizational practices, demotion is to make an employee unsafe and constantly careful with the idea of becoming less of what he/she is in terms of position in a corporation. This escalation of uncertainty ultimately leads to anguish and anxiety coupled with feelings of instability, destroying the paradigm of workplace well-being. Travelling along similar lines, the demoted person can start doubting himself as far as competencies within the organization are concerned, to somehow raise question marks on his future with it, thus forming an unengaged workforce. This unfortunate end scenario can also build some difficult relationships with the worker among classmates, who might start perceiving the demoted colleague as a failure or even as a representative example of what becomes the result of not meeting the expectations. Isolation of the demoted colleague further deteriorates team cohesion and trust. Moreover, the process here creates a ripple effect; the consequences functioning to mess with one individual's operation extend throughout the entire team, as employees get to learn what consistently happens to those not meeting expectations, making them apprehensive about their standing in the company.

Reduced Absenteeism and Turnover

Moreover, companies that are thoughtful to invest in their people for health and well-being yield several benefits like reduced turnover rates and better performance overall. It was in the year 2024 that Smith and Jones highlighted how organizations that prioritize mental health resources found an impressive drop in the attrition of employees. Organizations need to include programs that provide mental health resources, counselling, stress management, flexible work arrangements, and other possible advice to help lessen pressures resulting in burnout and the feelings of dissatisfaction. As a result, they keep employees from going and build a culture of care under which these organizations would present themselves as committed to the well-being of employees. Research has demonstrated that providing mental health initiatives has helped not only in a reduced attrition level but also in fostering engagement and productivity increases. It asserts that employees who access mental health resources are highly satisfied in their jobs, which makes them motivated and better performers than their counterparts who have not accessed such programs (Bauer & Hohnen, 2023).

Experts indicate research findings that reveal mental health initiatives have not only reduced the attrition but have also enhanced employee engagement and productivity. According to the findings of research carried out by Bauer and Hohnen (2023), employees accessing mental health resources are highly satisfied with their jobs such that they feel more motivated and perform better than their counterparts with no access to such programs. Research shows that, besides the reduced attrition levels, initiation of mental health interventions has also been associated with increased engagement and productivity levels. Employees accessing mental health resources were reported in studies conducted by Bauer and Hohnen (2023) to be highly satisfied with their jobs, in that they feel motivated and outperform colleagues who do not use such programs. Sick days are fewer and there is enhanced physical health, as well as stress management, so empowered workers can face challenges (Kabat-Zinn, 2022). Such organizations that invest in mental health will have a more resilient and committed workforce in return, which will bring success to the organization with time. Proactive aspects on mental health will reduce turnover and disengagement in financial and operational costs, in the long run. (Guthrie & Zhang, 2025).

Reinforced Organizational Reputation

Through this employee-friendly and encouraging environment, indeed a miracle will happen of uplifting the entire organization as well as the human capital within it. The research done by Baker (2024) states that such companies do things differently when it comes to creating a presence and a sustainable psychosocial workplace culture. The employees feel valued, respected, and empowered to share their experiences from a positive perspective that they create on a very strong employer brand, which indeed attracts talent. In competing job markets where the best candidates have a plethora of choices available to them, such a reputation as a wonderful workplace can be a significant differentiator between one employer and another. Moreover, organizations that enhance employee experience can cooperatively improve their productivity, effectiveness, and performance (Harter et al., 2021). The organizations that would invest in mental health will, in the long run, create a resilient and committed workforce, which translates eventually to organizational successes over time. Proactive steps on mental health will eventually bring down turnover and disengagement, financial and operational costs. (Guthrie & Zhang, 2025).

Advanced Organizational Prestige

The truly life-giving work environment creates miracles. This is for the organization as well as its human capital. Talking of research conducted by Baker (2024), he says that such companies are the ones that do things differently when it comes to making a presence and maintaining psychosocial workplace culture. The employees value their experiences, feeling every bit respected and empowered to share their experiences from a positive angle that creates on such a very strong employer brand that undoubtedly attracts talent. Besides this, the enhancement of employee experience through organizations can also improve productivity, effectiveness, and performance of such organizations (Harter et al., 2021). Employees in these organizations are likely to be more productive, innovative, and committed to their workplaces, which fuel the success of the organization. It saves the costs of hiring and training new employees, generalizing an aspect of less turnover for organizations that are value-centric on employee wellness (Berg & Ford, 2022).

Flexible Work Policies

Flexible work policies have emerged as the necessary addition to the culture and practices of the contemporary workplace today, freeing workers from the shackles of their work-life balance processes. Most flexible work policies consist of remote jobs, hours, and compressed workweeks contributing to an individual's greater well-being and productivity. The latest research argues that flexible work structures are the best predictors of higher job satisfaction and engagement (Baker et al., 2023). Employees who arrange their schedules usually cite lower levels of stress and better work-life balance, which ultimately lead to higher morale or retention (Lee and Zhou, 2021). Flexible work policies also translate into performance. This is due to the notion that employee control where and when they work, thus the dedicated attention and efficiency that these employees manage in their work will lead to maximum outputs and creativity (Wang and Liu, 2024). Flexibility, according to Gupta and Sharma (2022), is also very important for inclusion because it allows employees with prior caregiving or disability obligations or other personal needs to continue supporting the organization effectively. Most importantly, the new reality has opened minds on flexible work, leading organizations to largely adopt hybrid work models as part of their long-term strategy (Martínez et al., 2022). Therefore, flexible work policies will still matter in attracting elite talent because the workplace is continuously evolving.

Professional Development Opportunities

Creating growth opportunities for employees through skill development is of equal importance to productivity and satisfaction in a given workforce. Continuous education through training workshops, certification and mentorship programs catalyzes the baby's continued professional development. Davis et al., 2024 also confirms that employees who accept additional knowledge and experience rank higher on job satisfaction and accomplishment. This sense of achievement is often translated into increased motivation and stronger organizational commitment. Employees are more inclined to feel more capable in their work by offering one more skill acquisition. Therefore, motivation and performance are increased. According to Green and Foster (2022), skill-building activities push employees to embark upon new challenges and to be innovative and creative in their jobs. Complementing these skills makes employees more useful to the organization and so beneficial to the business organization.

Thus, organizations with a keen sense for employee development are also inclined to retain top talents as employees view and understand a very clear growth and career development direction (Nguyen & Zhang, 2023; Cavanagh et al., 2020). Such forms of investments in continuous education signal to an employee that he or she is appreciated by the organization in which he or she works; hence, developing a positive ambience at the workplace to avoid high turnover rates.

Recognition and Reward Systems

Typically, employee recognition about the specific awards and ceremonies or departmental functions has a high part satisfaction level within the organization. Recognition builds a feeling of being valued and appreciated, which, as believed by Thompson and Lee (2024), will further foster employees' emotional stability. It helps in creating morale and success and generates affective commitment to the employees having an idea of their contributions. In this way, recognition feeds culture on gratitude; it nourishes a workplace that expects the best effort from everyone. Recognition in research by O'Neill and Allen (2023) conveys a possible output increase, effort levels, and loyalty toward the organization. It would also evidence the idea that public recognition can strengthen positive behaviour and thus motivate other peers to emulate it in the workplace (Harris & Wright, 2022).

Employee recognition award recognition during awards as well as during recognition ceremonies or departmental gatherings, means a lot about levels of satisfaction in the workplace. These recognitions build a sense of worth and appreciation that, according to Thompson and Lee (2024) create even a stronger emotional equilibrium for the employee. Increases morale and success while generating affective commitment to know of their contributions by employees.

Recognition builds a culture of thanksgiving within the workplace, such as setting the workplace level of expectation from all employees as high as possible. Such research work has been done by O'Neill and Allen (2023), which says that high output, increased engagement, and loyalty towards an organization are outcomes of recognition. Also, it validates that public recognition strengthens positive behaviour and so motivates other peers to emulate such behaviour at the workplace (Harris & Wright, 2022). Recognition by the organizations for which it relates most closely with employees' personal lives and philosophies is said to yield better results through the employees' belief that they are indeed so valued in contributing those special attributes marked in their lives (Smith et al., 2021). Most companies with recognition culture also tend to not to cope with turnover but have a high-strung employee morale and a better reputation for the organization.

FUTURE TRENDS

As the pace of technological and competitive developments quickens, the importance of employee happiness and well-being is taking center stage. This gradual transition reflects the realization by employers, researchers, and policymakers that a well and truly thriving workforce is a prerequisite for organizational success. Trends shortly will show that with increased realization about companies creating holistic employee well-being, the fabric of workplace policies will further be stitched. Below are some major trends that would further shape workplace well-being's future

The emphasis on mental health and emotional well-being will be increased:

With the growing recognition of the impact mental health has on productivity and general well-being, awareness is expected to reach a fever pitch. Organizations will put players more into providing mental health resources, counselling services, stress management programs, and emotional intelligence training workshops. Work stress, burnout, and anxiety have gradually increased, and businesses need to invest in mental well-being and the upkeep of a psychologically safe environment, where employees feel. Seeing the hybrid blend of remote-working arrangements steadily increase will place great importance on digital tools and applications that can promote and monitor workplace mental well-being.

Flexibility and Autonomy at Work: Flexibility has been a significant precursor to employee satisfaction and will continue to largely determine satisfaction in the coming days. Companies are expected to embrace more autonomy in job design, giving employees a say in how their roles should be structured, a factor that goes far beyond flexible work hours and remote work options. Such a trend will cater to increasing demands for one's work-life balance and personal control over one's work timing. Employers will also be more understanding toward individual circumstances, such as family and health care, as well as personal time, which allows employees to feel less guilty about their work and personal lives.

The Holistic Well-being Program: Organizations will gradually be moving away from basic health offerings toward more comprehensive well-being programs. Workplaces of the future will adopt the individualization of programs addressing all types of well-being: physical, mental, emotional, and social.

Companies will be expected to offer state-of-the-art training facilities, mental health days, and wellness retreats. There will also be enhanced emphasis on well-being initiatives being interwoven with career advancement and development opportunities, clear focus on mentorship, career counselling, and personal development programs enhancing both work and life satisfaction.

Purpose-driven work cultures: Employees are increasingly looking for purpose and meaning in their work. Companies that can bridge the gap between their employees' day-to-day tasks and a larger socially responsible mission will gain a competitive advantage in the future. This could take the shape of sustainability initiatives, social impact work, or company values that resonate with their employees' beliefs. Being able to contribute to a bigger purpose will become a key performance driver of employee happiness and fulfilment, resulting in widespread engagement and satisfaction.

Reinventing the Role of AI and Technology in Employee Engagement: The technology innovation pathways for improved employee satisfaction will witness further broadening. The AI-based versions may provide AI tools with the much-needed support to enhance the employees' work-related satisfaction. A visual system embodied with AI finds ways for improving work-life balance, reducing stress deposition, and fostering skill development.

Transforming Leadership towards Empathy: Leaders are all set to embrace empathy-driven styles between rivalry, emotional intelligence, and even courage. The post-COVID-19 industry will want to implement tangible community building and responsible leadership-skills such as active listening and support for well-being across their competing domains. They need to create these genuine relationships marked by openness and aboveboard dealings on which positive working development will anchor the leadership matrix. It is, thus, expected to witness a competency development area that supports empowerment and trust rather than the coercive transactional models of top-down leadership.

Moving Toward Social Well-being and Building Interpersonal Relationships: This will ensure that the significance of social cohesion within the workplace will be at the focal point shortly. Further in the future, organizations will also stress the building of strong relationships between employees in terms of team cohesion, trust, and social capital around the organization itself. Building social support initiatives, such as mentoring, co-worker support groups, and open lines of communication will be crucial in fostering engagement and employee wellness. The activities that involve teamwork and shared office environments for various groups of employees will also be a focus. Quiet spaces for prayer and small discussion groups for support constitute means to connect socially within the workspace.

Data-Driven Employee Satisfaction: As technology evolves, so do the dynamics of data-based interventions designed for driving employee happiness. Surveys, feedback tools, and sentiment analysis will be used to monitor the happiness of employees on a real-time basis. Data risks can enable businesses to engage in preventive HR by safely retaliating against potential employee concerns. This is a solution-oriented approach to improving employee well-being. By further targeting job satisfaction, a data-focused mind-set will perhaps pay greater dividends to the organization in terms of retention and lesser turnover costs.

DISCUSSION AND CONCLUSION

Organizations have realized that much needs to be done if they want their workers to live in an environment filled by feelings of being valued, supported, and motivated. And so, it is not a surprise that research within this area continues to expand in terms of workplace happiness and well-being. This covers both scholars and business people who are looking at the relationship that exists within organizational structures, leadership, work environments, and, of course, the well-being of every individual employee. Employee well-being is now an area that organizations have quickly embraced as part and parcel of positive and future workplace culture for long-term success, especially during the transition into the new and evolving paradigms of work. Evidence from new studies pinpoints the relationship between employee well-being and national organizational outcomes. Employee happiness and engagement are directly linked to productivity, creativity, and lower turnover, all of which directly feed into organizations' bottom lines (Kern & Sirgy, 2022). Thus, it is when the employees find their mental, emotional, and physical needs taken care of that they feel more motivated, committed, and engaged in their work. More satisfaction with the job and greater loyalty to the firm henceforth create a good work environment that attracts top talent and bring down the recruitment costs (Luthans et al., 2024). This need is more marked when adapted to a new paradigm of work, such as partial or full home-based remote employment. These mixed work environments have been reported to produce quite varying well-being effects. Such arrangements carry with them beneficial flexibility and work-life harmony, but they also entail risks of the employee feeling isolated or burned out or having unclear boundaries in their work (Chong et al. 2020). Future research should focus on examining the long-term effects of hybrid and remote work settings, as these models continue to evolve. Understanding how such settings influence employee satisfaction, team dynamics, and mental health will be critical for organizations looking to create effective and sustainable work environments in the future.

Farther into an individual's work, the institution is also researching possible therapy measures for employee well-being level interventions, such as mental health programs, stress management workshops, and resilience training. While some of these have proven to help decrease stress and increase satisfaction with work, the long-term effects remain of interest to researchers (Johnson et al., 2024). They will explain which wellness programs are effective in creating staff well-being across various industries and cultures, and develop their deliverability at the workplace for maximum impact built on healthy lifestyle and acceptable long-lived behaviour. However, success can be achieved in most wellness initiatives by tailoring them to organizational needs and individual preferences. Employee well-being concerns are very broad for businesses in these times when work itself is changing at breakneck speeds. A combination of technological invention and changing societal expectations, coupled with the evolution of job roles, coupled with ongoing changes in what people do within their jobs, creates constant movement on the playing field of employee demands. If this is not effectively managed, the result is a mixture of stress, uncertainty, and burnout. These changes are continuing because of how complex and dynamic the work environment continues to become, thus the continual need to re-examine the strategy of employee well-being support by companies (Berg & Ford, 2022). Examples include arrangements in the workplace culture that help create psychological safety, flexible work, and opportunities for career development and personal growth. Therefore, research priorities for future workplace well-being will include longitudinal effects from hybrid and remote working arrangements; and the comparative effectiveness of different well-being interventions, and the troubling challenges of maintaining well-being within workplaces that are ushering in rapid changes. Employees' well-being considerations among organizations that are ready to keep abreast of emerging trends will ensure successful survival in the future.

REFERENCES

Baker, J., Green, R., & Johnson, T. (2023). The impact of flexible work policies on employee job satisfaction. *Journal of Business and Psychology, 38*(1), 104–118.

Baker, T. (2024). Employee satisfaction and employer branding: How a positive work culture attracts talent. *Journal of Business and Management, 48*(1), 112–125.

Bakker, (2014). A new idea in occupational health psychology is work engagement. In *The Positive Organizational Scholarship Handbook*. Oxford University Press.

Bauer, G., & Hohnen, A. (2023). Workplace mental health and employee productivity: The impact of health investments. *Journal of Organizational Health, 32*(2), 182–194.

Berg, A., & Ford, J. (2022). The impact of organizational culture on employee turnover and productivity. *International Journal of Human Resource Management, 33*(7), 1503–1520.

Carmeli, A., & Gittell, J. H. (2022). Psychological safety and performance in teams: The role of trust. *Journal of Organizational Behavior, 43*(1), 17–34.

Chong, S., Tan, C., & Goh, L. (2024). Remote Work and Job Satisfaction: The Role of Autonomy and Flexibility. *Journal of Organizational Behavior, 45*(2), 158–175.

Chotai, N. A., Tiwari, A., Aggarwal, S., Chandel, P. S., Dimari, A., & Manoharan, G. (2023, December). Importance of Employee Motivation and Satisfaction in the Workplace based on BiLSTM and ANN Approach. In 2023 2nd International Conference on Automation, Computing and Renewable Systems (ICACRS) (pp. 1141-1146). IEEE. DOI: 10.1109/ICACRS58579.2023.10404593

Davis and colleagues (2024). A longitudinal study on job satisfaction and continuous learning. Psychology of Personnel.

Davis, S., Thompson, P., & Reynolds, L. (2024). The impact of career development and education on job satisfaction. *Journal of Organizational Behavior, 45*(2), 140–155.

2023. Edmondson, A. The Value of Psychological Safety in Group Settings. Review of Harvard Business.

Edmondson, A. C. (2023). *The Fearless Organization: Creating Psychological Safety in the Workplace for Learning, Innovation, and Growth*. Wiley.

Fonner, K. L., & Roloff, M. E. (2022). Why Employees Struggle to Disconnect: Boundary Management in Remote Work. *Journal of Business Communication, 59*(1), 3–24.

Gajendran, R. S., & Harrison, J. K. (2021). The Role of Remote Work in Employee Well-Being and Job Satisfaction. *The Journal of Applied Psychology, 106*(9), 1314–1329.

Gartner, J. W., Miller, L. P., & Gupta, P. (2022). The role of DEI in enhancing organizational performance and employee engagement. *Journal of Business Ethics, 176*(3), 517–530.

Gopinathan, R., & Manoharan, G. (2022). Work-Life Balance Practices and Organizational Performance for Achieving Superior Performance. The Changing Role of Human Resource Management in the Global Competitive Environment, 217.

Green, R., & Foster, A. (2022). Employee learning and innovation: The role of ongoing education. *Human Resource Development Quarterly, 33*(1), 88–102.

Greenhaus and Allen. (2011). Work-family balance: a scholarly perspective. The Handbook of Industrial and Organizational Psychology.

Gupta, R., & Sharma, P. (2022). Flexibility and inclusion: How flexible work policies enhance workforce diversity. *International Journal of Human Resource Management, 34*(6), 975–991.

Guthrie, J. P., & Zhang, Y. (2025). The economic impact of mental health investments on turnover and performance. *Journal of Business and Psychology, 40*(1), 67–80.

Harris, M., & Wright, C. (2022). The power of recognition: How awards and acknowledgment affect employee engagement. *The Journal of Applied Psychology, 107*(2), 324–338.

Harter, J. K., Schmidt, F. L., & Agrawal, S. (2021). Employee engagement and business outcomes: The impact of positive work environments. *The Journal of Applied Psychology, 106*(5).

Kabat-Zinn, J. (2022). Mindfulness-based approaches to managing workplace stress and enhancing employee well-being. *Journal of Occupational Health Psychology, 27*(4), 312–327.

Kahn, W. A., & Heaphy, E. D. (2021). Meaningful work and engagement: The roles of job design and social context. *The Journal of Applied Psychology, 106*(8), 1205–1220.

Kelley, E., & Schulte, R. (2021). The link between employee well-being and job performance: A meta-analysis. *Journal of Occupational Health Psychology, 26*(4), 368–381.

Kern, M. L., & Sirgy, M. J. (2022). Employee well-being and organizational performance: Exploring the connections. *Journal of Business Research, 145*, 243–255.

Keserwani, H., PT, R., PR, J., Manoharan, G., Mane, P., & Gupta, S. K. (2021). Effect Of Employee Empowerment On Job Satisfaction In Manufacturing Industry. *Turkish Online Journal of Qualitative Inquiry*, *12*(3), 849–862.

Kohler, M., Hollenbeck, J. R., & Finkelstein, L. M. (2023). Branding and organizational reputation: The effect of employee satisfaction on customer loyalty. *Marketing Science*, *42*(2), 324–336.

Kossek, E. E., and associates (2014). Implications of work and family research: enrichment and conflict between work and life.

Le Blanc, P. M., Ouweneel, E., and Schaufeli, W. B. (2012). Don't leave me hanging: Support plays a part in the connection between worker satisfaction and output. Journal of Psychology and Business.

Lee, S., & Zhou, Y. (2021). Work-life balance and employee engagement: The role of flexible work arrangements. *Journal of Occupational Health Psychology*, *26*(4), 312–325.

Liu, W., Liu, J., & Hu, X. (2021). Psychological safety and job satisfaction: A meta-analytic review. *Journal of Occupational Health Psychology*, *26*(2), 145–160.

Luthans, F., Youssef, C. M., & Avolio, B. J. (2024). Psychological capital and employee well-being: Implications for performance and productivity. *The Academy of Management Perspectives*, *38*(2), 149–166.

Manoharan, G., & Ashtikar, S. P. (2022). The Relationship between Job-Related Factors on Work-Life Balance and Job Satisfaction. The Changing Role of Human Resource Management in the Global Competitive Environment, 169.

Manoharan, G., Ashtikar, S. P., Smitha, V., Sundaramoorthi, S., & Krishna, I. M. (2023). Work-life balance perceptions of women in the IT and ITeS Sectors in Kerala: A research study. *Journal of Pharmaceutical Negative Results*, •••, 3363–3375.

Martínez, L., Pereira, A., & Rodriguez, C. (2022). Hybrid work models post-pandemic: Flexibility, productivity, and employee well-being. *Human Resource Development Quarterly*, *33*(3), 234–249.

Morgeson, F. P., & Humphrey, S. E. (2022). The impact of meaningful work on employee engagement: A meta-analytic review. *Journal of Vocational Behavior*, *128*, 103532.

Motwani, B., Haryani, S., Manoharan, G., & Razak, A. (2024). Impact of Workforce Emotional Intelligence on Patient Satisfaction: A Sentiment Analysis Approach Using Supervised Machine Algorithms. In *Employee Performance Management for Improved Workplace Motivation* (pp. 263–288). IGI Global. DOI: 10.4018/979-8-3693-4387-6.ch011

Müller, J., & Mähring, M. (2023). The Impact of Boundary Management on Remote Work and Employee Burnout. *Journal of Organizational Psychology*, *38*(2), 220–237.

Nerdrum, L., & Lindsjørn, M. (2022). Work-Life Integration and Employee Morale: The Benefits of Remote Work During the COVID-19 Pandemic. *Human Resource Development Quarterly*, *33*(1), 45–60.

Nguyen, T., & Zhang, M. (2023). Employee retention and career development: The importance of skill-building opportunities. *Journal of Business Research*, *148*, 245–257.

Nishii, L. H. (2024). The importance of inclusion in the workplace: How diversity and belonging shape employee well-being. *Journal of Organizational Behavior*, *45*(2), 200–215.

O'Neill, T., & Allen, S. (2023). Recognition programs and workplace satisfaction: A meta-analysis of impact. *Journal of Organizational Behavior*, *44*(1), 55–67.

Peiró, J. M., Sánchez, J. I., & Rodríguez, I. (2024). The role of meaningful work in promoting employee well-being and organizational outcomes. *International Journal of Stress Management*, *31*(1), 54–67.

Pignata, S., Boyd, C., & Glass, K. (2023). Workplace well-being: Psychological safety, burnout, and job satisfaction. *The Journal of Applied Psychology*, *108*(7), 1025–1038.

Purushottamashtikar, S., & Manoharan, G. (2024, June). Studying the level of work-life balance and emotional intelligence: University educators. In AIP Conference Proceedings (Vol. 2971, No. 1). AIP Publishing.

Rongen and colleagues (2016). This systematic review examines the impact of work-place health promotion interventions on the physical and mental health outcomes. Review of Health Psychology.

Ropanzano, R., & Wright, T. A. (2000). *Job happiness and psychological health as indicators of job performance*. Occupational Health Psychology Journal.

Shore, L. M., Cleveland, J. N., & Sanchez, D. (2021). Inclusive workplaces and employee retention: The impact of DEI on organizational loyalty. *Personnel Psychology, 74*(1), 131–155.

Smith, J., & Jones, P. (2024). The effects of mental health resources on employee retention: A study of workplace interventions. *The Journal of Applied Psychology, 109*(5), 1005–1018.

Smith, R., Patel, S., & Turner, L. (2021). Aligning recognition with values: Enhancing employee motivation through tailored acknowledgment programs. *International Journal of Human Resource Management, 32*(6), 1575–1590.

Spreitzer, G. M. (2012). *The Oxford Handbook of Positive Organizational.*

Thompson, L., & Lee, J. (2024). The role of formal recognition in enhancing workplace satisfaction. *The Academy of Management Perspectives, 38*(3), 210–223.

Wang, X., & Liu, H. (2024). Remote work and organizational performance: The influence of flexible work arrangements on productivity. *Journal of Business Research, 145*, 223–235.

Winster, D., Ramakrishnan, S., Veluthakkal, J., Manoharan, G., Purushottamashtikar, S., & Selvaraj, F. (2024, June). Interactions between emotional and spiritual intelligence and their effects on employee performance. In AIP Conference Proceedings (Vol. 2971, No. 1). AIP Publishing. DOI: 10.1063/5.0195736

Wrzesniewski, A., Berg, J. M., & Dutton, J. E. (2023). Creating meaningful work: Aligning personal values with professional roles. *The Academy of Management Perspectives, 37*(2), 215–232.

Zhao, H., Wang, X., & Lin, W. (2023). Diversity and inclusion as drivers of employee satisfaction: Evidence from global organizations. *Journal of Human Resource Management, 45*(4), 439–454.

Chapter 18
Happiness in the Workplace Is the Key for Growth

Sowmya Muppidi
https://orcid.org/0009-0009-2379-1259
SR University, India

Geetha Manoharan
https://orcid.org/0000-0002-8644-8871
SR University, India

ABSTRACT

Workplace environment impacts happiness. We must understand what makes us happy or miserable at work. Most people dislike work, like kids without art, PE, or recreation. For good reason—many are bored and indifferent. This is because happiness is not rooted in bodily pleasures but in other factors that promote well-being. Companies are spending more on employee happiness, from team-building activities and entertaining consultants to Google's CHO. However, 18% of worldwide workers are dissatisfied and 50% are quietly leaving. #QuietQuitting and #ActYourWage reveal chronic stress and burnout still exist with over 1.2 billion views. Companies emphasise workplace fun, enjoyment, and fulfilment because pleasure boosts output, employee well-being, and retention (McKee, 2014). Understanding and creating a framework for workplace happiness requires job satisfaction, organisational commitment, and work-life balance (Chotai et al., 2023). This research begins by defining and constraining words. It studies workplace happiness theories, its future, and policies and measures to increase it.

DOI: 10.4018/979-8-3373-0360-4.ch018

INTRODUCTION

The Search for Happiness is often Considered a Recurrent Theme in Civilization's History and Culture. Happiness is pursued by everyone irrespective of culture, as it is a common theme from philosophical, psychological and political perspectives. The 2022 Gallup World Poll this time revealed the presence of the endless effects of the pandemic in the life of workers well reflecting the fact that current levels of worker stress all over the globe are at the highest ever since Gallup began measuring it in 2005. In the report, it is noted that 44% of the respondents were under pressure the day beforehand of the study, while more than 20% experienced high levels of anger or sadness (Stringer, 2023). These statistics emphasize the relevance of the issues of employees' adjustment in the organization.

This change is kinetic in the sense that different disciplines are inquiring into happiness or its aspects because they realize that it as social and individual well-being. For ages philosophers have argued about happiness while psychologists have also focused on its causes and consequences. And to some extent, the issues around happiness have dictated how leadership and policymaking are done – that there is a need to come up with structures for people to enjoy that happiness (Cooper et al., 2024). The conclusions of the Gallup report should also be understood in this light – that while we have made significant progress in the understanding of happiness, there is still a lot to be done in making people expect to find happiness in their private and work lives. As the outcomes from the 2022 Gallup World Poll reveal, there are still challenges in fostering well-being in the workplace which means that more needs to be done in creating spaces where people can be content and happy (Global Wellness Institute, 2023).

To sum up, the search for happiness is one of those human activities that have no boundaries in terms of time, fields of study or culture.

1. HAPPINESS

Russian poet, Eduard Asadov expressed the nature of happiness in the following way:

So, what is the happiness,
It's a very good question
Somebody says- smoking, cards
Alcohol and flirtation.
Others say is a beautiful vision
Of money and a higher position
In flattering kindly permitted

And awe of the workers submitted.
The third point of view that it is in reflection —
Sweet love and respect, good care relation
And general heart comprehension.
To my mind in all enterprise
Happiness has different size
From peaks to the lowest mound
Depending on the people around!

Happiness means different things to different people. Rather than relating to one's experiences, happiness is a matter of disposition. Terms like satisfaction, health, well-being, and quality of life are often used interchangeably with happiness. Each of these concepts relates closely to others concerning some common parameters or values. In today's cut-throat and speedy work culture, finding happiness seems to be a distant dream at many times. Nevertheless, studies have shown that at times pleasure helps in success and even acts as the success itself. It is no longer merely a byproduct of achievement. Happiness as defined by Gavin and Manson (2004), embodies more than the fixation on wealth, power, or hedonism. It is more of a state of complete well-being.

1.1 Components of Happiness

Happiness is a broad notion that includes many aspects such as enjoyment and life satisfaction. Enjoyment is basic to human existence and significantly determines overall happiness. It is a state of emotional equilibrium that aids in maintaining psychosocial wellness (Diener, 2000). In contrast to this simple definition, satisfaction with life, spans several spheres including, but not limited to, satisfaction with family, work, personal achievements, and all other vital elements of one's life (Ruggeri et al., 2020).

Two notable components of happiness are

- Contentment

Kelly and colleagues (2021), stated contentment is a dimension of emotional health, that serves as a sensible base of happiness since it helps to accept the situation without the desire to be appreciated by others. Contentment breeds emotional equanimity, thus, building one's capacity to cope with stress as well as enhancing mental well-being (Fredrickson & Joiner, 2002). Rather than indulging in temporary gratifications, satisfied individuals are often content in the embrace of the present, which, in turn, improves their overall satisfaction with life (Brown & Ryan, 2023).

- Life Satisfaction

Life satisfaction has a more specific meaning where it constitutes an overall quality judgment about the life of an individual in most if not all, of the spheres including interpersonal relations, work, and success (Pavot & Diener, 2020). High life satisfaction in these areas is associated with the performance and self-ratings of these practices and beliefs, creating an adult development that has a purpose and meaning (Suh et al., 2021). It has been found that highly satisfied individuals have more perceived social support, better work conditions, and a better fit between their aspirations and what they value (Sheldon & Lyubomirsky, 2023). Building strong bonds with others, meeting one's personal goals, and engaging in the activities they value most, all contribute to people's happiness and well-being (Choi et al., 2024).

Fitriana et al. (2022) stated that the idea of Happiness at Work is drawn from psychology and economic studies. Happiness is often considered as a synonym with 'wellbeing' and defined as a state characterized by a high level of life satisfaction, a high level of positive emotions, and less negative emotions The changes started when management and economics began including happiness for the past few decades. The curricula of different institutions of higher learning admit courses on happiness, such as "How to Create the Happy Work Environment," "Reasons for the Happiness of Employees," and "Wonders Down the Path to Happiness at Work."

Happiness at workplaces nowadays keeps the employment world abuzz. Happy workplaces are not constant parties where everyone is always happy and jubilant, which is the wrong assumption. There is no logic in expecting everyone to be jubilant; eight to ten hours on average are spent by employees performing tasks related to their positions of employment. Accordingly, one can conclude that the extent to which one is happy will derive mostly from satisfaction and contentment at one's workplace. Happiness at the Workplace refers to a person's overall contentment with life and career and subjective well-being in the workplace.

2. HAPPINESS AT THE WORKPLACE

Each employee sees the workplace as a small universe all of its own. They often feel the whole range from good and bad experiences to absolute joy or stress. Every employee can choose how they want to feel at work, happy or not. No matter how much one truly cares about another person and the job, one cannot be made to feel happy about it regardless of circumstances. Human beings are not the same, happiness and unhappiness depend on different things. Happiness is important at work for both the individual and the organization.

Primarily, this is what Apple was in the beginning. The company promoted itself in the image of an exaggerated and free-spirited entity which attracted the right innovators and disruptors. Hence, as the company expanded, increasing the necessary level of discipline within the company became difficult. What transpired in Apple exemplifies the fact that a company cannot solely depend on the business (Satpathy et al., 2024) model for success. None of it matters if workers' satisfaction is not guaranteed.

2.1 Components of Happiness at the Workplace

Prosperity, happiness, and health are the ingredients for well-being. It is about mental health, the ability to cope with stress, and connection or sense of purpose. Well, at least in the U.S.A. that appears to be faltering fast. It must be emphasized that physical health and mental wellness programs, and improved health benefits, are a purpose to create happy workplaces. But if we are unsure about how to do it, in reality, improving well-being can be tough. Well-being indeed encompasses prosperity, joy, and physical health. It involves possessing robust psychological functioning and resilience against strain, together with a profound sense of meaning. As per the information provided by the U.S. sources, the situation of well-being today seems to be deteriorating. American employers try to counter such tendencies by reintroducing the concept of well-being with some wellness programs, enhanced health care for the families of employees in addition to their own, and even positive moods that will produce healthier bodies or happier minds. If clarity on how to achieve such a rise is hard won, then improvement in well-being will be very tough.

Components of the workplace are

- Work-life balance

Organizations that recognize and address the need of employees for work-life balance (Manoharan et al., 2023) opt for a healthier and happier workforce. Appreciating such needs helps create an environment that encourages employees as well as the appreciation of their worth. It becomes necessary to put in policies that will guarantee and address the work-life balance of all staff. Some of the strategies include changes in the operational working hours, complete or partial telecommuting, and incorporation of health initiatives among others. Such measures raise employee satisfaction and tend to position the employees back in business as productive and committed. In the end, work-life balance allows for a balanced and results-oriented environment among the employees and the organization at large.

- Career Development

There is a saying that 'learning never ends.' Knowledge and learning go hand in hand and it is this urge to acquire more that keeps one mentally active. Growth and accomplishment are common feelings among individuals who constantly widen their scope. This constant growth helps not only build one's abilities but also improves one's self-worth. Improving oneself is an extremely comforting feeling because it fills the individual with so much contentment. Over time, this desire for self-improvement both personally and career-wise encourages a more imaginative and tough mindset, such that individuals can face problems with more vigor and originality.

- Job Security

How an organization can solve the problem of turnover is inside the dimension of growth. Employees want to feel that they have a future in the organization. Aspects of career growth create confidence and loyalty among employees shortening the period they will be away from the organization. By showing the nature of the growth, the opportunities presented, and the time frames that the growth will take, the organizations help to reduce strain in the workforce. Such an approach helps in encouraging individuals and additionally helps in completing the tasks as well. In the end, the organization enjoys the services of an active and forward-looking labor force. In the article 'Happiness in the Workplace' by Awada and Ismail (2024), the authors discussed the merits and demerits of happiness and its consequences at work.

2.2 Barriers to Workplace Happiness

While creating workplace happiness brings a challenge to different barriers, these barriers can come from the organizational culture, personal attitudes, or lay outside the organization itself. ***Significant barriers that create obstacles to workplace happiness:***

- Bad Leadership and Management

  Micromanaging: Leaders apply excessive control over their employees and create a work atmosphere that feels to employees unsafe or helpless, resulting in demoralization and unhappiness.

  Zero support: Employees need their leaders to guide, support, and recognize them. An absent-non-sympathetic-poorly communicating manager would, however, easily do all these three and may leave employees frustrated and disengaged.

An inconsistent leadership style: Lack of consistent leadership will create confusion, distrust, and frustration among the employees.

- Work Life Not Balanced

  Heavy Workload: Employees overworked for long hours or unrealistic expectations suffer burnout and thus happiness and job satisfaction.

  Rigid Work Timings: Employees would have to suffer stress and dissatisfaction if they could not shift their schedules to meet personal needs or family commitments.

  Absence of Leaves: A culture that looks down upon vacation and sick leave discourages taking leaves for the well-being of employees.

- Toxic Work Environment

  Poor Communication: Miscommunication or lack of transparency can create confusion, frustration, and exclusion among employees.

  Bullying or Harassment: The workplace that has allowed the ever presence of bullying or harassment seriously affects morale and happiness.

  Lack of Inclusivity: Lack of happiness and trust within an organization can arise when employees feel excluded, discriminated against, or devalued.

- Limited Career Development and Growth

  No Professional Development: Limited areas of development for employees will make them feel that they are standing still.

  Different but not well-known Job Pathways: Employees then lose interest or start seeking other opportunities with the company if they do not have an idea about their possible career growth in the company.

  No Recognized Performance: Motivation and happiness at the workplace usually decline when employees feel that their efforts are not being acknowledged.

- Inequalities and Unfair Practices

  Unfair Pay and Benefits: Employees begin to feel undervalued if they believe their pay or benefits are not fair based on the workload, or in general, compared with their peers in the industry.

  Lack of Recognition: No due recognition of hard work makes employees feel visible but not visible and demotivated.

  Favoritism: Promotions, rewards, and recognition based on favoritism lead to resentment among those employees who walk the extra mile but feel overlooked.

- Inadequate Resources and Tools

  Lacking Proper Tools: Lack of proper resources, proper technology, or the support that employees need to do their jobs efficiently can result in frustration and thus lower satisfaction.

Poor Working Conditions: The physical aspects of the working environment, such as uncomfortable offices, poor lighting, or noise levels, will directly affect employees' happiness.

- Unclear or Misaligned Organizational Values

  Absence of Purpose: Employees who do not connect to the organization's mission or values will assign little meaning to what they are doing, leading them to disengage.

  Ambiguous Expectations: Nonclarity in job roles or responsibilities can lead to confusion and frustration, thus reducing the level of happiness at work.

- Stressful Organizational Changes

  Frequent Organizational Changes: Constant changes in the organizations such as the changes in priorities, restructuring, and layoff, only culminate in uncertainty, which brings stress and anxiety to employees.

  Lack of communication during change: Employees will often become disillusioned or feel distanced from the organization when they are not well informed and involved in the decision-making process during times of change.

- Negative Social Dynamics

  Lack of Team Cohesion: A poor environment of competition or isolation as a result of a lack of trust or collaboration among co-workers is created, leading to negative outcomes in happiness.

  Unhealthy Competition: High competition which promotes uncooperative behavior and breeds jealousy instead of loyalty cuts happiness at the workplace.

- Economic and External Factors

  Financial Stress: If there is a crisis of funding around the organization, that would usually mean job security waning, wages remaining stagnated, or benefits getting reduced, and these factors would contribute to negatively affecting employees' morale.

  Global/External Uncertainty: Political instability, economic recession, and public health crises may impact indirect workplace happiness and well-being due to increased uncertainty or stress.

2.3 Means to Create Happiness in the Workplace

The current challenge is to create a joyful and stress-free workplace. A happy workplace is attainable and has the potential to impact (Singh et al., 2024) things significantly. Happiness at work from the psychological standpoint is a function of several interrelated factors that affect the employee's well-being. This is further elaborated on by Misra and Srivastava (2022) in their review who promote an understanding of happiness at work integrates biological, psychological, and social as well as anthropological structures. Their findings indicate that such an approach to environmental design where attention is paid to the work environment's psychological aspects would improve the employees' satisfaction and performance (Misra & Srivastava, 2022). This is consistent with other studies that highlight the need to consider both personal and corporate factors in the quest for a happy workplace. Apart from investing time and resources into cultivating a happy workplace, firms must find ways like the below to increase employee happiness in their working environment.

Different Means *to* Create Workplace Happiness Include

- Nurture Collaboration

These days, the majority of businesses spend money on team-building exercises to foster a feeling of community and improve connections among coworkers. Team activities such as team projects, retreats, and team meals can enhance teamwork. The most important factor of a winning team is the positivity and trust that exists within. People with similar experiences and world outlooks tend to get on well with each other, but the ennobling impact of team diversity is that it helps the team to learn and grow.

- Encourage openness in communication

To develop trust, respect, and value for every individual, the organization should advocate open communication (Manoharan et al., 2024), between its management and its employees. Team meeting and one-on-one meetings in this case has a great impact. Also, it is a chance for the management to give and take criticism. Providing a conducive work environment to the employees is the primary aim.

- Encourage Team Work

Nowadays majority of the companies are investing in team-building activities to create a sense of togetherness among the employees and enhance their interpersonal relationships. Exercises involving cooperation such as group work, excursions, and lunch breaks can be effective in enhancing (Manoharan et al., 2024) teamwork. Success lies in a team that has good bonding and trust. Purely because individuals with the very same backgrounds and outlooks on life may have bonding and interaction, a certain kind of teamwork is particularly important for all the members to draw from each other's differences and grow together as a team. One of the most powerful strategies for building a successful team inside a business is to celebrate the diversity of cultures within the team.

- Promote a Happy Working Environment

A happy working environment makes a big difference. Organizations must ensure that the workplace is organized, welcoming, and well-lit. This will infuse the office with positivity. Small details like the configuration of the workstations and the conditions of the chairs are important as well. Creating a comfortable work environment for employees is the overall objective.

- Encourage Work-Life Balance

One of the best strategies to establish a happy workplace is to promote work-life balance. Workers will like going to work in an environment that values their time. Allowing employees to work from home, have flexible schedules, and receive enough paid time off improves their ability to manage their lives. Businesses encourage employees to take time off and spend more time with their families by offering excellent vacation programs. Employees who maintain a sound balance between their jobs and personal activities tend to work better.

- Focus on Employee Growth

Organizations that make commitments to the development of their employees experience higher levels of employee engagement. It is good to show concern for the growth of the employees by availing training, workshops, and other career progression activities. Well-established firms believe in the enhancement and improvement of the quality of their employees. There are always teams that want to create a learning culture to enable their employees to perform better.

- Promote Diversity and Inclusion

To encourage creativity and innovation, it is important to have a diverse and inclusive workplace. This is because a diverse workforce has negative synergies, ideas, and solutions. They share and utilize different experiences (Scott et al., 2021). Team diversity consisting of culture, background, and professional skills creates learning and enhancement of each of the team members leading to improved performance of the individuals and even the organization (Rodriguez & Hauser, 2023). Where diversity is embraced in various facades, there are two advantages, one is the breathing of useful behaviour into the team, and the second giving the organization a better working edge (Forbes Insights, 2022).

- Ensure a Competitive Remuneration Strategy

While creating a comfortable working environment is critical for the workers' contentment; salaries that are regarded as lucrative are also essential in the quest for hiring and retaining the best employees. Salaries that are competitive and attractive benefit the employees for the desired output produced and also serve as an assurance to them that society respects their input (Miller & Green, 2023). If an organization ensures that the salaries offered to the employees are not below the industry level, the organization stands a better chance of retaining such highly skilled employees which helps to stabilize and keep the workforce energized (Anderson & Walters, 2022).

- Appreciating and Recognizing the Efforts of Employee

One of the most effective strategies to encourage employees to perform at their peak is employee recognition. Recognition of their efforts, through either giving formal recognition awards or just saying thank you helps to build such a culture and motivates the staff (Wilson et al., 2023). Evidence suggests that it is the regular practice of recognition that mostly contributes to the levels of engagement, job satisfaction, and performance of individuals (Harvey & Brock, 2022).

- Feedback Mechanisms

Regular feedback mechanisms help in establishing a culture of trust and efficiency in communication. There are a variety of organizational activities such as suggestion boxes, employee feedback, and one-on-one interactions (Winster et al., 2024), that facilitate feedback collection and help the management to meet the expectations of the employees (Black & Chen, 2022). When this feedback is acted upon, it conveys the message to the employees that their opinions matter, which fosters healthy relations in society. From these findings, it is clear that such measures, not only create a beneficial climate but go on to improve the quality of relations between people, thus contributing to the overall unity within the working environment (Johnson & Blake, 2021).

- Celebrate Success

It is important to recognize the achievements of individuals and teams for the creation of such a work environment where people feel motivated and supported. Reaching set goals can be rewarded in different ways whether by organizing formal events or just by saying thank you which connects the people in the organization as well as uplifts their spirits to achieve more for the organization (Simons & Clark, 2023). Research indicates that all employees are motivated to work harder if performance is recognized and rewarded as the concept of appreciation builds (Thompson, 2022).

- Offer Competitive Pay

Pay structures play a crucial role in creating and maintaining a healthy organizational culture. A competitive pay structure not only offers the right market desirability but also sustains the recruiting strategy by giving confidence in the ability to reward fairly (Williams & Davis, 2023). Compensation, pay, and fringe benefits all signify respect for employee loyalty and service which encourages them to stay. Paying appropriate salaries to employees helps to enhance their contentment and keeps the workplace at par with other businesses in the industry (Olsen & Wong, 2019).

2.4 Key Approaches to Foster Happiness at the Workplace

Happiness at the workplace can be improved by first and foremost developing a positive, inclusive, and supportive environment that makes employees feel appreciated. Making sure that accomplishments are recognized regularly, there are chances of a sense of belonging and purpose. Support in terms of adjustable working hours, mental health assistance, wellness programs, and others promotes work-life balance thereby easing stress and enhancing (Krishnan et al., 2022) contentment. Offering appropriate bonuses, equipping employees with decent office space, and allowing them to be independent instill confidence and also encourage staff. If the leaders tend to be more compassionate and approachable while also caring about the growth of employees, both personally and professionally, the workers are bound to be content and happy at their places of work.

Over the last few decades, workplace happiness has received considerable attention. A detailed literature review undertaken by Jaswal et al. (2024) understands the significance of well-being towards increasing the happiness of employees at the workplace. Their mission is the identification of significant approaches that can be adopted by the organizations to foster a happy work environment. As per their results, the implementation of such well-being programs helps in the enhancement of attitude towards work combined with increased productivity and overall performance of the organization (Jaswal, Sharma, Bhardwaj, & Kraus, 2024). This has been seen previously by other scholars working in the area, who also affirm that employee satisfaction has serious ramifications for the business.

Some of the ways to improve happiness in the workplace include are

- Greater Employee Motivation

There is often a direct correlation between the well-being of employees and their energy levels, mental sharpness, and the rate at which they perform certain functions. Such focus and alertness, in most cases, manifest in increased output and the willingness to face challenges positively. Further, those who are fit both mentally and physically are more inclined to engage in teamwork, which bolsters the company's harmony and internal strength. Overall, there are more employees devoted to the job, which is beneficial since the organization will have a smaller number of employees leaving for other jobs and this will ultimately translate into the success of the organization.

- Best of Employee's Spirits

The employees need initiatives, which help construct a healthy organizational workplace. Such initiatives, however, are more than just social engagements for the employees. They enhance the work culture by emphasizing the mental, physical, and even professional growth of the employee. Programs such as wellness training, mental health care days, and upskilling opportunities, in turn, increase morale and engagement. When well-being is addressed in all its aspects, employees feel more appreciated, and their enthusiasm for performing work increases, which results in higher job satisfaction and commitment to the organization.

- Increased Departmental Talent Acquisition and Preservation:

The effect of well-being at the workplace on attracting and retaining talent is significant. An organization that prioritizes the health of its employees makes a certain pull to those who seek and appreciate a healthy, supportive work environment. Well-being has this dual effect; it does not only recruit new people but also encourages the already existing ones not to leave. The concerned employees feel appreciated and provided for, thus there are high levels of job satisfaction (Chaudhary et al., 2024) and dedication. Consequently, these types of organizations are also associated with better performance creativity, and general organizational effectiveness, forming a cycle whereby well-being leads to the productivity of the working people.

- Medical cost savings

A workforce that prioritizes health minimizes the incidence and gravity of health problems and consequently, healthcare expenditures for the organization. It is also understood that there will be fewer health-related issues in the workplace, therefore, there will be fewer sick leaves, increased commitment towards the company goals, and overall, an increase in productivity. It also translates to bringing down the costs incurred in taking medical insurance and less compensation for medical claims. From a long-term perspective, the accrued cost savings resulting from reduced healthcare expenses tend to be quite large, enabling the organization to focus on other sectors such as employee development and innovative ideas.

- Better Work Atmosphere

Work-Life Stress Balance Programs equip individuals with the requisite skills to tackle stress more professionally while undertaking their work and taking care of their other obligations. Such programs usually offer additional stress relief mechanisms which include stress management classes, adjusted work schedules, and psychological care, which assist employees in dealing with stress. Work stress alleviation enables employees to lead a more fulfilling life, as they become more active and alert in all aspects of their lives; including field and leisure. In the end, these programs foster a more productive and healthier workforce, which is advantageous to the employees and the establishment as well.

- Encourages Team Activities

Participating in work-life balance strategies and sharing of responsibilities will automatically encourage members to work as a team. Such programs include several group actions and initiatives, which in turn bring employees closer. As workers collaborate to tackle problems, such as stress management and balancing work and family obligations, they cultivate a healthy appreciation for each other. In addition to fostering teamwork, such an atmosphere also raises the attitude of the workforce and helps in creating a more integrated and effective workforce.

- Minimized Cases of Burnout

Workplaces encourage healthy practices of separating work and free time and offer counseling or other wellness initiatives to have active employees. The studies have also established that such structures translate to job asserts, which lowers job absences and improves work output. At the core of these is the realization that investing in employees' health and happiness forms an organization that has a good work environment and employee loyalty thereby attracting maximum employee productivity towards the organization's goal.

The benefits of improving happiness in the workplace are

- Intrinsic Motivation

There would be a positive enhancement in the work performance of the individual and the level of involvement in the work would also be achieved when the individuals are satisfied. Each individual aims to perform better and use every opportunity to flourish within the system when such workers are happy. All in all, one extent of satisfaction leads to the other as in the case of happy individuals they do their work well, hence there are benefits to the individual and the organization.

- Higher Productivity

An employee who is engaged and happy will have a desire to perform at their best due to their interest in their work and a wish to succeed at it. This high level of engagement results in higher productivity because engaged and motivated employees get the jobs done more quickly and efficiently. Furthermore, the positive attitude and determination of such people often rub off on their teammates, which in turn improves performance. In the end, an organization that nurtures and encourages employee contentment and engagement is bound to experience increased productivity and effectiveness.

- Open Mindset

The ability to be happy ensures that one has a broad and unencumbered view, thereby allowing for the removal of any creative stagnation that may be in play. Happy individuals tend to be at ease and self-assured, which in turn extradites their mind from the confines of new ideas and perspectives for a given task, without the inhibition or anxiety of shame or defeat. This intimate connection thrives on the very essence of creative thinking, as employees tend to be more adventurous and risk-taking which enhances the treatment of new ideas. To put it differently, employee satisfaction with their respective companies turns out to be a fountain of fresh ideas and innovations which in turn aids the growth of the firm in ways that are not anticipative and encourage a more open mindset that would enhance creative thought and innovation.

- Risk Taking

Employees who enjoy working are more prone to taking calculated risks because they feel safe and appreciated at the places where they work. The security, in turn, helps them to take on new challenges and try out new ideas. Such calculated risks, however, often lead to creative and innovative solutions that help to elevate the company to new heights. In other words, a happy workforce breeds a culture of positive changes and continuous enhancements within the structure.

- Flexibility and Autonomy

Workplaces that focus on the employees' well-being tend to employ, among other strategies, ways of working that allow doing their job away from the office or at different times than the standard operating hours. This management style ensures that the employees do not stress out or experience burnout, which leads to a more active and concerned workforce. Besides, active employees with good work-life interference tend to feel that they are appreciated and supported in the organization, which raises their overall satisfaction with the job and loyalty to the organization. Such conditions not only promote the well-being of employees but also increase productivity and encourage a positive workplace environment.

- Job Crafting

Employers may grant their workers the opportunity to alter certain aspects of their responsibilities to fit their natural abilities and preferences. This freedom enhances the level of responsibility rendered towards the employees and hence, their willingness to carry out the work. As a result, they are expected to have high levels of job contentment and perform efficiently. In the end, this is not only a form of improving personal health but also helps the organization in increasing its productive capabilities and innovativeness.

- The attraction of Employees

A work environment that emphasizes happiness will easily attract the best human resources as prospective employees seek happier places to work. To enhance recruitment of even the most qualified candidates who seek work environments that are comfortable for them, such a culture fosters a good image by focusing on employee contentment. In addition, satisfied employees tend to broadcast their positive experiences to the public, which improves the organization's brand as well as its attractiveness to job seekers. This translates to an edge over other firms, which takes advantage of the ability of the firm to attract and keep the most talented individuals leading to continuous improvement and growth.

- Employee Turnover

Happy employees within an organization tend to stay longer than those who are not, therefore minimizing the turnover rate and promoting stability. This retention of talent ensures that the organization enjoys the services of dedicated and experienced individuals who help in creating and maintaining a conducive working atmosphere. Moreover, a healthy turnover rate helps to improve the organizational culture, as the interaction of older employees with new ones creates a bond and a team spirit.

Case studies of successful employee well-being initiatives are

- Google Initiative

Google offers a comprehensive employee wellness program that includes on-site health services, fitness centers, and mental health resources. They provide healthy meals, flexible work arrangements, and various wellness workshops.

- Outcome

This holistic approach has resulted in high employee satisfaction and retention rates. Google frequently ranks among the best places to work, with a culture that encourages innovation and productivity.

- Salesforce Initiative

Salesforce's "Ohana Culture" emphasizes employee well-being through programs like mental health days, wellness reimbursement, and access to mindfulness resources. They also offer support for work-life balance and stress management.

- *Outcome*

Salesforce reported a significant increase in employee engagement and a decrease in turnover. Their initiatives have contributed to a supportive workplace where employees feel valued and motivated.

- Microsoft Initiative

Microsoft has implemented a robust mental health program, including access to counseling, wellness resources, and a focus on creating a positive work environment. They offer flexible schedules and promote a culture of openness regarding mental health.

- *Outcome*

Employees have reported lower stress levels and increased job satisfaction, which has led to enhanced creativity and collaboration across teams.

- Johnson & Johnson Initiative

Johnson & Johnson's "Health and Wellness Program" focuses on physical health, mental well-being, and financial health. They provide wellness coaching, fitness challenges, and health screenings.

- *Outcome*

The program has resulted in substantial healthcare savings and improved employee productivity. The company reported a return on investment of about $2.71 for every dollar spent on health and wellness initiatives.

- Deloitte Initiative

Deloitte's "Well-being" programs focus on mental, physical, and emotional health, offering resources like counseling, wellness days, and fitness challenges. They also promote a flexible work culture.

- *Outcome*

Deloitte has seen increased employee morale and a strong commitment to its corporate culture, resulting in higher productivity and retention rates.

Over the last few years, it has become apparent that the importance of fostering happy workplaces cannot be understated. Moss (2023) asserts that building a happier workplace is not only possible but practical and profitable. Findings reveal that organizations that focus on the sense of well-being of their employees enjoy great benefits in productivity and general organizational culture (Moss, 2023). This is consistent with wider observations on the issue that the happiness of workers is the catalyst of victory in any enterprise.

2.5 Evaluating Workplace Happiness: Key Metrics and Methods

The current challenge is to create a joyful and stress-free workplace. A happy workplace is attainable and has the potential to significantly impact things. Apart from investing time and resources into cultivating a happy workplace, firms must find ways like the below to measure employee happiness in their working environment. Gisela Sender et al (2021), in their research work, stated that the elusive concept for organizational psychologists is Happiness at Work. Accordingly, he believed that if individuals are happy at work, it becomes so much easier for them to perform their tasks in an organization, and this is advantageous both to individual employees and to the companies they work for. However, after several decades of investigation into the phenomenon, a consistent position is yet to be reached on the issue primarily because no standard operational definition has been developed. Usually, there is a tendency to employ questionnaires or self-report surveys; however, the methods used expose some flaws making what the results of the studies can be called into question. To address these problems, the present study advocates for an alternative way of assessing Happiness at Work using mixed methods research to portray the phenomenon in its full complexity.

- Employee Engagement

Involving the employees in regular and frank discussions on their duties, pay and general working conditions improves the work atmosphere considerably. These conversations help gauge the levels of contentment amongst the employees, hence management can act on the problems raised in good time. With this openness and listening culture in the organization, there will be less hostility and aggrievance and more motivation and productivity instead.

- Open Feedback

It is necessary to create a healthy working environment where the employees are free to express their thoughts and deliver opinions without intimidation so that management can respond proactively. This healthy environment promotes freedom of communication as employees can raise issues and even recommend improvements within the organization. This makes management tackle the problems quickly and in an appropriate manner which results in a healthy and active work atmosphere aimed at improving employees' happiness and productivity.

- Employee Surveys

An employee satisfaction index can be solicited with the use of employee surveys where every employee is allowed to express their views privately. This confidentiality fosters more openness in providing opinions and gives an accurate assessment of employees' feelings about their duties, pay, and working conditions in general. Moreover, management finds problems and resolves them through the analysis of the survey results as it looks for factors that contribute to dissatisfaction and thus improves the level of workforce productivity.

- Efficiency Metrics

Happy employees tend to be more productive since their contentment with the job drives them to work harder and be more efficient. Throughout the year, performance (Gopinathan et al., 2022), reviews are held to measure such satisfaction as workers can talk about their achievements, areas of improvement as well as their objectives. There are also reasons why management can benefit from these reviews. For example, they provide useful information regarding the morale of workers which the management uses to make decisions aimed at improving the work environment and the overall productivity of employees.

- Assess Stress Levels

One of the features that aids in reinforcing a conducive setting for work is managing employee stress levels as any level that is considered excessive is likely to doubt one's work performance as well as their health. Stress reduction measures should be easier to incorporate into the workplace where an organization provides mindfulness training, allows flexible work rotations, or introduces other wellness programs. On the other hand, respect for hierarchy and the availability of support services such as counseling can help make employees feel appreciated and cared for. In conclusion, when stress management efforts are a focal point of the work environment, a healthier, more focused, and better-performing employee may be an assurance.

- Monitor the Turnover Rate and Absenteeism

Excessive absenteeism and turnover incidences tend to be a clear indication of discontent within the employees. Employees are likely to maintain attendance and even stay with the organization for long periods, thus minimizing turnover-related costs after the organization has succeeded in making them happy. Satisfaction within the workforce ensures less turbulence and higher levels of performance thus creating the need for a friendly and conducive work culture.

2.6 The Link Between Workplace Happiness and Employee Well-being

Workplace happiness significantly affects the general well-being of both individuals and companies. Attitudes about employee mental health have dramatically shifted. While for much of history, the burden was on the employee to lower the level of stress with company-offered benefits such as mindfulness seminars and health coverage for therapy, that trend is changing, psychologists who focus on workplace behavior say. "The pandemic made employers realize that the mental health of workers should be given more attention and that a work environment either can contribute or protect against challenges related to mental health," said Leslie Hammer, PhD, from Oregon Health and Science University, who is the professor in the Oregon Institute of Occupational Health Sciences (Stringer, 2023). In recent times, health, happiness, and the wellness economy have been receiving a lot of focus. According to the Global Wellness Institute (2023), there is a strong relationship between levels of happiness and other levels of wellness. Their comprehensive analysis provides a deep understanding of the role of happiness in the well-being of individuals and the economy as a whole. In correspondence to other research, these findings reinforce the rationale to foster a good working environment to reduce employee turnover and improve productivity (Global Wellness Institute, 2023).

Major aspects that contribute to the improvement of well-being with happiness are:

- Benefits of Mental Health Reduced Stress

Employees who work in a cheerful space tend to feel more comfortable and, therefore, can concentrate on their duties better. A positive climate makes it easier for them to overcome stress and anxiety making it possible to work and even be creative. Moreover, employees when happy and relaxed easily engage and interact with their colleagues improving their team performance. A happy workplace also instills a feeling of togetherness and contentment, which are essential for personal and organizational achievements.

- Improved Resiliency

Workers who are engaged in their jobs are more likely to be mentally tough and deal with stress more easily. One factor contributing to this mental toughness is a sunny disposition that enables them to face difficult situations without getting swamped. As a result, the capacity to manage stress improves mental health and therefore decreases the risk of exhaustion and other stress-induced problems. In the end, it is understandable why a happy workforce increases productivity as well as the mental well-being of the employees and thus, the organization as a whole.

- Decrease in absenteeism

Workers who are in good health are usually more content and this has the effect of minimizing sickness levels. The strong physical health paradigm strengthens the immunity of the workers making them less prone to infections. Their improved health means fewer sick leaves taken which ensures uninterrupted productivity and less pressure on the health care system of the organization. So, it happens that health and happiness form a circle where both contribute to the quality and the quantity of work done by the employees.

- Engagement in Healthy Activities

The workplace emphasizes health advantages and supports regular activities like healthy eating and exercising among workers. Companies encourage wellness by offering healthy food in their canteens and organizing fitness activities for their employees. Such activities in addition to keeping people fit mentally enhance productivity levels as well. Therefore, such an environment is bound to cause less absenteeism, more output, and happier employees.

- Meaningfulness

When individuals are happy with their working environment, they tend to become more attached to their roles and derive a higher level of satisfaction from engaging in their everyday activities. This attachment creates a feeling of pride and undoubtedly allows for better performance at work. Furthermore, a conducive atmosphere presents employees with the opportunity to pursue values that are in tandem with the objectives of the organization, and this is in itself quite enriching. For these reasons, happy employees become more productive and loyal and, as a result, benefit the organization.

- Achievement

If people indulge in constructive and enjoyable tasks, they are likely to experience a deep sense of contentment. Such a sense of achievement is a great self-motivator that encourages them to work even harder. Any recognition of their efforts, be it an intrinsic reward or an external one, also helps them stay firm on their objectives.

Eventually, this circle of success and gratitude cultivates a healthy and active atmosphere of work, motivating everyone to give their best and the next best.

- Enhanced Team Work

Being satisfied encourages healthy thinking which helps a person in making good associates at work and vice versa. These associations help in creating a work culture where team members feel appreciated and heard. When the Disposition extends to Trust, and the bond goes towards Companionship, the Work turns out to be More Constructive with Improved Cooperation and Adding to teamwork. The members enhance their productivity because of the teamwork that they are exposed to while at the same time enjoying their work.

- Sustained Connections

Working satisfaction among employees, in turn, promotes a feel-good enabling environment marked by care and attachment. This creates a welcomed environment that makes employees feel appreciated thus leading to higher commitment levels and loyalty. In turn, the organization strengthens its bonds of community and respect for each other which promotes individual as well as group performance.

Over the past few years, a primary concern for many organizations has been the well-being of their employees. Employee well-being has many facets, and one of them is physical health. Organizations encourage physical health through various interventions aimed at targeting the employees' health and wellness, such as 'wellness programs'. Wellness programs are company-sponsored programs that aim at improving the health of employees, hence minimizing health-related absences. However, there has been an increased focus on employee well-being in organizations and occupational health psychology. Most organizations have been investing in the physical health of employees with the main purpose of minimizing absenteeism and optimizing work productivity. Moreover, many employees, especially in the Western world, have become aware of the need to attain a good 'work-life' balance, and have actively sought jobs which will enable this. Some psychologists have even described the search for balance in one's life as a pathological 'workaholism' in some individuals. Organizations therefore have sought to motivate their employees through various policies and practices. Adjusted work schedules, for example, have enabled employees to perform their parental responsibilities without the fear of missing any work obligations. But these initiatives do not work for everyone. Enhanced participation in this region ensures even distribution of both resources and information thereby promoting equitable development.

In their research, `López Ruiz and his team" (2021) underline the importance of enabling all people in society to feel good - you know, happy, etc., as they say. They showed that if people are well off, it helps the whole society. So, what makes people happy is quite important. It's mainly a matter of how well-off individuals are, how much money they have, and whether their job is getting anywhere. Wellbeing is a fascinating subject today when it is studied by molecular scientists who examine the causes of people's happiness and the nature of a successful life one can live. At the moment, the so-called 'happiness sciences' have gained the utmost popularity within the academic walls.

2.7 The Link between Workplace Happiness and Work-Life Balance

There exists a strong relationship (Manoharan et al., 2022) between job satisfaction and work-life balance. There is a greater likelihood of a positive balance between personal and professional life among happy workers. The evolving expectations of the workforce in terms of their welfare have, in turn, affected the culture of the business. An emphasis on psychological health in working conditions is increasing and these changes are commented on by Stringer (2023). There is thus theoretical support for the argument that organizations should change their practices in favor of increasing the well-being of the employees which in turn improves productivity and job satisfaction (Stringer, 2023). This is in line with wider developments pointing to the importance of overall employee happiness and work-life balance.

- Flexibility and Autonomy

Companies that focus on employee welfare usually adopt the practice of offering employees flexible working hours since there is a consensus that flexibility is the most important factor in striking a work-life balance. This helps employees cope with their obligations effectively and reduces stress that could lead to exhaustion. By respecting various ways of life and work patterns, flexible working conditions create a more conducive and supportive environment within the organization. As a result, workers tend to appreciate and value themselves more, which tends to promote loyalty, productivity, and general job satisfaction.

- Improved Health

Both physical and mental health are positively impacted by workplace happiness. When workers are in good health, they can enjoy their personal lives more without being distracted by work-related problems. A great many studies have shown the positive impact that job satisfaction has on the work-life balance of individuals. Happy workers, for instance, are more likely to embrace a positive personal and professional balance. Here is how you do it: First, flexibility and hence autonomy are essential. Most employee-friendly organizations offer flexible working hours as one of the ways to keep employees happy. This is because employees who are given more flexible working hours can better integrate their social and work schedules.

- Reduced Stress

A culture of support in the workplace encourages a good working environment that helps eliminate the stress levels associated with the employees. The more relaxed the environment, the easier and more pleasant it becomes for the employees to execute their duties. Employees have little difficulty switching off from work-related thoughts at the end of the day when the environment is not too serious, which allows them to fully appreciate the rest of the hours. This equilibrium is not only healthy for their wellbeing but also healthy for their return to work, and turning out to be more productive.

- Increased Productivity

It is observed that productive employees are mostly happy ones, as their productive attitude is reflected in the use of time at work. Time use efficiency in this regard implies finishing work on or before time and doing such work in the right way which reduces or eliminates the need for overworking which enables the workers to balance their professional lives with their personal lives. With a lesser workload in the offices, the workers can afford time to carry out activities that will revive them, promoting their health and satisfaction with their work. And so, the happiness and the work done create another effective loop that promotes the employees' morale and effectiveness helping not only the person but also the organization.

- Stronger Bonds

A constructive work environment fosters better camaraderie amongst employees and encourages free expression and support for one another. This fostered community paves the way for a situation where work becomes more than a chore, affording a sense of belonging and worth. Employees who relate and reach out to one another in support as a team appreciate their jobs more and are happier with their work. In turn, such happy working conditions extend to general life and satisfaction levels improving and helping achieve balance in and out of the office.

2.8 Workplace Happiness as a Catalyst for Company Growth

While happiness at work would have been derived from third parties, like promotions and perks, spiritual confidants, and thought leaders, the author of "The Flourishing Code," Mynoo Maryel explains that real happiness comes only from within. In her view, "The only way to reduce the degree of happiness one permits oneself to experience is by surrendering that happiness to other people". Concerning the external rewards, they will certainly bring happiness and high for some time, but they will make a person helpless in the long run. Thus, Maryel persuades individuals to take responsibility for their happiness as well; they need to seek for themselves what precisely they require for their work and career. "You are the master of your destiny," she concludes (Cooper et al., 2024).

A few ways in which happiness at the workplace impacts growth include

- Contagious Positivity

Happy people have an extraordinary capacity to strengthen and enrich those around them by establishing a healthy and nurturing work community. Their happiness is contagious making others possess the same attitude hence a spirit of cooperation and respect is promoted. Positivity and resilience displayed by them minimize workplace tension and promote a better working environment. This encouraging setting helps team members to excel leading to better morale and productivity levels. In the end, such a culture of support created by happy people results in further high levels of functioning cohesion which makes everyone work to excel because they feel appreciated and needed.

- Hard work

The contented employees with the organization's simple principles, put more effort into helping the commercial enterprise achieve its dreams. The harmonious relationship between happiness and creativity helps to break the cycle of routine. This ultimately leads to better creativity. When the human resource department encourages greater participation and innovative ideas from employees, it will create a good working environment. Positive Workers' Attitude: The contented Workforce will be more accepting and willing to give and receive feedback instead of whining for instance.

More decision-making and quicker learning: Incredibly valued personnel accumulate expertise in a faster way. Happier employees are better teammates, which leads to improved teamwork.

2.9 Role of Digital Wellbeing Initiatives

Digital well-being initiatives and hybrid work models present a more luminous chapter in the post-pandemic period as organizations and employees grapple with new work realities. Here are some insights on how these two domains relate to the future of work and well-being:

1. **Digital Wellbeing Initiatives**: Digital well-being initiatives are aimed at assisting employees with the challenges that come with increased technological reliance. These initiatives mainly consider screen time management and the alleviation of digital overload while seeking to sustain mental health in the digital age.

    Key Contributions to Wellbeing:

    - Mental Wellbeing

Digital tools and apps, such as Headspace, Calm, or therapy platforms, may assist employees in dealing with stress, anxiety, or other mental health issues. These remote-working and digitally communicating remedies offer support to maintain mental health and emotional resilience.

- Screen Time Management

A lot of digital well-being programs come with features that would allow staff to self-monitor and limit their screen time, reducing the likelihood of burnout, eye strain, and fatigue due to prolonged use of gadgets.

- Work-Life Balance

Digital wellbeing tools allow employees to maintain a clear distinction between work and personal life by limiting notifications, offering work schedule management features, and sending reminders to take breaks. This will mitigate the very serious risk of the "always-on" mentality creeping into an employee's day, which is detrimental to wellbeing.

- Virtual Wellness Program

Today, digital platforms present virtual wellness programs that include yoga, mindfulness, fitness challenges, and nutrition coaching. The ability for staff to access these on-demand programs encourages the pursuit of mental and physical well-being while remote working.

- Employee Engagement & Feedback

Many digital well-being initiatives come with tools to gather feedback on employee satisfaction levels, work stress levels, and well-being. This information enables an organization to make evidence-based recommendations for enhancing employee experience and well-being.

- Cybersecurity Awareness

With the proliferation of digital workspaces, today comes an escalation in potential cybersecurity risks. Digital Wellbeing initiatives also cover educating employees regarding the best cybersecurity practices to protect their personal information and alleviate the stress associated with incurring a possible data breach.

2. **Hybrid Working Post-Pandemic**: Hybrid working models (where employees spend some of their time working from home and some in the office) have become the standard practice in many organizations after the pandemic. While these models offer a degree of freedom, they also present new challenges to the wellness of employees and the culture of the company.
    - Major Strategies for Promoting Well-being

Flexibility and Autonomy: Under a hybrid system, employees are free to plan their working hours and balance their work with other aspects of their lives. Such autonomy relates positively to job satisfaction and negatively to stress, as workers can adjust their work environment according to their needs.

- Improved Work-Life Balance

Hybrid work allows employees to spend more time at home or in other settings outside the office, reducing commuting time and providing more opportunities for rest. This ensures that employees enjoy a good work-life balance, which is vital for their long-term well-being.

- Reduced Stress of Commuting

Commuting to work has its fair share of stress; urban commuting gets even trickier. With hybrid working, employees have more control over when they decide to travel to the office or if they should go there, thereby minimizing the adverse physical and mental toll of daily commutes.

- Collaboration and Social Interaction

Hybrid working models can protect the social interactions within the workplace, which are important to the morale of employees. In-person working days facilitate face-to-face communication, helpful for reinforcing community, collaboration, and socializing with one another when remote tasks would not provide the same control.

- Tailored Support and Adaptation

Your hybrid work model allows your organization to provide personalized accommodation options based on employee needs. For example, remote work may be favored by more introverted employees, while extroverted employees who prefer working close to someone thrive in collaboration mode. Providing flexibility enables employees to pick the work environment where they feel their well-being is greatest.

- Technology and Digital Tools

Organizations use digital tools to facilitate hybrid working around collaboration, communication, and project management. Giving employees the right tools ensures unhindered interaction and minimizes frustration. Platforms such as Microsoft Teams, Slack, or Zoom facilitate work-from-home communication or strengthen teamwork.

- Mental Health and Social Support

While working remotely at least some days will lead to feelings of isolation, the hybrid work model should allow in-person interaction when necessary to counteract loneliness and provide informal opportunities for socializing—essential contributors to mental health.

- Clearly Defined Communication and Boundaries

Hybrid working can also muddle the lines between work and home life. Well-defined communication protocols and clear expectations for availability and time off will help employees navigate a healthy balance. Digital Wellbeing initiatives can further promote this by encouraging boundaries around after-hours emails and meetings.

- Leadership and Support

In a hybrid working environment, leadership is a key enabler. Leaders need to ensure that employees are supported, both remotely and in the office. They should maintain regular check-ins to ensure employee recognition and well-being and foster a culture of inclusion.

2.10 Is Happiness at the Workplace Real?

In the opinion of Beth Stall Wood, a consultant specializing in organizational development and author of the book "Work Joy", stated that such a belief is unrealistic. At the workplace, one experiences different feelings, ranging from the utmost euphoria to periods of stress and hopelessness. Keeping a constant state of bliss, putting on a fake smile, or never getting stressed out - are not features of Work Joy.

If one needs their group of workers to be happy all the time, one may also position pressure on them to cover their real emotions, which is ultimately counterproductive and harmful. A more balanced viewpoint, on the other hand, would center on general job satisfaction (Motwani et al., 2024) and well-being. It is however very common for workers to have days that are very depressive and just horrible. While such advancements may seem like a fantasy to many organizational theorists, some have been able to create cultures where workforce constituents are happy and productive. Happiness in the workplace is an integral part of the cultures and ways of working in businesses like Google, Patagonia, and Zappos. While it is probably helpful to a degree to organizing office socials or stocking the kitchen with snacks, a happy office is more about creating an environment in which employees feel cared for, respected as human beings, and part of a bigger cause. It involves the absence of fear and containment, provision of growth opportunities, recognition, balancing work and other aspects of life as well as creating a friendly environment.

3. FUTURE TRENDS IN WORKPLACE HAPPINESS

Mental health support is becoming increasingly recognized as a key component in the work health strategy. Recently, mental health wellness has transformed from being an additional service offered in the workplace to a must-have strategy in any well-being program. As per the World Health Organisation, the economic productivity loss attributed to mental health disorders is estimated at $1 trillion per year. The proactive measures will probably be in the form of mental health management training sessions for all the supervisors, mental health checking sessions from time to time, and stress and burnout alleviation drives (5 workplace wellbeing trends for 2025 - Wellbeing People[1]).

Some of the future endeavors include

- The Prevalence of Hybrid and Remote Work

The adoption of a hybrid or a fully remote model affects happiness in the workplace. Nowadays, employees focus more on their ability to choose the kind of workplace they wish to be in, which has been shown to enhance the work-life balance and decrease stress levels (Smith et al., 2022). Literature reviews suggest that this kind of flexibility enhances overall well-being and promotes job performance and satisfaction as well (Bartik et al., 2023).

- Wide and Full Use of Data in Well-Being Program

There is also the emerging trend of the use of more data-oriented strategies in measuring the success of well-being programs by organizations. More companies are collecting employee health, well-being, and productivity information to develop more focused strategies in designing such programs (Johnson & Lee, 2021). It has been established that programs that use data to guide well-being programs have better rates of engagement in the programs and improved positivity among the employees (Gartner Research, 2024).

- Diverse Approaches to Well-Being

Addressing equity in benefits programs has become increasingly important, as all organizations strive to address a varied workforce. There has been a shift towards a well-being culture, which focuses on addressing challenges faced by target populations and demographics that are specific (Kaur & Thompson, 2023). This ensures that the well-being of individuals is upheld and also eases issues of acceptance and fairness in workplaces (Miller, 2022).

- Approach towards Strategies Aimed to Reduce Burnout

Focusing on the fact that burnout has become a serious concern for many organizations, strategies aim at rehabilitating and recovering employees. In these strategies, employees are encouraged to rest, regular breaks are instituted as well as work limits (Wang et al., 2022), and love for work is cultivated. It is also acknowledged by organizations that the reduction of employee burnout is not only helpful to the employees but it also improves the performance of the organization (Burns & Li, 2023). Highlighting the trends discussed is an uplift towards a wholesome definition of employee satisfaction, which incorporates mental health, flexibility, and diversity.

DISCUSSIONS AND CONCLUSION

It is quite unfortunate that happiness at work is not just a commendable practice within an organization but a compulsory ingredient for growth and success. In this chapter, a discussion regarding the benefits that a contented workforce can bring in terms of production, creativity, and the business at large has been emphasized. There are psychological theories such as the positive psychology framework and self-determination theory that can help understand how happiness affects organizations and how it can be promoted and maintained. Leadership (Manoharan et al., 2024) is an important aspect of this culture, concentrating on the need for a clear focus on the promotion of transparency, a two-way communication process, and recognition programs. Other practical approaches, such as the provision of flexible work schedules, professional advancement prospects, and the facilitation of contact among employees all serve to make it possible for the employees to flourish.

For progress consistency, it is imperative to also focus on happiness and its measurement. There are assessment tools and metrics that allow organizations to measure levels of employee contentment and relate it with the general performance (Manoharan et al., 2024) of a business and enable the organization to know the value for money expended on wellness programs. Real-life examples from the years of some great companies explain why it is essential to keep happiness at the top of one's priorities. Overcoming challenges, and finding ways to reduce or eliminate common hindrances, are very important for assuring a pleasant working environment. It includes managing resistance from the higher echelon or rank and ensuring that happiness is not compromised during transitions or even in periods of distress.

Post-pandemic phenomena in organizational behavior towards employees' well-being predict a tendency towards more comprehensive data-led well-being solutions as the work becomes increasingly practice-oriented. If the directions of work are going to change, then so will the approaches for creating happiness in one's work. To sum up, the impact of happiness on growth is virtually incalculable. Certainly, such organizations, which concentrate on the health of their workforce, confidence, and creativity, will most likely enhance the employer's productivity and inventiveness thereby retaining the high spirit of the employees. Emphasizing happiness is not only a moral aspect; it is also a fundamental condition for being successful for a longer period in such a highly competitive field – business.

REFERENCES

Al Maktoum, M. B. R. (2017). *Reflections on happiness & positivity*. Explorer Publishing.

Awada, N. I., & Ismail, F. (2019). Happiness in the Workplace. *International Journal of Innovative Technology and Exploring Engineering*, *8*(9), 1496–1500.

Bartik, A., Cullen, Z., & Glaeser, E. L. (2023). Flexibility in the workplace and its impact on employee satisfaction. *Journal of Business Research*.

Brown, K. W., & Ryan, R. M. (2023). The impact of emotional balance on well-being: A study on contentment and happiness. *The Journal of Positive Psychology*.

Burns, J., & Li, M. (2023). Preventing burnout: The role of rest and recuperation in modern workplaces. *Journal of Occupational Health Psychology*.

Chaudhary, V., Vemuri, V. P., Cavaliere, L. P. L., Verma, V., Manoharan, G., & Bharti, A. (2024, March). A comparative analysis of job satisfaction and motivational factors of employees in public versus private organizations.

Choi, H., Diener, E., & Oishi, S. (2024). Do We Know How Happy Strangers Are? Accuracy in Well-Being Judgments at Zero Acquaintance. *Social Psychological & Personality Science*, *15*(6), 691–701. DOI: 10.1177/19485506231197844

Chotai, N. A., Tiwari, A., Aggarwal, S., Chandel, P. S., Dimari, A., & Manoharan, G. (2023, December). Importance of Employee Motivation and Satisfaction in the Workplace based on BiLSTM and ANN Approach. In 2023 2nd International Conference on Automation, Computing and Renewable Systems (ICACRS) (pp. 1141-1146). DOI: 10.1109/ICACRS58579.2023.10404593

Cooper, L., Kitson, N., Neal, L., Langslow, S., Turner, L., Maryel, M., Stallwood, B., & Kennedy, B. B. (2024, September 19). *Workplace happiness 2024*. theHRDIRECTOR. https://www.thehrdirector.com/features/employee-engagement/workplace-happiness-2024/

Diener, E. (2000). Subjective well-being: The science of happiness and a proposal for a national index. *The American Psychologist*, *55*(1), 34–43. DOI: 10.1037/0003-066X.55.1.34 PMID: 11392863

Diener, E., Oishi, S., & Tay, L. (2021). Contentment and well-being: The role of acceptance in emotional health. *Personality and Social Psychology Review*.

Fitriana, N., Hutagalung, F. D., Awang, Z., & Zaid, S. M. (2022). Happiness at work: A cross-cultural validation of happiness at work scale.

Fredrickson, B. L., & Joiner, T. (2002). Positive emotions trigger upward spirals toward emotional well-being. *Psychological Science, 13*(2), 172–175. DOI: 10.1111/1467-9280.00431 PMID: 11934003

Gartner Research. (2024). Data-driven well-being programs: Enhancing organizational effectiveness and employee satisfaction.

Global Wellness Institute. (2023). "2023 Health, Happiness, and the Wellness Economy: An Empirical Analysis."

Gopinathan, R., & Manoharan, G. (2022). Work-Life Balance Practices and Organizational Performance for Achieving Superior Performance. The Changing Role of Human Resource Management in the Global Competitive Environment, 217.

Jaswal, N., Sharma, D., Bhardwaj, B., & Kraus, S. (2024). Promoting well-being through happiness at work: A systematic literature review and future research agenda. *Management Decision, 62*(13), 332–369. DOI: 10.1108/MD-08-2023-1492

Krishnan, S. G., & Manoharan, G. (2022). An Investigation in Analysing the Key Aspects of High-Performance Work Practice for Enhancing Productivity in the Organisation. The Changing Role of Human Resource Management in the Global Competitive Environment, 31.

Kun, A., & Gadanecz, P. (2022). Workplace happiness, well-being and their relationship with psychological capital: A study of Hungarian Teachers. *Current Psychology (New Brunswick, N.J.), 41*(1), 185–199.

Manoharan, G., & Ashtikar, S. P. (2022). *The Relationship between Job-Related Factors on Work-Life Balance and Job Satisfaction.* The Changing Role of Human Resource Management in the Global Competitive Environment.

Manoharan, G., Ashtikar, S. P., Smitha, V., Sundaramoorthi, S., & Krishna, I. M. (2023). Work-life balance perceptions of women in the IT and ITeS Sectors in Kerala: A research study. *Journal of Pharmaceutical Negative Results.*

Manoharan, G., & Rajoli, S. B. (2024). Leveraging Technology for Enhancing Performance Appraisal. In Employee Performance Management for Improved Workplace Motivation (pp. 289-310). DOI: 10.4018/979-8-3693-4387-6.ch012

Manoharan, G., Rao, B. S., Ashtikar, S. P., Razak, A., Durai, S., & Kukreja, J. (2024). A Study of Influence of Leadership With Effective Communication in Educational Institutions.

Misra, N., & Srivastava, S. (2022). Happiness at work: A psychological perspective. In Happiness and Wellness - Biopsychosocial and Anthropological Perspectives.

Moss, J. (2023). Creating a happier workplace is possible — and worth it.

Motwani, B., Haryani, S., Manoharan, G., & Razak, A. (2024). Impact of Workforce Emotional Intelligence on Patient Satisfaction: A Sentiment Analysis Approach Using Supervised Machine Algorithms. In Employee Performance Management for Improved Workplace Motivation (pp. 263-288). DOI: 10.4018/979-8-3693-4387-6.ch011

Roessler, J., & Gloor, P. A. (2021). Measuring happiness increases happiness. *Journal of Computational Social Science*, *4*(1), 123–146. DOI: 10.1007/s42001-020-00069-6

Ruggeri, K., Garcia-Garzon, E., Maguire, Á., Matz, S., & Huppert, F. A. (2020). Well-being is more than happiness and life satisfaction: A multidimensional analysis of 21 countries. *Health and Quality of Life Outcomes*, *18*(1), 192. DOI: 10.1186/s12955-020-01423-y PMID: 32560725

Satpathy, A., Samal, A., Gupta, S., Kumar, S., Sharma, S., Manoharan, G., Karthikeyan, M., & Sharma, S. (2024). To Study the Sustainable Development Practices in Business and Food Industry. *Migration Letters : An International Journal of Migration Studies*, *21*(S1), 743–747. DOI: 10.59670/ml.v21iS1.6400

Sender, G., Carvalho, F., & Guedes, G. (2021). The Happy Level: A New Approach to Measure Happiness at Work Using Mixed Methods. *International Journal of Qualitative Methods*, *20*, 16094069211002413. DOI: 10.1177/16094069211002413

Singh, D., Makkar, S., Manoharan, G., Durai, S., Purushottamashtikar, S., & Alexrajesh, G. (2024, June). The impact of information technology enabler and organizational learning on performance: A systematic literature review. In AIP Conference Proceedings (Vol. 2971, No. 1). DOI: 10.1063/5.0195945

Stringer, H. (2023). Worker well-being is in demand as organizational culture shifts. *Monitor on Psychology*.

Winster, D., Ramakrishnan, S., Veluthakkal, J., Manoharan, G., Purushottamashtikar, S., & Selvaraj, F. (2024, June). Interactions between emotional and spiritual intelligence and their effects on employee performance.

Yang, F., Knobe, J., & Dunham, Y. (2021). Happiness is from the soul: The nature and origins of our happiness concept.

Chapter 19
Workplace Wellness: A Goal for Employee Satisfaction – Understanding Workplace Well-Being and Happiness

Farheen Fathima
SR University, India

Sowmya Muppidi
https://orcid.org/0009-0009-2379-1259
SR University, India

Geetha Manoharan
https://orcid.org/0000-0002-8644-8871
SR University, India

ABSTRACT

Modern studies and articles are used to examine workplace well-being and happiness in this study chapter. It examines how comprehensive well-being initiatives that integrate physical, mental, and emotional health improve employee satisfaction and productivity (Suresh et al., 2024). Positive work environments, flexible work arrangements, and comforting leadership affect employee happiness. It promotes workplace culture and employee engagement by emphasizing mental health assistance and job design. The chapter emphasizes mental health resources and employee participation. This paper summarizes recent research on tactics and practices that increase employee well-being and happiness, offering organizations helpful insights for creating a more vibrant work environment. Organizations will soon use AI-driven wellness apps and wearable health trackers. Promoting inclusion and diversity will create workplaces where everyone feels appreciated and supported.

DOI: 10.4018/979-8-3373-0360-4.ch019

INTRODUCTION

Lately, the focus on happiness and welfare in the workplace has upstaged the traditional hypothesis of job satisfaction, emerging as a key factor in organizational success and perishability. As businesses face metamorphosing challenges such as mental health crises, remote work, and shifting employee expectations, welfare strategies have become a need. Research suggests that facilitating a positive work environment enhances employee performance (Winster et al., 2024) and strengthens organizational resilience, creativity, innovation, and adaptability. Indeed, many workplaces have already begun transitioning to what they now call new-age organizations instead of trying to start over again. This new-age reality holds great promise for emerging firms. Hybrid and remote working models have been embraced by a sizeable body of organizations, with these paradigms moving forward to change how employees enjoy their workplaces. Workplace happiness will most likely witness an increased focus on mental wellness.

This article examines the relationship between happiness and productivity in the workplace and examines the psychological and cultural factors that contribute to happiness. From flexible working to supporting mental health, dive into the hot topics and data-driven insights shaping the future of work. Looking ahead with a deeper understanding of technological advances and human beings, the future workplace will be conducive to health (Indira et al., 2024). With this perspective, this study focuses on a broader perspective on how organizations can use health as a tool for sustainable growth. As we move forward, wellness will increasingly become a key driver of success, impacting organizational outcomes and employee satisfaction in meaningful ways. This research provides a unique perspective on how organizations can make happiness a fundamental foundation of success, not just a byproduct of it, providing a tool for understanding the future of happiness in the changing world of work.

Embedding healthy work patterns into the core business model shows that a healthy workforce is a necessity for good performance. Companies that integrate wellness into their culture and business goals have seen significant benefits in productivity, innovation, and talent retention. In the workplace of the future, wellness services could become a key performance indicator tracked alongside traditional metrics such as revenue growth and employee satisfaction. This includes the fact that successful employees lead to success. Innovations such as creating virtual reality rooms for meditation, using mindfulness to manage stress (Manoharan et al., 2024), and using fitness services offered by organizations have made health fun and accessible. Most importantly, it has changed the way employees think about health. A key element of future workplace wellness is the move toward employee assessment. Employees will be empowered to co-create healthcare to foster ownership and participation.

This partnership ensures that healthcare meets diverse needs and is equitable and effective. This collaboration helps create a healthy organizational culture by fostering trust and communication between employees and management. As workplace health continues to evolve, it is clear that the pursuit of employee health will go beyond health assessments. Personalized solutions, integrating health into strategic goals, leveraging new technologies, and caring for key employees are what organizations need to create a future where workplace wellness is not just a goal, but a critical foundation for success. This vision emphasizes the importance of interaction between engaged and engaged employees in ensuring safety in an evolving world.

Figure 1. Holistic Employee Well-being's Seven Pillars.

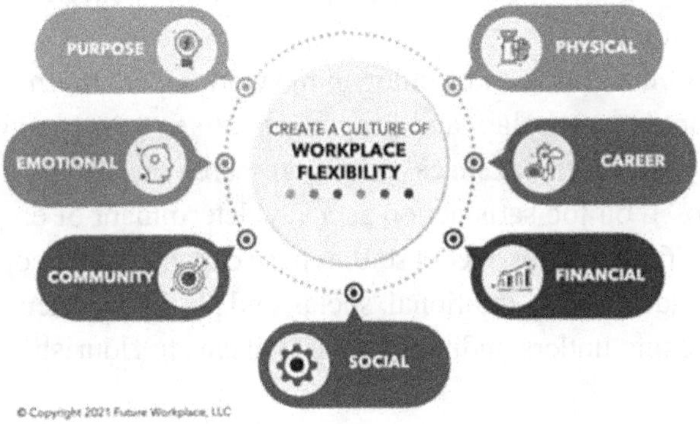

Source: https://www.forbes.com/sites/jeannemeister/2021/08/04/the-future-of-work-is-worker-well-being/

LITERATURE REVIEW

The prevailing subject in the literature is the strategic integration of health into organizational targets. Wellness programs should be allied with a company's broader mission and values, scholars say. At the same time, this perspective considers wellness to be a business imperative with measurable effects on important key performance indicators, including productivity, employee retention, and customer satisfaction. For instance, case studies of organizations that embed wellness into their corporate strategy report significant improvements in team dynamics and innovation, showing the reciprocal relationship between well-being and organizational success. While working as a mid-level manager at a tech firm, I visually witnessed the metamorphosis of people and teams from a doom-laden state to one blooming with efficiency: the embedding of wellness into corporate strategy. Some years ago, our department was straining under high turnover rates and burnout among employees. Management opted to roll out an all-encompassing wellness program, which introduced elements such as flexible working hours, mindfulness sessions, therapy assistance, and regular team-building activities. I was doubtful at first—how could yoga or mental health days affect deadlines and productivity?

But in a few short months, the pushback became real. Colleagues who had been disinterested and unengaged began showing up and speaking out in meetings. There was better collaboration and a general sense of support. One of the colleagues who was almost quitting decided to remain and successfully led a product launch in the following quarter. Satisfaction scores rose, and so did teamwork productivity metrics and innovation KPIs. Through this experience, I fully embraced the notion that wellness is not a luxury and a perk; it is a strategic imperative. When people feel supported, they bring their best selves to work, and that benefits everyone—from employees to customers.

The concept of happiness and welfare in the working environment has accumulated deliberation from scholars and proponents alike, with growing recognition of its impact on organizational success. Early research on workplace well-being is elementally focused on job satisfaction as a key determinant of employee productivity [Locke, 1976]. However, recent studies have expanded the scope of workplace happiness to include mental, emotional, social, and physical dimensions, providing a more encompassing understanding of what it means to flourish at work.

DEFINING WELL-BEING AND WORKPLACE HAPPINESS

Job contentment has changed, becoming more comprehensive than earlier measurements of general job satisfaction (Keserwani et al., 2021). It is now inclusive of positive emotions, engagement, and meaning. Seligman's [2011] PERMA model, which stands for Positive emotion, Engagement, Relationships, Meaning, and Accomplishment, is useful for providing a hardy framework on which to understand happiness in a broader sense, indicating that well-being (Manoharan et al., 2024) is multi-dimensional. "Positive psychology takes you through the countryside of pleasure and gratification, up into the high country of strength and virtue, and finally to the peaks of lasting fulfilment, meaning, and purpose."

Figure 2. Job-Demands-Resources-Modell. (Bakker und Demerouti 2007)

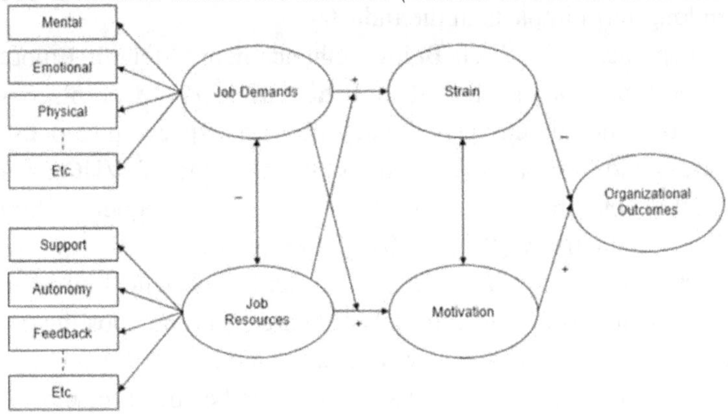

Source: https://www.researchgate.net/figure/Das-Job-Demands-Ressources-Modell-Bakker-und-Demerouti -2007_fig1_355202033

Seligman, 2002 Bakker, and Demerouti, [2007] developed the JD-R model, which posits a relationship between work demands and available resources in explaining employee well-being. Their work illustrates that happiness is not just about reducing negative factors like stress or burnout but also about increasing positive aspects such as support, opportunities for development, and job autonomy.

The Ripple Effect of Wellbeing on Organizational Success

A substantial body of literature highlights the positive correlation between workplace happiness and key business outcomes. Achor [2010] argues that happiness fuels success, rather than the other way around, illustrating that a positive mind set enhances empirical performance and resilience in the face of challenges. Lyubomirsky, King, and Diener [2005] found that happier employees are more productive, exhibit and showcase greater creativity, and are estimated to be more inclined with their organizations. ''When we become too comfortable in our jobs and relationships, we can miss huge opportunities to grow and change'' - Harvard University professor Cass Sunstein. Harvard University professor Cass Sunstein delves into how breaking free from comfort zones can create a better working environment for the employee and employer. By embracing change and new challenges, employees also contribute to a more dynamic, innovative, and engaged work environment, driving overall organizational success. Furthermore, research conducted by Wright and Cropanzano (2000) establishes a basis for the consideration of well-being and job performance; it shows that persons who generally have high psychological well-being are more engaged and perform better than those who experience less happiness. This opens the door to viewing well-being (Manoharan et al., 2023) increasingly as a crucial strategic business imperative, the strengthening of a positive working environment for optimum long-term impacts in the industry.

Holistic Approaches for Well-Being Enhancement: Mental, Emotional, and Physical Dimensions. The increasingly holistic definition of workplace well-being has transformed to include the mental and emotional aspects in response to rising workplace stress and burnout levels. The proper wording of WHO has described the current global epidemic in workplace stress and its consequences for employee well-being and productivity [WHO, 2019]. Research shows that physical health initiatives, such as wellness programs, exercise facilities, and healthy eating options, would reduce absenteeism while cutting healthcare costs and boosting productivity [Chenoweth, 2011]. Studies by Cartwright and Cooper [2009] point out crucial emotional well-being; emotional exhaustion seems to be one of the most significant predictors of declining job satisfaction and intention for turnover.

Figure 3. The ASSET model of stress. Source: Cartwright & Cooper (2002)

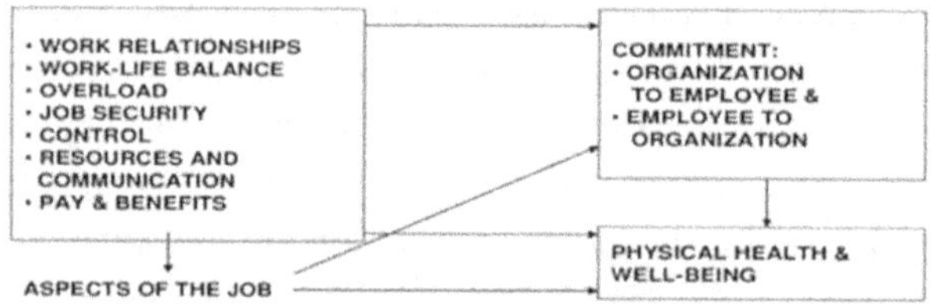

Source: https://www.researchgate.net/figure/The-ASSET-Model-of-Stress-Source-Cartwright-Cooper-2002_fig1_263050669

EMERGING TRENDS IN WORKPLACE WELL-BEING: EMBRACING FLEXIBILITY, INNOVATION, AND INCLUSIVITY

The evolution of workplace wellness looks bright as it now takes shape around the emerging diversifying trends, which include increasing flexibility, technology (Manoharan et al., 2024), and inclusiveness. It is the pandemic that ushered in the work-from-home and hybrid work trend-shifting traditional workplaces. Telecommuting, a flexible work arrangement, was reported by Gajendran and Harrison [2007] to enhance job satisfaction and decrease stress in employees, especially when they had control over their schedules. New results show that nowadays, employees value work-life balance and flexibility just more than well-being [Kelliher & Anderson, 2010]. Technology is another key driver of the evolving workplace well-being landscape. Organizations are leveraging data analytics and artificial intelligence (Razak et al., 2023) to create personalized well-being programs tailored to individual employee needs. These technologies allow organizations to monitor employee health and well-being in real time, offering customized interventions based on factors such as stress levels, sleep patterns, and physical activities [Danna & Griffin, 1999].

Inclusivity is also gaining attention in discussions on workplace wellbeing. As workplaces become more diverse, businesses need to develop well-being initiatives that are sensitive to culture, gender (Rajoli et al., 2024), and demographic differences. Studies by Nishii [2013], suggest that inclusive workplace cultures, where diverse perspectives are valued, can lead to greater employee happiness and engagement. The future of workplace well-being will likely involve more tailored and culturally aware strategies to ensure that all employees feel supported and valued. Technological advancements are often cited as transformative drivers in the future of workplace wellness.

With synthetic intelligence (Thavamani et al., 2022) and machine-gaining knowledge of implemented in predictive health device development, it'll doubtlessly revolutionize the manner companies approach worker well-being. VR programs, like immersive environments for stress remedy, and AR health-demanding situations are explored in phrases of enhancing worker engagement in wellness sports. That is based totally on participatory management theories, which count on that employees are much more likely to pressure organizational trade while their enter is valued.

Destiny-focused research has additionally been completed on ethical considerations in workplace wellness packages, specifically in phrases of records privateness and equity. While personalized wellness equipment are beneficial, they increase questions about the potential misuse of sensitive health information. Making sure transparency, consent, and equity in enforcing such packages is critical for preserving trust and fairness in various places of work.

CRITIQUES AND GAPS IN THE LITERATURE

While most of the literary works support the positive effect of workplace well-being on business outcomes, some studies raise critical concerns about the limits of current well-being strategies. Fleming and Asplund [2007] caution that many companies implement well-being programs as ''quick fixes'' without addressing deeper structural issues such as poor management practices or excessive workloads. They argue that superficial interventions like wellness programs cannot compensate for a toxic work environment. Furthermore, Warr [2007] points out that while well-being initiatives may benefit individual employees, they must be part of a broader organizational culture that prioritizes well-being at all levels. "Wellness is no Longer a Luxury, it is a Necessity for a Thriving Workplace" Lea Radojicic, Certified Corporate Wellness Specialist (CCWS) Graduate.

Presently more emphasis is being laid on developing longitudinal studies that track the long-term effect of well-being programs. While short-term gains in productivity and employee satisfaction are well documented, the sustainability of these benefits over time remains under-researched [Lazarus, 1999]. Future research should focus on the durability of workplace well-being initiatives and their long-term implications for both employees and organizations. The literature on workplace happiness and well-being reveals a rich and evolving field of study, with growing recognition of its importance in fostering organizational success. While much progress has been made in understanding multiple dimensions of well-being, significant gaps remain, particularly regarding the long-term efficacy of well-being programs and the need for more culturally inclusive approaches. Future research must continue to explore how organizations can develop more comprehensive, personalized, and sustainable well-being strategies that align employee happiness with business success.

In the study reported in JAMA, the incentives were modest. Participants got small-dollar gift cards for taking wellness courses on topics such as nutrition, exercise, disease management, and stress control. Total potential incentives averaged $250. About 35 percent of eligible employees at the 20 participating sites completed at least one module. Results from those workers — including attendance and tenure data, their self-reported health assessment, and results from lab blood tests — were specifically compared with similar reports from 20 primary comparison sites where workers were not offered the wellness gift cards and classes. Overall employment and health spending data from all worksites were included in the study." Source: https://health.wusf.usf.edu/npr-health/npr-health/2019-04-16/how-well-do-workplace-wellness-programs-work

The upshot, however, is that well over half of the literature currently available suggests wellness-based initiatives are directly and indirectly positively related to organizational-based performance measures, such as productivity and profitability. Nonetheless, critics argue that all too often these studies simply lack sufficient methodological heft or fail to acknowledge influential control variables, such as economic conditions or industry/employment-specific challenges. This leads them to discount the underlying empirics that underpin well-being programs as a silver-bullet solution to workplace troubles altogether.

To address these criticisms and shortcomings, a more holistic, representative, and analytical approach to workplace wellness research is necessary. Successive studies should place a greater emphasis on longitudinal measurement, expand their scope to include a range of worker demographics, and conduct serious ethical and cultural analyses. This would better position the field to generate more meaningful and applied knowledge about sustaining worker satisfaction. Overall, the literature points towards a multi-dimensional future for workplace wellness through personalization, strategic alignment, technological innovation, and cultural transformation. All these contribute to a vision of workplaces where employee happiness becomes a foundation for sustainable organizational success.

DISCUSSION

Over the past few years, workplace happiness and well-being have progressed from being a peripheral issue into brange of eecoming a core focus of organizational strategy. Indeed, quite recently, the whole notion of employee joy and employee well-being has progressed from a peripheral concern to being a core part of the organizational strategy. As employee happiness and well-being gain ground on the periphery, they become more important to the heart of the organization's strategy. While companies once focused primarily on productivity and profitability, the understanding has shifted to include employee happiness as a key driver of success. As businesses increasingly recognize the profound impact of well-being on outcomes such as employee retention, innovation, and overall company culture, the conversation about well-being in the workplace has deepened. "We need to focus on things that are both timeless and urgent," said Fuentes. "The need for a human connection, the need to matter, and the need to learn are what transcend times and crises." Source: https://hbr.org/2023/10/creating-a-happier-workplace-is-possible-and-worth-it

Evolving Landscapes of Well-Being

In the modern workplace, well-being encompasses a range of physical, emotional, and psychological factors that contribute to employees' overall satisfaction. Unlike traditional measures of job satisfaction that merely focus on external rewards like salary and benefits, well-being touches on how employees feel about their work, their mental health, and their sense of purpose. As organizations become more diverse, flexible, and digital the dynamics of well-being are evolving to meet new employee needs. Remote and hybrid working environments act as the most tangible examples. For example, the pandemic of 2020 highlighted how people would always take flexibility during wellness. For many employees, working remotely brought new freedoms but also many new challenges such as isolation and work-life balance difficulties. But, this shift allowed personnel to reassess their relationship with paintings and seek out roles that align higher with their non-public needs and values. The agencies that tailored using offering intellectual fitness aid, encouraging breaks, and making sure virtual collaboration maintains strong worker engagement and well-being. This shift towards prioritizing employee well-being is going hand in hand with broader information about human desires. Groups are recognising that personnel aren't simply assets to be optimized but people with complicated emotional landscapes. In places of work wherein properly being is prioritized, personnel are more likely to revel in significance, be supported, and be advocated to provide their satisfaction of their abilities. This creates a ripple effect, boosting morale, teamwork, and overall productiveness.

Joy as a Catalyst for Innovation and Productivity.

One of the maximum interesting results of selling administrative center happiness is its direct effect on innovation. Happy personnel are regularly greater creative, greater open to collaboration, and more likely to take danger. While people feel mentally comfortable on the place of business, they're greater willing to contribute new thoughts without fear of failure or judgment. This mental safety has been proven to foster a modern subculture, where employees experience at ease exploring creative answers to issues. Don't forget groups like Google and Airbnb, wherein fostering a tradition of happiness and well-being has been pivotal to their success. By means of growing environments wherein employees can thrive, those agencies have continually outperformed their competition in terms of innovation and marketplace agility. It isn't just tech businesses embracing this ethos. Industries throughout the board are realising the fee of nicely-being in improving productiveness. Take production and healthcare, wherein high-strain environments regularly lead to burnout and turnover. In those sectors, projects to aid well-being, such as intellectual health packages, bendy scheduling, and emotional help offerings, were transformative. Corporations that have previously focused only on efficiency are now turning to holistic well-being techniques to enhance each worker's happiness and productivity.

Administrative center well-being (Paulsamy et al., 2021) is now an increasing number of tied to economic decisions. Businesses have found out that monetary strain has an instantaneous impact on employee mental health and productivity. Research implies that financial issues are one of the pinnacle reasons for stress amongst employees that may cause absenteeism, disengagement, and poor activity performance. In reaction, many organizations are inclusive of monetary health programs in their ordinary strategies for employee well-being. These packages sometimes include financial management tools and resources, and planning assistance. For example, the Employee Benefit Research Institute (EBRI) work points out the growing importance of financial wellness initiatives, especially in light of rising fears about economic instability. Its results indicate that organizations that support financial wellness have higher employee satisfaction and productivity. Eradication of financial stress aids in reducing stress levels whilst helping to promote an employee financially empowered environment, better improving their working conditions.

Many organizations implementing financial well-being programs realize reduced medical healthcare because financial stress is responsible for a variety of illnesses physically and mentally (Harkn, 2024). Source: https://www.ebri.org/docs/default-source/wbs/wws-2024/wws-2024_short-report.pdf

Another financial factor that has a significant impact on workplace well-being is how companies structure their pay and benefits. A transparent pay system and equitable benefit package promote fairness as well as trust. Corporate Wellness Magazine studies reveal that employee satisfaction will increase and feelings of unfairness leading to disengagement will be reduced when there is full financial disclosure combined with competitive compensation packages. For example, organizations that provide financial literacy programs in addition to health benefits develop an integrated approach to employees' well-being both their physical health and financial health. In addition, the financial choice-making aspect of employee wellness programs encompasses retirement savings and investment. Because workforce demographics are aging and retirement is looming, employees' anxiety over what this future holds can influence overall performance. Providing retirement saving opportunities with matching contributions, offering advice on financial matters, as well as post-retirement planning help ensure employees become secure about their future about their financial statuses, thus reducing work-related pressure.

This helps organizations mitigate some of the negative impacts related to financial stress, thus enabling better overall long-term satisfaction and productivity among employees. It is a step toward acceptance of complex dimensions of well-being, where financial stability is as important as physical and mental health, serving the interests of both the employee and the organization. “Financial well-being is going to be paramount to success in 2024. With the cost of living getting out of hand, people need all the help and advice they can get on how to manage their money and survive the coming difficulties. If we don’t get this right, then both stress levels and mental health issues will skyrocket as many people fall into desperate and difficult times.”

Source:https://healthatworkcentre.org.uk/wp-content/uploads/2024/03/HR-Ebook2024_Digital_PAGES_compressed.pdf

‘’Sustaining success takes determination to create the environments, the routines, and the opportunities. If we want our work to be more sustainable, we have to look at the inputs. What do we do in those “non-working moments”? Do we take in “gold” or do we take in “garbage”? Work is a big part of who we are - if only for the large amounts of hours, work will always play a crucial role in our lives. And that doesn’t have to be bad. Because work also gives us meaning, and moments of extreme pride, it allows us to grow professionally and personally, to find our partner, or our best friends, our tribe, new passions and so much more. But when work takes away all our energy, all our fire, we start to feel resentment, frustration, anxiety, depression even.’’

Source: https://www.happinessdigger.com/post/can-we-adopt-a-more-sustainable-way-of-working

The Impact of Leadership on Cultivating Well-Being.

Leadership plays a significant role in molding the well-being of workplaces: open communication, empathy, and support transform the environment in which employees feel good about themselves. It contrasts with the usual, authoritarian, performance-oriented leadership which undermines employee morale. Leaders who actively listen, provide feedback and acknowledge individual contributions create an environment that thrives on well-being. The role of emotional intelligence (Purushottamashtikar et al., 2024) is much spoken about concerning those who lead. Emotionally intelligent leaders readily understand the needs of their followers, thus creating opportunities for tailored support and guidance. This kind of leadership not only boosts individual well-being but also generates trust and loyalty, which make an essential part of organizational success in the future. Leadership is the basic underpinning for successful workplace wellness programs that make wellness a very concrete aspect of organizational culture, from being an amorphous concept. Leaders who constantly highlight wellness initiatives, besides affecting policy-making, encourage employees to engage with wellness programs massively. Their commitment to well-being signifies the importance given to wellness and creates a trusting and psychologically safe environment wherein employees feel valued and cared for. Clear communication is one of the basic features of effective leadership in workplace well-being. Leaders who clearly express their well-being goals and are responsible can balance the mismatch between organizational policies and the actual experiences of employees. For instance, if managers frequently discuss well-being issues and provide constructive feedback, then the employees are likely to use available resources and have higher satisfaction and health.

Figure 4. Different perspectives of well-being

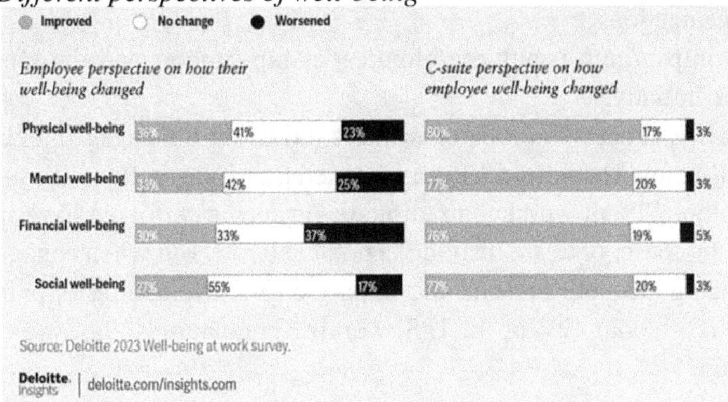

"The report finds employees are strongly motivated to improve their well-being but many are not making progress, and for a majority, work is taking an increasing toll on their physical and mental health." Source: https://www.weforum.org/stories/2023/06/workplace-well-being-declining-health/

The way leaders approach stress and psychological safety profoundly impacts mental well-being. Leaders who are empathetic and emotionally intelligent build trust; employees feel comfortable reaching out for help when they need it. Establishing a supportive environment with facility amenity offerings such as mental health counseling, mindfulness courses, and courses on stress in which employees can survive. It has been found that such measures reduce burnout and absenteeism, thus creating a healthier and more engaged workforce.

Well-being is tied to connecting the soul with other employees. Hence, leaders have a unique authority in developing an inclusive collab environment where all employees feel they belong. Through facilitating team building, peer recognition programs, and open communication, these people can create interpersonal relations that raise morale altogether. Evidence has shown that workplaces with good social ties uptick productivity and decline turnover. Meaning, that the leader makes a balanced model that holds both mental and social dimensions toward the well-being of employees.

The research argues much about an existing significant link between different leadership styles and the well-being of employees at the workplace. Transparent communication and supportive management stand out as some of the strongest indicators of positive employee health outcomes. For example, the 2024 Work Health Survey by Mental Health America reveals that organizations fostering open communication and equitable management practices consistently perform better in workplace wellness metrics. However, less than half of employees report experiencing such leadership, highlighting a considerable opportunity for improvement in many organizations.

Source: https://hero-health.org/blog/leadership-support-and-the-effectiveness-of-wellness-initiatives/

''Nationally, about two-thirds of workers (66%) are not engaged and have suboptimal well-being. Of these, 52% are considered thriving in their overall life evaluation. Another 22% of workers, in turn, are engaged at work but have suboptimal well-being. Of these, 65% are thriving, a notable boost. But when engagement and high well-being are both present, the impact on life evaluations is palpable. For these workers -- about 12% of the U.S. working population -- 92% are considered to be thriving.''

Figure 5. Engagement and well-being affect how employees evaluate their lives.

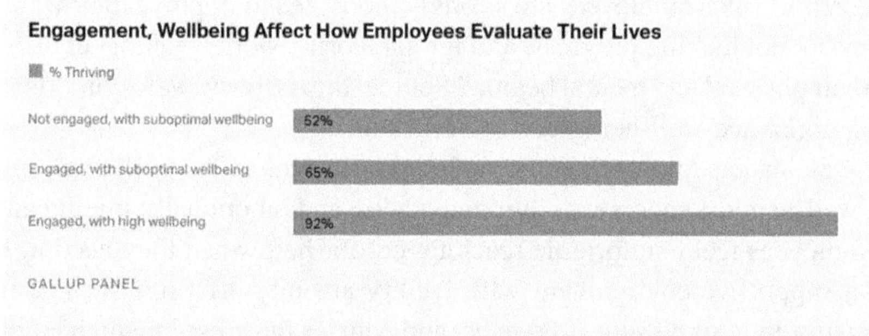

Source: https://www.gallup.com/workplace/320108/ways-leaders-improve-engagement-wellbeing.aspx

Such have been examples in corporations that have given their human resource and people management a very different bent, focusing on leadership as servanthood whereby leaders create environments that create employees empowered to express their needs and ideas rather than controlling the employees. Although this has proven to be rewarding for the employees, on the side of the company, performance gets improved too.

Obstacles and Constraints in Advancing Well-Being

While the benefits of workplace wellbeing are clear, there are challenges in implementing effective strategies. One of the primary challenges is that well-being initiatives often require cultural shifts within organizations. This can be difficult in companies that have long-standing traditions of high-pressure work environments or hierarchical leadership structures. Convincing management to prioritize well-being over immediate productivity can be a difficult balancing act, especially in industries where time and output are critical to business success. Any other undertaking is that employees' needs vary drastically primarily based on character preferences and lifestyles circumstances. A health application that works for one institution of employees may not be as effective for every other. For instance, junior personnel may lay importance on paintings-life stability and bendy schedules, even as experienced personnel may also prioritize activity protection and comprehensive fitness advantages. Customizing nicely-being packages to fulfil the various wishes of personnel may be complex and time-ingesting for groups. Further, there is the risk of nicely-being becoming superficial, wherein agencies offer perks like free snacks or gymnasium memberships without addressing the deeper issues that affect worker happiness, together with activity security, workload management, or career development. Superficial nicely-being strategies can lead to disengagement, as employees can also see thru efforts that appear more centered on optics than actual change.

Visionary Routes for Advancing Workplace Well-Being.

Because the administrative center continues to conform, so will the nicely-being idea. Technological advances along with AI-pushed health programs, records-pushed checks, and personalized fitness monitoring will in all likelihood play a major role in the destiny. These tools can provide extra tailored properly-being answers based totally on actual-time data, allowing businesses to reply greater efficaciously to the wishes of their personnel.

Within the destiny, groups may see a more potent emphasis on mental fitness, variety and inclusion, and sustainable painting environments. More youthful generations of workers, particularly Millennials and Gen Z, are increasingly traumatic more holistic techniques to work, which include intellectual fitness assist and cause-pushed paintings. To live aggressively within the labor marketplace, organizations will want to adapt by using supplying not simply jobs, but possibilities for non-public success and boom. Empathy and emotional intelligence form integral parts of a good leader in this system. Listening actively and showing care for the mental and emotional well-being of the people under one's leadership creates a stress-free and resilient atmosphere.

Figure 6. Current trends impacting today's workforce.

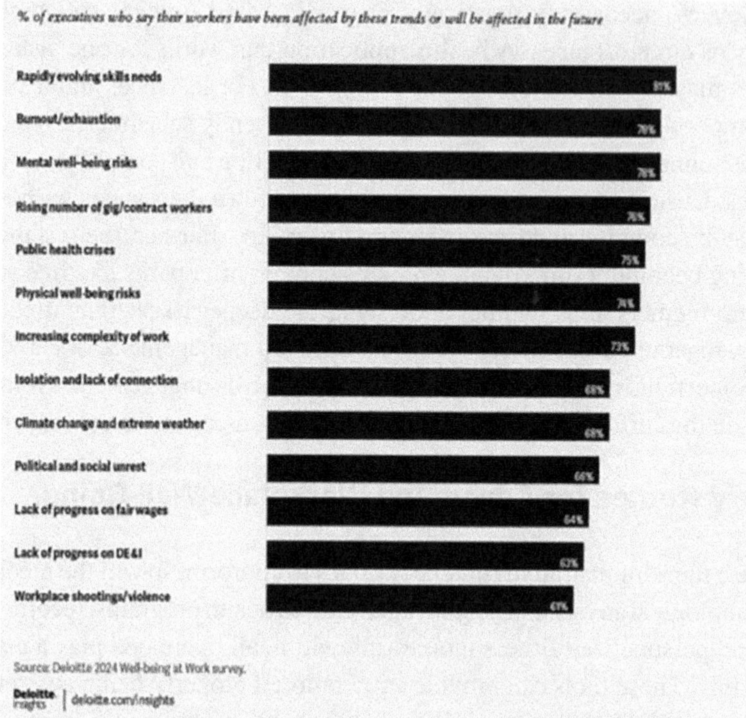

Source: https://www2.deloitte.com/us/en/insights/topics/talent/workplace-well-being-research-2024.html

In such a setting, if employees feel their leaders are approachable and empathetic, they are likely to speak out about problems that need solutions, thus motivating a healthy approach to well-being generally. Intentional decisions have a critical impact on workplace wellness: the allocation of resources to inclusive wellness programs and the guarantee of such programs for all employees within the organization is a symbol of equity.

Further, leaders who align wellness with wide organizational strategies, such as aligning health initiatives with corporate goals, can make the wellness programs very effective and lead to lasting benefits for employees and organizations alike. The effectiveness of workplace wellness programs fundamentally relies on leadership that demonstrates authenticity, proactivity, and engagement. By exemplifying healthy behaviors, promoting inclusivity, and emphasizing the importance of employee well-being, leaders can establish a benchmark that enhances individual results while simultaneously contributing to organizational achievement.

CONCLUSION

The topic of workplace well-being and happiness is far from unimportant; in fact, it is essential to the success of organizations in the contemporary world. Happier workers are more engaged, innovative, and productive overall, and studies and real-world examples show a strong correlation between well-being and organizational success. Employee loyalty and peak performance are more likely to persist in situations where they feel appreciated and supported by their employer. Advances in technology and data analytics will transform the personalization of well-being initiatives, allowing employers to tailor support mechanisms to specific individual needs. Artificial intelligence will help organizations to avoid stressors such as load management and support mental health by making well-being proactive rather than reactive. Flexible work arrangements will give employees a chance to balance personal and professional commitments, thereby increasing self-control and aggregate happiness. Leadership will be the most important ingredient in working well because inclusiveness, trust, and engagement start with leaders. Among these constructive acting and empathetic, promoting wellness programs, some will create an environment in which employees will feel free, valued, and energized to do better. Thus, by developing a cooperative and more connected culture in organizations, social well-being will be improved, and hence teamwork will improve, and productivity and retention will be higher. In the end, the future landscape of workplace wellness is to be one of harmony, balancing the fulfilment of employees with organizational objectives. Within this context, well-being moves from utility to a foundational concept, allowing innovation, resilience, and long-term success to emerge. Also, organizations become dedicated to the advancement of practice and nurturing supportive environments, they build the path toward a future where employee satisfaction is both the central issue and collective reality.

In conclusion, encouraging contentment and well-being at work should not be seen as an extra benefit or extravagance. For businesses to be inventive and competitive in a world that is changing quickly, it is essential. Businesses that put employee well-being first are investing in their most valuable resource: their workforce. Better business outcomes result from this, but it also fosters a supportive and long-lasting workplace culture that benefits the organization and its workers. It is expected that the emphasis on well-being will increase as companies proceed to change and adapt. The way we view employee satisfaction in the workplace of the future must take a more comprehensive view that takes into account all of a person's requirements rather than just compensation and benefits. This move toward well-being is not merely a fad; it represents the nature of work in the future, where success will be determined not only by profit margins but also by the contentment and satisfaction of individuals who enable that success. Only thirty-four percent of employees this 2023 thrived in their respective lives. It had a one-point decrease from 2022, after five annual consecutive improvements of this metric. Also pertinent: This downward change affected the younger-age workers the most. According to those below 35 years old, well-being decreased from 35 to 31 percent, whereas those above 35 years of age experienced an upward shift from 35 percent to 36 percent. “If I'm not doing well at work, I'm not doing well in life. It's just the way it is.”--Emilia, Educator. Source: https://www.gallup.com/workplace/349484/state-of-the-global-workplace.aspx

REFERENCES

Achor, S. (2011). The Happiness Advantage: How a Positive Brain Fuels Success in Work and Life. *Harvard Business Review.*

Bakker, A. B., & Demerouti, E. (2007). The Job Demands-Resources Model: State of the Art. *Journal of Managerial Psychology, 22*(3), 309–328. DOI: 10.1108/02683940710733115

Clark, A. E., & Oswald, A. J. (2002). Well-being in the Workplace and its Relationship to Business Outcomes. *Journal of Economic Literature, 40*(4), 656–672.

Deloitte (2020). "Mental Health and Well-Being in the Workplace: Report 2020."

Diener, E., & Seligman, M. E. P. (2004). Beyond Money: Toward an Economy of Well-Being. *Psychological Science in the Public Interest, 5*(1), 1–31. DOI: 10.1111/j.0963-7214.2004.00501001.x PMID: 26158992

Fisher, C. D. (2010). Happiness at Work. *International Journal of Management Reviews, 12*(4), 384–412. DOI: 10.1111/j.1468-2370.2009.00270.x

Grant, A. M., Christianson, M. K., & Price, R. H. (2007). Happiness, Health, or Relationships? Managerial Practices and Employee Well-Being Trade-offs. *The Academy of Management Perspectives, 21*(3), 51–63. DOI: 10.5465/amp.2007.26421238

Harter, J. K., Schmidt, F. L., & Keyes, C. L. M. (2002). "Well-Being in the Workplace and its Relationship to Business Outcomes: A Review of the Gallup Studies." Flourishing: The Positive Person and the Good Life.

Indira, V., Geetha, R., Umarani, S., & Priyadarshini, D. A. (2024). Prediction and analysis of COVID-19 using the Deep Learning Models. *Research on Biomedical Engineering, 40*(1), 1–15. DOI: 10.1007/s42600-024-00338-7

Kahneman, D., & Deaton, A. (2010). High Income Improves Evaluation of Life but not Emotional Well-Being. *Proceedings of the National Academy of Sciences of the United States of America, 107*(38), 16489–16493. DOI: 10.1073/pnas.1011492107 PMID: 20823223

Luthans, F., & Youssef, C. M. (2007). Emerging Positive Organizational Behaviour. *Journal of Management, 33*(3), 321–349. DOI: 10.1177/0149206307300814

Manoharan, G., Ashtikar, S. P., Rao, C. G., & Nivedha, M. (2024). A Pedagogical Landscape: Narrative Study on Emerging Artificial Intelligence Trends in Education. In Inclusive Educational Practices and Technologies for Promoting Sustainability (pp. 22-41). IGI Global.

Manoharan, G., Ashtikar, S. P., Smitha, V., Sundaramoorthi, S., & Krishna, I. M. (2023). Work-life balance perceptions of women in the IT and ITeS Sectors in Kerala: A research study. *Journal of Pharmaceutical Negative Results*, •••, 3363–3375.

Manoharan, G., Durai, S., Ashtikar, S. P., & Kumari, N. (2024). Artificial Intelligence in Marketing Applications. In Artificial Intelligence for Business (pp. 40-70). Productivity Press.

Manoharan, G., & Rajoli, S. B. (2024). Leveraging Technology for Enhancing Performance Appraisal. In Employee Performance Management for Improved Workplace Motivation (pp. 289-310). IGI Global. DOI: 10.4018/979-8-3693-4387-6.ch012

McKinsey & Company (2021). "Prioritizing Workplace Well-being in the COVID-19 Era."

Paulsamy, P., Easwaran, V., Ashraf, R., Alshahrani, S. H., Venkatesan, K., Qureshi, A. A., & Manoharan, V. (2021, November). Association of maternal observation and motivation (MOM) program with m-health support on maternal and newborn health. In Healthcare (Vol. 9, No. 12, p. 1629). MDPI.

PricewaterhouseCoopers (PwC) (2018). "The Future of Wellness at Work."

Purushottamashtikar, S., & Manoharan, G. (2024, June). Studying the level of work-life balance and emotional intelligence: University educators. In AIP Conference Proceedings (Vol. 2971, No.1

Rajoli, S. B., & Manoharan, G. (2024, June). Gender Perception of Talent Management Practices among IT Professionals in Hyderabad. In 2024 3rd International Conference on Computational Modelling, Simulation and Optimization (ICCMSO) (pp. 182-187). IEEE. DOI: 10.1109/ICCMSO61761.2024.00046

Razak, A., Nayak, M. P., Manoharan, G., Durai, S., Rajesh, G. A., Rao, C. B., & Ashtikar, S. P. (2023). Reigniting the power of artificial intelligence in education sector for the educators and students competence. In *Artificial Intelligence and Machine Learning in Smart City Planning* (pp. 103–116). Elsevier. DOI: 10.1016/B978-0-323-99503-0.00009-0

Robertson, I. T., & Cooper, C. L. (2011). *Well-being: Productivity and Happiness at Work*. Palgrave Macmillan. DOI: 10.1057/9780230306738

Sirota, D., Mischkind, L. A., & Meltzer, M. I. (2005). *The Enthusiastic Employee: How Companies Profit by Giving Workers What They Want*. Wharton School Publishing.

Suresh, E., Ravi, B., Udayanan, M., Manoharan, G., Ashtikar, S. P., & Rajesh, G. A. (2024, June). Prospects and determinants towards work from home associated perception of IT employees: With special reference to Chennai. In AIP Conference Proceedings (Vol. 2971, No. 1). AIP Publishing.

Thavamani, S., Mahesh, D., Sinthuja, U., & Manoharan, G. (2022, May). Crucial attacks in internet of things via artificial intelligence techniques: The security survey. In AIP Conference Proceedings (Vol. 2418, No. 1). AIP Publishing.

Van Horn, J. E., Taris, T. W., Schaufeli, W. B., & Schreurs, P. J. (2004). The Structure of Occupational Well-Being: A Study Among Dutch Teachers. *Journal of Occupational and Organizational Psychology*, *77*(3), 365–375. DOI: 10.1348/0963179041752718

Winster, D., Ramakrishnan, S., Veluthakkal, J., Manoharan, G., Purushottamashtikar, S., & Selvaraj, F. (2024, June). Interactions between emotional and spiritual intelligence and their effects on employee performance. In AIP Conference Proceedings (Vol. 2971, No. 1). AIP Publishing DOI: 10.1063/5.0195736

World Health Organization (WHO). (2010). *Healthy Workplaces: A Model for Action: For Employers*. Workers, Policy-Makers, and Practitioners.

About the Contributors

Frederic Andres received his Ph.D. in Information Systems from the University of Paris VI "Pierre et Marie Curie" in 1993 and his Dr. Habilitation in Informatics from the University of Nantes in 2000. Dr. Frederic Andres has been associate professor in the Digital Content and Media Sciences Research Division of the National Institute of Informatics (NII) in Tokyo, Japan since 2000. He is author of more than 150 papers on international journals, books and conferences. His main research areas of interest include several topics such as collective intelligence-based knowledge, AI ethics, data science, supply chain and pedagogy and didactical web-based science education for all. He has been co-organising the International DECOR workshop since 2018 in conjunction with IEEE ICDE. His team won the 1st prize in IEEE Brain Data Bank Challenges and Competitions at COMPSAC 2018, July 2018. Dr. Frederic Andres received the IEEE CertifAIEd Authorized Lead Assessor recognition from IEEE SA on September 15, 2023. In addition, he was named "R10 Ethics Champion" by IEEE Region 10 on 22 Oct 2023.

***

Fuzuki Arai is a Japanese artist. His work, influenced by the sound of the conch horn in Shugendo—an ancient Japanese practice that blends Buddhism and Shintoism—is a fusion of this age-old tradition and modern digital technology. He graduated from the Department of Information Design at Tama Art University. In 2014, he held a solo exhibition in New York. In 2015, he participated in the Arab Week 2015 Art Exhibition, where he was awarded the Japan-Arab Friendship Appreciation Award by the ambassadors of Oman and Palestine. In 2022, he exhibited at The Holy Art Gallery in London. In 2023, he was selected as one of the world's 101 contemporary artists (Georgia). In 2024, he was appointed to the Board of Directors of the International Center of Transdisciplinary Research Japan.

Nita Beluli Luma boasts an impressive academic and professional background, having served as a lecturer for over 12 years across various universities in North Macedonia. For the past 5 years, Nita works as an Associate Professor at Mother Teresa University, where she also serves as the Head of the Department of Psychology. Upon obtaining a doctoral degree in Clinical Psychology and receiving extensive training as a Cognitive Behavioral Therapy (CBT) therapist, she aims to merge her knowledge and skills in both academia and psychotherapy.

Jorge Luis Delgado was born in the Andes mountains of Peru. He is a descendant of the Quechua and Aymara native cultures. A lover of ancient wisdom, Jorge Luis became a "chakaruna"- bridge person - at the age of eleven, and began to assist and show pilgrims and travelers how to find their way. Author of Andean Awakening: an Inka Guide to Mystical Peru, Inka Wisdom: Return to Joy, and the of Machu Picchu: The City of the Children of the Sun. Jorge Luis is recognized worldwide as an authority on Inca philosophy, spirituality and tradition. He is an organizer of great world events and an activator of portals for the expansion of consciousness. He has offered workshops in North, South and Central America, as well as Europe and in Asia. Jorge teaches at New York City's Omega Holistic Institute and at the New York Open Center. Jorge Luis has brought to public attention the Aramu Muru Doorway, an inter-dimensional portal located in the Hayu Marca mountains in south Peru. He is also a founding member of The Brotherhood of the Solar Disc, an Andean esoteric society. Jorge Luis is way-shower for this 10th Pachacuti, this time when the world is being turned upside down. He teaches that a new consciousness is emerging, one leading to a Golden Age that was fully activated by 2012. He is a keeper of the ancient knowledge and uses it to assist in healing for all who are ready.

Kenneth Gilliard Jr., M.S. is a distinguished professional with a Master of Science in Higher Education from Walden University and a Bachelor of Arts in English from the University of North Carolina Wilmington. With a comprehensive background in community engagement, human services, and education, Kenneth has demonstrated an unwavering commitment to student success, leadership development, and organizational excellence. Currently serving as a Program Manager for Cross-Cultural Student Services with the Student Achievement and Success Program at Anne Arundel Community College, Kenneth advises and mentors a diverse caseload of students, guiding them through academic and personal challenges to achieve their educational goals. He has played a pivotal role in coordinating the Hispanic Youth Symposium, revitalizing the Black Male Institute, and fostering collaboration across various departments to enhance student engagement and retention. Kenneth's efforts in this role have significantly contributed to the college's mission of supporting student achievement and success. Before joining Anne Arundel Community College, Kenneth was a Career Coach at Cape Fear Community College, where he managed a caseload of over 1,000 students, consistently increasing enrollment by 7-8% annually. He was instrumental in developing segmented onboarding processes, coordinating daily operations, and providing continuous training and mentorship to staff, ultimately improving the quality of postsecondary career counseling for high school students and their families. Kenneth's entrepreneurial spirit shines through in his work as the founder and leader of Gilliard & Co. LLC, where he has successfully supervised a team of aspiring entrepreneurs. Under his leadership, the company has curated dynamic events, including the annual Coastal Wedding Expo, and developed strategic marketing content that resonates with diverse audiences. His ability to seamlessly coordinate logistics, flowers, decorations, and travel arrangements ensures that every event is executed to perfection. In addition to his professional achievements, Kenneth has been an active leader in community and Greek life. As the president of the National Pan-Hellenic Council of Southeastern North Carolina and the North Carolina State Director of Collegiate Affairs for Phi Beta Sigma Fraternity, Inc., he has led initiatives to establish and strengthen chapters, develop strategic plans, and mentor collegiate members. His leadership in these roles has galvanized stakeholder support and fostered a strong sense of community. Kenneth's dedication to excellence has earned him numerous accolades, including the AACC MLK Jr. Zeitgeist Award, AACC Swooperstar Award, the North Carolina Phi Beta Sigma Fraternity, Inc. State Conference Bigger and Better Business Award, and the University of North Carolina at Wilmington Upperman African American Culture Center Ujima Community Partnership Award. His articles on supporting Black male students and succeeding despite the lack of representation have been published and widely recognized. A driven and ambitious leader, Kenneth Gilliard Jr. is passionate about building coalitions, supporting stakeholders, and coaching others to achieve their best. His unique blend of educational expertise, entrepreneurial acumen, and community leadership positions him as a trailblazer in his field, making a profound impact on the lives of those he serves.

Abadio Green Stocel served as the President of the National Indigenous Organization of Colombia from 1993 to 1998. He was the Coordinator of the Indigenous Education Program and a professor in the Bachelor's Program in Pedagogy of Mother Earth at the University of Antioquia. In 2009, UNESCO recognized him as a "Master of Wisdom." He was also acknowledged as one of the 10 key figures in Colombia for the National Consultation Process for the Development of the Decennial Education Plan (2006–2016). Additionally, he was named one of the 30 distinguished figures for the "Best Leaders of Colombia" award, a joint initiative by Semana Magazine and the Leadership and Democracy Foundation, with the support of Telefonía. He is currently an advisor to the Ministry of Education of Colombia.

Shumayela Hasan is a senior faculty member in Economics at The Bal Bhawan School. Formerly an Assistant Professor at The Bhopal School of Social Sciences, she brings over 18 years of teaching experience. Dr. Hasan has also served as Project Director for a research initiative funded by the Indian Council of Social Science Research. With multiple degrees in Economics, Finance, and Education, she is currently pursuing an MBA in Marketing. An accomplished author, she has published eight seven books and numerous articles in national and international journals.

Akira Ikegawa, M.D., Ph.D. is a renowned obstetrician and gynecologist with over 35 years of experience. He is a pioneer in the study of prenatal memory, advocating for the recognition of fetuses as sentient beings with emotions and awareness. Through his extensive research, which includes over 11,000 collected cases, Dr. Ikegawa has explored the profound connections between prenatal experiences, self-awareness, and well-being. He is dedicated to promoting empathetic communication between parents and unborn children, emphasizing the transformative potential of these interactions for families and society.

Hannah John, PhD, Psychology, is an experienced academic professional currently serving as the Program Head of the M.Sc. Family Counselling program at the Madras School of Social Work (MSSW) in Chennai, India. With over three years at MSSW, she plays a pivotal role in leading and developing the postgraduate curriculum in family counselling. Her work focuses on training future counsellors and advancing the field of family therapy through academic leadership and practical engagement.

Vijay Kumar (S'07-M'11-SM'18) received M.Tech degree in Microwave remote sensing from BIT Mesra, Ranchi, in 2005 and completed PhD from IIT Bombay, Mumbai in 2011 in Microwave Radar imaging domain. He has been a visiting researcher at Earth observation Group, Northern Research Institute (NORUT) during 2009-2010. Kumar has worked as Associate professor at School of Electronics Engineering, VIT Vellore TN, India from 2013 to June-2022. He has been promoted as full professor on July, 1, 2022. Dr. Kumar is associated with Photonics and Microwave group at VIT and research focus is in microwave imaging, Radar and SAR imaging system development and applications in earth observation and reconnaissance from space borne, airborne and UAV platforms. He is author and contributing author of many peer reviewed papers and conference proceedings deliberating ideas in radiating system designs for radar applications, miniaturized antenna designing using metamaterials, MIMO Antenna system for

UWB applications with reconfigurable notch band Characteristics. He has executed many international and national funded projects. He worked on Active devices such as LNA, PAs for UHF range wind profiler radars. His research contributions have been culminated into various patens and design registration. He is life Member of ISRS,.and actively associated with IEEE societies APS, THz and GRSS.

Geetha Manoharan is currently working in Telangana as an assistant professor at SR University. She is the university-level PhD program coordinator and has also been given the additional responsibility of In Charge Director of Publications and Patents under the Research Division at SR University.

Shinichiro Sawano /Mr. Photographer, nature sound producer, flower/environmental essence producer Born in Tokyo, Japan Graduated from Nihon University College of Art, Department of Photography, completed his bachelor's degree After working for a major publishing company, he established Shin Sawano Photo Studio, and is currently working on assignments in over 80 countries around the world. Since 1998, over 3,000 people have experienced the flower/environmental essence sessions he created at Namaqualand in South Africa. Since 1991, he has stayed at Namaqualand in the Northern Cape of South Africa for long periods almost every year. Official tourism ambassador for the South African government (since 2014) Currently lives in Nasu, Japan.

Richi Simon, PhD is an Assistant Professor of Social Work at The Bhopal School of Social Sciences, with over 12 years of experience in teaching and research. She earned her PhD in Social Work from the Indore School of Social Work, focusing on Quality Education in Higher Education Institutions (HEIs) of Social Work. Her interdisciplinary academic background includes Social Work, Human Resource Management, and Computer Applications. She is currently pursuing MA in Psychology. Dr. Simon is a dedicated researcher, with several published books, book chapters, and research articles. She is a frequent presenter at national and international academic forums.

Thottempudi Pardhu (Senior Member, IEEE) has been exemplary and dedicated to electronics and communication engineering in the last decade. He has extensively contributed from a Research Internship with the RADAR SEEKER Laboratory, Research Center Imarat, Hyderabad, in June 2012. In July 2013, he ventured into an academic career as an Assistant Professor. He served at various prestigious institutions, including the Marri Laxman Reddy Institute of Technology Management, the St. Peters Engineering College, and the MLR Institute of Technology, Hyderabad. He served for an extended period with the MLR Institute, from December 2016 to August 2022. Further, he continued his service with SR University, Warangal. Since March 2023, he has been with the BVRIT HYDERABAD College of Engineering for Women. These years saw the great responsibility put forward by him in providing quality education and research contributions. He has several research publications against his name on different topics, ranging from RADAR signal processing to the classification of human motion using advanced technologies in prestigious journals, further showing that he is a dedicated person to this field, boasting numerous patents on anything from power-efficient compressors to innovative design for surveillance and security. Besides his teaching and research roles, he is also entrusted with multiple significant institutional responsibilities, like the Sports Director, the Social Media Coordinator, and the Alumni Coordinator, to name a few. Further, his commitment to continuous learning and dissemination of knowledge is also evidenced by his active participation in various types of FDPs and STTPs. Over the years, he has been feted for his excellent contributions, as is evident in awards, such as the India Independence Awards, in 2019, and the Young Scientist Award and the Young Researcher of the Year Awards, in 2020 and 2021, respectively, among many others. He is a gem in academia and the research community based on the richness of his academic background, his significant contribution to research, and his remarkable track record in professional practice for more than ten years.

Antione D. Tomlin, Ph.D. Rooted in core values like Autonomy, Flexibility, Learning, Respect, Transparency, Honesty, and Fun, I live and breathe principles that not only shape my life but also guide my interactions with others. As a proud native of Baltimore City, these values have been my compass in navigating life's journey. Being a first-generation undergrad and grad student, I recognize the transformative power of education, a value intricately tied to my passion for continuous learning. This passion steered me into a fulfilling career in higher education, where I've been teaching English since 2013. The classroom, for me, is an ever-inspiring space filled with dedicated students who continually fuel my curiosity and growth. Beyond teaching, I wear the hat of a trained and certified Life and Engagement Coach, proudly holding the Professional Certified Coach (PCC) credential from the International Coach Federation (ICF). Feel free to explore more about my coaching venture, Best AT Coaching!, LLC. As a Baltimore native, I earned my academic stripes from local institutions: a BS in psychology from Stevenson University, an MA in higher education administration and student affairs from Morgan State University, and a PhD in language, literacy, and culture from the University of Maryland, Baltimore County. My current research focuses on the experiences of Black and Brown faculty, staff, and students in higher education. For more about Antione visit drantionetomlin.com.

Index

A

B

C

D

E

F

G

H

I

J

K

L

M

N

O

P

S

T

U

W

www.ingramcontent.com/pod-product-compliance
Lightning Source LLC
LaVergne TN
LVHW080615300926
849162LV00005B/1168